BOARD BUSTER
STEP 2

BOARD BUSTER
STEP 2

Stanley Zaslau, MD

Assistant Professor

Section of Urology, Department of Surgery

West Virginia University School of Medicine

Morgantown, West Virginia

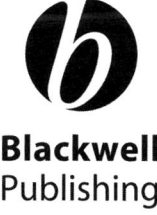

Blackwell
Publishing

© 2005 by Blackwell Publishing

Blackwell Publishing, Inc., 350 Main Street, Malden, Massachusetts 02148-5018, USA
Blackwell Publishing Ltd, 9600 Garsington Road, Oxford OX4 2DQ, UK
Blackwell Publishing Asia Pty Ltd, 550 Swanston Street, Carlton, Victoria 3053, Australia

04 05 06 07 5 4 3 2 1

ISBN: 1-4051-0385-X

Library of Congress Cataloging-in-Publication Data

Zaslau, Stanley.
    Board buster step 2/Stanley Zaslau.
        p. ; cm.
    Includes index.
    ISBN 1-4051-0385-X (pbk.)
    1. Medicine—Examinations, questions, etc.   2. Physicians—Licenses—United States—Examinations—Study guides.
    [DNLM: 1. Medicine—Examinations, Questions. W 18.2 Z38b 2005]   I. Title: Board buster step tow.   II. Title.

    R834.5.Z37 2005
    610'.76—dc22

                                                                                    2004013291

A catalogue record for this title is available from the British Library

Acquisitions: Beverly Copland
Development: Selene Steneck
Production: Debra Murphy
Cover design: Leslie Haimes
Interior design: Leslie Haimes
Typesetter: SNP Best-set Typesetter Ltd., Hong Kong
Printed and bound by Capital City Press in Berlin, VT

For further information on Blackwell Publishing, visit our website:
www.blackwellmedstudent.com

Notice: The indications and dosages of all drugs in this book have been recommended in the medical literature and conform to the practices of the general community. The medications described do not necessarily have specific approval by the Food and Drug Administration for use in the diseases and dosages for which they are recommended. The package insert for each drug should be consulted for use and dosage as approved by the FDA. Because standards for usage change, it is advisable to keep abreast of revised recommendations, particularly those concerning new drugs.

The publisher's policy is to use permanent paper from mills that operate a sustainable forestry policy, and which has been manufactured from pulp processed using acid-free and elementary chlorine-free practices. Furthermore, the publisher ensures that the text paper and cover board used have met acceptable environmental accreditation standards.

CONTENTS

Internal Medicine

1, 2, 8, 14, 17, 19, 24, 30, 34, 35, 37, 40, 41, 46, 49, 52, 56, 57, 62, 63, 64, 66, 70, 72, 77, 80, 82, 88, 94, 95, 99, 101, 104, 108, 118, 119, 125, 130, 132, 134, 137, 139, 140, 146, 147, 150, 153, 156, 161, 166, 168, 172, 176, 181, 184, 187, 197, 200, 201, 203, 204, 210, 213, 215, 218, 224, 227, 229, 233, 235, 241, 243, 246, 253, 258, 260, 263, 264, 266, 270, 273, 280, 285, 289, 291, 297, 300, 305, 308, 312, 321, 322, 323, 324, 325, 331, 334, 340, 341, 342, 344, 347, 354, 359, 360, 365, 367, 373, 376, 380, 381, 386, 387, 396, 400, 401, 406, 409, 413, 415, 418, 420, 421, 426, 435, 439, 440, 446, 449, 452, 455, 456, 458, 463, 470, 471, 475, 479, 482, 485, 491, 496, 497, 498, 499, 507, 509, 512, 514, 520, 522, 523, 529, 530, 538, 540, 542, 548, 550, 554, 556, 561, 566, 574, 578, 579, 580, 585, 587, 589, 591, 593, 596, 597, 604, 609, 612, 613, 617, 619, 620, 626, 629, 635, 638, 641, 648, 653, 654, 658, 662, 664, 666, 667, 672, 675, 677, 685, 687, 691, 694, 696, 700, 705, 708, 710, 713, 717, 718, 721, 722, 728, 731, 735, 737

Obstetrics and Gynecology

3, 6, 16, 21, 25, 31, 36, 42, 47, 53, 58, 61, 71, 78, 84, 90, 96, 103, 107, 120, 124, 129, 133, 135, 136, 141, 148, 155, 160, 169, 173, 178, 180, 185, 190, 199, 208, 212, 217, 220, 223, 228, 231, 237, 242, 247, 250, 256, 262, 267, 271, 272, 279, 283, 293, 298, 302, 306, 309, 313, 318, 326, 332, 336, 345, 350, 355, 361, 366, 370, 372, 378, 383, 389, 398, 403, 404, 408, 412, 422, 425, 433, 438, 444, 450, 453, 460, 462, 465, 469, 476, 483, 490, 492, 495, 501, 506, 513, 517, 524, 526, 536, 541, 543, 547, 553, 557, 563, 572, 577, 584, 588, 592, 598, 602, 603, 610, 615, 624, 632, 637, 642, 647, 652, 656, 660, 668, 674, 678, 684, 689, 693, 697, 706, 712, 715, 720, 724, 730, 734

Pediatrics

4, 9, 10, 11, 20, 26, 29, 33, 43, 48, 55, 65, 69, 79, 83, 87, 91, 98, 102, 105, 110, 121, 122, 127, 138, 143, 151, 158, 162, 163, 164, 174, 179, 186, 188, 196, 206, 211, 216, 221, 226, 236, 244, 251, 252, 257, 261, 269, 276, 284, 286, 290, 296, 301, 304, 307, 316, 327, 330, 338, 348, 349, 351, 356, 363, 371, 374, 377, 384, 390, 397, 407, 416, 423, 427, 436, 437, 443, 448, 459, 461, 464, 466, 474, 477, 486, 488, 493, 502, 516, 521, 525, 532, 533, 534, 546, 549, 558, 562, 564, 571, 576, 583, 594, 600, 606, 616, 623, 625, 630, 631, 636, 639, 645, 651, 659, 670, 680, 681, 682, 683, 688, 699, 707, 711, 719, 725, 729, 733, 740

Psychiatry

7, 12, 15, 22, 27, 28, 38, 44, 51, 59, 60, 68, 81, 85, 89, 92, 97, 111, 112, 113, 114, 115, 116, 117, 131, 142, 145, 154, 159, 167, 171, 177, 183, 189, 198, 205, 209, 214, 222, 225, 230, 232, 238, 239, 245, 248, 255, 265, 268, 274, 278, 281, 287, 292, 299, 310, 314, 317, 319, 328, 333, 339, 343, 353, 357, 362, 368, 369, 382, 388, 392, 393, 394, 395, 402, 411, 414, 417, 424, 434, 441, 445, 447, 451, 454, 468, 473, 480, 481, 484, 489, 494, 503, 505, 511, 518, 528, 531, 537, 544, 545, 551, 559, 567, 568, 569, 570, 581, 590, 599, 601, 605, 611, 618, 622, 627, 633, 640, 644, 650, 655, 661, 665, 671, 679, 686, 690, 695, 701, 709 714, 723, 727, 736, 739

Surgery

5, 13, 18, 23, 32, 39, 45, 50, 54, 67, 73, 74, 75, 76, 86, 93, 100, 106, 109, 123, 126, 128, 144, 149, 152, 157, 165, 170, 175, 182, 191, 192, 193, 194, 195, 202, 207, 219, 234, 240, 249, 254, 259, 275, 277, 282, 288, 294, 295, 303, 311, 315, 320, 329, 335, 337, 346, 352, 358, 364, 375, 379, 385, 391, 399, 405, 410, 419, 428, 429, 430, 431, 432, 442, 457, 467, 472, 478, 487, 500, 504, 508, 510, 515, 519, 527, 535, 539, 552, 555, 560, 565, 573, 575, 582, 586, 595, 607, 608, 614, 621, 628, 634, 643, 646, 649, 657, 663, 669, 673, 676, 692, 698, 702, 703, 704, 716, 726, 732, 738

CONTRIBUTORS

All of the contributors are students at West Virginia University School of Medicine in Morgantown, West Virginia.

Heather Bellotte
Class of 2004

Heather will receive her medical degree in 2004 from West Virginia University School of Medicine. As an undergraduate, she studied English, French, Visual Arts, and Biology. Heather is also pursuing a Bachelor of Music degree focusing on piano performance. When she finds free time, Heather has piano students and an equestrian riding program. Heather is also a certified scuba instructor.

Miranda Bosley
Class of 2004

Miranda is a 4th year medical student at West Virginia School of Medicine. She is originally from West Virginia and hopes to begin a residency in plastic surgery after she graduates. In her spare time, Miranda enjoys spending time with her pets and horseback riding.

Jill Kenamond Bradshaw
Class of 2004

Jill was born and raised in Wheeling, WV. She attended Butler University in Indianapolis, Indiana, where she played on the tennis team for four years. She then returned to WVU for medical school. In her free time, Jill enjoys spending time with her husband, John, running, and playing sports.

Thomas Alden Brown
Class of 2004

Tom was raised near Pittsburgh, PA, and then went to West Virginia University for a BS in Biology and research in Microbiology. He is currently a medical student at WVU and will graduate in 2004. On the side, he is a fanatical Ultimate Frisbee player, adores Jazz and Funk music, and tries to be a good environmentalist.

Matt Cindric
Class of 2004

Born and raised in Uniontown, PA, Matt completed undergraduate studies at WVU, where he graduated summa cum laude with a BS in Exercise Physiology. He remained at WVU while pursuing a medical degree and will graduate in 2004. At that point, several passionate lifelong journeys begin. Within allopathic medicine, he is excited to matriculate into a urology residency program at Geisinger Medical Center in July. In addition, he is interested in various modalities under the umbrella term "Energy Medicine," such as reiki, acupuncture, ayurveda, and craniosacral therapy. With an open mind, he challenges himself to explore the frontier of healing. When he has time, he enjoys running and the outdoors. He is also delighted to announce to the world his upcoming wedding with Angela Slampak . . . his truest love, best friend, biggest hero, and the most important person in his life.

Jennifer Defazio
Class of 2004

Jennifer is currently in her third year of medical school at West Virginia University. She is planning a residency in dermatology. In her free time, she enjoys running, skiing and spending time with her family.

Daniel DeLo
Class of 2004

Daniel was raised in Morgantown, WV, where he attended West Virginia University. He received a degree in Biology while helping conduct research on the process of damage to the Central Nervous System. He is currently in his fourth-year at WVU School of Medicine and is preparing to begin a medical residency.

Bahair Hussein Ghazi
Class of 2004

Bahair is currently a fourth year medical student at the West Virginia University School of Medicine. He grew up in WV and then left to attend the University of Vermont for undergraduate work. Research interests include wound closure, diabetic foot ulcers and muscle-based flaps. Bahair is interested in a career in plastic and reconstructive surgery. In his free time, Bahair enjoys playing outside in the sun!

Valerie Gouzd
Class of 2004

Valerie is a fourth year medical student at WVU School of Medicine. She graduated from WVU with a degree in Animal Science in 2000.

Rohit Goyal
Class of 2004

Rohit was born in Baltimore, MD. He graduated with a BA in Biology from West Virginia University. He currently is a fourth year medical student at West Virginia University and plans to pursue a career in Emergency Medicine.

Carl Robert Grey
Class of 2004

Carl is currently finishing his third year of medical school at West Virginia University. He enjoys playing the guitar and mountain biking.

B. Asher Louden
Class of 2004

Asher is currently a fourth year student at the West Virginia University School of Medicine. He earned his undergraduate degree from Princeton University and graduated cum laude in Molecular Biology. Following medical school, Asher hopes to further his training in Dermatology. Aside from school, Asher is looking forward to a May 2004 wedding to Stephanie Moore.

Ben Messinger
Class of 2004

Ben is currently in his fourth year of medical school at West Virginia University. He is pursuing a career in anesthesiology. When he's not working, Ben enjoys spending time with his wife, Kori, pursuing a number of outdoor activities in the beautiful mountains of West Virginia.

Chad J. Micucci
Class of 2004

Chad is originally from Follansbee, West Virginia. He graduated from West Virginia University in 1998 with a BS in Physical Therapy. Chad returned to WVU in 2000 and is currently in his fourth year of medical school; he plans to pursue a career in Orthopedic Surgery.

Gary James Miller
Class of 2004

Jamie received his undergraduate degree in Electrical Engineering and his medical degree from West Virginia University. He will continue his training in Ophthalmology at West Virginia University. He is happily married and enjoys many outdoor activities.

Justin Nelms
Class of 2004

Justin graduated from the University of Richmond with a BS in Biology. He will earn his medical degree from West Virginia University in 2004. In his free time, he enjoys playing hockey and soccer.

Brock J. Oliverio
Class of 2004

Brock received his Bachelor of Arts in Biology and Chemistry from West Virginia University and is currently completing his 4th year at his alma mater's school of medicine. He plans to enter a Pathology residency in 2004. Along with his scientific studies, he also plans to break into the electronic music scene with the release of his first two solo albums entitled "Sophistication" and "Out of Control."

John R. Orphanos
Class of 2004

John is currently a fourth year medical student at West Virginia University and will receive his medical degree in 2004. He will be doing a residency is neurological surgery at West Virginia University in Morgantown. In his spare time, John enjoys traveling, listening to music, and playing soccer.

Zeshan Rana
Class of 2005

Zeshan was born in Philadelphia, PA. He is currently a third year medical student at the West Virginia University School of Medicine. He is interested in the fields of Ophthalmology/Surgery. During his free time, he enjoys spending time with family and friends, playing sports/outdoor activities, and following up on current events. He aspires to be a great physician like the many before him.

Sara Kirsten Rasmussen

Class of 2004

Sara is an MD-PhD student at WVU. She did her doctoral research on retroviral reverse transcription and assembly. She got her BA in chemistry at University of Virginia in 1996. Her hobbies include scuba diving, mountain biking, watercolor, hiking, and photography.

John P. Renton

Class of 2004

Katrina Richards

Class of 2005

Kate is currently a 3rd year student at West Virginia University School of Medicine in Morgantown, West Virginia. She hopes to go on to do a residency in ENT/Head and Neck Surgery after graduation in 2005. In her spare time she enjoys playing soccer, skiing, and mountain biking.

Shon Patrick Rowan

Class of 2004

Shon will receive his medical degree in 2004 from West Virginia University. He attended WVU for undergraduate study, where he received his BS in Biology. He enjoys spending time with his wife, Holly, and their two dogs.

Dale A. Santrock

Class of 2004

After completing degrees in Biology and Psychology, Dale received a Masters in Exercise Physiology. He will complete a medical degree in 2004 and plans to pursue a career in orthopedic surgery.

Mark Schwab

Class of 2004

Mark graduated from Tulane University in 1999 where he majored in Biology and minored in French. He also focused on Spanish and rowed for Tulane Crew. He is interested in languages, travel, biking, rock climbing, surfing and house renovation. He will receive his medical degree from West Virginia University in 2004.

Geetha Vedula

Class of 2005

Geetha was born in Portsmouth, Ohio and raised in the suburbs of Washington, DC. She completed her B.A. in Biology and English at West Virginia University and then entered the M.D. program at WVU. Having completed her third year of medical school, she is currently pursuing a year of basic science and clinical research at Bascom Palmer Eye Institute. She will be returning to her fourth year of medical school this July at WVU. When she finds free time she enjoys dancing, swimming, and reading.

Robert Wilson

Class of 2004

Robert is currently a fourth-year student at the WVU School of Medicine. He will continue his medical training in the Department of Otolaryngology at the University of Kentucky Medical Center. During his free time, Robert enjoys golfing, skiing, traveling, and spending time with his wife, Dana, and airedale terrier puppy, Wylie.

Jill Yeager

Class of 2004

Jill was born in North Huntingdon, PA. She completed her undergraduate degree at Penn State University where she majored in Pre-Medicine and minored in Psychology. She is currently a fourth year medical student at West Virginia University.

REVIEWERS

Valérie Julie Brousseau

Med IV
McGill Medical School
Montreal, Canada

Kenneth Bryant, MD

Intern
University of Alabama Hospital
Birmingham, Alabama

Philip Chang

Class of 2004
New York University School of Medicine
New York, New York

Anand Deonarine

Class of 2004
Howard University School of Medicine
Washington, DC

Jennifer Kraschnewski

Class of 2004
University of Wisconsin
Madison, Wisconsin

Andrew Louie

Class of 2004
George Washington University School of Medicine
Washington, DC

Christopher Starnes, MD

Internal Medicine Resident
University of South Carolina School of Medicine
Columbia, South Carolina
University of Virginia
Charlottesville, Virginia

Katie Starnes, MD

Class of 2003
Eastern Virginia Medical School
Norfolk, Virginia

Brooke Burkart Thomas

Class of 2004
Eastern Virginia Medical School
Norfolk, VA

Lisa S. Usdan, MD

Resident Physician, Department of Internal Medicine
Thomas Jefferson University Hospital
Philadelphia, PA

PREFACE

One of the most challenging events in medical school is passage of the United States Medical Licensing Examination (USMLE). This three-step examination is not only required for licensure to practice medicine in the United States, but is also used by some residency programs to select applicants for interviews. Thus, demonstration of high scores on this examination can have major importance for students.

Question and answer study guides form an important framework to study for licensure examinations. These simulated clinical vignettes place students in nearly "real-life" and examination-like situations. Students using question and answer books effectively will learn not only the correct answer for each vignette, but also other pertinent information about why distracter choices (which are also possible answers but not the best one) are incorrect. Use of these question and answer books will also prepare students for situations that they will face on their clinical rotations. Patient presentations are the real-life form of the clinical vignettes in question and answer books.

The best question and answer books are written by students who have experienced these types of examinations first-hand. It is with these premises in mind that the ***Board Buster*** series has been created. All of the questions in this book have been written by medical students at West Virginia University School of Medicine. These questions were reviewed by ten other medical students, interns, and residents from programs throughout North America for level of difficulty, format, and accuracy. Additionally, the final, revised questions were given a final review by faculty.

We hope that you will find ***Board Buster Step 2*** to be both beneficial to your studies for your examination and a useful adjunct to your clinical rotations. We believe that this book of new vignettes will truly "bust the boards" for each user.

—Stanley Zaslau

ACKNOWLEDGMENTS

Board Buster Step 2 is the culmination of the efforts of many dedicated individuals. I would like to thank Beverly Copland for enthusiastic support and guidance. Selene Steneck has again stepped up to the plate and been a great editor and provided many helpful suggestions to the manuscript. A very special thanks to my West Virginia University medical students who served as contributing authors on this project. Thank you for your sincere interest, motivation and energy. I know that this book will be an important resource for your underclassman. Finally, a special thanks to my parents, David and Anne Zaslau, great role models, always supportive with love and understanding and truly devoted life-time educators.

TO THE READER

Board Buster Step 2 was written by students just like you. Students that had searched for an up to date, comprehensive, question review book based on the current USMLE exam.

This all new resource for USMLE prep was written by students who had recently taken the step 2 exam. It was developed to provide:

- A pre-test to determine which areas of study on which you need to focus your review

- A self-test of specific clinical content to enhance your weak areas

- A timed, full-length exam to simulate the challenge of answering 350 questions in 7 hours

Board Buster Step 2 HAS EVERYTHING YOU NEED! Use it to review during your clinical rotations and as a review prep for USMLE Step 2. Because it was written by students, it provides just what you want:

- Rationales for correct and incorrect answers

- 2 full length practice exams

- Tear-out answer sheets for timed self-test

- Clinical discipline index to review specific clinical content

Be prepared for the USMLE Step 2 with Blackwell's new *Board Buster Step 2*!

FIGURE CREDITS

BLOCK 1

Figure 14: Used with permission of Cedars-Sinai Medical Center, Los Angeles, California. (Originally appeared as Figure 8-2 in Davis RW, Komaiko MS, eds. Blueprints in Radiology. Malden, MA: Blackwell Science, 2003.)

Figure 34: Used with permission from Taylor GJ. 150 Practice ECGs: Interpretation and Review. 2nd ed. Malden, MA: Blackwell Science, 2002. (Originally appeared as Practice ECG 131.)

BLOCK 2

Figure 63: Used with permission of Cedars-Sinai Medical Center, Los Angeles, California. (Originally appeared as Figure 5-12 in Davis RW, Komaiko MS. Blueprints in Radiology. Malden, MA: Blackwell Science, 2003.)

Figure 82: Used with permission from Taylor GJ. 150 Practice ECGs: Interpretation and Review. 2nd ed. Malden, MA: Blackwell Science, 2002. (Originally appeared as Practice ECG 98.)

BLOCK 3

Figure 95: Used with permission from Taylor GJ. 150 Practice ECGs: Interpretation and Review. 2nd ed. Malden, MA: Blackwell Science, 2002. (Originally appeared as Practice ECG 4.)

Figure 125a: Used with permission of Cedars-Sinai Medical Center, Los Angeles, California. (Originally appeared as Figure 6-2a in Davis RW, Komaiko MS. Blueprints in Radiology. Malden, MA: Blackwell Science, 2003.)

Figure 125b: Used with permission of Cedars-Sinai Medical Center, Los Angeles, California. (Originally appeared as Figure 6-2b in Davis RW, Komaiko MS. Blueprints in Radiology. Malden, MA: Blackwell Science, 2003.)

BLOCK 4

Figure 140: Used with permission of Cedars-Sinai Medical Center, Los Angeles, California. (Originally appeared as Figure 4-4a in Davis RW, Komaiko MS. Blueprints in Radiology. Malden, MA: Blackwell Science, 2003.)

Figure 158: Used with permission from Marino BS, Fine KS, McMillan JA. Blueprints Pediatrics. 3rd ed. Malden, MA: Blackwell Publishing, 2004. (Originally appeared as Figure 19-2.)

BLOCK 5

Figure 203a: Used with permission of Cedars-Sinai Medical Center, Los Angeles, California. (Originally appeared as Figure 5-2 in Davis RW, Komaiko MS. Blueprints in Radiology. Malden, MA: Blackwell Science, 2003.)

Figure 203b: Used with permission of Cedars-Sinai Medical Center, Los Angeles, California. (Originally appeared as Figure 5-1 in Davis RW, Komaiko MS. Blueprints in Radiology. Malden, MA: Blackwell Science, 2003.)

Figure 215: Used with permission of Cedars-Sinai Medical Center, Los Angeles, California. (Originally appeared as Figure 4-3 in Davis RW, Komaiko MS. Blueprints in Radiology. Malden, MA: Blackwell Science, 2003.)

BLOCK 6

Figure 243: Used with permission of Cedars-Sinai Medical Center, Los Angeles, California. (Originally appeared as Figure 3-3 in Davis RW, Komaiko MS. Blueprints in Radiology. Malden, MA: Blackwell Science, 2003.)

Figure 263: Used with permission of Cedars-Sinai Medical Center, Los Angeles, California. (Originally appeared as Figure 4-2a in Davis RW, Komaiko MS. Blueprints in Radiology. Malden, MA: Blackwell Science, 2003.)

BLOCK 7

Figure 291: Used with permission of Cedars-Sinai Medical Center, Los Angeles, California. (Originally appeared as Figure 3-1 in Davis RW, Komaiko MS. Blueprints in Radiology. Malden, MA: Blackwell Science, 2003.)

Figure 305a: Used with permission of Cedars-Sinai Medical Center, Los Angeles, California. (Originally appeared as Figure 8-9 in Davis RW, Komaiko MS. Blueprints in Radiology. Malden, MA: Blackwell Science, 2003.)

Figure 305b: Used with permission of Cedars-Sinai Medical Center, Los Angeles, California. (Originally appeared as Figure 8-10 in Davis RW, Komaiko MS. Blueprints in Radiology. Malden, MA: Blackwell Science, 2003.)

BLOCK 4 (cont.)

Figure 172: Used with permission of Cedars-Sinai Medical Center, Los Angeles, California. (Originally appeared as Figure 5-4 in Davis RW, Komaiko MS. Blueprints in Radiology. Malden, MA: Blackwell Science, 2003.)

BLOCK 8

Figure 347: Used with permission of Cedars-Sinai Medical Center, Los Angeles, California. (Originally appeared as Figure 2-8 in Davis RW, Komaiko MS. Blueprints in Radiology. Malden, MA: Blackwell Science, 2003.)

Figure 359: Used with permission of Cedars-Sinai Medical Center, Los Angeles, California. (Originally appeared as Figure 8-4 in Davis RW, Komaiko MS. Blueprints in Radiology. Malden, MA: Blackwell Science, 2003.)

BLOCK 9

Figure 381: Used with permission of Cedars-Sinai Medical Center, Los Angeles, California. (Originally appeared as Figure 5-3 in Davis RW, Komaiko MS. Blueprints in Radiology. Malden, MA: Blackwell Science, 2003.)

Figure 409: Used with permission of Cedars-Sinai Medical Center, Los Angeles, California. (Originally appeared as Figure 8-14 in Davis RW, Komaiko MS. Blueprints in Radiology. Malden, MA: Blackwell Science, 2003.)

BLOCK 10

Figure 439: Used with permission of Cedars-Sinai Medical Center, Los Angeles, California. (Originally appeared as Figure 4-5c in Davis RW, Komaiko MS. Blueprints in Radiology. Malden, MA: Blackwell Science, 2003.)

Figure 452: Used with permission of Cedars-Sinai Medical Center, Los Angeles, California. (Originally appeared as Figure 5-5 in Davis RW, Komaiko MS. Blueprints in Radiology. Malden, MA: Blackwell Science, 2003.)

BLOCK 11

Figure 463: Used with permission of Cedars-Sinai Medical Center, Los Angeles, California. (Originally appeared as Figure 5-6 in Davis RW, Komaiko MS. Blueprints in Radiology. Malden, MA: Blackwell Science, 2003.)

Figure 485: Used with permission of Cedars-Sinai Medical Center, Los Angeles, California. (Originally appeared as Figure 4-8 in Davis RW, Komaiko MS. Blueprints in Radiology. Malden, MA: Blackwell Science, 2003.)

BLOCK 12

Figure 522: Used with permission of Cedars-Sinai Medical Center, Los Angeles, California. (Originally appeared as Figure 5-8 in Davis RW, Komaiko MS. Blueprints in Radiology. Malden, MA: Blackwell Science, 2003.)

Figure 542: Used with permission of Cedars-Sinai Medical Center, Los Angeles, California. (Originally appeared as Figure 4-11 in Davis RW, Komaiko MS. Blueprints in Radiology. Malden, MA: Blackwell Science, 2003.)

BLOCK 13

Figure 579: Used with permission from Taylor GJ. 150 Practice ECGs: Interpretation and Review. 2nd ed. Malden, MA: Blackwell Science, 2002. (Originally appeared as Practice ECG 10.)

Figure 593: Used with permission of Cedars-Sinai Medical Center, Los Angeles, California. (Originally appeared as Figure 5-13 in Davis RW, Komaiko MS. Blueprints in Radiology. Malden, MA: Blackwell Science, 2003.)

BLOCK 14

Figure 619: Used with permission of Cedars-Sinai Medical Center, Los Angeles, California. (Originally appeared as Figure 7-5 in Davis RW, Komaiko MS. Blueprints in Radiology. Malden, MA: Blackwell Science, 2003.)

Figure 641: Used with permission from Taylor GJ. 150 Practice ECGs: Interpretation and Review. 2nd ed. Malden, MA: Blackwell Science, 2002. (Originally appeared as Practice ECG 83.)

BLOCK 15

Figure 667: Used with permission from Taylor GJ. 150 Practice ECGs: Interpretation and Review. 2nd ed. Malden, MA: Blackwell Science, 2002. (Originally appeared as Practice ECG 69.)

Figure 691: Used with permission of Cedars-Sinai Medical Center, Los Angeles, California. (Originally appeared as Figure 7-2 in Davis RW, Komaiko MS. Blueprints in Radiology. Malden, MA: Blackwell Science, 2003.)

BLOCK 16

Figure 721: Used with permission of Cedars-Sinai Medical Center, Los Angeles, California. (Originally appeared as Figure 8-13 in Davis RW, Komaiko MS. Blueprints in Radiology. Malden, MA: Blackwell Science, 2003.)

Figure 735: Used with permission from Taylor GJ. 150 Practice ECGs: Interpretation and Review. 2nd ed. Malden, MA: Blackwell Science, 2002. (Originally appeared as Practice ECG 12.)

NORMAL LABORATORY VALUES

Blood, Plasma, Serum

Alanine aminotransferase (ALT, GPT at 30°C)	8–20 U/L
Alpha-fetoprotein (AFP)	0–10 ng/ml
Amylase, serum	25–125 U/L
Aspartate aminotransferase (AST, GOT at 30°C)	8–20 U/L
Bilirubin, serum (adult) Total/Direct	0.1–1.0 mg/dL/0.0–0.3 mg/dL
Calcium, serum (Ca^{2+})	8.4–10.2 mg/dL
Cholesterol, serum	Recommend: <200 mg/dL
Cortisol, serum	0800h: 5–23 ng/dL/1600h: 3–15 ng/dL/ 2000h: ≤50% of 0800h
Creatine kinase, serum	Male: 25–90 U/L Female: 10–70 U/L
Creatinine, serum	0.6–1.2 mg/dL
Electrolytes, serum	
Sodium (Na^+)	136–145 mEq/L
Chloride (Cl^-)	95–105 mEq/L
Potassium (K^+)	3.5–5.0 mEq/L
Bicarbonate (HCO_3^-)	22–28 mEq/L
Magnesium (Mg^{2+})	1.5–2.0 mEq/L
Ferritin, serum	Male: 15–200 ng/mL Female: 12–150 ng/mL
Follicle-stimulating hormone, serum/plasma	Male: 4–25 mIU/mL Female: premenopause 4–30 mIU/mL midcycle peak 10–90 mIU/mL postmenopause 40–250 mIU/mL
Gases, arterial blood (room air)	
PH	7.35–7.45
PCO_2	33–45 mm Hg
PO_2	75–105 mm Hg
Glucose, serum	Fasting: 70–110 mg/dL 2-h postprandial: <120 mg/dL
Growth hormone-arginine stimulation	Fasting: <5 ng/mL Provocative stimuli: >7 ng/mL
Human chorionic gonadotropin (hCG)	<5 mIU/mL
Iron	50–70 ug/dL
Lactate dehydrogenase, serum	45–90 U/L
Luteinizing hormone, serum/plasma	Male: 6–23 mIU/mL Female: follicular phase 5–30 mIU/mL midcycle 75–150 mIU/mL postmenopause 30–200 mIU/mL
Osmolality, serum	275–295 mOsmo/kg
Parathyroid hormone, serum, N-terminal	230–630 pg/mL
Phosphate (alkaline), serum (p-NPP at 30°C)	20–70 u/L
Phosphorus (inorganic), serum	3.0–4.5 mg/dL

Prolactin, serum (hPRL)	<20 ng/mL
Proteins, serum	
Total (recumbent)	6.0–7.8 g/dL
Albumin	3.5–5.5 g/dL
Globulin	2.3–3.5 g/dL
Prostate specific antigen	0–4 ng/mL
Testosterone, serum	300–1000 ng/dL
Thyroid-stimulating hormone, serum or plasma	0.5–5.0 nU/mL
Thyroidal iodine (^{123}I) uptake	8–30% of administered dose/24 h
Thyroxine (T_4), serum	5–12 ng/dL
Triglycerides, serum	35–160 mg/dL
Triiodothyronine (T_3), serum (RIA)	115–190 ng/dL
Triiodothyronine (T_9), resin uptake	25–35%
Urea nitrogen, serum (BUN)	7–18 mg/dL
Uric acid, serum	3.0–8.2 mg/dL

Hematologic

Bleeding time (template)	2–7 minutes
Erythrocyte count	Male: 4.3–5.9 million/mm^3
	Female: 3.5–5.5 million/mm^3
Erythrocyte sedimentation rate (Westergren)	Male: 0–15 mm/h
	Female: 0–20 mm/h
Hematocrit	Male: 41–53%
	Female: 36–46%
Hemoglobin A_{1c}	≤6%
Hemoglobin, blood	Male: 13.5–17.5 g/dL
	Female: 12.0–16.0 g/dL
Leukocyte count and differential	
Leukocyte count	4500–11,000/mm^3
Segmented neutrophils	54–62%
Bands	3–5%
Eosinophils	1–3%
Basophils	0–0.75%
Lymphocytes	25–33%
Monocytes	3–7%
Mean corpuscular hemoglobin	25.4–34.6 pg/cell
Mean corpuscular hemoglobin concentration	31–36% Hb/cell
Mean corpuscular volume	80–100 nm^3
Partial thromboplastin time (activated)	25–40 seconds
Platelet count	150,000–400,000/mm^3
Prothrombin time	11–15 seconds
Reticulocyte count	0.5–1.5% of red cells
Thrombin time	<2 seconds deviation from control
Volume	
Plasma	Male: 25–43 mL/kg
	Female: 28–45 mL/kg
Red cell	Male: 20–36 mL/kg
	Female: 19–31 mL/kg

Urine

Calcium	100–300 mg/24 h
Chloride	varies with intake
Creatine clearance	Male: 97–137 mL/min
	Female: 88–128 mL/min
Osmolality	50–1400 mOsmoL/kg
Oxalate	8–40 ng/mL
Potassium	varies with diet
Proteins, total	<150 mg/24h
Sodium	40–220 mEq/24h
Uric acid	210–750 mg/24h

Urinalysis

Color	clear
Odor	none
Glucose	none
Ketones	none
Protein	<150 mg/24h
pH	4.5–8.0
Specific gravity	1.001–1.035
Red cells	0–3/HPF
White cells	0–3/ HPF
Bacteria	negative
Crystals	negative
Epithelial cells (?)	not significant

Seminal Fluid Analysis

Appearance	Opaque, gray-white, highly viscid
Volume	2–5 mL
Liquefaction	complete within 30 minutes
pH	7.2–8.0
Leukocytes	occasional or absent
Count	20–250 million/mL
Motility	50–80% with progressive active motility
Morphology	50–90% with normal forms

TEST 1

Board Buster Step 2 was developed to give you the experience of a day of testing. Plan to set aside the time the real examination will take so that you may learn to pace yourself on answering the questions. Each block of questions should be completed in 60 minutes. While working on each block, you may answer the items in any order, review your responses, and change answers. After time expires, you may no longer review test items or change answers.

This section contains a full-length practice test for USMLE Step 2. To simulate the real examination, the test is divided into eight blocks and contains a total of 370 all-new board-format test questions. For your convenience, tear-out answer sheets on which you may record your answers are included in the back of the book.

The Answer Key for Test 1 is listed on p. 76. Complete explanations for each correct and incorrect answer option follow.

1. A 39-year-old black woman with a long history of progressive burning epigastric pain 2 hours after meals, often nocturnal and relieved by food, presents for evaluation. She states that her symptoms improve when she takes calcium carbonate (Tums®). She believes that she has peptic ulcer disease and brings you an article about this condition. Physical examination reveals a palpable thyroid gland without masses. Cardiac examination reveals no evidence of rubs, murmurs, or gallops. Pulmonary auscultation reveals no evidence of wheeze or rhonchi. Gastrointestinal examination reveals mild tenderness in the mid-epigastric region without focal peritoneal signs. Rectal examination reveals small internal nonprolapsing hemorrhoids, guaiac negative with stool in the vault. Modern views on the etiology of this condition relate to which of the following factors in the pathogenesis?

    A. *Helicobacter pylori*
    B. Impaired gastric blood flow
    C. Impaired gastric epithelial turnover
    D. Prostaglandin inhibition
    E. Thinning of mucous layer

2. A 28-year-old man presents to the ambulatory care clinic complaining of fever and a productive cough. He states that he has always been sick, particularly with fevers with productive coughs. He does not appear to be in any acute distress. Head and neck examination is remarkable for mild erythema of the pharynx. Cardiac examination yields a regular rate and rhythm without murmurs, rubs, or gallops. Pulmonary examination reveals bilateral rales more prominent on the left side. Chest x-ray demonstrates bilateral cystic lesions with fluid levels in middle and lower lung zones. What is the most appropriate treatment for this patient?

    A. Antibiotics and drainage
    B. Bronchoscopy
    C. Lung transplantation
    D. Respiratory isolation
    E. Surgical resection

3. A 29-year-old G5P2 woman is 20 weeks pregnant. She has a long history of intermittent bloody and watery diarrhea. Her symptoms have remained stable during the current pregnancy. Cardiac examination reveals a regular rate and rhythm. Pulmonary evaluation reveals clear lungs bilaterally without rales or rhonchi. Abdominal examination reveals normoactive bowel sounds with a fundal height 22 cm from the pubis. Anorectal evaluation reveals evidence of a healed left and right lateral anal fissure. What is the most likely diagnosis?

    A. Appendicitis
    B. Gastroesophageal reflux
    C. Hepatitis
    D. Hyperemesis gravidarum
    E. Inflammatory bowel disease

4. You are paged to evaluate a male neonate who was born 26 hours ago. The nurse explains to you that he has been doing well, but has not passed any meconium. The neonate has stable vital signs, with clear lungs and no murmur on auscultation. On palpation of the abdomen, you discover a mass and order an abdominal x-ray. The film shows a "ground-glass" appearance within the bowel, and you order a Gastrografin enema, which removes the meconium. What is the next most appropriate step in the evaluation of this neonate?

    A. No further evaluation is necessary
    B. Perform a transrectal biopsy
    C. Perform genetic analysis
    D. Repeat abdominal radiography
    E. Perform exploratory laparotomy

5. A 27-year-old man complains of a painless lump in his right groin. He has a prior surgical history of right orchiopexy at age 4. He has no other medical conditions and takes no medications. Cardiac examination reveals a regular rate and rhythm. Pulmonary auscultation reveals no rales, rhonchi, or wheezing. Gastrointestinal examination reveals normoactive bowel sounds. The right testis has a 1.5-cm area of induration on the posterior surface. The right epididymis and vas deferens are palpable. The left testis has no areas of induration. The left epididymis and vas deferens are palpable. Chest x-ray reveals no evidence of effusions, masses, or infiltrates. Results of laboratory studies are shown below:

Blood, plasma, serum

Alanine aminotransferase (ALT)	10 U/L
Alpha-fetoprotein	5 ng/mL
Amylase, serum	50 U/L
Aspartate aminotransferase (AST)	10 U/L
Calcium, serum	9 mg/dL
Glucose, serum	100 mg/dL
Hematocrit	33%
Human chorionic gonadotropin	Normal
Urea nitrogen, serum (BUN)	10 mg/dL

Urinalysis

Urine pH	6.0
RBC count	2/HPF
WBC count	2/HPF
Nitrates	Negative
Bacteria	Negative

Which of the following is the most likely diagnosis?

    A. Embryonal carcinoma
    B. Endodermal sinus tumor
    C. Seminoma
    D. Teratocarcinoma
    E. Teratoma

6. A 25-year-old woman presents for evaluation of a lobular, firm, well-circumscribed 2-cm breast mass in the left upper outer quadrant. Prior medical and surgical history are unremarkable. The patient does note that her mother had multiple bilateral breast cysts that were followed with annual mammographic studies. There is no known family history of breast cancer. Physical examination reveals no evidence of dimpling, skin retraction, or axillary adenopathy. Examination of the right breast reveals no evidence of dimpling, skin retraction, or axillary adenopathy. What is the most likely diagnosis?

   A. Fibroadenoma
   B. Fibrocystic change
   C. Fibrosarcoma
   D. Infiltrating ductal cell carcinoma
   E. Intraductal papilloma

7. A 29-year-old man presents to his primary care physician complaining of chronic back pain. He states that he fell off a ladder 3 years ago and broke his back. Since that time he has been unable to work and has only been able to function when taking a combination of pentazocine and meperidine. He walks slowly and carefully, and is unable to flex or extend his lumbar spine because of pain. He points to the L3 area as the point of maximum pain. He states that he does not like to take drugs but has to do so in order to function. What is the most likely diagnosis?

   A. Chronic lumbar pain syndrome
   B. Deformity of the lumbar spine with fractures
   C. Drug abuse
   D. Prior lumbar spine fractures
   E. Somatiform pain disorder

8. A 32-year-old man is hospitalized following a motor vehicle accident in which he suffered head trauma. He is currently tracheally intubated in the surgical intensive care unit (SICU). On day 8 of admission, he develops hemoptysis. Chest x-ray reveals poor inspiratory effort, is underpenetrated, and suggests a large lobar infiltrate. Gram stain reveals numerous white blood cells and gram-positive cocci in clusters. Results of laboratory studies are shown below:

Leukocyte count	14,000/mm^3
Segmented neutrophils	75%
Bands	6%
Eosinophils	3%
Basophils	1%
Lymphocytes	24%
Monocytes	4%

   What is the most likely explanation of these findings?

   A. Aspiration pneumonia
   B. *Haemophilus influenzae* pneunonia
   C. *Mycobacterium tuberculosis* pneumonia
   D. *Staphylococcus aureus* pneumonia
   E. *Streptococcus pneumoniae* pneumonia

Questions 9–11:
   A. Alport syndrome
   B. Autosomal-dominant polycystic kidney disease
   C. Focal segmental glomerulosclerosis
   D. Hemolytic-uremic syndrome
   E. IgA nephropathy
   F. Neonatal hydronephrosis
   G. Nephrotic syndrome
   H. Primary vesicoureteral reflux
   I. Posterior urethral valves
   J. Renal hypoplasia
   K. Sponge kidney (cystic collecting tubule dilation)

For each child with renal disease, select the most likely diagnosis.

9. A 2-year-old boy with a history of deafness presents to his pediatrician with gross hematuria. Physical examination findings of the heart, lungs, and abdomen are within normal limits. Serum creatinine is 1.9 mg/dL. Urine analysis reveals microscopic hematuria and proteinuria. Renal biopsy reveals abnormalities in the glomerular basement membrane.

10. A newborn male with prenatal hydronephrosis on screening fetal ultrasonography has a poor, intermittent, dribbling urinary stream. Physical examination of the heart and lungs is within normal limits. A palpable lower abdominal midline mass is noted. Voiding cystourethrography reveals elongation and dilation of the posterior urethra with a prominent bladder neck.

11. A 3-month-old boy is evaluated by his pediatrician for failure to thrive. He weighs 10 pounds. His mother reports that for the last 3 weeks he has had decreased urine output and she has changed his diapers an average of twice daily. The mother is of Scandinavian descent and has renal problems. Review of records from birth reveal that the placenta was enlarged. Physical examination findings of the heart, lungs, and abdomen is unremarkable. Serum creatinine is 1.5 mg/dL. Urine dipstick reveals +3 proteinuria.

12. A 22-year-old man presents to the emergency room complaining of progressive weakness in both of his lower extremities. He states that he first noticed an abnormality earlier in the week when he began experiencing abnormal sensations in both of his feet. Soon after, he noticed difficulty standing on his toes. Since that time, he states he has had trouble rising from a seated position. Now he claims that it is difficult for him to walk. He has also noticed a similar progressive weakness of his upper extremities. His past medical history is positive for an episode of gastroenteritis a few weeks ago. On review of systems, the patient revealed a recent onset of palpitations and unexplained periods of sweating. He has not had a bowel movement for the past 4 days, which is abnormal for him. Physical examination reveals increased respiratory effort and absent deep tendon reflexes in all four extremities. Muscle strength is decreased most prominently

in the distal musculature. The patient is admitted to the hospital. Nerve conduction testing shows marked slowing of motor and sensory conduction velocities. Cerebrospinal fluid analysis reveals a normal cell count and elevated protein. The patient is treated for an acute idiopathic polyneuropathy. Which of the following treatment options has been shown to decrease the likelihood of persistent neurologic deficits while enhancing the possibility of a faster recovery?

A. Intravenous immunoglobulin

B. Antibiotics for infection with *Clostridium jejuni*

C. Fluids, pressors, and heparin

D. Plasmapheresis

E. No treatment has shown to influence the natural history of this disease

13. A 38-year-old man has a 1-year history of tenesmus, intermittent diarrhea, and constipation. He admits to tearing pain with defecation and bright red bleeding per rectum noted on the toilet tissue for the past 6 months. His prior medical history is notable for irritable bowel syndrome. Current medications include dicyclomine. Physical examination reveals descended testicles bilaterally without masses and palpable inguinal lymph nodes. Anoscopy reveals a split in the anoderm at the posterior midline. He also has evidence of a skin tag, chronic ulceration, and hypertrophied anal papillae. Which of the following is the most appropriate treatment?

A. Ampicillin (intravenous)

B. Metronidazole (oral)

C. Rubber band ligation

D. Sitz baths and dietary bulking agents containing psyllium

E. Surgical excision and lateral anal sphincterotomy

14. An 82-year-old woman presents to her primary care physician with right wrist pain after falling 1 hour ago. She has a history of osteoporosis and coronary artery disease. Physical examination reveals point tenderness over the right distal radius and over the ulnar styloid. The right wrist is severely edematous, but the skin is intact. Anteroposterior and lateral radiographs of the right wrist are ordered and are presented below (Figure 14). What is the most likely diagnosis?

A. Colles fracture

B. Greenstick fracture

C. Smith fracture

D. Torus fracture

E. Type IV fracture (Salter Harris) of the right distal radius

Figure 14

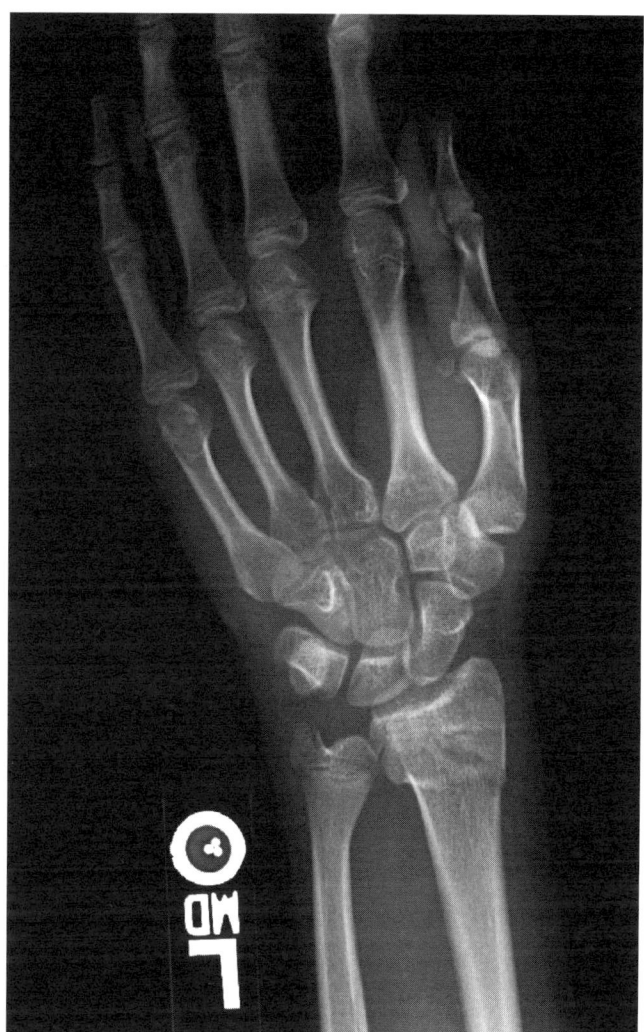

15. A study is performed to look at the number of false-positive results found in exercise stress tests. Two groups of people are included in the study. The control group consists of men in their thirties who do not smoke. The second group consists of men in their sixties who do not smoke. There will obviously be a higher prevalence of heart disease in the older group simply because of their age. What happens to the specificity and the positive predictive values (PPV) of a test such as an exercise stress test when the prevalence of a disease increases in the population you are looking at?

   A. Both stay the same

   B. Specificity increases, PPV decreases

   C. Specificity stays the same, PPV increases

   D. Both decrease

   E. Unable to determine with the information given

16. A 26-year-old postpartum woman presents to her primary care physician complaining of increase in redness and tenderness of her right breast. She states she is breast-feeding, but states her breast has felt different over the past few days. Physical examination reveals her temperature is 38.5°C. There is increased erythema and cracking of her right nipple when compared with the left. Results of laboratory studies are shown below:

Electrolytes, serum

Na, serum	143 mEq/L
Cl, serum	100 mEq/L
K, serum	3.7 mEq/L
Bicarbonate, serum	24 mEq/L
Magnesium, serum	2.0 mEq/L
Creatinine, serum	1.0 mg/dL

Leukocyte count and differential

Leukocyte count	12,000/mm^3
Segmented neutrophils	75%
Bands	7%
Eosinophils	3%
Basophils	1%
Lymphocytes	27%
Monocytes	4%

What is the most appropriate treatment for this condition?

   A. Antibiotics and continue breast-feeding

   B. Antibiotics, ice, and stop breast-feeding

   C. Antibiotics, warm compresses, and stop breast-feeding

   D. Condition is self-limiting and requires observation

   E. Warm compresses, tight bra, oral analgesics, and stop breast-feeding

17. A 67-year-old man presents to his primary care physician complaining of a 6-month history of cough productive of sputum and pain on inspiration. He complains of rhinorrhea, occasional bloody nasal discharge, and sinus pain. He denies having a sore throat, hoarseness, nausea, vomiting, diarrhea, frequency, urgency or dysuria. Physical examination of the

eyes reveals mild injection bilaterally. Cardiac, abdominal, and neurologic examinations are unremarkable. Pulmonary auscultation reveals poor air movement consistent with pleuritic pain. Laboratory studies reveal a leukocyte count of 13,000/mm^3 with 70% segmented neutrophils, hemoglobin of 16 g/dL. Urinalysis reveals 25 RBCs per HPF and 3 WBC per HPF. What is the most likely diagnosis?

   A. Alveolar hemorrhage

   B. Anti–glomerular basement membrane disease

   C. Churg-Strauss syndrome

   D. Pulmonary abscess

   E. Wegener granulomatosis

18. A 19-year-old woman complains of a 12-hour history of intense rectal pain. The pain was precipitated by straining during a bowel movement, after which a small amount of bright red blood was noted on the toilet tissue. Her prior medical history is notable for seasonal allergic rhinitis and hyperthyroidism (currently on no medications). Physical examination reveals a regular rate and rhythm without rubs, murmurs, or gallops. Pulmonary auscultation reveals no rales, rhonchi, or wheezes. Abdominal examination reveals no evidence of peritoneal signs. Anoscopy reveals a small tear in the mucosa of the anorectum in the posterior midline approximately 1.5 cm from the anal verge. There is no evidence of hypertrophied anal papillae or skin tags. What is the most likely diagnosis?

   A. External hemorrhoids

   B. Fissure-in-ano

   C. Fistula-in-ano

   D. Internal hemorrhoids

   E. Proctitis

19. A 38-year-old obese woman presents to her primary care physician for a routine evaluation. She has no prior medical or surgical history. Physical examination of the heart, lungs, and abdomen are unremarkable. Results of laboratory studies are shown below:

Na, serum	123 mEq/L
Osmolarity, serum	305 mOsm/kg

What is the most likely explanation of these findings?

   A. Dehydration

   B. Hyperglycemia

   C. Hyperlipidemia

   D. Nephrotic syndrome

   E. Syndrome of inappropriate antidiuretic hormone secretion (SIADH)

20. A 9-month-old male infant is brought to the emergency department for evaluation of fever and many superficial bullae. Yesterday there were no lesions present, only areas of diffuse erythema. The bullae are rupturing shortly after they appear. Physical examination reveals that light rubbing leads to separation of the epidermis. What is the most likely explanation for these findings?

A. *Haemophilus influenzae*
B. *Staphylococcus aureus*
C. β-hemolytic streptococcus
D. *Sarcoptes scabiei*
E. *Strongyloides* species

21. A 13-year-old girl presents to the gynecologist because of abdominal pain. She has not yet had menarche; however, she had thelarche 4 years ago. Physical examination findings of the heart, lungs, and abdomen are within normal limits. Pelvic examination reveals a bulging wall just inside her vagina with purple-red discoloration. What is the most likely diagnosis?

A. Bartholin gland cyst
B. Imperforate hymen
C. Rectocele
D. Sexual abuse
E. Uterine prolapse

22. A 22-year-old schizophrenic man is brought to the thought disorder clinic by his wife. She says that his symptoms were fairly well controlled until the past couple of weeks, when he started to send large numbers of letters to people she has never heard of before. He often doesn't write anything to them, but he does send them coupons that he cut out of the Sunday paper. She feels he may need a medication change, and hands you his bottle of thioridazine. One adverse reaction of this medication is:

A. Agranulocytosis
B. Delayed ejaculation
C. Hypertension
D. Pigmentary retinopathy
E. Weight gain

23. A 91-year-old man who is wheelchair bound and in a nursing home has a urinary catheter placed because of a prolonged history of enuresis and daytime urinary incontinence. His current medical problems include diabetes mellitus, hypertension, and congestive heart failure, and he has a history of myocardial infarction 2 years ago. His current medications include glyburide, atenolol, and furosemide. On a recent urine culture in the nursing home the patient is noted to have 75,000 colony-forming units of *Escherichia coli*. Laboratory studies sent with the patient from the nursing home are as follows:

Globulin, serum	2.1 g/dL
Thyroxine, serum	4 μg/dL
Triiodothyronine, serum	130 ng/dL
Iron, serum	95 μg/dL
Hematocrit	29%
Cholesterol, serum	210 mg/dL

In which of the following scenarios should the patient receive antibiotic therapy?

A. After removal of the urinary catheter
B. Gross hematuria develops
C. Pyuria develops
D. The patient develops fever and chills
E. Urine culture reveals a second organism

24. A 36-year-old male physics professor presents to his primary care physician with complaints of painful, swollen joints and hematuria. Upon further questioning the patient recalls a bout of nausea and bloody diarrhea that occurred 2 weeks prior to the presenting symptoms. Physical examination reveals several tender, swollen, and erythematous joints, shallow painless ulcers on the penis, and a hyperkeratotic papular rash on the soles of both feet. Urinalysis reveals microhematuria. What additional abnormality would you expect in this patient?

A. Bamboo spine on lumbar film
B. *Chlamydia* on Gram stain
C. Conjunctivitis
D. Mitral valve stenosis
E. Pleural effusion

25. A 32-year-old G2P1 female well-controlled diabetic presents to her obstetrician at 39½ weeks' gestation. She reports no significant contractions and no vaginal discharge. Physical examination of the heart, lungs, and abdomen are unremarkable. Pelvic examination reveals 10% effacement and 1 cm cervical dilatation. What is the most appropriate treatment for this patient?

A. Bed rest for remainder of pregnancy
B. Check hemoglobin A1C levels and obtain pelvic ultrasound study
C. Continuing current diabetes management and follow up in 1 week
D. Immediate cesarean section
E. Induction of labor and vaginal delivery after verifying fetal lung maturity

26. A 6-month-old African-American infant is brought to the emergency department by his parents. The child is irritable, has a fever, and seems to have nonspecific pain. Physical examination reveals symmetric swelling on the dorsal surface of his hands and feet along with splenomegaly. A systolic ejection murmur is noted in the pulmonic region. Skin is jaundiced. Hemoglobin electrophoresis is abnormal. What is this patient's most likely diagnosis?

A. Anemia of chronic disease
B. Ferratin deficiency
C. Hereditary spherocytosis
D. Sickle cell anemia
E. Transient erythroblastopenia

27. You are the rotating intern working with the liaison psychiatry team when your attending physician is called to the emergency department. She is annoyed because it is "another drunk" and asks you to go work the patient up. When you arrive, the patient is lying on the bed and is dry heaving in the trash can. His wife is with him; she is too upset to talk to you. He tells you that he is 42 years old and has been sick for 2 days. He has had vomiting and diarrhea for "at least a couple of days" and has not been able to keep anything down. He has been unable to get out of bed due to the nausea and muscle aches. He says that he was also sweating day and night, but that seems to have gotten better. You notice that he keeps wincing and looking around the room. You ask if he has been taking drugs, he says he has not, and that he used to drink. His wife gives a chuckle and informs you that he "used to drink" for the past 15 years and stopped a couple of days ago. When asked how much, she replies that he was up to two fifths of vodka a day. She mentions to you that she only brought him in because he started shaking all over earlier that morning. On physical examination, the patient has dry mucous membranes, poor capillary refill, and orthostatic hypotension. His laboratory values are:

Na, serum	148 mEq/L
K, serum	5.0 mEq/L
Cl, serum	110 mEq/L
Creatinine, serum	1.1 mg/dL

The patient has been given 50 mg of phenothiazine for nausea. You decide that he is dehydrated and needs some fluids and nutrients. However, before you start his fluids, the first thing you should do for the patient is:

   A. Give carbamazepine for his withdrawal symptoms
   B. Give folic acid
   C. Give haloperidol for hallucinations
   D. Give sodium bicarbonate for metabolic alkalosis
   E. Give thiamine

28. A 22-year-old man had been obese since grade school when his friends used to call him names. He presents to his primary care physician for evaluation. He dieted many times throughout high school and lost a significant amount of weight. His current body mass index (BMI) is 21.5, but several times a week for the past 8 months he has been eating 3000 calories at a time. He often hides himself in his dorm room and eats whatever he can find. He feels that he has no control once he starts to eat, and then spends an hour in the bathroom forcing himself to vomit. He is obsessed with his weight and often spends hours at a time at the gym after he vomits. He realizes he has a problem and really wants to seek help. What is the most likely diagnosis?

   A. Anorexia nervosa
   B. Bulimia nervosa
   C. Eating disorder not otherwise specified
   D. Kluver-Bucy syndrome
   E. This patient does not meet DSM-IV criteria for any specific disorder

29. A 2-week-old African-American neonate presents to the pediatric clinic with jaundice, which is apparent from the head to the lower trunk and thighs. In addition, the child appears somewhat lethargic and agitated. The mother reports that the child has decreased bottle feeding but has no symptoms of gastrointestinal distress. History reveals that the child was born at 36 weeks with a birth weight of 1450 g. Both the labor and delivery were uneventful. Laboratory studies reveal a total bilirubin of 15 mg/dL and conjugated bilirubin of 1 mg/dL. Hematocrit is 28% and Coombs test is negative. What is the most likely diagnosis?

   A. ABO blood group incompatibility
   B. Biliary atresia
   C. Dubin-Johnson syndrome
   D. Hemolysis secondary to sickle cell disease
   E. Unidentified malignancy

30. A 6-year-old boy is brought to the emergency department after being bitten on the right hand by a stray cat that he was chasing. He has a prior medical history of attention deficit hyperactivity disorder. His prior surgical history is notable for tonsillectomy and hypospadias repair. Physical examination of the right hand reveals an open wound measuring approximately 2.5 cm and involves the thenar eminence. The wound is thoroughly cleaned and irrigated. What is the next step in the treatment of this patient?

   A. Suture the wound and give dicloxacillin
   B. Suture the wound and give penicillin V
   C. Suture the wound and give no antibiotics
   D. Leave wound open and give ampicillin/sulbactam
   E. Leave wound open and give penicillin V

31. A 28-year-old G1P1 woman had recently given birth to a healthy baby girl. She had developed preeclampsia during this pregnancy at 38 weeks; labor was induced, and she had an uncomplicated, vaginal delivery. You are seeing this patient at a postnatal visit and she asks if she would be at increased risk for developing preeclampsia during subsequent pregnancies. Which of the following is the most appropriate statement to make to this patient?

   A. She is not at an increased risk compared with the general child-bearing population
   B. She is at 25% to 30% increased risk, but will be given prophylactic antihypertensives and magnesium sulfate during her pregnancy
   C. She is at 25% to 30% increased risk, and low-dose aspirin has been shown to decrease risk
   D. She is at 50% to 60% increased risk and at a high likelihood of requiring cesarean section
   E. She is at a decreased risk for developing preeclampsia on subsequent pregnancies

32. A 55-year-old white man presents to the emergency department after having an episode of burning substernal chest pain while watching television earlier in the day. The patient

also complained of dyspnea earlier in the day but has no complaints on arrival. The patient has a past medical history of hypertension, diabetes mellitus, 60 pack per year history of smoking, and gastroesophageal reflux disease. Family history is significant for gallstones. Vital signs reveal a pulse of 90 beats/min and blood pressure of 130/70 mm Hg. Physical examination findings of the heart, lungs, and abdomen are unremarkable. The resting ECG reveals inverted T-waves. Serial values for creatinine kinase (CK) and isoenzyme of creatinine kinase with muscle and brain subunits (CK-MB) were 192 U/L and 2 U/L, respectively. Ventilation-perfusion (V/Q) scan shows a low probability for pulmonary embolism. What is the most appropriate next step in the management of this patient?

A. Cardiac echocardiography

B. Chest radiography

C. Coronary angiography

D. Exercise stress test

E. Right upper quadrant ultrasonography

33. A 13-year-old boy is brought to the emergency room after having a seizure that lasted 20 minutes. The patient has a history of grand mal seizures that have been successfully controlled by medication, which his mother believes he has not been taking regularly. His pulse is 85 beats/min, blood pressure is 118/72 mm Hg, temperature is 37.3°C, and oxygen saturation is 96% on room air. Physical examination reveals no evidence of cyanosis, clear lungs bilaterally, and good bilateral peripheral pulses. What is the most appropriate management for the patient?

A. Intravenous lorazepam and a loading dose of phenytoin

B. Intravenous phenobarbital and a loading dose of phenytoin

C. Intravenous ethosuximide and a loading dose of phenytoin

D. Intravenous valproic acid and a loading dose of phenytoin

E. Observation, with continuous monitoring of vital signs

34. A 62-year-old man has the sudden onset of chest pain while in the waiting room of your clinic. He says the pain is sharp, does not radiate, and is located just to the left of the lower sternum. He says sitting forward makes it worse. On examination he is febrile, his blood pressure is 150/90 mm Hg, and his pulse is 105 beats/min. Cardiac examination reveals a pericardial friction rub. ECG shows the following (Figure 34). What is the next best step in the management of this patient?

A. Aspirin

B. Chest x-ray

C. Echocardiogram

D. Pericardiocentesis

E. Pericardial biopsy

35. A 31-year-old woman presents to her primary care physician complaining of a 4-day history of fever, chills, vomiting, watery diarrhea, sore throat, and myalgias. Physical examination reveals a fever of 39.2°C, blood pressure of 90/60 mm Hg, pulse of 90 beats/min, and a diffuse macular erythematous rash with some minor skin peeling. What is the most likely diagnosis?

A. Botulism

B. Kawasaki disease

C. Lyme disease

D. Rocky Mountain spotted fever

E. Toxic shock syndrome

36. A 43-year-old G2P2002 smoker has used oral contraceptive pills between her pregnancies for 20+ years. Her husband has taken an early retirement, and they plan to travel extensively now that their youngest child has entered college. She has tried several methods for smoking cessation, without success. Which one of the following contraceptive methods should be avoided at this point?

A. Combined oral contraceptive pill

B. Condoms

C. Diaphragm

D. Intrauterine device

E. Progestin-only oral contraceptive pill

Figure 34

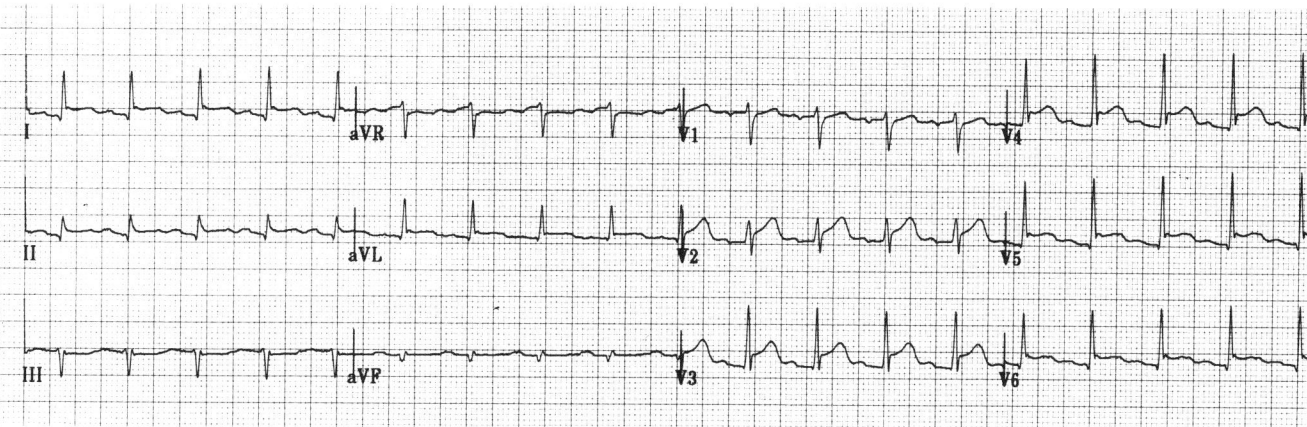

37. A 68-year-old man presents to his primary care physician with a 4-month history of lower back pain that is worse with movement. He also reports shortness of breath, productive cough, and fever for the past 2 weeks. Physical examination reveals rhonchi in the left lower lung fields, normal heart sounds, no abdominal tenderness, no hepatosplenomegaly, and no lymphadenopathy. A chest x-ray reveals lytic lesions of multiple ribs and left clavicle and consolidation of the left lower lobe. CBC reveals pancytopenia. Urinalysis is normal. Serum electrolytes are normal except for elevated serum calcium and an elevated BUN and creatinine. What is the most likely diagnosis?

    A. Chronic myelogenous leukemia
    B. Hyperparathyroidism
    C. Lymphoma
    D. Multiple myeloma
    E. Waldenström macroglobulinemia

38. An 18-year-old man was in an automobile accident 3 weeks ago after he and his friends were out drinking on a Friday night. His best friend was driving and was killed in the accident. Since that time, he has been horrified and cried continuously. He has not been able to go to school and has locked himself in his room since that time. He has not spoken with his parents or friends. When his mother confronted him, he was unable to recall anything about the accident and spoke as if nothing had occurred. He has had nightmares every night and whenever he has heard any loud noise he has jumped up terrified. What is the most likely explanation of these findings?

    A. Acute stress disorder
    B. Generalized anxiety disorder
    C. Major depressive episode
    D. Panic disorder
    E. Posttraumatic stress disorder

39. A 20-year-old man is involved in a car wreck in which he was thrown from the vehicle. Paramedics inform you in the emergency department that the man was found with both of his lower extremities trapped beneath the vehicle. The estimated time of entrapment was 50 minutes. The lower extremities are extremely bruised but no fractures are immediately evident and distal pulses are strong bilaterally. A Foley catheter is placed in the patient, and smoky brown urine is found collecting within the Foley bag. What is the appropriate treatment regimen for this patient?

    A. Catheter removal
    B. Intravenous hydration
    C. Intravenous hydration and calcium gluconate
    D. Intravenous hydration and mannitol
    E. Intravenous hydration, mannitol, and sodium bicarbonate

40. A 65-year-old woman with hypertension undergoes renal ultrasonography for worsening renal function. The results show mildly enlarged kidneys without stenosis or hydronephrosis. Two months pass, and unexplained nephrotic range proteinuria develops and a renal biopsy is performed. The biopsy reveals large nodular eosinophilic masses. The sample is stained with Congo red and demonstrates apple-green birefringence under polarized light. Immunofluorescence microscopy is also conducted and reveals a slight increase in immunoglobulin light chains. Results of laboratory studies are shown below:

Electrolytes, serum

Na, serum	145 mEq/L
Cl, serum	101 mEq/L
K, serum	3.9 mEq/L
Bicarbonate, serum	24 mEq/L
Magnesium, serum	1.8 mEq/L
Creatinine, serum	1.4 mg/dL

Leukocyte count and differential

Leukocyte count	9700/mm^3

What is the most likely diagnosis?

    A. Amyloidosis
    B. Hypersensitivity nephropathy
    C. Multiple myeloma
    D. Renal vascular hypertension
    E. Waldenström macroglobulinemia

41. A 95-year-old man is brought to the emergency department from a nursing home where he is supervised most of the time. The staff tells you he has had difficulty breathing for the past week and that it is worsening. He has a history of asthma for which he takes a leukotriene inhibitor and inhaled steroids as needed. Physical examination reveals an oral temperature of 99.4°F, respirations are 14 breaths/min, blood pressure is 110/74 mm Hg, and pulse is 88 beats/min. He appears mildly uncomfortable with retractions. Auscultation reveals inspiratory stridor and expiratory wheezing in the left chest. No rubs or rales are appreciated. No lymphadenopathy is present. Which of the following x-ray findings would be consistent with this patient's diagnosis?

    A. Atelectasis of the left lung
    B. Diffuse infiltrates bilaterally
    C. Hyperinflated left lung
    D. Mediastinal shift toward the left
    E. Normal x-ray

42. A 25-year-old woman presents to her primary care physician because of inability to conceive a child with her husband. They have been having unprotected sexual intercourse for 18 months. She has no prior medical history. However, questioning reveals that she has never had a sense of smell. Further review of her medical records indicates that she underwent renal ultrasonography that revealed left-sided renal agenesis. Physical examination is significant for flat-chestedness. The remainder of the gynecologic examination is normal. What is the most likely explanation for these findings?

A. Anorexia nervosa
B. Brain tumor
C. Constitutionally delayed puberty
D. Kallmann syndrome
E. Swyer syndrome

43. A child with known insulin-dependent diabetes mellitus presents to the emergency department with polyuria, polydipsia, headache, emesis, and abdominal pain. He appears dehydrated and moderately confused. Vital signs reveal a blood pressure of 90/60 mm Hg and respirations of 40 breaths/min. Arterial blood gas reveals a pH of 7.17. What is the next most appropriate step in the treatment of this patient?

A. Bicarbonate infusion
B. Carbohydrate snack
C. Glucagon infusion
D. Insulin bolus of 0.2 units/kg/h
E. Replacement of fluids

44. A 55-year-old man presents to his primary care physician complaining of excessive daytime sleepiness. A nighttime polysomnogram (total monitoring time 450 minutes) reveals that the apnea/hypopnea index is within normal limits, but his periodic limb movement index is significantly elevated. When the patient is asked about such movements, he is unaware that they have occurred. First-line pharmacologic treatment for this disorder affects which neurotransmitter?

A. Acetylcholine
B. Dopamine
C. GABA
D. Glutamate
E. Norepinephrine

45. A 34-year-old man presents to the ambulatory care outpatient clinic for a follow-up evaluation of his impotence. Two weeks ago, when the patient established care here, you focused on the problem at hand and performed a thorough physical examination, noting apparently normal neurologic and vascular functions. Without much time at that visit, you simply listed the patient's problem list: anxiety (untreated), chronic constipation, chronic fatigue, recurrent peptic ulcers, chronic pain "all over," and history of three documented kidney stones. You believed an arterial cause to be unlikely (nonsmoker, no diabetes, normal blood pressure and lipids) and assumed a psychogenic etiology. Accordingly, you gave the patient "strips" to monitor nocturnal penile tumescence and ordered a toxicology screen, which came back negative. Today, the patient reports he has had no nocturnal erections (the circumferential "strips" did not break). Among the following, what is the most likely diagnosis?

A. Factitious disorder
B. Impotence with psychogenic etiology
C. Multiple endocrine neoplasia type I

D. Multiple sclerosis
E. Somatization disorder

46. A 79-year-old farmer accompanied by his wife presents to your office with a large 3-cm nodule on his right cheek. He says it has been there for over 10 years. He also has multiple other rough areas on his face, neck, and forearms that are slightly hyperkeratotic. Each of them is variable in size and no one is larger than 1 cm. The 3-cm nodule appears to be ulcerating without evidence of discharge with other areas of crusting. He says he has never used sunscreen in his life and his wife recalls that he was always fair skinned.

Recent laboratory values are shown below:

Electrolytes, serum

Na, serum	143 mEq/L
Cl, serum	100 mEq/L
K, serum	3.7 mEq/L
Bicarbonate, serum	24 mEq/L
Magnesium, serum	2.0 mEq/L
Creatinine, serum	1.0 mg/dL

Leukocyte count and differential

Leukocyte count	12,000/mm^3
Segmented neutrophils	75%
Bands	7%
Eosinophils	3%
Basophils	1%
Lymphocytes	27%
Monocytes	4%

Blood, plasma, serum

Alanine aminotransferase (ALT)	10 U/L
Amylase, serum	50 U/L
Aspartate aminotransferase (AST)	10 U/L
Calcium, serum	9 mg/dL
Glucose, serum	100 mg/dL
Hematocrit	32%
Urea nitrogen, serum (BUN)	10 mg/dL

Urinalysis

Urine pH	6.0
RBC count	2/HPF
WBC count	2/HPF
Nitrates	Negative
Bacteria	Negative

What is the most likely diagnosis of the 3-cm nodule?

A. Actinic keratosis
B. Basal cell carcinoma
C. Malignant melanoma
D. Rosacea
E. Squamous cell carcinoma

47. A 25-year-old woman complains of vulvar itching, burning, and vaginal discharge with rancid odor for 2 weeks. She has a prior medical history of gestational diabetes mellitus and asthma for which she takes no medications. She lives alone and has had unprotected sexual intercourse with multiple male partners during the past several weeks. The vaginal discharge is yellow-green in color, frothy, and has a pH of 7.0. Vulvovaginal examination reveals vulvar edema and erythema and petechia on the cervix. The vaginal vault has no evidence of mass lesions. Wet smear reveals large numbers of mature epithelial cells, WBCs, and a fusiform protozoan organism. What is the most appropriate treatment for this patient?

  A. Amoxicillin
  B. Ampicillin
  C. Metronidazole
  D. Miconazole
  E. Terconazole

48. A 4-year-old boy is brought into the emergency room for evaluation. His mother explains that her son fell while playing in the house. The mother gives a history of prior fractures, and also notes that her son has bilateral hearing loss. Physical examination reveals that the right arm is erythematous and swollen, and extremely tender to palpation. X-rays demonstrate a fracture of the radius, as well as characteristics of old, healed fractures. What is the most likely explanation for the pattern of fractures?

  A. Abnormal fibroblast growth factor (FGF) receptor
  B. Abnormal synthesis of type I collagen
  C. Abuse by the caregivers
  D. Deficiency in vitamin D
  E. Underlying bone tumor

49. A 49-year-old premenopausal woman presents to her primary care physician for angina occurring with exertion for 2 months. Upon cessation of activity, pain does not immediately go away. She reports having taken her husband's sublingual nitroglycerin without relief. She is a nonsmoker and drinks a couple of glasses of wine on weekends. Physical examination reveals:

Temperature	36.7°C
Pulse	82 beats/min
Blood pressure	125/85 mm Hg
Respirations	20 breaths/min
Body mass index	27

Physical examination of the heart, lungs and abdomen are unremarkable. Exercise stress testing reveals ST segment depression. Coronary arteriography is normal. Ergonovine provocation is unremarkable. What is the most likely explanation for these findings?

  A. Acute myocardial infarction
  B. Costochondritis
  C. Esophageal dysmotility
  D. Mitral valve prolapse
  E. Syndrome X

50. A 42-year-old man has a calculated resting energy expenditure of 1800 kcal/day (basal energy expenditure plus 10%). He suffered third degree burns of approximately 50% of his body surface area while attempting to cook dinner on a camp stove. He is taken to the university burn center and admitted. What is his daily energy requirement?

  A. 1600
  B. 2000
  C. 2500
  D. 3000
  E. 3600

51. A 25-year-old man has a history of manic-depression. He also has a history of hypercalcemia secondary to parathyroid adenoma and a prior history of renal stones that were treated with shock-wave lithotripsy. Multiaxial evaluation of this individual with regard to hyperparathyroidism is included on

  A. Axis I
  B. Axis II
  C. Axis III
  D. Axis IV
  E. Axis V

52. A 31-year-old woman presents to her primary care physician because of progressive visual disturbances. She notes that she has compromised distance and near vision. Prior history is notable for HIV disease. She does not know her last CD4 count. Funduscopic examination reveals large white areas proximal to the macula with perivascular exudates and hemorrhages. Shotty cervical adenomathy is noted bilaterally along the sternocleidomastoid muscle. What is the most appropriate treatment for this patient?

  A. Erythromycin
  B. Ganciclovir
  C. Penicillin VK
  D. Prednisone
  E. Prednisolone

53. A 24-year-old G2P1 woman is 20 weeks pregnant. She complains of a 10-hour history of anorexia, nausea, vomiting, and right lower quadrant pain. Physical examination reveals a woman in acute distress. Temperature is 101.5°F. Cardiac examination reveals a regular rate and rhythm. Pulmonary auscultation reveals no evidence of rhonchi or rales. Gastrointestinal examination reveals tenderness to soft palpation in the right lower quadrant with localized guarding and rebound tenderness. Rectal examination reveals the presence of external hemorrhoids. Tenderness is noted during bi-manual examination of the right lower quadrant. WBC count is 16,500 cells/mm³. What is the most likely diagnosis?

A. Appendicitis
B. Gastroesophageal reflux
C. Hepatitis
D. Hyperemesis gravidarum
E. Perforated tuboovarian abscess

54. Surgical resection of 15 cm of terminal ileum is undertaken in a 29-year-old man with a long history of intermittent diarrhea, crampy abdominal pain, and weight loss. Cardiovascular examination prior to surgical intervention showed tachycardia and a regular rhythm. Pulmonary auscultation revealed good inspiratory effort bilaterally. Gastrointestinal examination revealed the presence of a mass lesion in the right lower quadrant. Bowel sounds were normoactive. Peritoneal signs were absent. Rectal examination revealed the presence of a perianal fistula with an exit tract in the midline of the posterior anal wall lateral to the external sphincter. Several anal fissures were noted in various stages of development, as well as several hypertrophied anal papillae with skin tags nearby. Pathologic report indicates mucosal edema with aphthous ulcers in some areas; in other areas, transmural inflammation with mononuclear cell infiltration were noted. Which of the following physiologic consequences may result from surgical resection?

A. Constipation
B. Fat malabsorption
C. Increased reabsorption of bile salts
D. Increased vitamin B$_{12}$ absorption
E. Increased vitamin D absorption

55. A 4-year-old boy presents to his pediatrician for evaluation of several days of right otalgia, fever, and generalized discomfort. Right otoscopic examination reveals a hyperemic, opaque tympanic membrane that has poor mobility on pneumatic ostoscopy. Left otoscopy reveals no evidence of bulging or retraction. Pneumatic otoscopy reveals good mobility of the tympanic membrane. Cultures of middle ear fluid aspirate would most likely yield which of the following organisms?

A. *Haemophilus influenzae*
B. *Moraxella cateralis*
C. *Streptococcus pneumoniae*
D. *Streptococcus pyogenes*
E. No isolate

56. A 95-year-old man is brought to the emergency department from a nursing home where he is supervised most of the time. The staff tells you he has had difficulty breathing for the past week, and that it is worsening. He has a history of asthma

for which he takes a leukotriene inhibitor and inhaled steroids as needed. Physical examination reveals an oral temperature of 99.4°F, respiration of 14 breaths/min, blood pressure of 110/74 mm Hg, and pulse of 88 beats/min. He appears mildly uncomfortable with retractions. Auscultation reveals inspiratory stridor and expiratory wheezing in the left chest. No rubs or rales are appreciated. No lymphadenopathy is present. What is the most appropriate next step in the evaluation/management of this patient?

A. Antibiotics
B. Blind finger sweep
C. Intubation for airway control
D. Observation
E. Rigid bronchoscopy

57. A 21-year-old male college student presents to the university student health center complaining of a 3-day history of dysuria and urethral discharge. Physical examination findings of the heart, lungs, and abdomen are within normal limits. The testes are descended bilaterally and without masses. He has a left-sided grade I varicocele and a small right hydrocele. Prostate is 15 grams in size and is slightly tender to palpation. Gram stain of the urethral discharge reveals gram-negative diplococci inside polymorphonuclear leukocytes. Results of laboratory studies are shown below:

Leukocyte count	10,000/mm³
Segmented neutrophils	65%
Bands	5%
Eosinophils	3%
Basophils	1%
Lymphocytes	29%
Monocytes	7%

What is the most appropriate treatment?

A. Ceftriaxone
B. Ceftriaxone and doxycycline
C. Ciprofloxacin
D. Doxycycline
E. Penicillin and acyclovir

58. A 19-year-old woman who looks to be her stated age presents to her physician with concerns about never having had a period. She has never been sexually active. She denies having pelvic pain. Physical examination reveals a short vagina, and the cervix is not palpable. Which of the following is the most appropriate explanation for the clinical findings?

A. She has an imperforate hymen
B. She is an infertile female
C. She is 46XY
D. She is 47XXY
E. She is 45XO

59. A mother presents with her 5-year-old child to the pediatric clinic for a well-child check. Up to this point, the child had been meeting most of his developmental milestones with few exceptions. However, he was late in learning to walk, and recently he has had difficulty keeping up with his peers. The mother states that she has noticed him using his arms when attempting to stand up from a seated position. The mother denies observing similar symptoms in any of the child's immediate family. She was unable to comment on the boy's father, as she did not maintain a relationship with him. Physical examination reveals that the child's calves are disproportionately large in comparison to the rest of his body. Muscle weakness is more prominent in the proximal muscle groups. Creatine kinase levels are elevated. Muscle biopsy reveals dystrophic features. Which of the following statements pertaining to the likely etiology of this child's clinical presentation is correct?

A. The disease equally effects both men and women

B. The patient will most likely die from respiratory insufficiency in his twenties

C. The patient's father is likely to have a similar complex of symptoms and clinical course

D. The disease is known to exhibit the phenomenon known as anticipation

E. The patient is likely to have pathologic changes only in skeletal and not cardiac muscle

60. A 39-year-old schizophrenic male returns to his primary care physician for follow-up. It has been difficult to get his symptoms under control with medication, and many dose adjustments have been made. He states that the voices are under control, but he has started to develop a tremor in his right hand. His wife states that it looks like he is always chewing gum because he keeps smacking his lips. What is an appropriate treatment for this patient?

A. Benztropine

B. Betamethasone

C. Cannabis

D. Lorazepam

E. Propranolol

61. A 25-year-old G1P0 woman at 37 weeks' gestation has been found to have a blood pressure of 160/110 mm Hg, and urinalysis reveals +2 protein. After inducing labor, the medical team had administered hydralazine and magnesium sulfate. A few hours later, the patient's oxygen saturation was noted to be 89%, respiratory rate is 8 breaths/min, and there was absent patellar reflexes on examination. What is the next most appropriate step in the management of this patient?

A. Administer calcium gluconate intravenously and continue close monitoring

B. Administer oxygen by face mask and monitor closely

C. Perform immediate cesarean section

D. Perform immediate intubation

E. Watchful waiting initially, then administer calcium gluconate by continuous infusion

62. A 24-year-old female graduate student presents to the student health clinic with a 3-day history of sore throat, coryza, cough, and temperature of 38.5°C. Physical examination reveals that the tympanic membranes are erythematous bilaterally with bullous lesions. The oropharynx is erythematous. A smear of sputum shows no organisms but has WBCs and monocytes. Laboratory values reveal a hematocrit of 33%, reticulocyte count of 4%, and increased IgM cold agglutinins. Chest x-ray shows bilateral patchy lower lobe infiltrates. What is the most likely diagnosis?

A. *Chlamydia* pneumonia

B. *Mycoplasma* pneumonia

C. *Pneumocystis carinii* pneumonia

D. Rubeola

E. *Streptococcus* pneumonia

63. A 61-year-old man complains of intermittent bouts of rectal bleeding. He presents to his primary care physician for evaluation. These episodes of bleeding have produced blood in the toilet bowl. Now he complains of 2 days of left lower quadrant pain, nausea, and vomiting. He has a history of benign prostate enlargement and erectile dysfunction. His current medications include terazosin and sildenafil. Physical examination reveals tenderness to palpation in the left lower quadrant without evidence of guarding or rebound tenderness. Colonoscopy reveals no evidence of colorectal inflammation. CT scan of the abdomen is shown below (Figure 63). What is the most likely diagnosis?

Figure 63

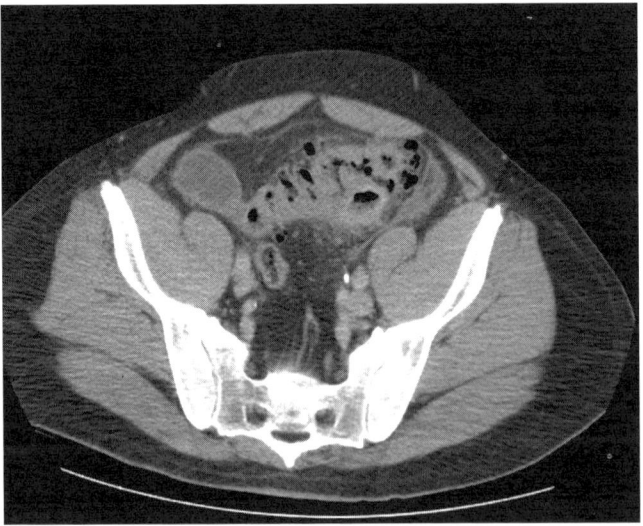

A. Abscess

B. Diverticulitis

C. Regional enteritis (Crohn disease)

D. Ulcerative colitis

E. Ulcerative proctitis

64. A 30-year-old white man presents to the emergency department complaining of intermittent episodes of severe right flank pain. The pain begins as mild but progresses to severe pain after 20 to 60 minutes. The pain radiates to his testicle on the ipsilateral side. He also admits to nausea and describes gross hematuria. Physical examination reveals normal cardiac and pulmonary findings. There is mild right costovertebral angle tenderness. Urinalysis reveals microhematuria without leukocytes or nitrates. CT scan without contrast reveals a 3-mm stone in the right distal ureter without evidence of hydronephrosis. There is a 1-cm simple cyst in the lower pole of the left kidney. What is the most appropriate treatment of this patient?

A. Analgesics and aggressive hydration
B. External nephrostomy tube placement
C. Shock-wave lithotripsy
D. Ureteroscopic removal followed by a course of antibiotics
E. Urology consultation for ureteral stent

65. A 3-year-old child is brought to the clinic with a 2-week history of intermittent diarrhea and weight loss. The patient's parents are strict vegetarians and have been trying to instill the same dietary habits in their child over the past couple of months. The parents also noted that their child has become increasingly clumsy and that his gait is ataxic. The physical examination reveals glossitis and some vitiligo. A peripheral blood smear shows ovalocytosis, neutrophils with hypersegmented nuclei, nucleated RBCs, basophilic stippling, and Howell-Jolly bodies. What is the most appropriate management of this patient?

A. Corticosteroid therapy
B. Folate supplementation
C. Iron
D. Vitamin B_{12} injections
E. Watchful waiting

66. A 21-year-old college student is going to be taking the Medical College Admission Test (MCAT) in 2 days. She has been studying with increasing intensity since the beginning of summer 3 months ago. While writing on a particularly vague essay topic she suddenly develops sharp abdominal pain and the urge to defecate. She passes nonbloody diarrhea along with significant flatulence. These symptoms persist through the day of the test and until 6 weeks later when she received the test results. Results of laboratory studies are shown below:

Electrolytes, serum

Na, serum	143 mEq/L
Cl, serum	100 mEq/L
K, serum	3.7 mEq/L
Bicarbonate, serum	24 mEq/L
Magnesium, serum	2.0 mEq/L
Creatinine, serum	1.0 mg/dL

Leukocyte count and differential

Leukocyte count	5000/mm^3
Segmented neutrophils	55%

Blood, plasma, serum

Alanine aminotransferase (ALT)	10 U/L
Amylase, serum	50 U/L
Aspartate aminotransferase (AST)	10 U/L
Calcium, serum	9 mg/dL
Glucose, serum	100 mg/dL
Hematocrit	38%
Urea nitrogen, serum (BUN)	10 mg/dL

Urinalysis

Urine pH	6.0
Red blood cell count	1/HPF
WBC count	1/HPF
Nitrates	Negative
Bacteria	Negative

What is the most likely diagnosis?

A. Crohn disease
B. Gastroenteritis
C. Irritable bowel syndrome
D. Peptic ulcer disease
E. Ulcerative colitis

67. A 52-year-old woman presents to the emergency department with a 30-hour history of hemoptysis (estimated to be 500 mL). She denies having chest pain (dull or pleuritic) but says she now feels "more tired and short of breath than usual." She has a 50 pack/year history of smoking. She has seen a pulmonologist occasionally during the past 6 years for recurrent infections. This time, however, she is coughing up mostly blood, with whitish mucus. Physical examination reveals mild tachypnea with increased tidal volume and mild retractions. The chest is nontender. Auscultation reveals decreased breath sounds over the entire lung fields anteriorly and posteriorly, worse on the right. Percussion yields no focal areas of dullness or effusion, but loose secretions in the upper airways are audible without the stethoscope. What is the most appropriate next step in the workup/evaluation of this patient?

A. Admit. Give the patient 24 hours of "watchful waiting," to see if it resolves, keeping an eye on her hematocrit and hemoglobin and transfusing if necessary. Type and screen; skin test for tuberculosis (TB).
B. Skin test for TB; CT scan; sputum culture; +/− blood cultures; type and screen.
C. Skin test for TB; chest x-ray; sputum culture; +/− blood cultures; type and screen.
D. Chest x-ray; bronchoscopy; type and screen.
E. Bronchoscopy; skin test for TB; HIV testing; sputum cultures; type and screen.

68. A 20-year-old male college student presents to his primary care physician with a complaint of excessive daytime sleepiness. He explains that he is always falling asleep during his lectures, and his grades are suffering as a result. He also tells you that he occasionally loses the ability to hold his head up and even slumps over when he laughs or gets angry. He tries to avoid these situations as a result of these uncomfortable experiences. He later explains to you that he frequently is unable to move on awakening in the morning. First-line treatment for this disorder is similar to that for which of the following conditions?

A. Amyotrophic lateral sclerosis
B. Attention deficit hyperactivity disorder
C. Major depressive disorder
D. Restless leg syndrome
E. Stiff man syndrome

69. A mother brings her 3-week-old neonate to the pediatrician for a well-child visit. She explains that this is her first child, and she wants to know the appropriate amount of 20 kcal/ounce formula to feed her infant each day. The child weighs 5000 g and is healthy and growing, but was born preterm at 37 weeks' gestation. What is the minimum amount of formula this mother should feed her infant per day?

A. 20 ounces/day
B. 30 ounces/day
C. 40 ounces/day
D. 60 ounces/day
E. 80 ounces/day

70. A 32-year-old man presents to his primary care physician because of a fever of 101°F for the past month. He has a prior medical history of seasonal allergies. He has no prior surgical history. Physical examination reveals bilateral shotty adenopathy along the course of the sternocleidomastoid muscle. After obtaining routing laboratory studies and blood cultures, what is the next step in the workup?

A. Barium enema
B. Chest x-ray
C. Echocardiogram
D. Lumbar puncture
E. Positron emission tomography (PET) scan

71. A 9-year-old girl is brought to her pediatrician for her well-child check-up by her parents, who have questions regarding her physical development. They are interested in the changes that will occur during puberty. In educating her parents, what phenotypic change should they expect to occur first?

A. Development of breast buds
B. Increase in sebaceous gland secretions
C. Onset of growth of pubic hair
D. Onset of menstruation
E. Peak height velocity in growth rate

72. A 35-year-old white female school teacher presents to her primary care physician because of amenorrhea for 3 months. She states that she has had regular 28-day cycles since she was 16 years old. The onset of puberty was at age 12. She has never been pregnant. She has not developed hot flashes or any other symptoms of menopause. She also complains of milky discharge from both breasts that causes her to wear pads throughout the day to keep from having to change her shirt. Past medical and social history are unremarkable. Physical examination reveals that her breasts are nontender and without nodules, but milky discharge is noted bilaterally. What would be the most helpful laboratory finding to confirm the diagnosis?

A. Decreased dopamine
B. Decreased Na
C. Elevated carcinoembryonic antigen protein (CEA)
D. Elevated growth hormone
E. Elevated luteinizing hormone
F. Elevated prolactin

Questions 73–76:

A. Associative
B. Cardiogenic
C. Communitive
D. Distributive
E. Hypovolemic
F. Obstructive
G. Postobstructive
H. Septic (nonbacterial) shock
I. Uremic shock

For each of the following critically ill patients, select the most appropriate form of clinical shock.

73. A 28-year-old man who has sustained several gunshot wounds to the abdomen and lower extremities is left in the field for 2 hours before being brought to the emergency room.

74. A 51-year-old man had a myocardial infarction 4 weeks ago and suddenly falls to the ground while walking in front of his home. As emergency personnel arrive on the scene, he is apneic and pulseless. Electrocardiography reveals asystole. Autopsy studies later reveal rupture of the intraventricular septum.

75. A 39-year-old woman with a history of diabetes mellitus and hypertension presents with left-sided chest pain that improves when she sits up. A presumed diagnosis of pericarditis is made.

76. A 41-year-old man with a history of chronic pancreatitis is readmitted to the hospital with recurrent abdominal pain and persistent vomiting. His mucous membranes appear dry.

77. A 40-year-old man presents to his primary care physician complaining of progressive shortness of breath. He admits to a 25 pack/year history of cigarette smoking. Physical examination is significant for an obese man with distant heart sounds (S_1 and S_2) and decreased breath sounds bilaterally. Abdominal examination fails to reveal peritoneal signs. Chest x-ray demonstrates the presence of air within the pericardial sac. What is the most likely finding associated with this condition?

   A. Jugular venous distention and a P2
   B. Pericardial rub
   C. Positional change of x-ray findings
   D. S_3 or S_4 gallop
   E. Subcutaneous emphysema

78. A 23-year-old G1P0 woman is 30 weeks pregnant. She complains of dizziness and fatigue. Both of her parents have insulin-dependent diabetes. Her mother has diabetic retinopathy. Results of her physical examination are normal. Urine analysis reveals glucosuria. Serum glucose is 180 mg/dL. Other laboratory values are shown below:

Blood, plasma, serum

Alanine aminotransferase (ALT)	15 U/L
Amylase, serum	40 U/L
Aspartate aminotransferase (AST)	13 U/L
Calcium, serum	9.2 mg/dL
Creatinine, serum	1.2 mg/dL
Glucose, serum	180 mg/dL
Hematocrit	37%
Urea nitrogen, serum (BUN)	11 mg/dL

Which of the following is the appropriate time for an initial ocular examination for this patient?

   A. At the time of diagnosis of diabetes
   B. Within 1 year of the diagnosis of diabetes
   C. Within 5 years of the diagnosis of diabetes
   D. Within 10 years of the diagnosis of diabetes
   E. Within 15 years of the diagnosis of diabetes

79. A 5-year-old boy presents to the pediatrics clinic for his annual evaluation. He has been in good health, but his mother states she has noticed him becoming progressively clumsier. She says she has also noticed him walking funny for a few months. Physical examination reveals some proximal muscle weakness, calf muscle pseudohypertrophy, and a positive Gower sign. What is the most appropriate confirmatory test to be performed next in this patient?

   A. DNA analysis
   B. EMG
   C. Creatinine kinase
   D. Muscle biopsy
   E. No further testing is required

80. A 25-year-old woman presents to her primary care physician with a 10-day history of malaise, myalgia, fever, and sore throat. Physical examination reveals an erythematous oropharynx without exudate, and cervical adenopathy. The liver span is 14 cm in the midclavicular line. Peripheral blood smear shows atypical lymphocytes. The remainder of laboratory studies obtained are shown below:

Electrolytes, serum

Na, serum	141 mEq/L
Cl, serum	100 mEq/L
K, serum	3.9 mEq/L
Bicarbonate, serum	26 mEq/L
Creatinine, serum	1.0 mg/dL

Leukocyte count and differential

Leukocyte count	9700/mm^3

What is the next most appropriate step in the evaluation of this patient?

   A. Admit patient and begin intravenous antibiotics
   B. Chest x-ray
   C. Heterophile antibody
   D. Rapid streptococcus test
   E. Weil-Felix titer

81. A 55-year-old man presents to the emergency department for a "place to sleep." He is a known alcoholic and has had hallucinations in the past. You decide to investigate the patient's mental status examination due to the auditory hallucinations. If the patient were having classic alcoholic hallucinosis, what other findings would be present on the mental status examination?

   A. Clear sensorium
   B. Flat affect
   C. Flight of ideas
   D. Inability to write
   E. Loss of abstract thought

Figure 82

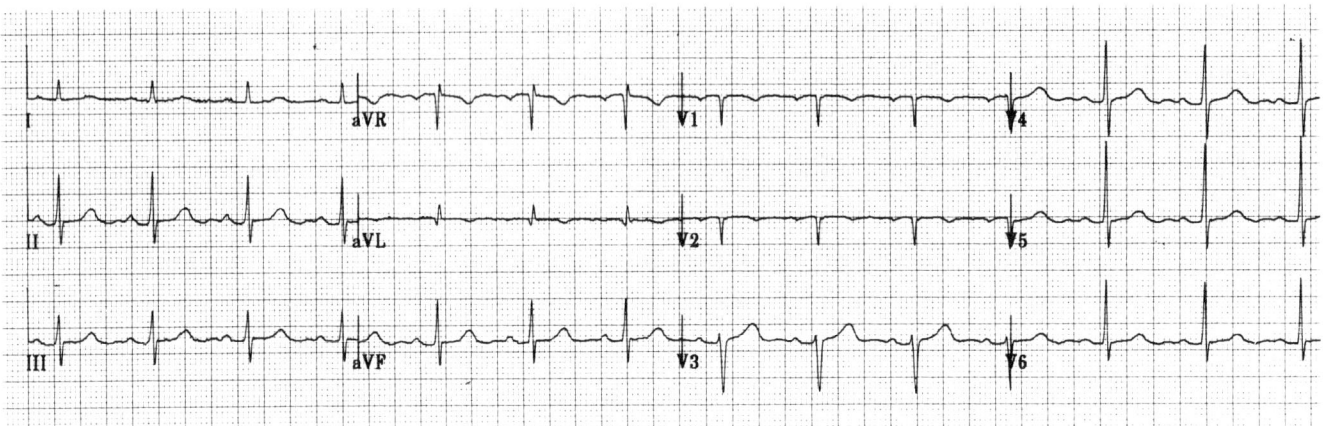

82. A 79-year-old woman with advanced Alzheimer disease presents with her caregiver for a 1-month follow-up appointment with her primary care physician. Her caregiver believes she has been having increased episodes of moaning and agitation. Routine follow-up ECG is shown above (Figure 82). Which coronary artery was most likely occluded to produce this ECG pattern?

   A. A branch of the right coronary artery
   B. A terminal branch of the left coronary artery
   C. Circumflex branch of the left coronary artery
   D. A terminal branch of the right coronary artery
   E. Left anterior descending artery

83. A 14-year-old girl presents to the pediatric clinic with her parents. The family is concerned with the girl's proportional short stature and absence of pubertal development. Otherwise, she is healthy. She is at the fifth percentile for her age with normal growth velocities. Her parents are of average height. Her mother does admit to being short for her age until high school and her menarche occurred at 15. What is the most likely cause for this patient's short stature?

   A. Achondroplasia
   B. Constitutional delay
   C. Cushing disease
   D. Familial short stature
   E. Growth hormone deficiency

84. A 26-year-old woman started a triphasic oral contraceptive 6 weeks ago. She presents to her primary care physician because she "missed" her period last month. She says she did not miss any pills and has no other complaints other than some anxiety regarding her missed menses. She is currently sexually active with her boyfriend of 6 months. They use condoms about half the time. Which one of the following measures is most appropriate at this point?

   A. Add more progesterone to her oral contraceptive regimen.
   B. Discontinue the use of her oral contraceptive.
   C. Increase the androgenic potency of the progestin component of her oral contraceptives.
   D. Increase the estrogen dose of her oral contraceptive.
   E. Perform a pregnancy test. If the result is negative, continue her current oral contraceptive regimen for another month.

85. A 29-year-old man comes in to see his primary care physician. He tells you that for a long time he has suspected that his wife has been unfaithful. You ask him what makes him think that, and he replies, "If I say anything, you'll probably just run and tell my wife." He also experiences difficulties at work, stating that he dislikes his co-workers and that they all attempt to make him look bad in front of the boss so that they will be promoted sooner than him. He tells you that one of his co-workers complimented his new car, but that "what he really meant to tell me was that I am selfish." You tell him that you would like to schedule an appointment to discuss these issues further and help him to sort them out. He responds by saying: "Why? You don't think I'm doing well enough on my own?" Under which axis does this patient's condition fall?

   A. Axis I
   B. Axis II
   C. Axis III
   D. Axis IV
   E. Axis V

86. A 30-year-old man has a long history of intermittent abdominal pain, diarrhea, and recurrent perianal fistulization that has required surgical intervention. He notes a 20-pound weight loss over the past 3 months. Physical examination reveals a regular rate and rhythm without evidence of rubs, murmurs, or gallops. Pulmonary auscultation reveals no evidence of wheezes, rhonchi, or rales. Gastrointestinal examination reveals tenderness to palpation in the right lower quadrant with a mass lesion palpable to superficial palpation. Anorectal examination reveals evidence of healed anterior and posterior fistulas with no evidence of new fistula formation. Small bowel barium studies reveal a nodular contour and luminal narrowing with linear ulcerations and clefts. Results of laboratory studies are presented below:

Na, serum	132 mEq/L
Cl, serum	99 mEq/L
K, serum	3.3 mEq/L
Bicarbonate, serum	22 mEq/L
Magnesium, serum	1.5 mEq/L
Creatinine, serum	0.7 mg/dL
Albumin, serum	3.3 g/dL
Hematocrit	32%
Hemoglobin, blood	10.2 g/dL
Leukocyte count	11,000/mm^3
Platelet count	280,000/mm^3

What is the most likely diagnosis?

A. Crohn disease
B. Small bowel leiomyoma
C. Small bowel lipoma
D. Tuberculous enteritis
E. Villous adenoma

87. A 6-month-old boy is brought to the emergency department for acute onset of dyspnea and fever. Past medical history is significant for numerous hospitalizations secondary to recurrent pyogenic infections as well as enteroviral infections. Physical examination reveals that the child is febrile and tachypneic. Chest x-ray is suspicious for pneumonia. What is the most likely underlying cause of this patient's recurrent infections?

A. Chronic granulomatous disease
B. Common variable immunodeficiency
C. DiGeorge syndrome
D. Selective IgA deficiency
E. X-linked (Bruton) agammaglobulinemia

88. A 32-year-old black woman with Raynaud disease treated with calcium channel blockers presents to her primary care physician with complaints of dysphagia. Physical examination reveals long thin fingers, telangiectasia on the face and thighs, and subcutaneous nodules on the forearms. Barium swallow studies reveal significant esophageal dysmotility without nodules or lesion. Aspirate from the nodules reveals calcium deposits. Routine laboratory studies show normocytic anemia, decreased albumin, and elevated globulin. The most specific marker of this syndrome is?

A. Antinuclear antibody
B. Anticentromere antibody
C. Anti–double-stranded DNA (anti-dsDNA) antibody
D. Anti-Jo immunoglobulin
E. Anti-Smith antibody

89. A 38-year-old woman with a history of schizophrenia requiring chronic therapy presents for a follow-up examination. At her visit today she is making noticeable repetitive movements of her face, including lip smacking. What is true about this condition?

A. Benztropine is unlikely to be effective
B. Clozapine is indicated for treating this condition
C. Haloperidol is not known to cause this condition
D. Intervention is required to make this condition improve
E. This patient's condition is likely a primary manifestation of her schizophrenia

90. You are the intern covering the labor and delivery floor. You are called by the nurse because a 28-year-old woman who is 5 days postpartum from a cesarean section develops a fever of 101°F. Physical examination reveals the wound to be non-erythematous and healing well. Cardiac examination reveals a regular rate and rhythm without murmur. Lungs are clear bilaterally. Abdominal examination reveals suprapubic tenderness with mild guarding. There is no calf tenderness. Results of laboratory studies are shown below:

Electrolytes, serum

Na, serum	143 mEq/L
Cl, serum	100 mEq/L
K, serum	3.9 mEq/L
Bicarbonate, serum	26 mEq/L
Magnesium, serum	2.1 mEq/L
Creatinine, serum	1.1 mg/dL

Leukocyte count and differential

Leukocyte count	12,900/mm³
Segmented neutrophils	71%
Bands	7%
Eosinophils	3%
Basophils	1%
Lymphocytes	27%
Monocytes	4%

Blood, plasma, serum

Alanine aminotransferase (ALT)	10 U/L
Amylase, serum	50 U/L
Aspartate aminotransferase (AST)	10 U/L
Calcium, serum	9 mg/dL
Glucose, serum	100 mg/dL
Hematocrit	33%
Urea nitrogen, serum (BUN)	10 mg/dL

Urinalysis

Urine pH	6.0
Red blood cell count	2–4/HPF
WBC count	2–4/HPF
Nitrates	Negative
Bacteria	Negative

What is the most likely diagnosis for this patient?

A. Atelectasis
B. Endomyometritis
C. Renal calculi
D. Urinary tract infection
E. Wound infection

91. A 6-year-old boy is hospitalized with a fever for several days because of bilateral conjunctivitis, strawberry tongue, erythema of palms and soles, membranous desquamation from fingertips, and rash primarily on his trunk along with cervical lymphadenopathy. What is the most serious complication of the patient's illness?

A. Aseptic meningitis
B. Coronary vasculitis
C. Gastroenteritis
D. Testicular torsion
E. Uveitis

92. A 65-year-old man has a 1-year history of ceaseless pacing and a shuffled gait. His wife notes that he has had some noticeable changes in his personality and social skills. He has a decreased emotion and desire to partake in his usual activities, although he states that he is just fine. Immediate and recent memory loss have also occurred. During the past 2 months he has become progressively withdrawn. He has no prior medical or surgical history. He currently takes no medications. He is a nonsmoker and nondrinker. Which of the following findings are most likely to be noted on an electroencephalogram of this patient?

A. Diffuse slowing
B. Global rapid activity
C. Intermittent rapid and slow activity
D. Partial slowing
E. Normal activity

93. A 34-year-old man who works as a teacher is changing school districts. Because of his job change, he is required to have a complete physical examination. His social history is notable for occasional drinks on weekends. He is a non-smoker. Physical examination reveals no evidence of pharyngeal erythema. There is no cervical adenopathy. The thyroid gland is palpable. Cardiac examination fails to reveal evidence of rubs, murmurs, or gallops. Pulmonary auscultation reveals no evidence of wheeze, rhonchi, or rales. Gastrointestinal examination notes some mild tenderness to deep palpation in the left lower quadrant without focal peritoneal signs. Bilateral inguinal lymph nodes are palpable but without tenderness. Anorectal examinations reveals small internal hemorrhoids that do not prolapse. Results of laboratory studies are listed below:

Magnesium, serum	2.1 mg/dL
Total protein, serum	7 g/dL
Na, serum	147 mEq/L
Urea nitrogen, serum (BUN)	11 mg/dL
K, serum	3.5 mEq/L
WBC count	7000/mm³
Hematocrit	39%
Chest x-ray	2-cm solitary nodule in the right lower lobe

What is the most likely diagnosis?

A. Adenocarcinoma
B. Arteriovenous malformation
C. Bronchogenic tumor
D. Granuloma
E. Hamartoma

94. A 63-year-old man presents to his primary care physician after an episode of syncope 3 days ago. He has experienced no further episodes since that time. Further history reveals that other presyncopal episodes occurred when he wore tight-fitting collars. The patient is a retired mechanic. He has a 35 pack/year history of smoking. He has a prior medical history of hypercholesterolemia, hypertension, and diabetes mellitus. His current medications include Lipitor, metoprolol, metformin, and a daily aspirin. Physical examination reveals a mildly obese man. Pulses are equal, and no murmur is appreciated. Pulmonary and abdominal examination are within normal limits. Testicular and prostate examinations fail to reveal any pathology. What is the next most appropriate step in the evaluation of this patient?

A. Cardiac catheterization
B. Carotid massage with careful monitoring
C. Gentle compression of the carotid artery
D. Observation as an inpatient
E. Observation as an outpatient

95. A 57-year-old man with diabetes and hypercholesterolemia presents for a 1-year follow-up examination. He reports no problems in the past year except a 1-day episode of chest tightness about 2 to 3 months ago. He does not remember much about the episode except that it was gone the next day. Electrocardiography is ordered and the results are shown in Figure 95. What is the most likely diagnosis?

A. Normal study
B. Acute inferior myocardial infarction
C. Acute lateral myocardial infarction
D. Inferior myocardial infarction, age undetermined
E. Lateral myocardial infarction, age undetermined

Figure 95

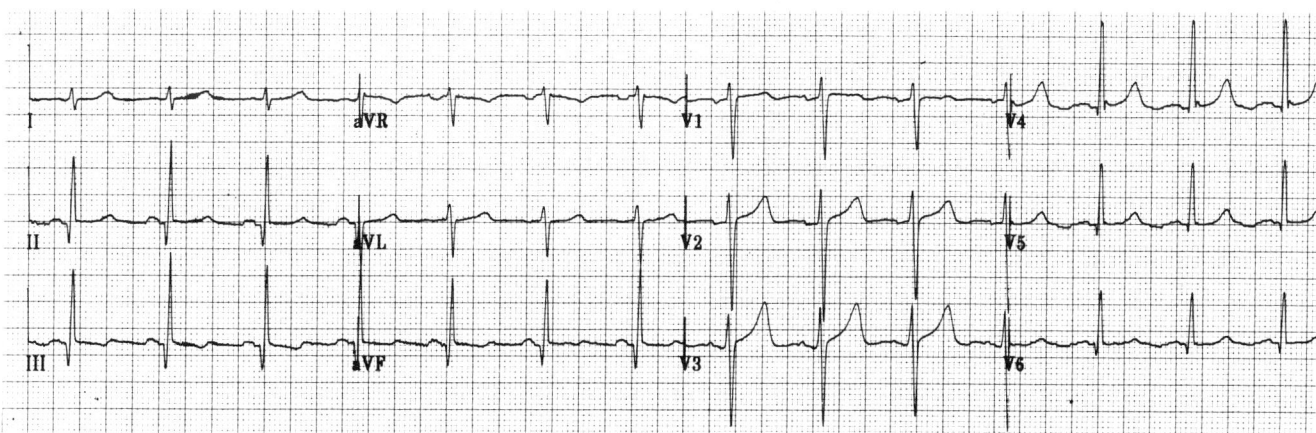

96. A 29-year-old G3P3 woman is 24 weeks pregnant. She complains of daily craving for ice, and lately she desires to eat laundry starch. Her symptoms have remained stable during the current pregnancy. Cardiac examination reveals a regular rate and rhythm. Pulmonary evaluation reveals clear lungs bilaterally without rales or rhonchi. Abdominal examination reveals normoactive bowel sounds with a fundal height 24.5 cm from the pubis. Anorectal evaluation reveals evidence of external hemorrhoids.

What is the most appropriate explanation for these findings?

A. Hyperemesis gravidarum

B. Manic depression

C. Obsessive-compulsive disorder

D. Oral contraceptive use during pregnancy

E. Pica

97. A 39-year-old woman has a history of mental retardation, insomnia, and hyperthyroidism. She often uses defense mechanisms such as displacement and rationalization to deal with the stresses of her life. Mental status examination reveals depressed mood and insomnia. The patient generally functions well with some meaningful interpersonal relationships. Multiaxial evaluation of this individual with regard to psychosocial and environmental problems is indicated on

A. Axis I

B. Axis II

C. Axis III

D. Axis IV

E. Axis V

98. A first-time mother brings her 4-week-old daughter to the pediatric clinic for routine evaluation. The mother explains that the birth was full-term with breech presentation. She reports that the child is having no difficulties with feeding or sleeping. No heart murmur is heard on auscultation, and all primitive reflexes are present. When performing the Ortolani maneuver, a click is noted. What is the most appropriate intervention?

A. Closed reduction with hip adducted and flexed

B. Maintain hip abduction and flexion with the use of a harness

C. Observation only with reevaluation in 4 weeks

D. Open reduction and internal fixation of the abnormality

E. Pharmacotherapy with intravenous antibiotics

99. A 72-year-old woman with a history of metastatic renal cell carcinoma underwent cytoreductive left nephrectomy 6 months ago. She now presents to her primary care physician for evaluation of a 1-month history of chronic constipation. She also notes occasional left lower quadrant pain that is relieved with passage of bowel movements. Physical examination reveals a regular rate and rhythm. Pulmonary auscultation reveals no evidence of rales or wheezes. Gastrointestinal examination reveals tenderness along the left sigmoid colon without evidence of peritoneal signs. Anorectal examination reveals no evidence of fissure or gross neoplasm. CT scan of the chest, abdomen, and pelvis reveals evidence of metastatic foci in the liver, lumbar spine, and right hip. Which of the following is a plausible cause for this patient's constipation?

A. Hypercalcemia

B. Hyperkalemia

C. Hypoglycemia

D. Hypoparathyroidism

E. Thyrotoxicosis

100. A 44-year-old woman presents for evaluation of painful breasts. She has a prior medical history of panic disorder, which is controlled with propranolol. Her family history is notable for colon cancer in her father and breast cancer in her mother that was diagnosed at age 39 and treated with radical mastectomy with postoperative radiotherapy. Physical examination of the right breast reveals no evidence of mass, dimpling, skin retraction, or nipple inversion. The right axilla reveals small palpable lymph nodes. The left breast reveals a 1.5-cm mass in the left upper outer quadrant. An asymmetric contour is noted overlying the mass when the patient is sitting upright. The left axillary fossa is notable for palpable lymph nodes. Cardiovascular examination reveals a regular rate and rhythm with no evidence of rubs, murmurs, or gallops. Pulmonary auscultation reveals good breath sounds bilaterally, and gastrointestinal examination reveals no evidence of peritoneal signs. Mammographic findings include architectural distortion of the left breast and a 1.7-cm mass with increased density and stippled microcalcifications. Which of the following is the most likely diagnosis?

A. Fibroadenoma

B. Fibrocystic change

C. Fibrosarcoma

D. Infiltrating ductal cell carcinoma

E. Intraductal papilloma

101. A 43-year-old poorly kempt man is brought to the emergency department by police after being found in an alley. His clothes smell of alcohol and cigarettes. He admits to a 4-week history of vomiting. A recent episode of vomiting also included blood and clots. Cardiac examination reveals a regular rate and rhythm. Pulmonary examination notes no evidence of wheeze, rhonchi, or rales. Gastrointestinal examination reveals mild midepigastric tenderness without evidence of peritoneal signs. Rectal examination reveals stool in the vault and is guaiac positive. Laboratory values are as follows:

Hematocrit	31%
Hemoglobin	11.1 g/dL
WBC count	10,500/mm^3
Platelet count	299,000/mm^3
Urinalysis	Heme negative
	Leukocyte esterase negative
	Nitrate negative

What is the most likely diagnosis?

A. Esophagitis (fungal)

B. Esophagitis (viral)

C. Mallory-Weiss tear

D. Peptic ulcer disease

E. Tuberculosis

102. A 6-year-old girl is brought to the emergency department because of a 4-week history of intermittent vaginal bleeding. Which of the following is the most useful tool or diagnostic test to confirm your suspicions in the evaluation of this patient?

A. Diagnostic hysteroscopy

B. Vaginal speculum examination

C. Diagnostic culposcopy

D. Observation of verbal and nonverbal clues when speaking with the patient and family members

E. CBC and serum electrolytes

103. A 66-year-old woman complains of vaginal itching for approximately 1 year. She has a prior medical history of hypertension and diet-controlled diabetes. She takes atenolol daily. Physical examination reveals no evidence of murmur or gallop. Pulmonary auscultation reveals clear lungs bilaterally with good inspiratory effort. Gastrointestinal examination reveals stool in the vault without evidence of hemorrhoids. She is guaiac negative. Vaginal speculum examination reveals no evidence of cervical or vaginal masses with a closed cervical os. A 1.5-cm red ulcerative exophytic area is found on the right labia majus. What is the most likely diagnosis?

A. Malignant melanoma

B. Paget disease

C. Squamous cell hyperplasia

D. Vaginal carcinoma

E. Vulvar carcinoma

104. A 42-year-old man develops profuse diarrhea and occasional vomiting shortly after eating 2-week-old hamburger casserole he warmed up in his microwave oven. The symptoms resolve in 4 days. He is diagnosed with *Clostridium perfringens* infection. What is the most likely pathogenesis?

A. Enterotoxin transmits impulses to medullary center by acting on receptors in the gut

B. Epithelial necrosis of colon cause by enterotoxin

C. Hypersecretion in the small intestine caused by enterotoxin produced in food

D. Superficial gut infection with little invasion

E. Toxin blocks acetylcholine at neuromuscular junction

105. A neonate who suffered in utero from meningoencephalitis is evaluated at birth with microcephaly, chorioretinitis, and seizures. Maternal social history reveals employment as a veterinary technician. Physical examination of the child reveals jaundice, diffuse petechiae, a maculopapular rash, and generalized lymphadenopathy. What is the most appropriate treatment for the child?

A. Acyclovir

B. Immunoglobulin

C. Penicillin

D. Pyrimethamine plus sulfadiazine

E. Trimethoprim-sulfamethoxazole

106. A 54-year-old, 210-pound woman with a history of stroke is admitted to the hospital after falling and fracturing the right femur. Ten days after a prosthetic hip replacement, the nursing staff points out that the febrile patient has developed a decubitus ulcer on her sacrum, slightly left of midline. On examination, the wound's central ulcer (2.5 × 2.0 cm) is weeping a thin, green-yellow exudate. There is marked swelling and some erythema irregularly around the ulcer. Probing the wound reveals the tissue is macerated and friable. What is the best treatment option for this patient?

A. Débridement of all necrotic tissue; allow to heal by secondary intention

B. Débridement of all necrotic tissue; muscle or musculocutaneous flap from donor site

C. Débridement of all necrotic tissue; primary closure of cutaneous tissue if possible, full-thickness skin graft if not

D. Débridement of all necrotic tissue; primary closure of cutaneous tissue if possible, split-thickness skin graft if not

E. Wet-to-dry dressing changes twice per day; positional changes every 2 hours

107. A 25-year-old woman presents to her primary care physician because of concerns of heavy periods that occur every 15 days. Through evaluation and follow-up you determine that she has approximately 70 mL of blood loss with each period. What is the most likely diagnosis?

A. Menorrhagia

B. Menometrorrhagia

C. Metrorrhagia

D. Oligomenorrhea

E. Polymenorrhea

108. A 27-year-old Mexican immigrant presents to the ambulatory care center after being seen in the emergency department 3 weeks ago for abdominal pain. A diagnosis of viral gastroenteritis was made. The patient is currently asymptomatic. After a complete history is obtained, the patient reports that she has never received a tetanus shot. Physical examination findings of the heart, lungs, and abdomen are within normal limits. Results of laboratory studies are shown below:

Urinalysis

Urine pH	6.0
RBC count	1/HPF
WBC count	2/HPF
Bacteria	Negative
Nitrates	Negative
Leukocyte esterase	Negative

What is the next step in the management of this patient?

A. Give the patient a tetanus booster and suggest she receive another every 10 years
B. No vaccine should be given because this patient is too old
C. Give diphtheria-pertussis vaccine now and two more doses 1 to 2 months apart
D. Give two doses of tetanus 1 to 2 months apart and a booster in 6 to 12 months
E. Give tetanus immune globulin

109. A 60-year-old man who has not seen a physician in 15 years presents to the emergency department with progressively worsening dyspnea over the past 4 months. He also is complaining of chest pain that is dull and intermittent in nature. His past medical history is significant for arthritis. He is a nonsmoker. Physical examination reveals a grade III midsystolic ejection murmur that is best heard at the second intercostal space. What is the most likely diagnosis of this patient?

A. Aortic dissection
B. Aortic regurgitation
C. Aortic stenosis
D. Mitral regurgitation
E. Mitral stenosis

110. A previously healthy 2-year-old boy is brought to the pediatric clinic for evaluation of an abdominal mass. His mother states that she noticed the mass last week while giving him a bath. He has had no change in bowel habits. He has been afebrile and without hematuria. Physical examination reveals a 4.0-cm solid mass in the left upper quadrant of the abdomen. Cardiac and pulmonary examinations are unremarkable. CBC and serum electrolytes are within normal limits. Urine studies reveal elevated vanilmandelic acid and homovanillic acid levels. What is the most likely explanation for these findings?

A. Autosomal-dominant polycystic kidney disease
B. Autosomal-recessive polycystic kidney disease
C. Neoplasm of embryonal renal cells of the metanephros
D. Neoplasm of primitive neural crest cells
E. Remnant of the omphalomesenteric duct

Questions 111–117

A. Dyspareunia
B. Exhibitionism
C. Fetishism
D. Frotteurism
E. Hypoactive sexual desire disorder
F. Inhibited male orgasm
G. Paraphilia
H. Sexual aversion disorder
I. Transsexualism
J. Vaginismus
K. Voyeurism

For each patient with a psychosexual disorder, select the most likely diagnosis.

111. A 23-year-old homosexual man with a history of bipolar disorder becomes sexually aroused by exposing his genitals to unsuspecting females. He is not aggressive and often masturbates during the exposure. A shock reaction from the female concludes his behavior.

112. A 23-year-old woman complains to the police after being touched and briefly fondled by a young man in a crowded shopping mall. He briefly touched her breasts while she pushed him away. He appeared to be aroused by the situation and escaped in the mall minutes later.

113. A 31-year-old woman with a history of depression and anxiety is under emotional stress in her relationship with a 29-year-old man. She is afraid to become intimate with this man and is unable to become excited sexually and achieve an orgasm. She does admit to a fear of pregnancy in addition to strong religious beliefs.

114. A 27-year-old woman who was involved in a hostile marital relationship 2 years ago is now involved in a relationship with a new partner with whom she is quite happy. She complains of being unable to accept penile penetration during sexual relations with this new partner. Physical examination reveals no evidence of anatomic abnormalities of the vaginal vault.

115. A 33-year-old woman complains of a 5-month history of pain with intercourse. She has a history of cervical carcinoma, which has been treated with chemotherapy and radiation. Her last cycle of therapy was 6 months ago. Results of physical examination of the heart, lungs, and abdomen are unremarkable. Pelvic examination reveals immobility of the cervix and fibrosis with inflammation of the vaginal vault.

116. A 59-year-old man with a long history of urinary hesitancy and decrease in his force of stream undergoes a transurethral resection of the prostate. Four months after the surgery, he is able to obtain an erection and has the sensation of ejaculation despite visualization of the emission. Physical examination of the abdomen is unremarkable. Both testes are descended without masses. The penis is circumcised and the urethral meatus is patent. The prostate is nontender.

117. A 34-year-old man with a history of schizoid personality disorder becomes sexually aroused in the presence of colored fish in an aquarium. In the presence of this stimuli, he will masturbate to a rapid orgasm. Psychosocial evaluation reveals a man who is troubled by his desires with feelings of depression, guilt, and anxiety.

118. A 50-year-old woman presents to her primary care physician with complaints of fatigue, shortness of breath, and several presyncopal episodes. She is a nonsmoker and denies alcohol use. She admits to not exercising due to lack of time, but she does avoid saturated fats. Her family history is unremarkable. Current medications include a daily calcium tablet and a multivitamin. She is 5'4" and weighs 146 pounds. She has a blood pressure of 130/80 mm Hg, pulse of 77 beats/min, and respirations of 15 breaths/min. Neck examination reveals jugular venous distention. There is 1+ pitting edema on the lower extremities. Cardiovascular examination reveals a systolic ejection murmur and narrow pulse pressure. Urine dipstick shows 3+ protein. What is the most likely diagnosis?

A. Air embolism
B. Budd-Chiari syndrome
C. Congestive heart failure
D. Cor pulmonale
E. Primary amyloidosis

119. A 22-year-old woman is found to have hypertension, angiokeratomas of the skin, opacity of the lens, painful dysesthesias of the extremities, and arthropathy of the terminal interphalangeal joints. Urinalysis reveals lipiduria, proteinuria, nephrotic syndrome, and progressive renal insufficiency. Urine also reveals glycosphingolipids and elevated alpha-galactosidase levels of peripheral leukocytes. What is the most likely diagnosis?

A. Alport syndrome
B. Fabry disease
C. Lecithin-cholesterol acyltransferase deficiency
D. Lipodystrophy
E. Nail-patella syndrome

120. A 33-year-old woman presents to her primary care physician for her routine prenatal appointment. She is currently 24 weeks pregnant with a single fetus. She has no pertinent prior medical or surgical history. Examination results of the heart, lungs, and abdomen are within normal limits. Laboratory results are shown below:

Blood, plasma, serum

Alanine aminotransferase (ALT)	11 U/L
Amylase, serum	55 U/L
Aspartate aminotransferase (AST)	14 U/L
Glucose, serum	100 mg/dL
Hematocrit	37%
Urea nitrogen, serum (BUN)	12 mg/dL

Urinalysis

Urine pH	7.0
RBC count	1–3/HPF
WBC count	2–4/HPF
Nitrates	Negative
Bacteria	Negative

What is her expected fundal height?

A. 4 cm below the umbilicus
B. 20 cm above the symphysis pubis
C. 24 cm above the symphysis pubis
D. 24 cm below the xiphoid process
E. 28 cm above the symphysis pubis

121. A worried first-time mother brings her 3-year-old daughter to the pediatric clinic for evaluation of a persistent fever. The mother states that the child has had a fever of 39°C for 2 weeks and has not improved. She also says there has been a rash present "all over her" for the past 5 days. Physical examination reveals clear tympanic membranes bilaterally. No rhinorrhea is present. The spleen is palpable and the inferior liver edge is 2.5 cm below the costal margin. There are petechiae dispersed throughout the skin, and concentrated mainly on the extremities. A CBC shows WBC count 3000/mm³, hemoglobin 7.5 g/dL, hematocrit 23.5%, and platelet count of 26,000/mm³. What is the appropriate next step to confirm the diagnosis?

A. Aspiration of bone marrow
B. Chest radiography
C. CT scan
D. Cytogenetic studies for Philadelphia chromosome
E. Peripheral blood smear

122. A 14-year-old boy presents to the pediatric clinic with complaints of progressive weakness of his legs for 2 days. He states that he also has some paresthesias of both legs. There is no recent fever or chills, but he says he had a viral illness approximately 3 weeks ago. Physical examination reveals the lungs are clear bilaterally with no lymphadenopathy. Strength of lower extremity is 4/5 bilaterally with 1+ patellar and 1+ ankle reflex. Strength of the upper extremity is 5/5, and triceps reflex is 2+. Lumbar puncture reveals WBC count 2/mm^3, protein 60 mg/dL, and glucose 70 mg/dL. What is the most appropriate treatment for this disease?

A. Acyclovir
B. Antibiotics
C. Anticholinesterase therapy (intravenous)
D. Immunoglobulin
E. Intubation

123. Three days after undergoing a right hip arthroplasty, a 73-year-old man complains of being unable to catch his breath for 1 hour. He states that his breathing is difficult. He is febrile and tachycardic. Physical examination reveals a friction rub with clear breath sounds. What is the next most appropriate step in the treatment of this patient?

A. Chest x-ray
B. CT scan without contrast
C. Pulmonary arteriogram
D. Ventilation/perfusion scan
E. Vascular study (duplex Doppler ultrasonography) of the lower extremities

124. A 51-year-old woman presents to her primary care physician with complaints of a 3-month history of menstrual irregularities marked by multiple episodes of spotting each month for 2 to 4 days. She describes symptoms of dyspareunia, difficulty sleeping, and uncharacteristic mood swings for the past 6 months. Physical examination findings of the heart, lungs, and abdomen are unremarkable. Pelvic examination reveals thinning of the vaginal and urethral mucosa. There is a grade I cystocele and grade II rectocele. What diagnostic test should be performed to confirm the diagnosis of menopause?

A. Blood serum estrogen levels
B. Blood serum follicle-stimulating hormone levels
C. Blood serum testosterone levels
D. Ovarian tissue biopsy to establish primary ovarian failure
E. Papanicolaou smear

125. A 40-year-old woman with a history of recurrent urinary tract infections presents to her primary care physician complaining of right flank pain, nausea, and vomiting for 1 month. She has been taking levofloxacin for her recurrent infections. She also has a history of diabetes mellitus and takes glucophage. Physical examination reveals mild right costovertebral angle tenderness. Radiologic studies are obtained and shown below. Figure 125a is a plain abdominal x-ray and Figure 125b is a noncontrast CT scan of the abdomen. What is the most likely diagnosis?

Figure 125a

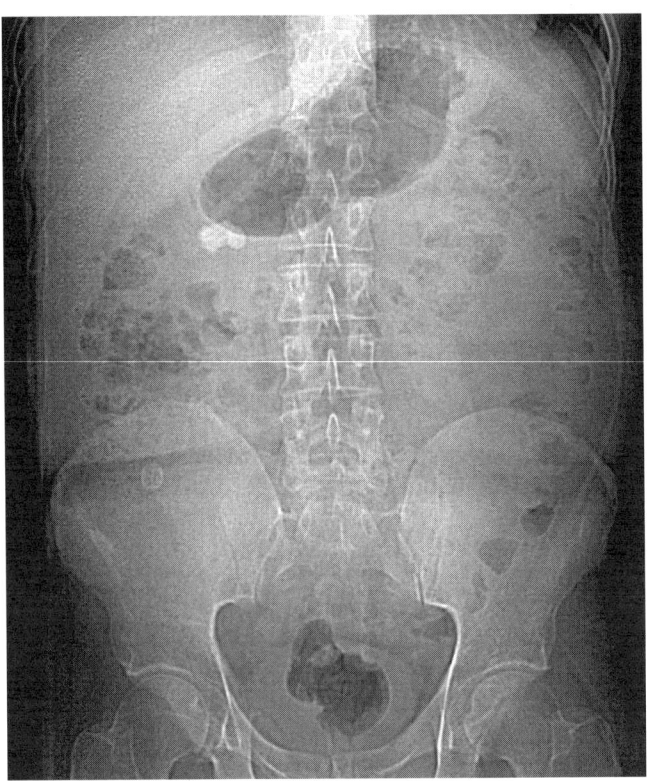

Figure 125b

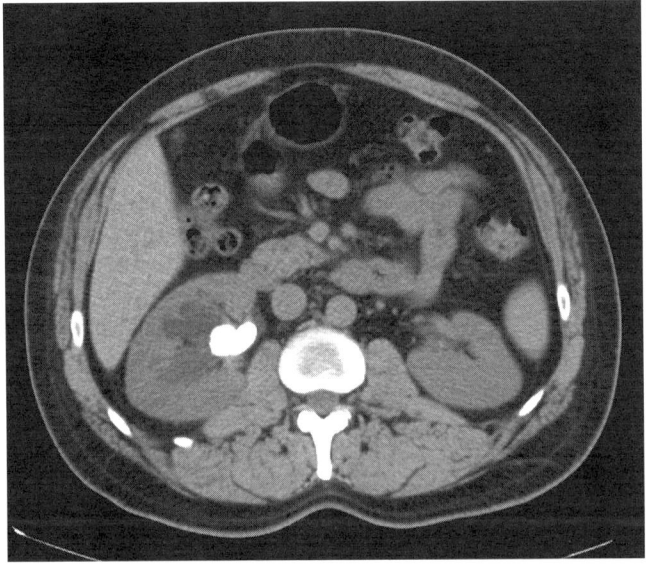

A. Cholecystitis
B. Cholelithiasis
C. Phlebolith
D. Renal stone
E. Transitional cell carcinoma

126. A 53-year-old man with hypertension, asthma, and a 45 pack/year history of smoking is rushed to the hospital by ambulance, accompanied by his wife. Upon arrival, the patient becomes unresponsive. His spouse provides some history. "He was standing over the sink washing dishes, suddenly dropped a glass, and shouted. When I asked him what was the matter, he said his head was pounding. As I called 911, he began vomiting and sunk to the floor. After that, he stopped vomiting, but he kept covering his eyes and saying how bad his head hurt." What is the best way to evaluate this patient?

A. Immediately perform a CT scan, with and without contrast.
B. Perform a lumbar puncture. If negative for blood, immediately get a CT scan.
C. Perform a lumbar puncture. If positive for blood, immediately get a cerebral angiogram.
D. Perform an immediate cerebral angiogram.
E. Watchful waiting.

127. A 2-year-old girl has a history of polyuria, polydipsia, and increased thirst. She is admitted to the hospital because of hypernatremic dehydration. Further workup reveals an elevated serum osmolality, and a normal blood glucose. A DDAVP [1-deamino(8-D-arginine) vasopressin] test dose is given without change in urine output. What is the most likely diagnosis?

A. Central diabetes insipidus
B. Diabetes mellitus
C. Glomerulonephritis
D. Nephrogenic diabetes insipidus
E. Renal tubular acidosis

128. A 60-year-old man with a history of diabetes mellitus and hypertension complains of progressive dysphagia, weight loss of 25 pounds over 2 months, coughing, choking, and generalized malaise. He also has a 20-year history of gastroesophageal reflux that has been treated with sucralfate and antacid therapy. Physical examination reveals a regular rate and rhythm. Pulmonary auscultation reveals decreased breath sounds at the bases bilaterally without wheeze or rhonchi. Gastrointestinal examination reveals tenderness to palpation in the midepigastric region. Results of laboratory studies are shown below:

Hematocrit	29%
Mean corpuscular volume	70 μm³

Which of the following is the most likely pathologic entity implicated in this condition?

A. Adenocarcinoma
B. Leiomyoma
C. Lymphoma
D. Sarcoma
E. Squamous cell carcinoma

129. A 26-year-old pregnant woman presents to her primary care physician complaining of burning when she urinates. She states the symptoms started 2 days ago and denies having a history of similar symptoms. Physical examination reveals no evidence of abdominal guarding or peritoneal signs. There is no evidence of costovertebral angle tenderness.

Results of laboratory studies are shown below:

Urinalysis

Color	Cloudy
Urine pH	6.0
RBC count	50–100/HPF
WBC count	50–100/HPF
Nitrates	Positive
Bacteria	Positive

What is the most appropriate next step in the management of this patient?

A. Order an intravenous pyelogram to rule out pyelonephritis
B. Start patient on oral trimethoprim/sulfamethoxazole
C. Start patient on intravenous ampicillin/gentamicin
D. Start patient on oral ciprofloxacin
E. Start patient on oral tetracycline

130. A 65-year-old man has developed sepsis. Eighteen hours later he develops severe dyspnea, coughing, and wheezing. The patient seems distressed and using accessory muscles to breathe. Respiratory rate is 27 breaths/min. Rales are present to auscultation in both lung bases. Chest x-ray reveals diffuse infiltrates bilaterally with sparing of the costophrenic angles. An alveolar and an interstitial pattern are noted. What is the most likely explanation of these findings?

A. Centrally mediated decrease in respiratory drive
B. Damaged type I pneumocytes decreasing production of surfactant
C. Decreased alveolar-arterial gradient
D. Neutrophil-mediated injury of the lung tissue with widespread atelectasis
E. Respiratory alkalosis with compensation

131. A 55-year-old woman is brought to her family physician because of several months of increasingly erratic behavior. She was found wandering the neighborhood looking for her cat, which had died 8 years ago. She also has been increasingly forgetful of everyday tasks, and recently got lost driving around her neighborhood. Last week, her neighbors found her in her yard, watering the hedges in her winter coat despite the fact that it was a sunny 90°F day. What is the most appropriate treatment for this patient?

A. Anticholinergic agent

B. Cholinesterase inhibitor

C. Electroconvulsive therapy

D. Reassurance

E. Selective serotonin reuptake inhibitor

132. A 24-year-old woman presents with an 8-day history of a slowly progressing purulent, erythematous lesion over her mandible. She reports minimal pain. Physical examination results of the heart, lungs, and abdomen are within normal limits. Microscopic examination of exudate shows sulfur granules. Results of laboratory studies are shown below:

Electrolytes, serum

Na, serum	143 mEq/L
Cl, serum	100 mEq/L
K, serum	3.7 mEq/L
Bicarbonate, serum	24 mEq/L
Magnesium, serum	2.0 mEq/L
Creatinine, serum	1.0 mg/dL

Leukocyte count and differential

Leukocyte count	12,000/mm³
Segmented neutrophils	75%
Bands	7%
Eosinophils	3%
Basophils	1%
Lymphocytes	27%
Monocytes	4%

Urinalysis

Urine pH	6.0
RBC count	2/HPF
WBC count	2/HPF
Nitrates	Negative
Bacteria	Negative

What is the most likely diagnosis?

A. *Actinomyces israelii*

B. *Listeria monocytogenes*

C. *Haemophilus influenzae*

D. *Providencia stuartii*

E. *Streptococcus viridans*

133. A 30-year-old woman with a history of five dilation and curettages for unwanted pregnancy presents to her primary care physician with complaints of not being able to conceive. She has also stopped having periods. She has been trying to conceive for 14 months without success. Abdominal and pelvic ultrasonography reveals bridging in the middle of the uterus. What is the most likely diagnosis?

A. Asherman syndrome

B. Luteinizing hormone:follicle-stimulating hormone (LH:FSH) ratio greater than 2.5:1

C. Premature ovarian failure

D. Stein-Leventhal syndrome

E. Swyer syndrome

134. A 42-year-old white woman with no significant medical history presents to her primary care physician for a 6-month history of severe low back pain worsened by straining or coughing. She denies having urinary or fecal incontinence or a history of trauma. Physical examination reveals pain radiating below the knee with straight leg raise on the left and is negative on the right. No sensory or motor deficits are noted. What is the most appropriate initial treatment of this patient?

A. Bed rest for 6 weeks, ibuprofen and reevaluation

B. Bed rest for 1 to 3 days, ibuprofen, physical therapy, and local heat

C. Encourage patient to seek permanent disability

D. Referral to pain clinic

E. Surgical removal of disk

135. A 32-year-old G2P1 woman at 35 weeks' gestation was found to have a blood pressure of 142/90 mm Hg on routine visit. She has not reported contractions or vaginal discharge at this time. She also denies having any noticeable edema. Fundal height correlates with gestational age. Urinalysis and 24-hour urine collection reveal protein to be +1 and 245 mg, respectively. Repeat blood pressure measured 136/88 mm Hg. What is the next most appropriate step in this patient's treatment?

A. Administer hydralazine and monitor blood pressure for 4 to 6 hours

B. Bed rest for the remainder of the pregnancy

C. Cervical examination to assess effacement

D. Immediate induction of labor

E. Watchful waiting, follow up at next scheduled appointment

136. Two patients are seen in the primary care clinic. Both patients have complaints of anovulation. The differential diagnosis of both patients includes polycystic ovarian syndrome and Stein-Leventhal syndrome. Which of the following findings is associated with neither of these conditions?

A. Decreased estrogen

B. Increased incidence of type II diabetes mellitus

C. Increased LH:FSH ratio

D. Increased testosterone

E. Normal FSH:LH ratio

137. An obese 50-year-old male inpatient has been hospitalized for 2 weeks after a motor vehicle accident in which he sustained multiple fractures of the lower extremities. He complains of right leg pain with swelling and warmth of the right calf. He also complains of dyspnea and mild chest pain. Which of the following is an ominous finding of impending demise?

A. Bradycardia

B. Cellulitis

C. Homan sign negative

D. Hypocoagulability

E. Venous markings distally

138. A 6-month-old boy is brought to the emergency department for acute onset of dyspnea and fever. Past medical history is significant for numerous hospitalizations secondary to recurrent pyogenic infections as well as enteroviral infections. Physical examination reveals that the child is febrile and tachypneic. Chest x-ray is suspicious for pneumonia. What is the appropriate treatment for this patient?

A. Appropriate antibiotic therapy

B. Appropriate antibiotic therapy and periodic intravenous immune globulin

C. Thymic and bone marrow transplantation

D. Daily prophylactic doses of trimethoprim

E. Watchful waiting

139. A healthy 15-year-old white girl presents to her primary care physician with new-onset fever, malaise, weight loss, and arthralgias. She also complains of two recent episodes of syncope. She denies having headaches or visual disturbances. Physical examination reveals a blood pressure of 142/88 mm Hg, a pulse of 86 beats/min, temperature of 99.2°F, height of 64 inches, and weight of 51 kg. Radial pulses are equally diminished bilaterally. Laboratory studies are significant for an erythrocyte sedimentation rate of 110 mm/hr and normochromic, normocytic anemia. Angiography of the subclavian arteries reveals irregular vessel walls, with stenosis, and poststenotic dilatation. What is the next most appropriate step in the evaluation of this patient?

A. Antineutrophil antibody studies

B. Blood cultures

C. Chest x-ray

D. CT of the head

E. Joint aspirate cytology

F. Temporal artery biopsy

140. An 18-year-old man complains of difficulty breathing and cough of 1 hour's duration. This started while attending a soccer game with his friends. He is brought to the emergency department for further evaluation. The patient says he has always had some difficulty breathing, especially during the springtime, but this was the first severe episode he has ever had. He reports no weight loss but fatigue since the episode began. He also has had a runny nose. Physical examination reveals expiratory wheezes throughout the posterior chest. His cough is dry. His oxygen saturation is 80% on room air. His temperature is 37°C, pulse 99 beats/min, and blood pressure 125/85 mm Hg. Chest x-ray is ordered and shown below (Figure 140). What is the most likely diagnosis?

Figure 140

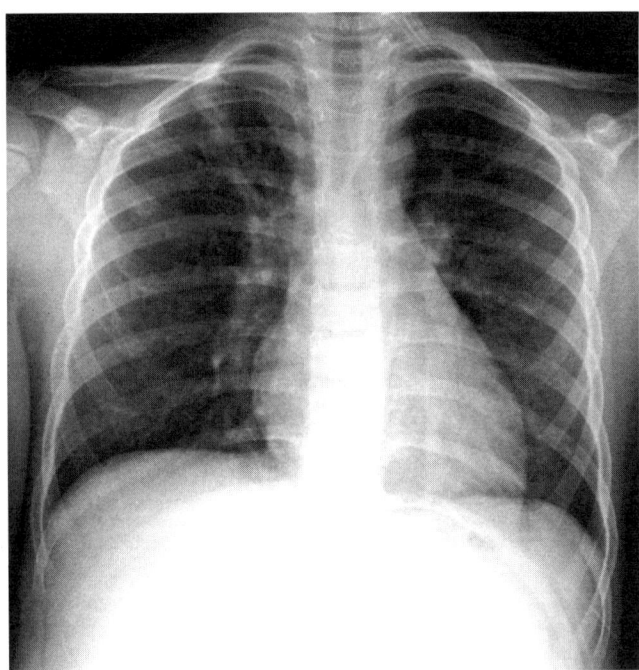

A. Adenocarcinoma
B. Allergic rhinitis
C. Asthma
D. Rhinovirus infection
E. Small cell carcinoma

141. A 26-year-old G2P1 woman is 25 weeks pregnant. She complains of annoying excessive salivation that has occurred throughout her pregnancy. She feels as if she produces gallons of saliva each day. However, her symptoms have remained stable during the past 2 weeks. Cardiac examination reveals a regular rate and rhythm. Pulmonary evalua-

tion reveals clear lungs bilaterally without rales or rhonchi. Abdominal examination reveals normoactive bowel sounds with a fundal height 24.5 cm from the pubis. Anorectal evaluation reveals no evidence of external hemorrhoids. What is the most likely diagnosis?

A. Appendicitis
B. Gastroesophageal reflux
C. Hepatitis
D. Hyperemesis gravidarum
E. Ptyalism

142. A 65-year-old man presents to the office for a routine examination. His past medical history is notable for hypertension and asthma. The patient was intubated for his asthma approximately 15 years ago and was hospitalized for 10 days. At the present visit, the patient reports that his wife died last week after battling a long illness. She was diagnosed with breast cancer 5 years ago and underwent modified radical mastectomy with chemotherapy and radiation. However, she succumbed to her disease with liver metastasis noted at autopsy. Upon further discussion with the patient, he reports a 5-pound weight loss, decreased appetite, and a lack of pleasure in his life at the present time. He seeks your guidance and advice. What is the most likely diagnosis?

A. Adjustment disorder
B. Brief reactive psychosis
C. Depression (atypical)
D. Depression (major)
E. Schizoaffective disorder

143. A mother presents to the community health center with her 5-year-old son for a well-child check-up. She reveals that her son has been diagnosed as having moderate mental retardation. While taking a careful birth history, it is revealed that he was born at 38 weeks and was 11 pounds 1 ounce. Physical examination reveals that the boy has large ears, macrognathia, and macroorchidism. It is likely that he has a genetic disorder due to which of the following:

A. Autosomal-dominant disease
B. X-linked disease
C. Sex chromosome abnormality
D. Autosomal trisomy
E. Y-linkage

144. A 55-year-old man with progressive gait abnormality is referred for evaluation. He is a retired painter whose job entailed weight bearing on his knees for prolonged periods during the past 15 years. He smokes two packs of cigarettes per day and drinks approximately 1 can of beer per day. His prior medical history is notable for hiatal hernia repair via an endoscopic approach and postoperative gastroesophageal reflux disorder, which responds to H2 blockers. Physical examination reveals decreased range of motion of the right femur with muscle strength reduced to 20% when compared with the left lower extremity. MRI reveals a metaphyseal cartilagenous mass. A similar lesion is also seen in the pelvis. What is the most likely diagnosis?

A. Adamantinoma
B. Aneurysmal bone cyst
C. Chondrosarcoma
D. Metastatic tumor of bone
E. Unicameral bone cyst

145. A woman presents to her physician because she has had progressive onset of dementia, accompanied by psychomotor slowing and difficulty swallowing. She cannot complete difficult tasks, and shows significant distress over the decline of her condition. Others in her family have had the same condition. Where is the primary pathology of this disease located?

A. Caudate nucleus
B. Cerebellar cortex
C. Corpus callosum
D. Diffuse cortical involvement
E. Substantia nigra

146. A 53-year-old overweight black man presents to his primary care physician for an annual check-up. He has no significant past medical history. A nurse checks his vital signs and finds a temperature of 36.8°C, pulse of 80 beats/min, blood pressure of 190/126 mm Hg, and a normal respiratory rate. Physical examination reveals an overweight black man in no apparent distress. Cardiac, pulmonary and abdominal examinations are within normal limits. Results of laboratory studies are shown below:

Electrolytes, serum

Na, serum	145 mEq/L
Cl, serum	102 mEq/L
K, serum	3.9 mEq/L
Bicarbonate, serum	26 mEq/L
Magnesium, serum	1.9 mEq/L
Creatinine, serum	1.3 mg/dL

Leukocyte count and differential

Leukocyte count	6000/mm^3
Segmented neutrophils	65%
Bands	6%
Eosinophils	2%
Basophils	1%
Lymphocytes	27%
Monocytes	4%

Blood, plasma, serum

Alanine aminotransferase (ALT)	15 U/L
Amylase, serum	55 U/L
Aspartate aminotransferase (AST)	14 U/L
Calcium, serum	9.2 mg/dL
Glucose, serum	110 mg/dL
Hematocrit	43.2%
Urea nitrogen, serum (BUN)	10 mg/dL

Urinalysis

Urine pH	7.0
RBC count	1/HPF
WBC count	0/HPF
Nitrates	Negative
Bacteria	Negative

What is the best management of this man's hypertension?

A. Measure blood pressure again tomorrow
B. Modifications of lifestyle
C. Stress management therapy
D. Treatment with an angiotensin-converting enzyme inhibitor
E. Treatment with sodium nitroprusside

147. A 65-year-old man has developed sepsis. Eighteen hours later he develops severe dyspnea, coughing, and wheezing. The patient seems distressed and uses accessory muscles to breathe. Respiratory rate is 27 breaths/min. Rales are present to auscultation in both lung bases. Chest x-ray reveals diffuse infiltrates bilaterally with sparing of the costophrenic angles. An alveolar and interstitial pattern is noted. What is the most appropriate treatment for this patient?

A. Corticosteroids
B. Expectant management
C. Mechanical ventilation
D. Positive end-expiratory pressure (PEEP)
E. Tracheotomy

148. Advocates in a large community are concerned about the development of osteoporosis among area residents. Which of the following profiles of individuals would be most likely to develop this condition?

A. A 38-year-old white male marathon runner with a history of diabetes mellitus
B. A 47-year-old Asian woman who has a history of hyperthyroidism and weighs 95 pounds
C. A 48-year-old black woman with a history of sarcoidosis
D. A 36-year-old black woman who has four children
E. A 19-year-old white woman who binge eats frequently and weighs 150 pounds

149. A 42-year-old male patient with a solitary pulmonary nodule has a repeat chest x-ray taken 3 years later as a follow-up. X-ray revealed no change in the size of the nodule. Physical examination findings of the heart, lungs, and abdomen are within normal limits. Results of follow-up laboratory studies are as follows:

Magnesium, serum	2.0 mg/dL
Total protein, serum	6.8 g/dL
Na, serum	142 mEq/L
Urea nitrogen, serum (BUN)	11 mg/dL
K, serum	3.8 mEq/L
WBC count	8500/mm^3
Hematocrit	41%
Chest x-ray	2.2-cm solitary nodule in the right lower lobe

What is the most likely diagnosis?

A. Aspirated foreign body
B. Benign
C. Malignant (melanoma)
D. Malignant (metastatic carcinoma)
E. Malignant (primary foci)

150. A 15-year-old high school student is interested in volunteering at a local nursing home. Requirements for volunteering at this facility requires that each participant receive a PPD (purified protein derivative) test prior to beginning work. He has no known risk factors for tuberculosis (TB). Physical examination findings of the heart, lungs, and abdomen are unremarkable. A 7-mm area of induration is discovered within 48 hours of the test. What is the most appropriate intervention for this patient?

A. Isoniazid
B. Isoniazid and rifampin
C. Isoniazid, rifampin, and streptomycin
D. No treatment is needed
E. Termination from the workplace

151. Twenty-four hours after birth a neonate develops a rash on the trunk and face consisting of heterogeneous papules, pustules, and vesicles on an erythematous base. Gram stain of the vesicular contents is positive for eosinophils. What is the most likely diagnosis?

A. Cutis marmorata
B. Erythema toxicum neonatorum
C. Milia
D. Mongolian spots
E. Seborrheic dermatitis

152. In the middle of a soccer game, a 19-year-old man collides with another player. As he recalls, he made a diving slide to kick the ball while his opponent was getting ready for a "goal shot." As a result, the opponent ended up kicking the patient in the left, posterolateral leg, one-third the distance from the knee to the ankle. Two hours later, the patient is in the emergency department, complaining of relentless, severe leg pain. Physical examination reveals mild ecchymoses overlying the injury and mild swelling when compared with the right leg. Femoral, dorsal pedal, and posterior tibial pulses all seem normal. There is weakness in dorsiflexion, plantar flexion, and eversion of the ankle; knee flexion and extension are intact. The calf is tense; the Thompson test elicits plantar flexion, and the patient seems to have a positive Homan sign (pain with forced dorsiflexion). With light touch, he reports diffusely decreased sensation over the posterior leg, with the anterior and lateral aspects being mostly normal. X-ray fails to reveal fracture. What is the next step in the evaluation of this patient?

A. None needed—prepare patient for fasciotomy
B. None needed—serial physical examinations of the patient
C. None needed—take to operating room for Achilles tendon repair
D. Duplex ultrasonography, looking for thrombosis in deep veins
E. None needed—treat muscle contusion symptomatically; follow-up necessary to watch for development of traumatic myositis ossificans

153. A 24-year-old HIV-positive man presents to a local community health center complaining of muscle aches and abdominal cramps. He has lost approximately 10 pounds during the past 3 months. He has a prior surgical history of inguinal hernia repair. Physical examination of the heart, lungs, and abdomen are unremarkable. Results of laboratory studies are shown below:

Bleeding time	4 minutes
Erythrocyte count	4.3 million/mm^3
CD4 count	600/mm^3
Mean corpuscular volume	80 nm^3

Likely findings on physical examination that could explain this presentation may include which of the following?

A. Herpes vesicles
B. Lymphadenopathy
C. Kaposi sarcoma
D. Non-Hodgkin lymphoma
E. Oral thrush

154. A 23-year-old woman recently quit her first job in marketing and has been working at a bar to support herself while also interviewing for a new marketing position. She does not smoke and has no other health problems. She is also very concerned about her health. Two months ago in her first interview, she was speaking with a few members of the company when she suddenly felt her heart start to pound. Her hands were trembling by her sides and she felt like she was choking and unable to speak or breathe. She broke into a sweat and began to feel very faint. The symptoms did not last much longer than 5 minutes, but she was very embarrassed. She was also very worried about what happened because her mother had died of a heart attack when she was 52. She quickly left her interview and rushed to the hospital. Her electrocardiogram, chest x-ray, and cardiac enzymes were completely normal. Six weeks ago, the same symptoms occurred. However, she decided to finish the interview and she did not go to the hospital. Since that time, she has been very worried that this will continue to happen at each job interview and is worried that she is never going to find a job. What is the most likely diagnosis?

A. Agoraphobia
B. Obsessive-compulsive disorder
C. Panic disorder
D. Social phobia
E. Unstable angina

155. A 37-year-old woman presents with obesity and recent diagnosis of diabetes. She has an allergy to dogs and cats. She has a 15 pack/year history of smoking and is an occasional drinker of wine. Physical examination reveals a male hair distribution and frontal balding. She is interested in treatment for her "masculinized appearance" because it is distressing to her. She has a luteinizing hormone:follicle-stimulating hormone (LH:FSH) ratio of 3. What is the most appropriate treatment for this patient?

A. Combined oral contraceptive pill
B. Gonadotropin-releasing hormone agonists
C. Prednisone
D. Progestin
E. Spironolactone

156. A 16-year-old male high school athlete is brought to the emergency room by ambulance after collapsing on the football field during a practice session. Teammates told the paramedics that the individual was snorting cocaine approximately 1 hour prior to practice. Physical examination in the emergency room shows a blood pressure of 40/20 mm Hg, undetectable pulse, and absent respirations. Electrocardiography reveals asystole. What is the most likely explanation of these findings?

A. Aortic rupture
B. Hypotension
C. Mitral valve dysfunction
D. Pulmonary valvular atresia
E. Right ventricular dysfunction

157. A 23-year-old man was in a head-on automobile collision that rendered him unconscious at the site of the accident. Upon arrival to the emergency department, the patient was unresponsive, but breathing with a normal heart rate. Physical examination revealed a fixed, dilated right pupil. CT scan revealed a crescent-shaped hematoma. What is the most likely finding as surgical exploration?

A. Acute subdural hematoma
B. Chronic subdural hematoma

C. Diffuse axonal injury
D. Epidural hematoma
E. Subarachnoid hematoma

158. An 11-year-old boy is brought to the pediatric clinic for evaluation of right knee pain for 3 weeks. There is no history of trauma. The patient's father states he has recently noticed a limp when his son walks. The patient is 62 inches tall and weighs 193 pounds. Physical examination of the right knee reveals limited internal rotation and tenderness to palpation. Radiographs obtained are shown below (Figure 158). What is the most appropriate management of the patient?

Figure 158

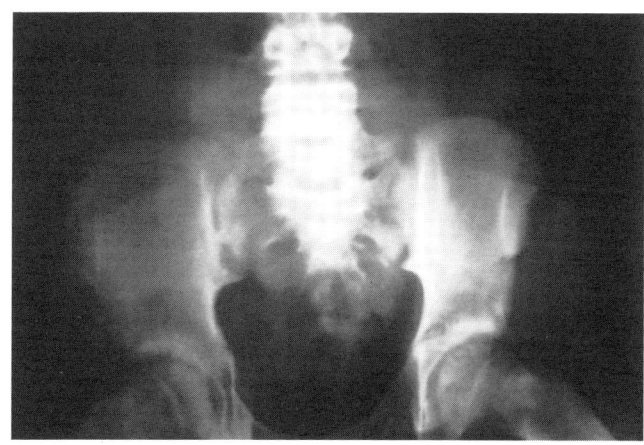

A. Enroll the patient in a physical therapy program
B. Manage pain with nonsteroidal antiinflammatory drugs and rest
C. Observation
D. Surgical treatment with pin fixation
E. Surgical treatment with arthroscopy of the hip joint

159. A mother brings her 2-year-old son to a pediatrician for evaluation. The child has a history of failing to develop a social smile or make eye-to-eye contact. He has not learned any words, but makes many repetitive sounds. Upon entering the room, the pediatrician sees the toddler sitting on the floor in the corner, ignoring his mother and making flapping motions with his hands. What is the most likely diagnosis?

A. Autistic disorder
B. Attention deficit hyperactivity disorder
C. Congenital deafness
D. Fragile X syndrome
E. Mental retardation

160. A 29-year-old woman has a positive pregnancy test result. She presents to her primary care physician for confirmation. She has a history of recurrent urinary tract infections, headaches, seizure disorder, and pulmonary embolus. Her current medications include acetaminophen, ciprofloxacin, warfarin, valproic acid, and methotrexate. Physical examination findings of the heart, lungs, and abdomen are within normal limits. Serum beta-human chorionic gonadotropin is elevated. Other laboratory studies obtained are shown below:

Electrolytes, serum

Na, serum	143 mEq/L
Cl, serum	99 mEq/L
K, serum	3.4 mEq/L
Bicarbonate, serum	24 mEq/L
Magnesium, serum	1.9 mEq/L
Creatinine, serum	1.1 mg/dL

Leukocyte count and differential

Leukocyte count	7000/mm^3
Segmented neutrophils	6%
Bands	6
Eosinophils	3
Basophils	2%
Lymphocytes	25
Monocytes	3

Which of the following medications that this patient is taking can be maintained at its current dosage during her pregnancy?

A. Acetaminophen
B. Ciprofloxacin
C. Methotrexate
D. Valproic acid
E. Warfarin

161. A 12-year-old boy with a history of rheumatic heart disease presents to his primary care physician complaining of fever, cough, chills, sweats, and back pain. Physical examination of the lungs are normal. Cardiac auscultation reveals a III/IV systolic ejection murmur. Echocardiography reveals an oscillating intracardiac mass on the mitral valve. What is the next most appropriate step in the evaluation of this patient?

A. Administer nafcillin, penicillin, and gentamycin
B. Chest x-ray
C. Obtain blood cultures
D. Transfusion of fresh frozen plasma
E. Valve replacement

The response options for items 162–164 are the same. You will be required to select one answer for each item in the set.

A. Trisomy 8
B. Trisomy 13
C. Trisomy 21
D. Triploidy (69 XXX)
E. 4p- syndrome
F. 5p- syndrome

G. 13q- syndrome
H. 18p- syndrome

For each live newborn with clinical findings, select the appropriate chromosomal disorder.

162. A 1-day-old boy who was born at 39 weeks via spontaneous vaginal delivery is found to have a small head and eyes. In addition, micrognathia is present. He also has large ears, small hands, and small feet.

163. A newborn girl is stillborn. Examination of the delivered placenta reveals hydatiform changes. Physical examination of the stillborn infant reveals microphthalmia with coloboma. Genitourinary examination reveals hypospadias and a left undescended testicle.

164. A newborn is evaluated by the pediatrics resident shortly after birth. Physical examination reveals thick lips, deep-set eyes, prominent ears, and permanent flexion of the interphalangeal joints.

165. A 56-year-old woman who underwent laparoscopic cholecystectomy presents to her primary care physician 5 days after the operation complaining of severe constipation. The patient has been using over-the-counter laxatives and has had some improvement in her symptoms. She ends the interview by asking you to refill her pain medication, stating, "It hurts so bad that sometimes I take twice the dose." What is the most likely etiology of her constipation?

A. Formation of postoperative adhesions
B. Iatrogenic damage to bowel during surgery
C. Ileus
D. Opioid-induced constipation
E. Postoperative inflammatory bowel disease

166. An unconscious 30-year-old black man is brought to the emergency department after being found lying on a jogging trail in the park. He is wearing jogging clothing and sneakers stained with vomit. Physical examination reveals that he is tachycardic and diaphoretic. His blood sugar is found to be 12 mg/dL; 5% dextrose intravenous fluids are administered. Soon into the infusion he begins to regain consciousness and is able to answer questions. He says he was jogging in the park and began to develop a headache with blurred vision. He kept running and became nauseated, but kept pushing himself and remembers collapsing. He did not stop because he was trying to get back into shape because he had gained weight over the past few months. He states that he had to eat more frequently beginning about 3 months ago because he would get headaches and become diaphoretic if too much time elapsed between meals. Physical examination of the heart, lungs, and abdomen are unremarkable. Laboratory studies reveal serum thyroid-stimulating hormone is within normal limits, but insulin and protein C are both elevated several times the normal limit. What is the most likely explanation of these findings?

A. Exertional

B. Injection of exogenous insulin to lose weight

C. Ingestion of exogenous thyroid hormone to lose weight

D. Pancreatic insulinoma

E. Undiagnosed type II diabetes

167. You are a medical student doing an elective rotation in a drug rehabilitation center. A woman and her 16-year-old son present for evaluation. The woman is tearful. When you ask her what is wrong, she shows you a bag of marijuana that she found in her son's room, along with some drug paraphernalia. She states that her son has a decreased interest in activities, lower grades, and is always borrowing money. He states that he was just holding the drugs for a friend. When asked for a urine sample, he finally confesses. After working with drug addiction for many years, you know that it is quite a large amount of marijuana. You tell him that you are worried that he may be dependent on marijuana. He gets angry and yells back that it is impossible to get addicted to marijuana. You tell him that according to the definitions of dependence and addiction, a person can be:

A. Addicted to and dependent on marijuana

B. Addicted but not dependent

C. Neither addicted nor dependent

D. Not addicted, not dependent

E. Unable to determine

168. An 8-year-old boy is referred to the cardiologist after presenting to the emergency department with tachycardia. He has had frequent episodes of dizziness with most activities. He has not been able to participate in school sports well due to impact causing his "heart to race." He has experienced concomitant nausea and vomiting. Review of the emergency department records indicate the patient's presenting pulse was 200 beats/min. He is currently stable at 80 beats/min. Physical examination findings of the head, eyes, ears, and throat are unremarkable. Cardiac and pulmonary examinations reveal no evidence of wheeze, rhonchi, or rales. The cardiac rate is normal. Electrocardiography reveals a shortened PR interval with a wide QRS complex with a slurred upstroke. What is the most appropriate management for this patient?

A. Beta blocker

B. Calcium channel blocker

C. Catheter radiofrequency ablation

D. Digoxin

E. Rehydration with intravenous 0.9% saline

169. A 43-year-old G2P2002 woman with no significant past medical history presents to her gynecologist for her annual health maintenance appointment. She complains of multiple episodes per week of involuntarily leaking small amounts of urine. She describes the episodes as occurring primarily when she laughs, coughs, or sneezes. Pelvic examination reveals a grade I cystocele with urethral hypermobility. What is likely associated with this patient's diagnosis?

A. Absence of bladder contractions leading to overdistention of the bladder

B. Neurogenic bladder secondary to underlying diabetes mellitus

C. Pelvic relaxation and displacement of the urethrovesical junction

D. Uninhibited bladder contractions

E. Urinary fistula resulting from pelvic surgery or pelvic radiation

170. A 57-year-old African-American man comes to the ambulatory care clinic for an annual physical examination. He reports no problems. Physical examination findings of the heart, lungs, and abdomen are within normal limits. Upon digital rectal examination, a 1.5-cm rock-hard discrete prostate nodule is palpated. Results of laboratory studies are shown below:

Electrolytes, serum

Na, serum	143 mEq/L
Cl, serum	100 mEq/L
K, serum	3.7 mEq/L
Bicarbonate, serum	24 mEq/L
Magnesium, serum	2.0 mEq/L
Creatinine, serum	1.0 mg/dL

Leukocyte count and differential

Leukocyte count	5000/mm^3
Segmented neutrophils	55%
Bands	5%
Eosinophils	2%
Basophils	1%
Lymphocytes	23%
Monocytes	3%

Blood, plasma, serum

Alanine aminotransferase (ALT)	15 U/L
Amylase, serum	55 U/L
Aspartate aminotransferase (AST)	12 U/L
Calcium, serum	9 mg/dL
Glucose, serum	110 mg/dL
Hematocrit	42%
Urea nitrogen, serum (BUN)	10 mg/dL

Urinalysis

Urine pH	6.0
RBC count	2–3/HPF
WBC count	2–3/HPF
Nitrates	Negative
Bacteria	Negative

What is the next appropriate step in the treatment of this patient?

A. Begin a course of flutamide

B. Begin a course of nilutamide

C. Measurement of prostate specific antigen (PSA)

D. Prostatectomy

E. Transrectal needle biopsy

171. A 25-year-old male university graduate student presents to the student health clinic for evaluation. He lives alone and has never had many friends, nor has he had any serious romantic relationships. He spends his time studying and playing computer games. When asked what he does for fun, he replies, "Nothing really . . . computer games I guess." He has never had sexual intercourse, and states that he simply has no interest in it. He seems emotionally detached, and he has a flattened affect. What is the most likely diagnosis?

   A. Autistic disorder
   B. Avoidant personality disorder
   C. Schizoid personality disorder
   D. Schizophrenia
   E. Schizotypal personality disorder

172. A 33-year-old man has a history of chronic diarrhea, nausea, poor appetite, and a 25-pound weight loss. He presents to his primary care physician for evaluation. Physical examination reveals a tender mass in the right lower quadrant. There is no evidence of guarding or rebound tenderness. CT scan with oral gastrograffin is undertaken and is shown below (Figure 172). What is the most likely diagnosis?

Figure 172

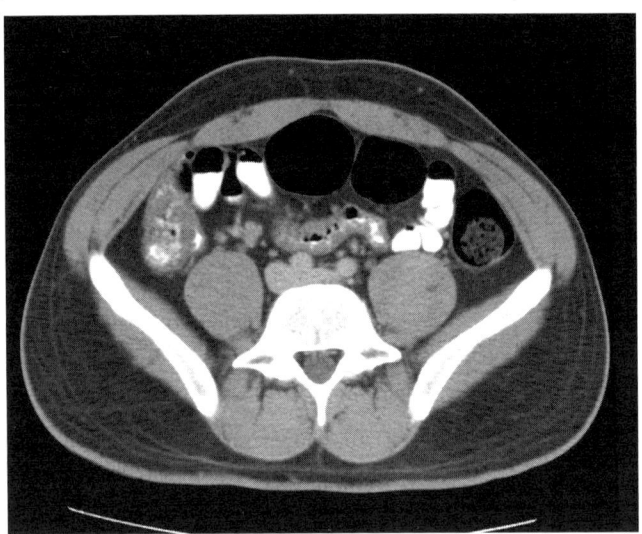

   A. Adenocarcinoma
   B. Crohn disease
   C. Meckel diverticulitis
   D. Mesenteric ischemia
   E. Ulcerative colitis

173. A 32-year-old G4P3 woman at 39 weeks' gestation presents to the labor and delivery floor for induction of labor. Previous ultrasonography showed a twin gestation in vertex positions. The patient is begun on epidural anesthesia. During the course of her prolonged labor, oxytocin is started and a few hours later she begins contracting. After another 12 hours, the patient develops a fever and fetal tachycardia.

Chorioamnionitis is suspected and antibiotics are administered. The patient delivers two babies 4 hours later. There is continuous hemorrhage from her vagina. What is the most likely diagnosis?

   A. Cervical laceration
   B. Placenta accreta
   C. Uterine atony
   D. Uterine rupture
   E. Vaginal laceration

174. A previously healthy 3-year-old boy is brought to the pediatric clinic for his annual evaluation. His mother states that he has been in good health. He has an occasional ear infection occurring no more frequently than every 9 months. His vitals signs reveal a blood pressure of 125/85 mm Hg, respirations of 18 breaths/min, and temperature of 38.5°C. Physical examination reveals a mass palpated in the right flank. What is the most appropriate next step in the treatment of this patient?

   A. Abdominal CT scan
   B. Abdominal ultrasonography
   C. CBC and urinalysis
   D. MRI of the abdomen
   E. Percutaneous biopsy of the mass

175. A 62-year-old woman with a history of perineal condyloma infections, chronic hemorrhoids, and proctitis presents with anorectal bleeding and pain. She has a prior medical history of perineal fistulas that were treated with surgical excision 3 and 5 years ago. Physical examination reveals a 2.5-cm cauliflower-like mass approximately 4 cm from the anal verge. Which of the following is the most appropriate next treatment for this individual?

   A. Chemotherapy (multiagent)
   B. Radiotherapy (external beam)
   C. Radiotherapy and chemotherapy
   D. Subtotal proctocolectomy
   E. Surgical resection

176. An 18-year-old Haitian woman presents to her primary care physician complaining of a 3-day history of runny nose, fever, cough, and irritated eyes. A red papular rash is noted on the head, neck, and trunk. The patient states that the rash was only on her face last night. The remainder of the physical examination findings, including cardiac, pulmonary, and abdominal examinations, are within normal limits. Results of laboratory studies are shown below:

Blood, plasma, serum

Alanine aminotransferase (ALT)	15 U/L
Amylase, serum	53 U/L
Aspartate aminotransferase (AST)	12 U/L
Calcium, serum	8.8 mg/dL
Glucose, serum	120 mg/dL
Hematocrit	38%
Urea nitrogen, serum (BUN)	11 mg/dL

Urinalysis

Urine pH	6.0
RBC count	2/HPF
WBC count	2/HPF
Nitrates	Negative
Bacteria	Negative

What is the most likely diagnosis?

A. Erythema infectiosum

B. Infective mononucleosis

C. Rubeola

D. Rubella

E. Varicella

177. A 35-year-old man with a history of schizophrenia returns for follow-up. He currently takes several medications. Most recently his symptoms have been well controlled on clozapine. You get the following laboratory results: WBC count 1200/mm^3, hemoglobin 14 mg/dL, and hematocrit 42%. What is the most appropriate next step in the treatment of this patient?

A. Add clonidine

B. Discontinue clozapine

C. Increase the dose of clozapine

D. Reduce the dose of clozapine

E. Switch to electroconvulsive therapy

178. A 32-year-old G2P2002 woman presents to her primary care physician with an arrest of her periods. She does not remember when her last period was, but she knows they used to be regular. She thinks it was more than 8 weeks ago. Physical examination findings of the heart, lungs, and abdomen are within normal limits. What is the next most appropriate diagnostic step in the evaluation of this patient?

A. Beta human chorionic gonadotropin level

B. CA 125 level

C. Luteinizing hormone and follicle-stimulating hormone levels

D. Percentage body fat analysis

E. Thyroid-stimulating hormone level

179. A 6-year-old boy presents to the pediatric clinic with a 4-week history of fever, fatigue, and bone pain. Physical examination reveals hepatosplenomegaly, petechiae, and pallor. A bone marrow aspirate reveals acute lymphocytic lymphoma. Before beginning chemotherapy, which of the following treatments is indicated?

A. Granulocyte infusion

B. Intravenous antibiotic therapy

C. Intravenous hydration, sodium bicarbonate, and allopurinol

D. Packed RBC transfusion

E. Platelet transfusion

180. A 31-year-old woman is seen in the emergency department because of secondary amenorrhea. She has no primary care provider. Physical examination findings of the heart, lungs, and abdomen are within normal limits. Laboratory studies obtained are shown below:

Electrolytes, serum

Na, serum	145 mEq/L
Cl, serum	104 mEq/L
K, serum	3.9 mEq/L
Bicarbonate, serum	25 mEq/L
Magnesium, serum	2.1 mEq/L
Creatinine, serum	1.1 mg/dL

Leukocyte count and differential

Leukocyte count	7000/mm^3
Segmented neutrophils	50%
Bands	6%
Eosinophils	3%
Basophils	1%
Lymphocytes	24%
Monocytes	4%

Blood, plasma, serum

Alanine aminotransferase (ALT)	13 U/L
Amylase, serum	52 U/L
Aspartate aminotransferase (AST)	16 U/L
Calcium, serum	9.2 mg/dL
Glucose, serum	130 mg/dL
Hematocrit	37%
Urea nitrogen, serum (BUN)	11 mg/dL
Prolactin	Normal
FSH	Elevated
LH	Elevated

Urinalysis

Urine pH	6.0
RBC count	2/HPF
WBC count	2/HPF
Nitrates	Negative
Bacteria	Negative

What is the most likely diagnosis?

A. Gonadotropin-releasing hormone (GnRH) overstimulation

B. Hypothalamic disorder

C. Ovarian failure

D. Pituitary disorder

E. Sheehan syndrome

181. A 24-year-old man develops recurrent pyogenic infections with *Staphylococcus aureus*, periodontal disease, and nystagmus. It is believed that he has a disease causing decreased chemotaxis and phagolysosome fusion in neutrophils and monocytes. What is the most likely disease?

A. Chédiak-Higashi disease

B. Chronic granulomatous disease

C. Drug-induced neutropenia

D. Felty syndrome

E. Myeloperoxidase deficiency

182. A 14-year-old boy complains of progressive right leg pain that is typically severe at night and is relieved by aspirin. He is otherwise healthy with no other medical problems. Physical examination reveals no evidence of erythema and edema overlying the right femur. Right lower extremity x-ray reveals a sharply demarcated radiolucent nidus of osteoid tissue surrounded by sclerotic femoral bone. What is the most likely diagnosis?

A. Aneurysmal bone cyst

B. Chordoma

C. Histiocytic lymphoma

D. Osteoid osteoma

E. Unicameral bone cyst

183. A 66-year-old man is brought for evaluation by his wife because she states that her husband is not acting like himself. According to his wife, he is unable to remember important personal information and other facts he knew in the past. However, he denies that he has a memory loss. He cannot remember simple things such as what he had for breakfast that day. He is very distractible and is unable to focus his attention to participate in a conversation. He has experienced some misperceptions such as believing that someone is climbing into his bedroom window. These described deficits vary in severity over hours and days. The patient exhibits no evidence of anhedonia or flattening of affect. He states that he sleeps poorly at night and that his symptoms are worse in the dark. He is usually drowsy during the day. The patient and his wife deny having any marital problems or recent evidence of psychosocial stress. Which of the following is the most likely diagnosis?

A. Delirium

B. Dementia

C. Depression

D. Normal aging

E. Normal grief reaction

184. A 52-year-old male construction worker presents to his primary care physician because of sudden onset of severe pain in the left first metatarsophalangeal joint 2 days ago. He states that he is unable to tolerate even a thin sheet lying over his left big toe. The patient has no kidney disease. Physical examination reveals that the left great toe is swollen, grossly erythematous, and exquisitely tender. There is no swelling, erythema, or tenderness in any other joints. Joint aspirate shows needle-shaped negatively birefringent crystals and an increased WBC count. Radiographs are normal. What is the most appropriate treatment of this patient?

A. Acetaminophen

B. Allopurinol and probenecid

C. Cephalexin

D. Choline

E. Hydrochlorothiazide

185. A 24-year-old G3P1 woman presents to her primary care physician complaining of amenorrhea. She has a history of two cesarean sections that produced two stillborn infants. She is a crack cocaine abuser and smokes two packs of cigarettes per day. Should this patient be given a progestin challenge, which of the following conditions is unlikely to produce a response?

A. Anorexia nervosa

B. Asherman syndrome

C. Hyperthyroidism

D. Hypothyroidism

E. Polycystic ovarian syndrome

186. A 7-year-old boy is brought to the pediatric clinic with a 3-month history of a limp while walking. No pain is described, and there is no history of trauma. Physical examination reveals limited right hip motion, mainly with internal rotation and abduction. Radiographs of the right hip and knee are normal. What is the most likely diagnosis?

A. Developmental dysplasia of the hip
B. Legg-Calve-Perthes disease
C. Osgood-Schlatter disease
D. Rickets
E. Slipped capital femoral epiphysis

187. A 36-year-old white woman complains of fever, fatigue, weight loss, arthralgia, and transient patchy alopecia during the past 3 months. Her review of systems is notable for occasional rhinorrhea and cough that responds well to oral decongestant therapy. A similar constellation of symptoms occurred 6 months ago during treatment for a cardiovascular disease. Results of antinuclear antibody testing were positive at her last visit 6 months ago and are still positive at the present time. Laboratory studies obtained are presented below:

Na, serum	144 mEq/L
K, serum	5.0 mEq/L
Hematocrit	33%
Sedimentation rate, erythrocyte	50 mm/h

Which of the following is a possible explanation for this patient's symptoms?

A. Erythromycin
B. Ferrous sulfate
C. Hydralazine
D. Penicillin
E. Procainamide

188. A mother of an 8-month-old girl comes to the clinic complaining that her infant does not seem to be gaining weight, is irritable, and appears to be easily fatigable. Physical examination reveals that the child is pale, has spooning nails, is tachycardic with a systolic ejection murmur, and has glossitis. What is the next appropriate laboratory test that should be ordered?

A. Hematocrit
B. Lead level
C. Thyroid-stimulating hormone cascade
D. Total iron binding capacity (TIBC), serum iron, and serum ferritin
E. Urinalysis

189. A 35-year-old man with a history of seizure disorder on carbamazepine lost his wife 2 years ago in a car accident when an oncoming truck hit them. After her death, he quit his job and isolated himself from all of his previous friends. He lost 20 pounds in the first 2 months after she passed away. However, after he moved to a different town 6 months after her death, he found a new job that he loved, met a lot of new friends, and felt very happy again. He felt a lot better about himself and his future, and set many new goals for his life. Two and a half weeks ago, he decided to quit his new job and stopped answering the phone or calling any of his friends. He lost any desire to go out and do anything. He stopped going to the gym because he felt that he never had any energy, and found himself sleeping nearly all day and night. He again started to lose weight, and had no desire to eat. He had nightmares about his wife's death, and began to feel that it was his fault. At times he feels hopeless. However, he didn't feel that his mood was depressed. What is the most likely explanation of these findings?

A. Bereavement followed by major depressive disorder
B. Bipolar I disorder
C. Cyclothymic disorder
D. Dysthymic disorder
E. Hypothyroidism

190. A 26-year-old G2P2 woman is 23 weeks pregnant. She complains of a 4-day history of nausea and vomiting four to eight times per day. She is unable to tolerate a diet except for ice chips. She notes a 5-pound weight loss during this time period. She appears ill with dry skin and parched oral mucous membranes. Cardiac examination reveals tachycardia and a weak pulse, with a regular rate and rhythm. Pulmonary evaluation reveals clear lungs bilaterally without rales or rhonchi. Abdominal examination reveals normoactive bowel sounds with a fundal height 22 cm from the pubis. Palpation of the right and left lower quadrant reveals mild pain without peritoneal signs. Anorectal evaluation reveals no evidence of external hemorrhoids. What is the most likely explanation for these findings?

A. Acute pyelonephritis
B. Endometriosis
C. Hyperemesis gravidarum
D. Peptic ulcer disease
E. Psychosis

The response options for items 191–195 are the same. You will be required to select one answer for each item in the set.

A. Atopic dermatitis
B. Basal cell carcinoma
C. Erythema multiforme
D. Malignant melanoma
E. Pityriasis rosea
F. Psoriasis
G. Scabies
H. Seborrheic dermatitis
I. Squamous cell carcinoma
J. Tuberculosis
K. Tuleremia
L. Uremic dermatitis

For each skin condition listed above, select the appropriate clinical scenario.

191. A 55-year-old man with a history of insulin-dependent diabetes mellitus has multiple erythematous plaques with silvery white surfaces over the knees, elbows, and buttocks. His hands have thickening of the nail plates with accumulation of subungual debris. Results of laboratory studies are shown below:

Blood, plasma, serum

Alanine aminotransferase (ALT)	18 U/L
Amylase, serum	45 U/L
Aspartate aminotransferase (AST)	16 U/L
Calcium, serum	9.2 mg/dL
Glucose, serum	107 mg/dL
Hematocrit	37%
Urea nitrogen, serum (BUN)	12 mg/dL

192. A 29-year-old physician has erythematous patches with greasy yellowish scale along the bridge of his nose and eyebrows. Lesions are also noted on the scalp, central chest, and posterior auricular area bilaterally. Results of laboratory studies are shown below:

Leukocyte count and differential

Leukocyte count	6000/mm³
Segmented neutrophils	58%
Bands	6%
Lymphocytes	24%
Monocytes	3%

193. A 41-year-old woman with a recent urinary tract infection was treated with trimethoprim. She develops erythematous papules and bullae as well as lesions that consist of concentric circles with a central vesicle on the palms and soles. Results of laboratory studies are shown below:

Urinalysis

Urine pH	6.0
RBC count	2/HPF
WBC count	2/HPF
Nitrates	Negative
Bacteria	Negative

194. A 59-year-old man presents with a pearly, translucent papule that measures 3×2.5 cm on the bridge of his nose. The edges are rolled, and surface telangiectases are noted. He has a history of exposure to pesticides in his former occupation as a gardener.

195. A 20-year-old woman presents with a 4-week history of skin changes and generalized pruritus. She is otherwise asymptomatic. Physical examination reveals multiple round erythematous patches with a peripheral rim of scale. These lesions appear along skin lines of the anterior chest wall and back. Laboratory studies obtained are shown below:

Electrolytes, serum

Na, serum	145 mEq/L
Cl, serum	101 mEq/L
K, serum	3.8 mEq/L
Bicarbonate, serum	25 mEq/L
Creatinine, serum	1.1 mg/dL

Leukocyte count and differential

Leukocyte count	7000/mm³
Segmented neutrophils	55%
Bands	6%
Eosinophils	4%
Basophils	2%
Lymphocytes	26%
Monocytes	3%

196. A neonate who suffered from polyhydramnios in utero is born prematurely at 35 weeks' gestation. At birth, it is found that the child's small bowel is contained in a translucent sac which has herniated through the umbilical wall. What is the most likely diagnosis?

A. Congenital diaphragmatic hernia
B. Duodenal atresia
C. Hypothyroidism
D. Gastroschisis
E. Omphalocele

197. A 67-year-old woman has been experiencing worsening shortness of breath and presents to the urgent care center of a local emergency department. She occasionally experiences a cough when trying to catch her breath. She is a nonsmoker and currently takes no medications. She denies dizziness or palpitations. Examination shows that she appears to be using respiratory effort. She has poor excursion of the diaphragm as well as decreased fremitus on the right side. Chest x-ray reveals a right-sided pleural effusion. Thoracentesis is performed and reveals a ratio of total protein in the fluid to that of the serum of 0.25, lactate dehydrogenase (LDH) level of 115 U/L, and a serum LDH ratio of 0.40. Urinalysis reveals a pH of 6.0 and trace microscopic hematuria. What is the most likely explanation for these findings?

A. Congestive heart failure
B. Mesothelioma
C. Pneumonia
D. Sarcoidosis
E. Tuberculosis

198. A 79-year-old woman is brought to the emergency department by her family following a sudden onset of stuporous behavior, after 4 days of feeling restless and fearful. She appears to be hallucinating. She has no history of depression and is taking a beta blocker for hypertension. She has never been known to drink alcohol. Which of the following is the likely cause of her delirium?

A. Acetaminophen overdose
B. Alcohol overdose
C. Alzheimer disease
D. Dehydration
E. Stroke

199. A 21-year-old female college student presents to the university health center because of a 2-week history of bleeding from her left breast nipple. She denies having experienced any breast trauma. Prior medical and surgical history are unremarkable. Physical examination of the right breast reveals no evidence of masses, dimpling, skin retraction, or axillary adenopathy. The left breast is tender to palpation in the areola with no evidence of masses, dimpling, or skin retraction. The left axilla is free of adenopathy. What is the most likely diagnosis?

A. Fibroadenoma
B. Fibrocystic breast disease
C. Fibrosarcoma
D. Infiltrating ductal cell carcinoma
E. Intraductal papilloma

200. A frail 82-year-old white woman suffered an embolic stroke affecting movement and light tough sensation in her left side below her neck. Three months later she had a left middle cerebral arterial stroke, which led to difficulty speaking. She was rushed to the emergency department and within 2 hours received thrombolysis to dissolve the clot. Her speech returned to normal. Nine months later her primary care physician is concerned when he notices she has been losing weight steadily for the past 3 months. She complains of no abdominal pain, but upon examination she has abdominal guarding. Abdominal x-ray reveals mild thumbprinting in the distribution of the right colon. The most likely explanation of her weight loss is:

A. Bowel infarction
B. Cholecystitis
C. Colon cancer
D. Depression
E. Hyperthyroidism

201. A 35-year-old black man presents to his primary care physician complaining of lethargy, dyspnea, and dizziness. He lives in low-income housing which has poor plumbing and no hot water. Physical examination reveals a man who appears to be his stated age. Mucous membranes are dry. Cardiac, pulmonary, and abdominal examinations are within normal limits. Laboratory studies reveal a hematocrit of 31% and a mean corpuscular volume (MCV) of 67 nm^3. Iron studies reveal low serum ferritin, high iron-binding capacity, and low serum iron. Peripheral smear shows hypochromia and anisocytosis. What is the most likely diagnosis?

A. Anemia-iron deficiency type
B. Anemia-neoplastic (chronic disease)
C. Hemolytic anemia
D. Megaloblastic anemia
E. Sideroblastic anemia

202. Colonoscopy is undertaken in a 48-year-old man who complains of occasional bright red blood per rectum. Family history is positive for colorectal carcinoma in the patient's mother, who was treated with anterior resection and primary anastomosis at age 53. The patient's father has had multiple lower gastrointestinal endoscopies that revealed adenomatous and hyperplastic polyps. The patient underwent colonoscopy. Findings include several 1.5-cm distal sigmoid colonic tubular glandular epithelial proliferations that are pedunculated. What is the most likely diagnosis?

A. Adenomatous polyps
B. Hyperplastic polyps
C. Juvenile polyposis
D. Peutz-Jeghers syndrome
E. Turcot polyposis

203. A 40-year-old man presents to the emergency department complaining of abdominal pain, nausea, and vomiting for 2 weeks. However, he also complains of not being able to "pass gas" for the past 24 hours. He has a prior medical history of a laparoscopic appendectomy and right inguinal hernia repair. Physical examination reveals tenderness throughout the abdomen without the presence of bowel sounds in any quadrant. X-ray films are shown below. Figure 203a is a supine kidney, ureter, and bladder (KUB) image and Figure 203b is an upright KUB image. What is the most likely diagnosis?

- **A.** Atalectasis
- **B.** Bezoar
- **C.** Small bowel obstruction
- **D.** Renal calculus
- **E.** Tumor thrombus

204. A 72-year-old man is hospitalized for unstable angina and undergoes cardiac catheterization. The procedure occurs without complication. In the recovery room later that evening, laboratory studies reveal a serum blood urea nitrogen (BUN) of 80 mg/dL and a serum creatinine of 7.8 mg/dL. Cardiac, pulmonary, and abdominal examinations are within normal limits. Urine output is 10 mL/h. What is the most likely explanation of these findings?

- **A.** Acute tubular necrosis
- **B.** Glomerulonephritis
- **C.** Malignant hypertension
- **D.** Pyelonephritis
- **E.** Renal artery stenosis

Figure 203a

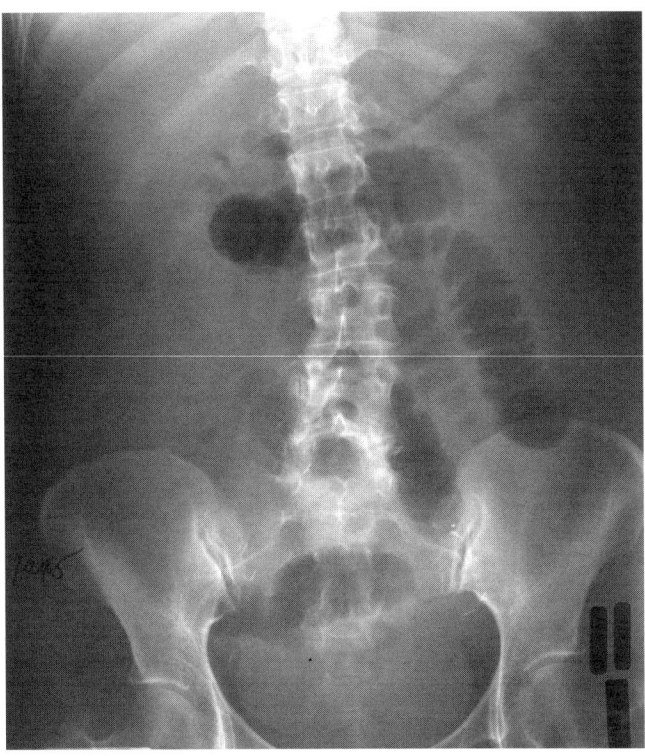

Figure 203b

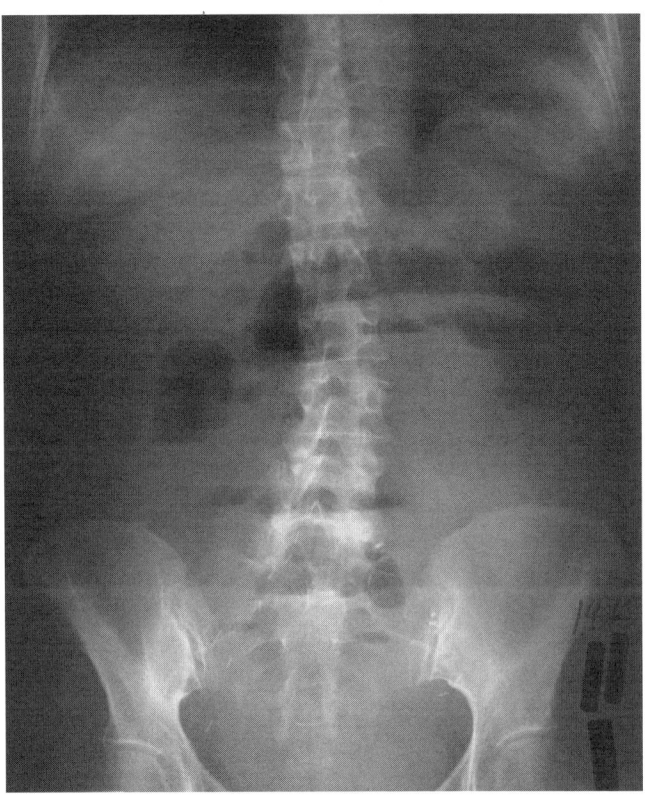

205. A 15-year-old boy presents to his pediatrician for evaluation of recurrent nightmares, difficulty sleeping, and terrible anxiety. Five months ago his sister was shot and killed at a party after a confrontation. He was standing by his sister's side and the bullet missed him by only a few inches. His sister died at the scene, and he was extremely scared and frantic and quickly ran home. Since that time he has been very agitated and anxious. He has told his family that he feels guilty for what happened to his sister. Recently, whenever he leaves his home and is in contact with strangers, he feels very agitated, and if someone makes a slight movement, he is very startled. He has stopped going to school or going out with his friends. He is reminded many times during the day of his sister and the trauma that occurred. He states he cannot get rid of the images from that night and it takes him hours at night to fall asleep. However, he doesn't like to talk to anyone about what happened because it is too painful. What is the most likely diagnosis?

A. Acute stress disorder

B. Borderline personality disorder

C. Generalized anxiety disorder

D. Malingering

E. Posttraumatic stress disorder

206. A 16-year-old boy presents to the pediatric clinic complaining of pain and swelling of his right upper leg for 3 weeks. He initially thought he hurt it playing basketball, but got worried when the pain failed to resolve. He has a family history of rheumatoid arthritis. Physical examination reveals a temperature of 38.1°C, his lungs are clear bilaterally, and cardiac rate and rhythm are within normal limits. Range of motion of the right hip joint is limited in all directions due to pain. A pelvis radiograph reveals a lytic bone lesion with calcified periosteal elevation. What is the most likely diagnosis?

A. Ewing sarcoma

B. Osteochondroma

C. Osteomyelitis

D. Osteogenic sarcoma

E. Rheumatoid arthritis

207. A 29-year-old black man is brought to the emergency room after jumping out of a third floor window (approximately 25 feet above ground level). His breath smells of alcohol. Blood pressure is 130/80 mm Hg, pulse 92 beats/min, and respirations 16 breaths/min. The patient is awake, alert, and oriented to time, place, and person. He complains of right upper quadrant pain. The following studies are taken in the emergency room:

Hematocrit #1	39%
Hematocrit #2	37%
Hematocrit #3	36%
Urinalysis	Trace microhematuria
CT scan of the abdomen	3-cm laceration of the right lobe of the liver with free blood in the peritoneal cavity

Exploratory laparatomy is performed and confirms the presence of the injuries mentioned. A small splenic laceration is also noted in the operating room. During mobilization of the liver, the anatomic landmark that divides the right and left hepatic lobes is

A. Falciform ligament

B. Gall bladder (body)

C. Gall bladder (fundus)

D. Left hepatic artery

E. Right hepatic artery

208. Two patients, a man and a woman, present to your office after they met on the Androgen Awareness Chatroom website. The woman is concerned because she has facial hair and frontal balding, and the man is concerned because he has gynoid fat distribution and a high-pitched voice. What is a single etiology that would account for both their presentations?

A. 3-beta-hydroxysteroid dehydrogenase

B. 11-beta-hydroxylase deficiency

C. 17-alpha-hydroxylase deficiency

D. 21-alpha-hydroxylase deficiency

E. Anabolic steroid use

209. A 21-year-old woman presents to her primary care physician because of difficulty sleeping. She has had frequent spells of screaming in the middle of the night. These episodes normally occur before 2:00 A.M. When asked about the episodes, she has no recollection. She has been told about them before and has noticed that they tend to occur when she has repeatedly lost sleep as a result of demanding academic requirements. What is the most appropriate treatment for this patient?

A. Amitriptyline

B. Diazepam

C. Diphenhydramine

D. Paroxetine

E. Zolpidem

210. A 64-year-old woman presents to her primary care physician with reports of dizziness and malaise for the past 2 months. She has a history of myocardial infarction 6 years ago and atrial fibrillation. The patient reports that 2 years ago she had a renal artery thrombosis leading to an episode of renal failure, for which she was hospitalized. The patient made an apparent full recovery with BUN and creatinine in the normal ranges thereafter. She denies dysuria or hematuria. Physical examination reveals normal lung sounds, and an irregularly irregular heart beat. She has no costovertebral angle tenderness, and no palpable bladder. Results or laboratory studies are provided below:

Urinalysis

Specific gravity	1.020
Glucose	Negative
Protein	Negative
Blood	Negative
Ketones	Negative
Microscopic	0–1 RBCs/HPF, significant hyaline casts
Na, urine	35 mEq/L
Creatinine, urine	80 mg/dL

Electrolytes

Na, serum	145 mEq/L
K, serum	4.0 mEq/L
Cl	100 mEq/L
Bicarbonate	25 mEq/L
Urea nitrogen (BUN)	110 mg/dL
Creatinine	6.0 mg/dL

What is the most likely diagnosis in this patient?

A. Acute tubular necrosis

B. Congestive heart failure

C. Pyelonephritis

D. Recurrent renal artery thrombosis

E. Urinary tract obstruction

211. A 6-year-old girl presents to the pediatric clinic with abrupt onset of ecchymoses, and petechiae appearing on her skin along with mucosal membrane bleeding. Her past medical history is unremarkable. She had a viral upper respiratory infection approximately 2 weeks ago. Physical examination reveals petechiae, ecchymoses, and bleeding. CBC reveals a platelet count of 60,000/mm³. Serology reveals antiplatelet antibodies. What is the most likely cause of this patient's symptoms?

A. Drugs

B. Hypersplenism

C. Idiopathic thrombocytopenic purpura

D. Leukemia

E. Sepsis

212. A 34-year-old G3P2 woman at 32 weeks' gestation presents to her primary care physician complaining of left calf pain and swelling. She denies experiencing any trauma. Review of systems is negative for fever, chills, chest pain, shortness of breath, or gastrointestinal complaints. Physical examination reveals that her left lower leg is edematous, erythematous, and tender to palpation. What is the next appropriate step in the management/treatment of this patient?

A. Leg elevation and bed rest

B. Physical therapy, including whirlpool treatments

C. Venous ultrasonography

D. X-ray studies of the left leg

E. Warm compresses, analgesics, and bed rest

213. An 18-year-old woman with type 1 diabetes mellitus presents to the emergency department with black necrotic lesions on her nose. Nasal endoscopy reveals black crust overlying necrotic tissue within the nasal cavity that extends to the soft palate. Results of laboratory studies are shown below:

Electrolytes, serum

Na, serum	143 mEq/L
Cl, serum	100 mEq/L
K, serum	3.7 mEq/L
Creatinine, serum	1.0 mg/dL

Leukocyte count and differential

Leukocyte count	17,000/mm³
Segmented neutrophils	80%

Blood, plasma, serum

Alanine aminotransferase (ALT)	10 U/L
Glucose, serum	155 mg/dL
Hematocrit	33%
Urea nitrogen, serum (BUN)	10 mg/dL

Urinalysis

Urine pH	6.0
RBC count	1/HPF
WBC count	0/HPF
Nitrates	Negative
Bacteria	Negative
Ketones	Positive

What is the most likely diagnosis?

A. *Aspergillus fumigatus* infection

B. Blastomycosis

C. *Cryptococcus neoformans* infection

D. *Histoplasma capsulatum* infection

E. Mucormycosis

F. Sporotrichosis

214. A woman brings her 23-year-old husband to his primary care physician because of some odd behavior he has been having lately. She began to notice his speech did not always make sense about 4 months ago. When she would question what he said, he would change the subject. About a month ago he began listening to radio in other languages, writing down page after page of what seemed like another language. He told her it was German, but he never took German in school. She said the most compelling information occurred the other evening when her neighbor called to tell her that Ralph came by to show her his new plan to stop the alien takeover that was going to happen next week. He has continued to work, and she has not heard any complaints from his boss. What is the most likely diagnosis?

A. Brief psychotic disorder
B. Delusional disorder, grandiose type
C. Schizophrenia
D. Schizophreniform disorder
E. Unable to diagnose at this time

215. A 61-year-old woman presents to the medical clinic with a 2-week history of dry cough. Physical examination reveals that she is febrile with stable vital signs. She has decreased breath sounds over the right posterior lung field along with mild rales. Chest x-ray is obtained and shown below (Figure 215). Sputum culture grows multiple gram-positive cocci in clusters, multiple gram-positive cocci in pairs, and multiple gram-negative cocci in pairs. What is the most likely diagnosis?

Figure 215

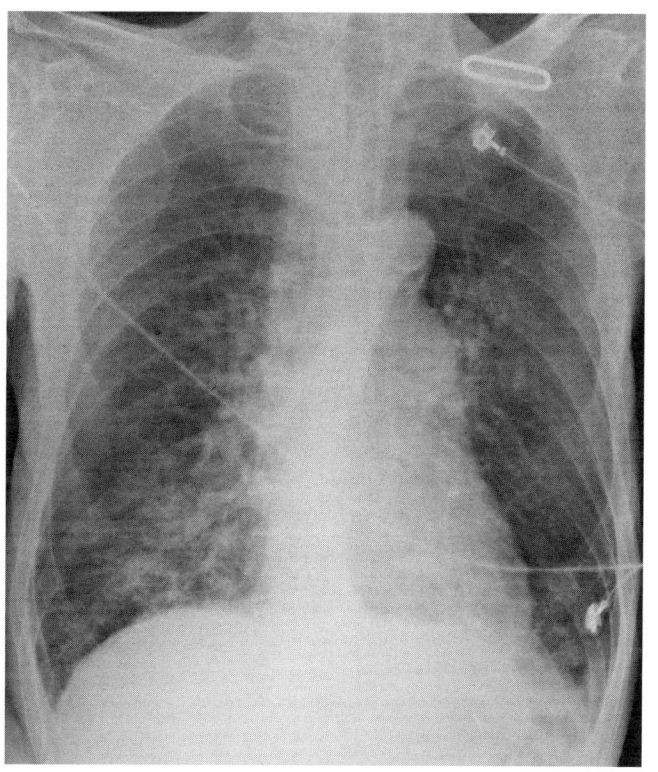

A. Adult respiratory distress syndrome
B. Asthma
C. Bronchopneumonia
D. Lobar pneumonia
E. Sarcoidosis

216. A 4-month-old boy is brought to the emergency department because of failure to thrive, anorexia, nausea, and vomiting. Laboratory studies reveal a low serum pH, low serum bicarbonate, and a normal anion gap. The K level is 5.8 mEq/L. Urine studies reveal a positive urine anion gap and a urine pH of less than 5.5. What is the most likely diagnosis?

A. Distal renal tubular acidosis (type 1)
B. Distal renal tubular acidosis (type 4)
C. Lactic acidosis
D. Proximal renal tubular acidosis (type 2)
E. Uremia

217. A 52-year-old perimenopausal woman presents to her gynecologist with complaints of night flushes, insomnia, and resultant irritability. She wants to discuss hormone replacement therapy as an option of treatment for her symptoms. As her physician informing her of the risks and benefits concerning exogenous estrogen replacement, you should tell her the following:

A. Exogenous estrogen replacement has been found to alter bone remodeling by way of increasing osteoblastic activity while decreasing osteoclastic activity
B. Exogenous estrogen replacement has been found to pose an additional risk in the development of ovarian cancer
C. Exogenous estrogen replacement has not been found to have an inhibiting effect on the natural progression of bone mineral density loss
D. Exogenous estrogen replacement has not been found to pose an additional risk in the development of endometrial cancer
E. Exogenous estrogen replacement has not been found to pose an additional risk in the induction of breast cancer

218. A 34-year-old man who is employed as a meat inspector presents to the emergency department for evaluation of 3 weeks of headache, weakness, 10-pound weight loss, arthralgia, and low-grade fever. Physical examination of the heart, lungs, and abdomen are unremarkable. Laboratory studies reveal a positive IgM assay. What is the most appropriate treatment for this individual?

A. Doxycycline and gentamycin
B. Penicillin
C. Penicillin and ceftriaxone
D. Streptomycin
E. No therapy needed

219. A 41-year-old woman with multiple myeloma treated with chemotherapy complains of a 3-month history of progressive low back pain. She denies having experienced any recent trauma. Her pain is unrelieved by rest and minimally relieved with oral antiinflammatory agents. Physical examination of the heart, lungs, and abdomen are unremarkable. Examination of the spine reveals no evidence of scoliosis. Her skin is intact without obvious abnormalities. Results of laboratory studies are presented below:

Serum

Erythrocyte sedimentation rate	20 mm/h
Hematocrit	38%
Hemoglobin	12 g/dL
WBC count	7500/mm^3
Alanine aminotransferase, serum	30 U/L
Creatinine, serum	1.0 mg/dL

Urinalysis

Urine pH	6.0
RBC count	2/HPF
WBC count	2/HPF
Nitrates	Negative
Bacteria	Negative

MRI is remarkable for sparing of the disk space. Which of the following is the most likely diagnosis?

A. Low back strain
B. Lumbar arachnoiditis
C. Metastasis
D. Spondylolisthesis
E. Vertebral osteomyelitis

220. A 35-year-old woman presents to her primary care physician with questions about the intrauterine device (IUD). She desires this as a form of birth control. Physical examination of the heart, lungs, and abdomen are unremarkable. Which of the following statements is most appropriate to make to this patient?

A. IUDs often affect ovulation, resulting in lengthened intervals between periods
B. Progesterone-containing IUDs can reduce sperm motility and capitation as well as thin the lining of the endometrium
C. There is a decreased incidence of ectopic pregnancy when an IUD is used
D. There is a decreased spontaneous abortion rate when an IUD is used
E. This is a safe method of birth control in a patient with a history of pelvic inflammatory disease

221. A 10-year-old girl is brought to the pediatric clinic to be evaluated for nasal congestion, profuse watery rhinorrhea, and sneezing that has been intermittent for the months of April and May. She had a similar episode the previous year

around the same time. Physical examination reveals stable vital signs and no evidence of tactile fever. The nasal mucosa is boggy, and dark circles are visible under her eyes. What type of hypersensitivity reaction is causing this patient's symptoms?

A. Type I hypersensitivity immune reaction
B. Type II hypersensitivity immune reaction
C. Type III hypersensitivity immune reaction
D. Type IV hypersensitivity immune reaction
E. This patient is not having a hypersensitivity immune reaction

222. A 29-year-old man is hospitalized in the psychiatric unit. He had been arrested 4 days ago for assault and battery of his wife. He has been arrested multiple times in the past for driving under the influence of alcohol, grand larceny, and racketeering. He has already been involved in an altercation with another prisoner since his arrest. When talking to his family, you learn that he had problems as early as fourth grade, when he would steal money and fight with his classmates. He also would run away from home frequently. When you ask him if he regrets the harm he has done to his wife, he shrugs, and states, "She had it coming anyway." What is the most likely diagnosis?

A. Antisocial personality disorder
B. Borderline personality disorder
C. Conduct disorder
D. Histrionic personality disorder
E. Narcissistic personality disorder

223. A 55-year-old woman with excessive uterine bleeding presents to the emergency department for evaluation. She states that she has been evaluated by a local gynecologist and determined to be normal. Blood pressure is 90/60 mm Hg and pulse is 130 beats/min. Examination of the heart, lungs, and abdomen are unremarkable. Laboratory studies reveal a CA 125 level of 20 U/mL. What is the most appropriate treatment of this patient?

A. Analgesics
B. Dilation and curettage
C. Endometrial ablation
D. Estrogen
E. Progesterone

224. A 65-year-old man has been receiving radiation treatments for the past 2 years following the development of debilitating ankylosing spondylitis. During the course of these treatments the patient's blood and reticulocyte counts were monitored periodically. The most recent laboratory results showed a marked reduction in the erythroid, granulocytic, and megakaryocytic cells of the blood, creating a pancytopenia as well as a low reticulocyte count. What is the most likely reason behind this phenomenon?

A. Acute myeloid leukemia
B. Aplastic anemia

C. Hereditary spherocytosis
D. Myelodysplastic syndrome
E. Polycythemia vera

225. You are called about a patient on your service in the hospital. The nurse tells you that Mr. B has a temperature of 42°C and blood pressure of 165/110 mm Hg, and that he cannot identify where he is, despite being fully oriented when you saw him on admission. You have the nurse take an immediate CBC, which shows a WBC count of 14,000/mm³ and a creatinine phosphokinase (CPK) level of 4500/mm³. What is the next step in the appropriate management of this patient?

A. Acetaminophen
B. Bromocriptine
C. Blood culture
D. Bicarbonate infusion
E. Dantrium

226. A 5-year-old boy presents to his pediatrician with complaints of recurrent headaches for the past 4 weeks. His mother states that the patient has awakened her at night complaining of his head hurting, and 2 nights ago vomited after a bout with headache. He has had no fevers, cough, or abdominal pain. Physical examination reveals papilledema. MRI reveals a lesion in the floor of the fourth ventricle. What is the most appropriate next step in the evaluation of this patient?

A. Cerebrospinal fluid examination
B. Chest radiograph
C. Preoperative chemotherapy
D. Preoperative radiation
E. Resection

227. A 23-year-old white male graduate student presents to his university student health service because he noticed the whites of his eyes have a yellowish hue. He has no prior medical history, takes no medications, and has an unremarkable social history. Physical examination shows the skin to be mildly jaundiced. The patient reports that his skin is usually that color or paler and has no noticeable pattern to when it is more or less yellow. Laboratory studies reveal elevated levels of conjugated bilirubin. What is the most likely diagnosis?

A. Crigler-Najjar syndrome type I
B. Crigler-Najjar syndrome type II
C. Dubin-Johnson syndrome
D. Gilbert syndrome
E. Rotor syndrome

228. A 27-year-old woman has just given birth to a healthy baby girl. She is interested in postpartum contraception. Physical examination of the heart, lungs, and abdomen are unremarkable. Results of laboratory studies are shown below:

Electrolytes, serum

Na, serum	145 mEq/L
Cl, serum	103 mEq/L
K, serum	3.8 mEq/L
Bicarbonate, serum	25 mEq/L
Magnesium, serum	2.1 mEq/L
Creatinine, serum	1.3 mg/dL

Leukocyte count and differential

Leukocyte count	7000/mm³
Segmented neutrophils	55%
Bands	6%
Eosinophils	3%
Basophils	2%
Lymphocytes	24%
Monocytes	4%

Blood, plasma, serum

Alanine aminotransferase (ALT)	15 U/L
Amylase, serum	52 U/L
Aspartate aminotransferase (AST)	15 U/L
Calcium, serum	9.1 mg/dL
Glucose, serum	115 mg/dL
Hematocrit	36%
Urea nitrogen, serum (BUN)	12 mg/dL

Urinalysis

Urine pH	6.5
RBC count	2–4/HPF
WBC count	2–4/HPF
Nitrates	Negative
Bacteria	Negative

She states that she wants to breast-feed her child. In addition to advising pelvic rest for 6 weeks, the most appropriate recommendation is

A. Breast-feeding alone will provide adequate contraception
B. Combination oral contraceptive pill
C. Intrauterine device
D. Progesterone-only contraceptive pill
E. She is physiologically unable to get pregnant again for at least 8 weeks

229. A 47-year-old woman presents to her primary care physician with dysphagia. On further questioning she reveals that she tires easily, has felt lethargic, and has lately lost some weight. Vital signs are taken and appear to be stable. Physical examination reveals a smooth, shiny red tongue and cracks at the corners of her mouth. Her fingernails have a spoon shape to them. What is the most likely diagnosis?

A. Achalasia
B. Cytomegalovirus infection
C. Esophageal adenocarcinoma
D. Mallory-Weiss syndrome
E. Plummer-Vinson syndrome

230. A 38-year-old woman notes a 4-year history of episodes of feeling short of breath, and shaking when she is in crowded places such as a concert hall. She states that these symptoms are also accompanied by nausea, abdominal pain, chills, and tingling sensations in her hands. During these episodes she feels as if she is going crazy. Physical examination reveals a well-developed, well-nourished woman in no apparent distress. Her thyroid gland is palpable without masses. Cardiovascular examination reveals a regular rate and rhythm. Pulmonary auscultation reveals no evidence of rales, rhonchi, or wheezing. Which of the following is the most appropriate treatment for this individual?

A. Alprazolam
B. Clonidine
C. Imipramine
D. Propranolol
E. Trazodone

231. A 27-year-old G3P1 woman is now 8 weeks pregnant with her second child. She has a history of one spontaneous abortion and one stillborn child. Her mother has diabetes mellitus. Her surviving child weighed 4500 g at birth and is currently 3 years of age and in good health. Physical examination at the present visit reveals a heart rate of 105 beats/min and a blood pressure of 130/80 mm Hg in the right arm and 120/80 mm Hg in the left arm. Cardiac examination reveals no murmurs. Pulmonary auscultation reveals no evidence of rhonchi or wheezes. Gastrointestinal evaluation fails to reveal evidence of peritoneal signs. Which of the following interventions is most appropriate?

A. 1-hour glucola screening at current visit
B. 1-hour glucola screening at 24 weeks' gestation
C. 1-hour glucose tolerance test at 24 weeks' gestation
D. 3-hour glucose tolerance test at 28 weeks' gestation
E. No further testing is necessary in this patient

232. A 34-year-old man has a 1-year history of emotional lability and looseness of associations. He is brought for evaluation by his wife who has noted a change in his behavior and personality. He is given a self-administered personality test that produces a general description of his personality characteristics. Which of the following is the most likely examination that was administered to this individual?

A. Bender-Gestalt test
B. Draw-a-person test
C. Minnesota multiphasic personality inventory
D. Rorschach test
E. Thematic apperception test

233. A 19-year-old woman presents to the emergency department after returning from a camping trip in North Carolina 1 week ago. After a few days of fever, severe headache, and muscle aches, she noticed a rash beginning on her palms and soles that is now spreading to her wrists and ankles. Results of physical examination of the heart, lungs, and abdomen are noncontributory. Recent female pelvic examination findings (by her gynecologist) were unremarkable. What is the most likely explanation for this condition?

A. *Borrelia burgdorferi*

B. Coxsackie A virus

C. *Rickettsia rickettsii*

D. *Rickettsia typhi*

E. *Treponema pallidum*

234. A 27-year-old woman complains of a 3-month history of abdominal distention and relief of abdominal pain with bowel movements. She notes increased frequency of stools with pain, and mucus in stools. The sense of incomplete evacuation has been apparent. She also notes a history of back pain, palpitations, and urinary frequency. Physical examination reveals a well-developed, well-nourished female in no apparent distress. Cardiac examination reveals a regular rate and rhythm. Pulmonary auscultation reveals no evidence of wheeze or rhonchi. Gastrointestinal examination reveals tenderness to deep palpation in the left lower quadrant. There is also some mild tenderness to deep palpation in the right lower quadrant. Rectal examination is guaiac negative with stool in the vault.

Laboratory studies obtained are as follows:

Na, serum	134 mEq/L
Cl, serum	101 mEq/L
K, serum	4.1 mEq/L
Bicarbonate, serum	25 mEq/L
Magnesium, serum	1.9 mEq/L
Creatinine, serum	1.3 mg/dL
Osmolality, serum	294 mOsmol/kg
Albumin, serum	4.1 g/dL
Urea nitrogen, serum (BUN)	19 mg/dL
Hematocrit	39%
Hemoglobin, blood	14 g/dL
Leukocyte count	9000/mm^3
Platelet count	278,000/mm^3

What is the most appropriate treatment for this patient?

A. Amitriptyline

B. Leuprolide acetate

C. Rowasa enemas

D. Support and reassurance

E. Tetracycline orally for 10 days

235. A 24-year-old male long distance runner presents to his primary care physician for evaluation of epigastric pain described as gnawing and not relieved with food. He reports using anti-inflammatory agents chronically the past 2 years since he has been focusing on running marathons. Stool tests positive for blood. An upper endoscopic examination is performed and areas of deep mucosal erosion are seen in the stomach surrounded by normal-appearing mucosa. A biopsy of these regions is performed, and *Helocobacter pylori* is cultured. He is treated appropriately and stops the use of oral analgesics and does not push his body so hard anymore. Unfortunately, he continues to develop more ulcers. Due to frustration and pain he eventually opts to have a vagotomy with a partial gastrectomy. Within 2 months he presents with more abdominal pain, this time associated with postprandial diarrhea, palpitations, and bloating as well. What is the most likely diagnosis?

A. Anesthetic side effects

B. Dumping syndrome

C. Duodenal ulcer

D. Mechanical obstruction

E. Short gut syndrome

236. During routine physical examination of a 12-year-old girl, a significant lateral curvature of her thoracolumbar spine is identified. She denies having any back pain. Her past medical history is significant for a fractured radius, which has completely healed. Anteroposterior radiographs of the spine indicate that the curve is approximately 21 degrees. What is the next most appropriate step in the treatment of this patient?

A. Bracing the patient

B. Daily antiinflammatory medication (ibuprofen)

C. Observation

D. Physical therapy and weight lifting

E. Surgical spinal fusion

237. A 55-year-old woman presents to her gynecologist for an annual examination. During the history taking, the patient reveals the recent loss of her husband in a tragic automobile accident. She is an otherwise healthy woman with no medical problems. She takes no medications. Pelvic examination reveals no evidence of cervical motion tenderness or adnexal tenderness. There is no pelvic floor prolapse. Regarding her grief management and therapy, which of the following strategies would be most successful?

A. Encourage internalization of feelings

B. Encourage open communication with former friends of the deceased

C. Encourage several long visits with her physician

D. Routine prescription of antianxiety medications

E. Routine prescription of antidepressant medications

238. A 24-year-old woman was hospitalized 3 weeks ago after being diagnosed with her first episode of major depression and suicidal ideation. She has a medical history significant only for asthma treated with an Albuterol inhaler and steroids as needed. She has taken prednisolone at least five times before and has tolerated it well without side effects. She has been on prednisolone for 2 days for a severe asthma exacerbation. Her father was an alcoholic but passed away when she was 4 years old. Her mother's medical conditions of hypertension, diabetes, and bipolar disorder are all well controlled with medication. She presents to her psychiatrist for evaluation. She was started on fluoxetine in the hospital and was discharged after 1 week. She was told to follow up with her psychiatrist a week later. She presented to her psychiatrist with her mother a week after her discharge. Her mother was angry, claiming that her daughter was arrested for three speeding tickets in the past week and totaled her car after running into a building near her house. She had also stolen her mother's credit card and purchased $2000 worth of items in addition to plane tickets to Paris and Hawaii. Her friends had become very concerned and angry because she began to tell them that she was smarter and more beautiful than all of them and they should try to be more like her. She told her mom she wanted to go back to school, and started making plans to build her own home. In a week's time, she had already hired a contractor using her mother's money. Her mother states that she never stops talking about her plans for her home, and how she is going to buy pets and plants and she is going to be the happiest person in the world. She has not slept more than 2 hours each night since she was discharged from the hospital. What is the most likely diagnosis?

A. Bipolar I disorder
B. Bipolar II disorder
C. Borderline personality disorder
D. Histrionic personality disorder
E. Substance-induced mood disorder

239. A 10-year-old boy has a 1-year history of recurrent eye blinking, head jerking, and facial grimacing. Recently he has progressed to multiple coughing attacks as well as grunting and sniffling. During the past week he has begun to repeat his own words and the words of his family members. Teachers in school have noted that the child has little attention span and occasionally hits himself and jumps up and down. Which of the following is the most likely diagnosis of this individual?

A. Elective mutism
B. Mood disorder of childhood
C. Schizophrenia of childhood
D. Tourette disorder
E. Undifferentiated attention deficit disorder

240. A 32-year-old female presents to the emergency department with a 24 hour history of right upper quadrant abdominal pain. This is accompanied by nausea, vomiting, and and a low-grade fever. She has had a similar attack within the last 6 months. On physical examination the patient has a temperature of 38.5°C. Blood pressure is 150/90 mm Hg and pulse is 80 beats/minute. Abdominal examination reveals tenderness to palpation in the right upper quadrant and voluntary guarding. Pain radiates to the scapula. Murphy sign is positive. What is the most likely diagnosis?

A. Acute cholecystitis
B. Ascending cholangitis
C. Biliary colic
D. Pancreatitis
E. Peptic ulcer disease

241. A 23-year-old woman presents to her primary care physician because of masses in her neck. The patient reports an 8-pound weight loss in the past month, pruritus, frequent night sweats, and lethargy. Physical examination reveals two nodes in the left anterior cervical chain that measure 3 and 4 cm, respectively. The nodes are firm, freely moveable, and nontender. Chest x-ray and CT scan of the chest, abdomen, and pelvis are all unremarkable. Which of the following is the most likely diagnosis?

A. Acute myelogenous leukemia
B. Infectious mononucleosis
C. Hodgkin lymphoma
D. Non-Hodgkin lymphoma
E. Sarcoidosis

242. A 33-year-old G4P2 woman is 24 weeks pregnant. She complains of an intermittent headache and fatigue during her pregnancy. Her blood pressure has been at least 150/110 mm Hg on three successive occasions. Cardiac examination reveals a regular rate and rhythm. Pulmonary evaluation reveals clear lungs bilaterally without rales or rhonchi. Abdominal examination reveals normoactive bowel sounds with a fundal height 23 cm from the pubis. Palpation of the right and left lower quadrant reveals mild pain without peritoneal signs. What is the most appropriate treatment of this patient?

A. Hydralazine
B. Labetalol
C. Methyldopa
D. Prazosin
E. Sodium nitroprusside

243. A 63-year-old man collapses while walking in a shopping mall. He is unresponsive and brought to the emergency department by local paramedics. He is unable to open his eyes, to have a motor response to commands, and to respond to verbal cues. Blood pressure is 90/60 mm Hg, pulse is 110 beats/min, and respirations are 12 breaths/min. He is brought immediately to the radiology suite for CT scan (Figure 243). What is the most likely diagnosis?

Figure 243

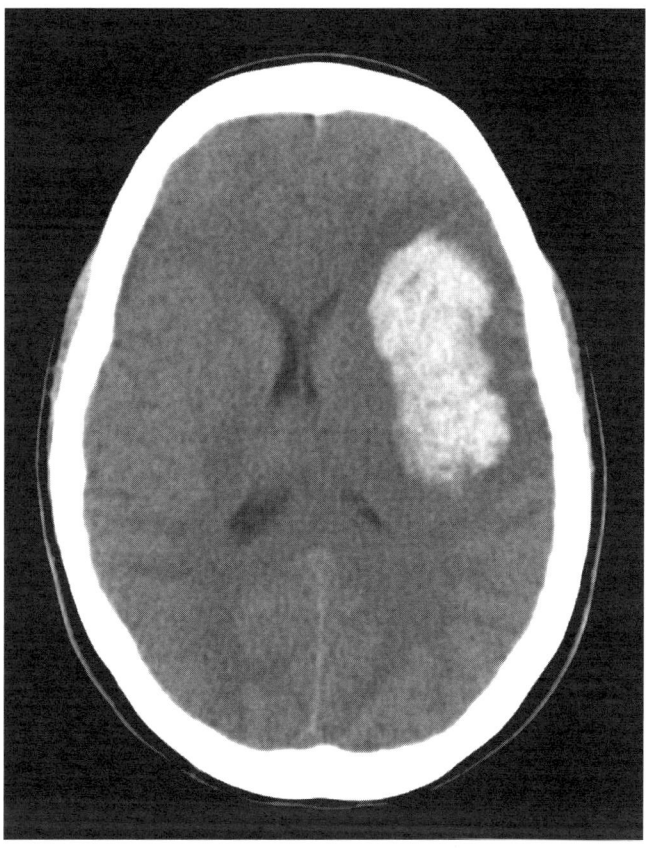

A. Brain abscess

B. Intracerebral hematoma due to arteriovenous malformation

C. Metastatic tumor to the brain

D. Multiinfarct dementia

E. Subdural hematoma

244. A mother of an 8-month-old girl comes to the clinic complaining that her infant does not seem to be gaining weight, is irritable, and appears to be easily fatigable. Upon physical examination, the child is pale, has spooning nails, is tachycardic with a systolic ejection murmur, and has glossitis. What is the most appropriate treatment for this infant?

A. Folate supplementation

B. Iron supplementation for a minimum of 3 months

C. Splenectomy

D. Thyroid hormone replacement

E. No treatment is required

245. A 46-year-old male chemist presents to his physician for evaluation. He reports that for the past 3 months his wife has been trying to poison him. He tells you that she is slipping arsenic into the meals she cooks for him. He knows this because occasionally he can smell traces of it. He denies any history of depression, anxiety, or alcohol or drug use. He is successful in his career, and has a good relationship with his friends and children. He has confronted his wife, but says that she denies everything. He feels as though he cannot trust her, and their relationship is suffering. What is his most likely diagnosis?

A. Brief psychotic disorder

B. Delusional disorder

C. Paranoid personality disorder

D. Schizophrenia

E. Schizophreniform disorder

246. A 45-year-old woman presents to the emergency department after experiencing weakness in the right upper extremity. She has a history of poorly controlled hypertension. Physical examination reveals blood pressure of 180/90 mm Hg, pulse of 90 beats/min, and respirations of 16 breaths/min. Cardiac examination reveals a regular rate and rhythm without murmurs, rubs, or gallops. Lungs are clear bilaterally. Results of laboratory studies are shown below:

Na, serum	149 mEq/L
K, serum	3.0 mEq/L
Bicarbonate, serum	31 mEq/L
Glucose, serum	125 mg/dL
Blood gas	
pH	7.48
P_{CO_2}	41 mm Hg
P_{O_2}	80 mm Hg

CT scan of the head reveals a small cerebral infarct. What is the most likely diagnosis?

A. Addison disease

B. Conn syndrome

C. Edema (pulmonary)

D. Pheochromocytoma

E. Renal tubular acidosis

247. A 63-year-old white woman presents to her gynecologist complaining of a long history of vulvar itching and vulvar pain. Physical examination reveals velvety red lesions on the skin of the labia. Biopsy of the lesion reveals it is carcinogenic embryonic antigen (CEA) positive on immunohistochemical staining. What is the most likely diagnosis?

A. Herpes genitalis

B. Melanoma

C. Paget disease

D. Vulvar intraepithelial neoplasia (VIN)

E. Vulvovaginal carcinoma

248. Anna is a 20-year-old woman. Her mother told Anna to go to her primary care physician because she was really concerned about Anna's behavior. Anna has a daily routine when she wakes up each morning. She always awakens 4 hours before she has to leave. She also always sets her alarm for 4:48 A.M. because she likes even numbers. After rising from bed, she walks to the bathroom and washes then dries her hands 12 times. Next, she showers for 48 minutes to make sure she has removed all germs, and washes her hair six times. After showering, she walks into her room, puts on gloves to stay clean, and brushes her hair 18 times. When she leaves her home, she always walks back in eight times to make sure she has turned off her coffee pot and to make sure the windows are all locked. She wears gloves to school and tries not to get close to any other classmates. She tells her physician that her thoughts of cleanliness and organization are ridiculous and that she has tried to resist without success. Which of the following is the best initial treatment for this patient?

- **A.** Clomipramine
- **B.** Clonazepam
- **C.** Lithium
- **D.** Phenelzine
- **E.** Venlafaxine

249. A 21-year-old man brings his 44-year-old mother with bipolar disorder (type 1) and alcohol dependence to the emergency department. The son reports that yesterday morning his mother woke up "hung over." He continues, "She thought she was going to vomit and tried to run to the toilet, but she tripped while turning into the bathroom and hit her head on the doorway." The patient's son witnessed a loss of consciousness lasting 5 seconds, and afterwards she was "typically how she is when hung over, but didn't remember hitting her head." The son rushed to summon the neighbor, a neurologist, who evaluated the mother and said that it was only a concussion, but to come to the emergency room if she does not get totally better in a day. Today the patient is still lethargic, irritable, and has memory problems, but the son denies any subsequent loss of consciousness or seizures. What is the most appropriate next step in the treatment of this patient?

- **A.** Complete physical examination, focusing on the neurologic aspect
- **B.** CT scan
- **C.** Lumbar puncture
- **D.** MRI
- **E.** Skull x-ray

250. A 27-year-old woman is interested in taking oral contraceptives for the prevention of pregnancy. She has no prior medical or surgical history. Physical examination findings of the heart, lungs, and abdomen are within normal limits. Results of female pelvic examination are within normal limits. The most likely benefit in terms of disease prevention from oral contraceptives is which of the following?

- **A.** Decreased risk for colorectal carcinoma
- **B.** Decreased risk for ectopic pregnancy
- **C.** Decreased risk for malignant breast disease
- **D.** Decreased risk for thyroid carcinoma
- **E.** Decreased risk for uterine teratoma

The response options for items 251–252 are the same. You will be required to select one answer for each item in the set.

- **A.** Acetaminophen
- **B.** Benzodiazepines
- **C.** Cyanide
- **D.** Digoxin
- **E.** Ethylene glycol
- **F.** Iron
- **G.** Isoniazid
- **H.** Lead
- **I.** Methanol

For each child below who has ingested a poison, select the most appropriate diagnosis.

251. A 5-year-old unresponsive boy is brought to the emergency department. His mother has a history of tuberculosis and takes multiple medications. Prior to becoming unresponsive, paramedics witnessed a bout of vomiting followed by a seizure.

252. A 6-year-old boy is brought to the emergency department because of vomiting and diarrhea. He was being cared for by his grandmother who has multiple medical problems, including diabetes, hypertension, and congestive heart failure. She takes multiple medications. The boy appears to be confused. His heart rate is 60 beats/min. Laboratory studies reveal a serum K of 5.5 mEq/L.

253. An 84-year-old man is brought to the emergency department after an apparent suicide attempt. He was found in his home with an open bottle of trimethoprim. According to the patient's wife, the bottle had approximately 50 pills earlier that day. At present time, 4 pills remain in the bottle. Electrocardiography reveals bradycardic cardiac arrest. What is the most appropriate treatment for this patient?

- **A.** Calcium gluconate
- **B.** Hydrochlorothiazide
- **C.** Increased dosage of bicarbonate
- **D.** Intravenous potassium chloride
- **E.** Spironolactone

254. A 16-year-old boy presents to the emergency department with acute onset of right testicular pain that began 2 hours ago. There was no history of trauma to the testicle, and the patient reports being in good health with no recent illness. Physical examination reveals that the right testicle is swollen, painful, and high riding with a horizontal lie. Elevation of the testicle by the examiner provided some relief of pain. What is the most likely diagnosis?

A. Acute epididymitis

B. Acute prostatitis

C. Henoch-Schonlein purpura

D. Testicular carcinoma

E. Testicular torsion

255. A 10-year-old boy presents to the pediatric clinic with a complaint of amnesia. His parents state that they frequently find him on the couch downstairs in the morning or in one of his siblings' bedrooms. On one occasion, the patient woke up on the floor in the kitchen, and he had a significant cut on his head. The patient never remembers how he ends up in these odd locations. His parents have wondered if he is lying to them and really sneaking around at night. His parents have also noticed that these episodes occur more frequently when the patient is sleep deprived. After ruling out the possibility of psychomotor epilepsy via electroencephalography, you are pretty certain of a diagnosis and suspect a nighttime parasomnia. During what stage of sleep do these episodes occur?

A. Delta sleep

B. Drowsiness

C. REM sleep

D. Stage I

E. Stage II

256. A 34-year-old G3P2 woman at 34 weeks' gestation presents to the emergency department with complaints of right lower leg pain and swelling. She states the pain has become increasingly severe and she is having difficulty walking. Doppler ultrasonography reveals a right deep vein thrombosis. What is the most appropriate management of this patient?

A. Begin coumadin, and follow-up with her obstetrician in 1 week

B. Begin heparin, admit to hospital, and consult with obstetrician

C. Begin oral pain medications, warm compresses, and bed rest

D. Begin subcutaneous heparin and start coumadin in 1 week

E. Watchful waiting at this time unless chest pain or shortness of breath develops; follow with serial ultrasonography through remainder of pregnancy

257. A 2-year-old boy is brought to the emergency department by his parents for evaluation of fever and a rash. Fevers have been as high as 103.1°F. The rash is maculopapular and is originating from the trunk and then spreading peripherally. Physical examination of the heart and lungs are within normal limits. Results of laboratory studies are shown below:

Leukocyte count and differential

Leukocyte count	4000/mm^3
Segmented neutrophils	60%
Bands	7%
Eosinophils	3%
Basophils	1%
Lymphocytes	27%
Monocytes	4%

What is the most likely diagnosis?

A. Fifth disease

B. Roseola infantum

C. Rubella

D. Rubeola

E. Syphilis

258. A 34-year-old man with known HIV presents to his primary care physician with complaints of dyspnea, dry cough, and fever of 6 days duration. The patient appears fatigued and has difficulty breathing. Physical examination reveals that the skin is warm and moist without lesions. Results of cardiovascular examination are unremarkable. Blood work demonstrates a CD4 count of less than 200/mm^3 and increased lactate dehydrogenase. PaO$_2$ is 70 mm Hg. Chest x-ray demonstrates a mild right pneumothorax and two small cavitations on the left. What is the most likely diagnosis?

A. Cytomegalovirus

B. Kaposi sarcoma

C. *Mycobacterium avium-intracellulare*

D. *Pneumocystis* pneumonia

E. Tuberculosis

259. A 23-year-old man who was an unrestrained passenger in a motor vehicle accident is seen in the emergency department. He is able to breathe on his own but tells you that each breath is extremely painful. Physical examination reveals that a segment of the chest wall appears to sink inwards with each respiration and when he exhales this same segment does not move with the rest of the chest wall. The patient has no other obvious traumatic injuries. The arterial blood gas reads as follows: 7.3/55/85/25. Which of the following is the most appropriate next step in the treatment of this patient?

A. CT scan of the abdomen

B. Endotracheal intubation and mechanical ventilation

C. Observe the patient an hour for change

D. Oxygen by nasal cannula

E. Place sand bags on both sides of chest for respiratory support

260. A 41-year-old man experiences massive trauma subsequent to a car accident. Following stabilization, the patient is found to be actively bleeding from joint injuries that were sustained during the accident. Laboratory results show thrombocytopenia, prolonged prothrombin, partial thromboplastin, and thrombin times, a reduced fibrinogen level, and elevated fibrin degradation products. The hemoglobin, hematocrit, and WBC count were within normal limits. What is the best treatment for this patient?

A. Antibiotics
B. Fresh frozen plasma
C. Heparin
D. Packed RBCs
E. Warfarin

261. A mother brings her 3-week-old infant to the pediatric clinic and complains that the child has had nonbilious, projectile vomiting that has progressively worsened since birth. Physical examination reveals visible peristaltic waves and a firm, palpable mass in the epigastric region. Laboratory studies reveal a metabolic alkalosis with decreased K and Cl. The WBC count is within normal limits. What is the most likely diagnosis?

A. Gastric ulcer
B. Gastroenteritis
C. Meconium ileus
D. Necrotizing enterocolitis
E. Pyloric stenosis

262. A 39-year-old G1001 woman presents to her gynecologist with a 10-month history of dysmenorrhea and menorrhagia. She has a prior medical history of hypertension. She takes no medications. Pelvic examination reveals an enlarged uterine fundus. Endometrial biopsy reveals the presence of endometrial glands within the endometrial stroma and myometrium. What is the most appropriate management for this condition?

A. An endometrial biopsy should be performed
B. A total abdominal or vaginal hysterectomy should be performed
C. Patient should be followed annually to monitor symptom progression
D. Patient should be started on a trial of mifepristone
E. Patient should be started on a trial of a gonadotropin-releasing hormone (GnRH) agonist

263. A 62-year-old man with a history of uncontrolled diabetes mellitus has undergone amputation of his left leg below the knee. While in the hospital on postoperative day 3, he complains of fever, chills, and nausea. He also complains of cough productive of yellow/green sputum. Physical examination reveals right lower lobe rhonchi and increased fremitus. He has a temperature of 38.1°C and diaphoresis. His urine output is normal. WBC count is 21,000/mm³. Sputum culture grows multiple gram-positive and gram-negative rods. Chest x-ray is shown below (Figure 263). What is the most likely etiologic agent of this condition?

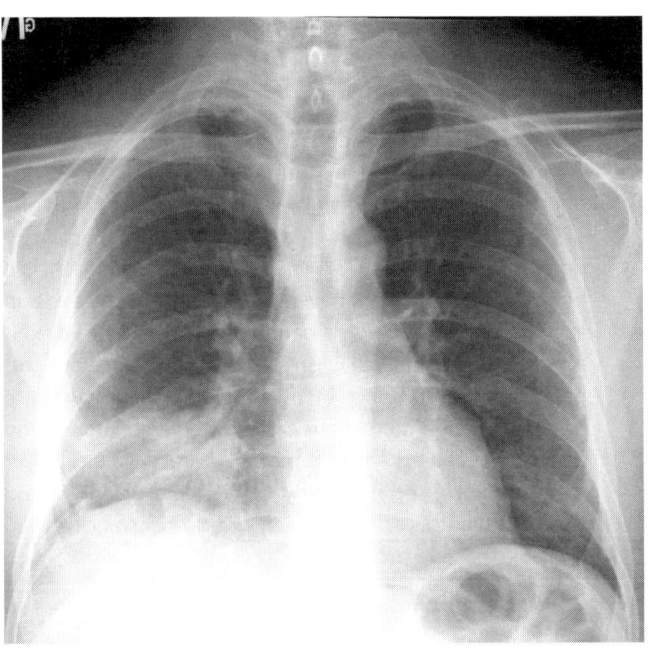

Figure 263

A. *Escherichia coli*
B. *Haemophilus influenzae*
C. *Legionella pneumophila*
D. *Staphylococcus aureus*
E. *Streptococcus pneumoniae*

264. A 40-year-old man presents to his primary care physician because he had his cholesterol checked at a pharmacy and the fasting total cholesterol was 210 mg/dL. His high-density lipoprotein (HDL) level was 40 mg/dL. Past medical history reveals no evidence of heart disease, diabetes, or hypertension. He has a 10 pack/year history of smoking. He is a social drinker. No male or female in his family have a cardiac history. What is the best management of this man's elevated total cholesterol?

A. Check low-density lipoprotein (LDL) cholesterol
B. Check triglycerides
C. Counsel and recheck in 12 months
D. Prescribe lovastatin
E. Prescribe niacin

265. You have been following a schizophrenic patient for more than 20 years. In the past, he had been famous for running for local office with a campaign promising to stop the gnomes from poisoning the water. He also had a couple of years where he stood still in strange poses for hours at a time. With the trial of a new antipsychotic drug, the past 7 years have been much better. He rarely has delusions or hallucinations, and when he does, he is able to ignore them. His relationship with his wife is much more productive than before. What is the most likely diagnosis?

A. Schizophrenia, catatonic type

B. Schizophrenia, paranoid type

C. Schizophrenia, undifferentiated

D. Schizophrenia, residual type

E. Schizophrenia, waxing type

266. A 43-year-old black man presents to his primary care physician for an annual check-up. He has a prior medical history of irritable bowel syndrome and lactose intolerance. He has no prior surgical history. He has a 20 pack/year history of smoking. Physical examination is undertaken. His blood pressure is found to be 154/94 mm Hg. His doctor tells him to return in a week to recheck his blood pressure, and it is 148/102 mm Hg. Again, his doctor tells him to return in a week, and when he does so his blood pressure is 136/80 mm Hg. Results of laboratory studies are shown below:

Electrolytes, serum

Na, serum	142 mEq/L
Cl, serum	99 mEq/L
K, serum	3.5 mEq/L
Bicarbonate, serum	24 mEq/L
Magnesium, serum	2.0 mEq/L
Creatinine, serum	0.9 mg/dL

Leukocyte count and differential

Leukocyte count	9000/mm^3
Segmented neutrophils	65%
Bands	5%

What is the best treatment option for this patient?

A. Angiotensin-converting enzyme inhibitor

B. Beta blocker

C. Calcium channel blocker

D. Diet/lifestyle modification

E. No treatment is necessary

267. A 25-year-old female patient presents with concerns about never having had menses. She has no reported health problems and has had no surgeries. Physical examination findings of the heart, lungs, and abdomen are within normal limits. Female genital examination reveals that she has no breast development and is without a uterus. What is the most likely explanation of these findings?

A. Müllerian inhibiting factor deficiency

B. 17-beta-hydroxylase deficiency

C. Defect in 17,20-desmolase

D. 17-alpha-hydroxyprogesterone deficiency

E. Surgical adhesions

268. A 34-year-old woman comes in to your clinic for the first time after being referred by her primary care physician. When you walk into the examination room, she gives you a hug, hands you a dozen roses, and tells you what a pleasure it is to meet you. She is wearing a short skirt with fishnet stockings. She tells you that she hates being alone, and is almost always spending time with friends, although she has never had a serious intimate relationship. After talking to her, you observe that she is emotionally labile, rapidly shifting between hysterical laughter and a somber, depressed affect. Her speech is rapid and tangential. What is this patient's most likely diagnosis?

A. Antisocial personality disorder

B. Borderline personality disorder

C. Dependent personality disorder

D. Histrionic personality disorder

E. Narcissistic personality disorder

269. A 15-year-old girl comes to the pediatric clinic because of a noticeable limp. She complains of left knee pain, and states she fell 2 weeks ago and believes this is the cause of her pain. Physical examination reveals that the left knee is edematous and tender to light palpation. Plain film knee x-rays reveals a "sunburst" pattern of periosteal reaction in the metaphysis of the distal femur. Which of the following is the most appropriate treatment?

A. Observation

B. Preoperative radiation therapy, then surgical resection

C. Surgical resection of the lesion

D. Surgical resection of the lesion, with chemotherapy

E. Surgical resection of the lesion, with radiation therapy

270. A 68-year-old ill-appearing patient with chronic obstructive pulmonary disease who smokes one pack of cigarettes per day presents to the emergency department with cough productive of purulent sputum, high fevers, and pleurisy. He is currently a visitor to this community and is staying in a local hotel. Several other hotel guests have the same symptoms and are being evaluated at this facility. Laboratory studies reveal elevation of serum IgG and IgM levels. Results of direct fluorescent antibody staining of sputum are positive. What is the most appropriate next step in the management of this patient?

A. Blood cultures

B. Culture on charcoal-yeast agar

C. MRI

D. Pulmonary function tests

E. Treat with steroids

271. A 19-year-old woman complains of vulvar itching, burning, and vaginal discharge with a foul smelling odor for 4 weeks. She presents to her primary care physician for further evaluation. She admits to heterosexual and homosexual relations. She uses cocaine and crack, and smokes marijuana. She describes the discharge to be yellow-green in color and frothy. The pH of the secretions is 7.0. Pelvic examination reveals vulvar edema and erythema and cervical petechiae. Wet smear reveals large numbers of mature epithelial cells, WBCs, and a fusiform protozoan organism. Which of the following is the most likely diagnosis?

- **A.** *Candida albicans* infection
- **B.** *Gardnerella vaginalis* infection
- **C.** Hidradenitis suppurativa
- **D.** Normal vaginal secretions
- **E.** *Trichomonas vaginalis* infection

272. A 24-year-old woman who is 20 weeks pregnant complains of headache and intermittent right upper quadrant pain. She is a G1P0 and weighs 160 pounds. Her prenatal care has been up to date to the present time. Social history is notable for occasional drinking of wine. She is a former crack cocaine abuser but denies usage of substances during the present pregnancy. Blood pressure is 140/90 mm Hg (as recorded on three separate occasions) with a pulse of 86 to 92 beats/min. Cardiovascular examination reveals a midsystolic click without gallops. Pulmonary examination reveals no evidence of wheezes or rales. Gastrointestinal examination reveals mild tenderness in the lower quadrants bilaterally. Bilateral 1+ pitting edema is also noted. Urinalysis reveals 1+ proteinuria with no evidence of hematuria or glucosuria. Which of the following is the most appropriate treatment plan for this patient?

- **A.** Bed rest
- **B.** Hydralazine (intravenous)
- **C.** Hydralazine (oral)
- **D.** Prazosin (oral)
- **E.** Thiazide (oral)

273. A previously healthy 45-year-old white male construction worker from New England presents to his primary care physician complaining of new onset of fever, malaise, weight loss, arthralgias, and rash on his lower extremities. He also complains of recurrent asthma attacks for the past 3 weeks without a prior history of asthma. He denies headache, vision changes, or hemoptysis. He denies participating in risky sexual behavior or having a recent tick bite. The patient also denies having hematuria or any change in urinary tract function. Physical examination reveals multiple red to purple raised lesions on bilateral lower extremities. Results of laboratory studies are shown below:

Electrolytes, serum

Na, serum	143 mEq/L
Cl, serum	100 mEq/L
K, serum	3.7 mEq/L
Bicarbonate, serum	24 mEq/L
Magnesium, serum	2.0 mEq/L
Creatinine, serum	1.0 mg/dL

Leukocyte count and differential

Leukocyte count	12,300/mm^3
Segmented neutrophils	70%
Bands	7%
Eosinophils	10%
Basophils	1%
Lymphocytes	25%
Monocytes	4%

Blood, plasma, serum

Alanine aminotransferase (ALT)	18 U/L
Amylase, serum	57 U/L
Aspartate aminotransferase (AST)	15 U/L
Calcium, serum	9 mg/dL
Glucose, serum	113 mg/dL
Hematocrit	38%
Sedimentation rate, erythrocyte	50 mm/h
Urea nitrogen, serum (BUN)	10 mg/dL
Creatinine, serum	1.1 mg/dL

Urinalysis

Urine pH	6.0
RBC count	2/HPF
WBC count	2/HPF
Nitrates	Negative
Bacteria	Negative

Chest x-ray reveals pulmonary infiltrates. The mediastinum is normal. What is the most likely diagnosis?

- **A.** Churg-Strauss syndrome
- **B.** Polyarteritis nodosa
- **C.** Rheumatoid arthritis
- **D.** Takayasu arteritis
- **E.** Temporal arteritis

274. A 6-year-old boy is brought to the pediatric clinic by his parents because he has been having "behavioral difficulties." He was recently sent home from school for setting fires in the boys' bathroom. His teacher complains because he cannot stay in his seat. At home, his father is weary of having to redirect his son to finish chores or complete homework. His grandmother reports similar problems with his father as a child. What is the most appropriate statement regarding the care of this patient?

A. This patient should be started on methylphenidate therapy

B. This patient will be helped best with cognitive therapy

C. This patient's fire-setting behavior should be ignored

D. This patient's condition most likely will be chronic and last into old age

E. This child has a normal risk for developing adult antisocial personality disorder

275. A 27-year-old man presents to his physician because of scrotal heaviness for 1 year. Physical examination reveals a right-sided scrotal mass measuring 6 cm with induration of the scrotal skin. Ultrasonography reveals homogeneous enlargement of the right testicle without evidence of hemorrhage or necrosis. Tumor markers are negative. Which of the following is the most appropriate initial step in the management of this condition?

A. Chemotherapy (cisplatin, bleomycin, and etopiside)

B. Inguinal orchiectomy

C. Interstitial radiotherapy with iodine 125

D. Radiotherapy and chemotherapy

E. Transcrotal orchiectomy and interstitial radiotherapy with iodine 125

276. A 14-month-old boy is brought to the pediatric clinic by his mother. She is complaining that her baby seems to "bruise very easily." The patient's mother reports that her child bruises with mild trauma. Past medical history is unremarkable. The mother does note that her brother also had a problem with easy bruising. Physical examination reveals multiple ecchymoses located diffusely over the trunk and abdomen. Laboratory studies reveal a prolonged partial thromboplastin time, a low factor VIIIC level, normal platelet aggregation, and normal prothrombin time. What is the most likely diagnosis?

A. Hemophilia A

B. Hemophilia B

C. Vitamin B_{12} deficiency

D. Vitamin K deficiency

E. von Willebrand disease

277. A 28-year-old man who is on a camping trip and sleeping outdoors awakens suddenly complaining of abdominal pain. He thinks he was bitten by a spider with a red hourglass mark on the abdomen. During the next 24 hours he complains of generalized muscle pains, nausea, vomiting, and headache. He is brought to the emergency department for evaluation. Physical examination reveals an area of erythema and edema on the left lateral thigh. Results of laboratory studies are shown below:

Leukocyte count and differential

Leukocyte count	12,000/mm³
Segmented neutrophils	75%
Bands	7%
Eosinophils	3%
Basophils	1%
Lymphocytes	27%
Monocytes	4%

Which of the following is the most appropriate primary treatment for this individual?

A. Ampicillin

B. Corticosteroids

C. Muscle relaxants

D. Plasmapheresis

E. Systemic administration of antivenin

278. A 39-year-old woman has a 2-week history of catatonic behavior, delusions, and auditory hallucinations after being fired from her job as an executive of a corporation. She appears to be in emotional turmoil and is confused. Conversations with her are notable for rapid shifts from one intense affect to another. She is emotionally labile with confused and incoherent speech. She appears to be transiently disoriented and cannot remember events from her recent past. Which of the following is the most likely diagnosis?

A. Brief reactive psychosis

B. Posttraumatic stress disorder

C. Psychotic disorder not otherwise specified

D. Schizoaffective disorder

E. Schizophrenia

279. A 50-year-old woman presents for evaluation of new-onset bloody vaginal discharge as well as urinary frequency and dysuria. She notes that sexual intercourse has become painful. Vaginal speculum examination reveals a mass lesion in the upper portion of the vaginal vault. Laboratory values are as follows:

Electrolytes, serum

Na, serum	143 mEq/L
Cl, serum	100 mEq/L
K, serum	3.7 mEq/L
Bicarbonate, serum	24 mEq/L
Magnesium, serum	2.0 mEq/L
Creatinine, serum	1.0 mg/dL

CBC, leukocyte count, and differential

Leukocyte count	9000/mm^3
Segmented neutrophils	62%
Bands	7%
Eosinophils	3%
Basophils	1%
Lymphocytes	27%
Monocytes	4%
Hematocrit	29%

The primary treatment option should include which of the following?

A. Chemotherapy (multiagent)

B. Intravesicular chemotherapy with bacillus Calmette-Guérin

C. Radiotherapy (focused, high-intensity)

D. Surgical excision

E. Watchful waiting with biopsy in 6 months

280. A 62-year-old woman who is hospitalized for treatment of enterococcal pyelonephritis develops fever and diarrhea. She is currently on day 7 of a 10-day regimen of intravenous ampicillin and gentamicin. The diarrhea is described as watery, voluminous, and without gross blood or mucus. Physical examination of the abdomen reveals mild tenderness in all four quadrants without evidence of guarding or rebound tenderness. Her stool is Gram stained and cultured and reveals *Clostridium difficile*. The best treatment is which of the following?

A. Change ampicillin to amoxicillin

B. Ceftriaxone

C. Metronidazole

D. Trimethoprim

E. Watchful waiting

281. A 28-year-old man is given a prescription of valproate for bipolar disorder, and the use, side effects, and importance of compliance for this drug are explained to him. The next step in the treatment of this patient would be

A. Obtain liver function tests at baseline

B. Obtain blood urea nitrogen (BUN) and creatinine levels at baseline

C. Obtain pulmonary function tests at baseline

D. Measure valproate levels in 3 months

E. Obtain an abdominal CT scan

282. A 29-year-old man with no prior medical history presents to the emergency room complaining of a 12-hour history of tearing pain with defecation and bright red bleeding per rectum noted on the toilet tissue. Blood pressure was 138/90 mm Hg, pulse 90 beats/min, and respirations 14 breaths/min, and the patient was afebrile. Urinalysis shows no evidence of microhematuria, glucosuria, or proteinuria. Cardiovascular examination reveals a regular rate and rhythm. Pulmonary auscultation reveals no evidence of rales, rhonchi, or wheezes. Good air exchange is noted bilaterally. Gastrointestinal examination reveals tenderness to deep palpation in the lower left quadrant with no localizing peritoneal signs. Anoscopy reveals a split in the anoderm at the posterior midline with fresh blood oozing from the site. What is the most appropriate treatment?

A. Ampicillin (intravenous)

B. Metronidazole (oral)

C. Rubber band ligation

D. Stool softeners, sitz baths, and bulking agents

E. Surgical excision and sphincterotomy

283. A 32-year-old G2P1 woman comes to her primary care physician for prenatal care. She has a history of delivery of a 4250-g baby. At 28 weeks' gestation, she had a 50-g glucose loading test (GLT); her blood glucose at 1 hour was measured at 155 mg/dL. What would be the next appropriate step in treating this patient?

A. Begin oral hypoglycemic

B. Check 3-hour glucose tolerance test (GTT)

C. Give patient betamethasone and prepare for cesarean section

D. Implement appropriate insulin regimen

E. Implement diabetic diet

284. You are called to the emergency room to evaluate an 18-month-old girl. Her parents state that she has been very irritable and has not been walking since yesterday. There is no history of recent trauma. However, the child did have a cold 4 weeks ago. Physical examination reveals that the right hip joint has limited range of motion, and the patient refuses to bear weight. Erythema and edema of the hip are also present. Aspiration of the synovial fluid is performed. What is the most likely diagnosis?

A. Avascular necrosis of the femoral head
B. Femoral neck fracture
C. Pelvis fracture
D. Septic arthritis
E. Toxic synovitis

285. A 63-year-old woman with long-standing cirrhosis secondary to hemochromatosis has become concerned about developing cancer. She has become an avid reader of *Prevention Magazine* and has embarked on a path toward cancer prevention with use of megavitamins. Physical examination of the heart and lungs are normal. However, she does have some palpable liver nodules. Which of the following tests is most likely to be elevated if the patient's suspicion of liver cancer is correct?

A. Alpha-fetoprotein (AFP)
B. CA-125
C. Carcinogenic embryonic antigen (CEA)
D. Human chorionic gonadotropin (hCG)
E. Prostate-specific antigen (PSA)

286. An 11-month-old infant of Mediterranean descent is hospitalized for failure to thrive and severe anemia. Physical examination reveals marked splenomegaly as well as some frontal bossing, maxillary hypertrophy, and a tower skull. Peripheral blood smear shows marked hypochromia, microcytosis, anisocytosis, and poikilocytosis. Hemoglobin electrophoresis reveals that hemoglobin A is markedly decreased. What is the genetic abnormality responsible for this infant's condition?

A. Alpha-thalassemia trait
B. Beta-thalassemia major
C. Beta-thalassemia minor
D. Fragile X syndrome
E. Hemoglobin Bart disease

287. A study looks at the effectiveness of performing a random nonfasting serum glucose test to detect diabetes. One thousand people are tested, but 200 are lost to follow-up. After a positive test result, a glucose tolerance test is performed to confirm the results. The following 2 × 2 table shows the results of the study (Table 287). What is the positive predictive value of the screening test?

Table 287	Diabetes	
SCREENING TEST RESULT	**PRESENT**	**ABSENT**
Positive	250	450
Negative	50	50

A. 0.62
B. 0.38
C. 0.25
D. 0.33
E. 0.5

288. An obese 54-year-old woman presents to the emergency department with a 3-hour history of severe left-sided back pain. Thrashing around in the bed, the patient tells you the pain is relentless and a "10 out of 10" in severity. Her last meal was 8 hours ago and last (normal) bowel movement 7 hours ago. However, the patient began vomiting 20 minutes after the pain abruptly began several hours ago. Past medical history includes cluster headaches, gout, and "hot flashes," but no prior surgeries. Physical examination reveals few bowel sounds and percussion yields little useful information. No masses are palpated. There is left-sided abdominal tenderness without guarding or rebound tenderness. Abdominal x-ray films reveal diffusely distended small and large bowels with multiple air-fluid levels. A urinalysis reveals 3 RBCs/HPF and 2 WBCs/HPF. What is the most likely diagnosis?

A. Bowel obstruction secondary to adhesions from Crohn disease
B. Diverticulitis
C. Pancreatitis
D. Prostatic calculi
E. Ureteral calculi

289. A 23-year-old man presents to his primary care physician with generalized malaise for approximately 3 months. He has been sexually active with multiple partners without use of contraception. Physical examination reveals hepatosplenomegaly and palpable inguinal lymphadenopathy bilaterally. Laboratory studies reveal detectable serum levels of anti–hepatitis B core antigen (HBcAg) IgM. What is the best initial management of this patient?

A. Administer the hepatitis B vaccine
B. Await detectable levels of anti–hepatitis B surface antigen (HBsAg) IgG
C. Await detectable levels of anti-HBcAg IgG
D. Await detectable levels of anti–hepatitis B e antigen (HBeAg) IgG
E. Administer interferon-alpha

290. One minute after birth, a neonate is assessed and found to have a weak cry and is pink in the torso and extremities. The child cries and withdrawals when tested for reflex irritability. Arms and legs are in a flexed position. Heart rate is 124 beats/min. The child weighs 3200 g. What is the initial Apgar score?

A. 6
B. 7
C. 8
D. 9
E. 10

291. A 19-year-old man is brought to the emergency department after being struck in the head with a baseball while attempting to catch a foul ball with his bare hands. He was conscious in the ambulance, but upon arrival in the emergency department became unconscious. Pupils are unequal but respond to light. CT scan of the head is performed and is shown below (Figure 291). What is the most likely diagnosis?

Figure 291

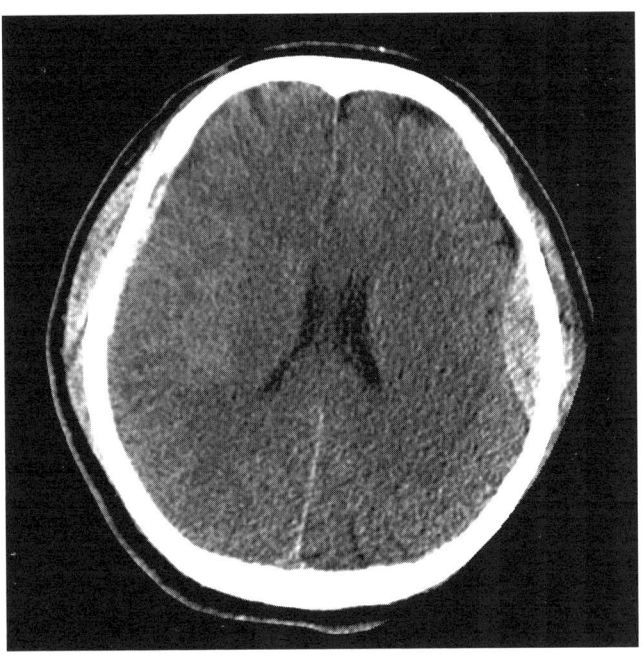

A. Brain abscess
B. Epidural hematoma
C. Meningioma
D. Subarachnoid hemorrhage
E. Subdural hematoma

292. A 16-year-old girl you have followed since birth comes to your office without an appointment. She has no prior medical or surgical history. She is about to graduate high school and is the valedictorian. She is very nervous about giving her speech and wonders if there is anything you can give her to calm her down during her speech. Physical examination findings of the heart, lungs, and abdomen are within normal limits. What is the most appropriate treatment for this patient?

A. Atenolol
B. Clonidine
C. Diphenhydramine
D. Methylphenidate
E. Propranolol

293. A 68-year-old woman presents to her physician complaining of itching and pain in her genital area. Physical examination findings of the heart, lungs, and abdomen are unremarkable. Female pelvic examination reveals a grade II cystocele, a grade I rectocele, and white plaque-like lesions on her labia and perineum. What is the most appropriate treatment for this patient?

A. Excision of lesions with postoperative pelvic radiation
B. Seven-day treatment with antifungal medication
C. Seven- to ten-day course of antibiotics
D. Surgical excision of lesions with pathologic examination of margins
E. Watchful waiting

294. A 50-year-old man has been treated for back pain for 6 months with analgesics and muscle relaxants. At work, upon lifting a heavy box of tubing, he suddenly feels excruciating pain in his lower back. He states that the pain shoots down his leg all the way to his big toe. Upon examination the patient has severe pain in his legs on straight leg testing, and a Valsalva maneuver causes the shooting pain down his leg. He has no weakness or paresthesias in his legs. What is the most likely diagnosis?

A. A lumbar vertebral fracture
B. Herniated lumbar disc at L3–L4
C. Herniated lumbar disc at L4–L5
D. Herniated lumbar disc at L5–S1
E. Herniated sacral disc at S3

295. A 33-year-old man presents to the emergency department with progressively worsening left upper quadrant abdominal pain and distention. Earlier that day he was an unrestrained driver in a motor vehicle accident. His chest and abdomen hit the steering column hard, but he did not feel bad enough to warrant a hospital trip. The patient complains of aching pain whenever he lies down. Physical examination reveals a blood pressure of 90/50 mm Hg and a pulse of 120 beats/min. There is tenderness and ecchymoses over the left ninth and tenth ribs. What is your next step in the treatment of this patient?

A. Administer fluids and blood
B. Administer pain medications and repeat examination
C. Immediate exploratory laparotomy with splenectomy
D. Order a transesophageal echocardiogram
E. Order serum blood alcohol levels

296. A 7-year-old girl patient presents to the pediatric clinic for her annual check-up. Her father states that she has been in good health, but is concerned that his daughter may have a learning disability. Her grades have fallen over the past year, and the teacher has noticed her not paying attention during class. Physical examination demonstrates an appropriate level of development. Electroencephalography reveals a generalized, symmetrical 3-per-second spike-and-wave pattern. What is the most appropriate treatment?

A. Carbamazepine

B. Ethosuximide

C. Methylphenidate

D. Observation

E. Phenytoin

297. A 48-year-old woman presents to the ambulatory care center because of sudden onset of rust-colored urine. She has no history of urinary problems. She has been complaining of a several day history of cough and sore throat. Physical examination shows a blood pressure of 150/96 mm Hg, pulse of 82 beats/min, and respirations of 12 breaths/min. There is no evidence of cardiac or pulmonary abnormalities on examination. There is no costovertebral angle tenderness. Urinalysis results are shown below:

Color	Red
Odor	Pungent
Glucose	None
RBC count	20/HPF and dysmorphic in appearance
Red cell casts	Numerous
Protein	>1000 mg/24 h

Which of the following is the most likely diagnosis?

A. Focal segmental glomerular sclerosis

B. Goodpasture syndrome

C. IgA nephropathy

D. Membranous glomerulonephritis

E. Postinfectious glomerulonephritis

298. A 23-year-old G1P0 African-American female presents to the ambulatory care clinic at 32 weeks' gestation. She reports no contraction or vaginal discharge at this time. However, she states she has noticed some difficulty putting on her rings and some swelling in her face. Which of the following would be an appropriate next step in working up this patient?

A. Adnexal and cervical examination

B. Echocardiography

C. Evaluation of blood pressure

D. Renal ultrasonography

E. Watchful waiting

299. A 39-year-old morbidly obese man presents to his primary care physician because of excessive daytime sleepiness. Physical examination of the throat reveals minimally obstructing tonsils. Physical examination findings of the heart, lungs, and abdomen are normal. Polysomnography reveals frequent apneic events, and a diagnosis of obstructive sleep apnea is made. What is the most appropriate treatment for this patient?

A. Continuous positive airway pressure

B. Nasal surgery

C. Sedative medications

D. Uvulopalatoplasty

E. Weight loss

300. A 60-year-old white man presents to his primary care physician for evaluation of a 2-cm white patch on his inner cheek. He has a 45 pack/year smoking history. He reports no shortness of breath, cough, or wheezing. He has been in a monogamous relationship for the past 20 years. The lesion is not painful but bleeds when he tries to pick at it. The patch is firm, rough, and ulcerated. What is the next most appropriate step in the treatment of this patient?

A. Antifungal therapy

B. Biopsy of the lesion

C. Chest x-ray

D. HIV testing

E. Reassurance

301. A 28-day-old girl who is being treated for sepsis as an inpatient on the pediatric ward begins to bleed profusely from venipuncture sites and around indwelling catheters. She is also noted to have hematochezia and hematuria. Results of laboratory studies reveal thrombocytopenia with prolonged prothrombin time, partial thromboplastin time, and thrombin time. Fibrinogen and factors V and VIII are low, and fibrin split products and D-dimer are high. What is the most likely diagnosis?

A. Aplastic anemia

B. Diamond-Blackfan syndrome

C. Disseminated intravascular coagulation (DIC)

D. Hemophila B

E. Idiopathic thrombocytopenia purpura (ITP)

302. A 34-year-old woman presents to her primary care physician because of unexplained infertility. She and her husband have been attempting to achieve pregnancy for 2 years. Her husband was evaluated by a urologist and was found to have bilateral subclinical varicoceles. His semen analysis was within normal limits. She has a history of recurrent pregnancy loss, heavy menses, and chronic pelvic pain. What is the most likely explanation of her unexplained infertility?

A. Endometriosis

B. Endometritis

C. Fibroids

D. Presence of intrauterine device

E. Presence of pelvic inflammatory disease

303. A 22-year-old man presents to the emergency department with a 12-hour history of an extremely painful left eye. He complains of blurred vision and seeing halos around lights. He states that this has occurred in the past but the attacks were milder. Physical examination reveals that the eye is tender and inflamed. The left eye is indurated as compared to the right eye. What is the most likely diagnosis?

A. Acute angle closure glaucoma

B. Acute episcleritis

C. Acute iridocyclitis

D. Bacterial conjunctivitis

E. Viral conjunctivitis

304. A mother brings her 4-year-old son to the pediatric clinic with concerns about his tea-colored urine. He also has a history of intermittent gross hematuria. Physical examination reveals bilateral pedal edema. Renal biopsy reveals crescent formations. What is the most likely diagnosis?

A. Acute poststreptococcal glomerulonephritis
B. Alport syndrome
C. Focal segmental glomerulosclerosis
D. IgA nephropathy
E. Rapidly progressive glomerulonephritis

305. An 8-year-old boy presents to the emergency department with left ankle pain after jumping out of his club house 2 hours ago. His parents believe he jumped about 7 feet before landing on the pavement, after which he cried out and began clutching his left ankle. Physical examination reveals significant swelling of the left ankle, but the surrounding skin is intact. Light touch, vibration, and pinprick are intact over the left foot, ankle, and leg. He can wiggle all 10 toes, although doing so on the left causes much pain. Anteroposterior and lateral radiographs of the left ankle are ordered (Figure 305a and b). What is the most likely diagnosis?

A. Salter-Harris epiphyseal fracture type I
B. Salter-Harris epiphyseal fracture type II
C. Salter-Harris epiphyseal fracture type III
D. Salter-Harris epiphyseal fracture type IV
E. Salter-Harris epiphyseal fracture type V

306. A 20-year-old woman presents who has never had menses but has breast development that occurred about the same time as her classmates. She is a virgin. Ultrasonography reveals no detectable uterus. Physical examination findings of the heart, lungs, and abdomen are within normal limits. Pelvic examination shows her to be at Tanner stage IV. What is the most likely explanation of these findings?

A. Mayer-Rokitansky-Kuster-Hauser syndrome
B. Savage syndrome
C. Swyer syndrome
D. Testicular feminization
E. Vaginal atresia

307. A 12-year-old girl presents to the clinic with a 2-month history of intermittent joint pain, swelling, and limitation of range of motion in her elbows, knees, ankles, and wrists bilaterally. She reports that her symptoms are worse in the morning. She has also has an intermittent low-grade fever associated with her joint pain. She denies having recently traveled outside her hometown in Florida and denies getting any recent insect bites. The patient also admits to feeling fatigue over the past couple of months. Laboratory values reveal an elevated erythrocyte sedimentation rate, and synovial fluid from joint space reveals a WBC count of 15,000/mm³, elevated protein, and low glucose and complement. What is the most likely diagnosis?

Figure 305a

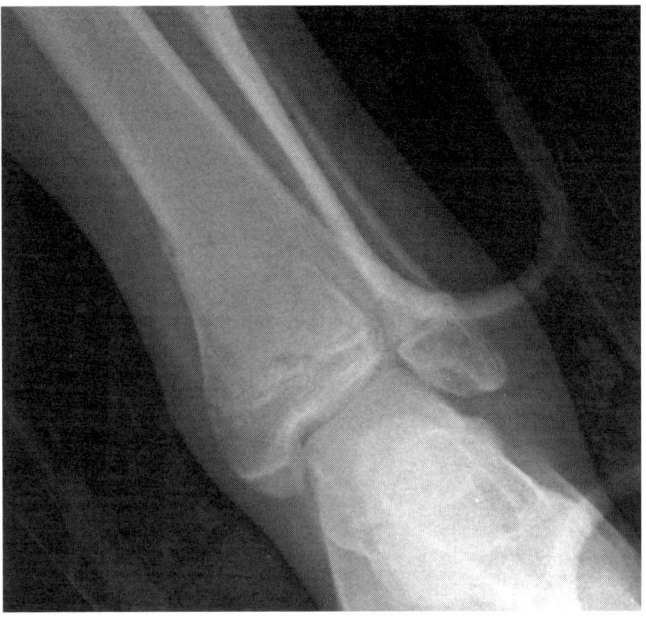

Figure 305b

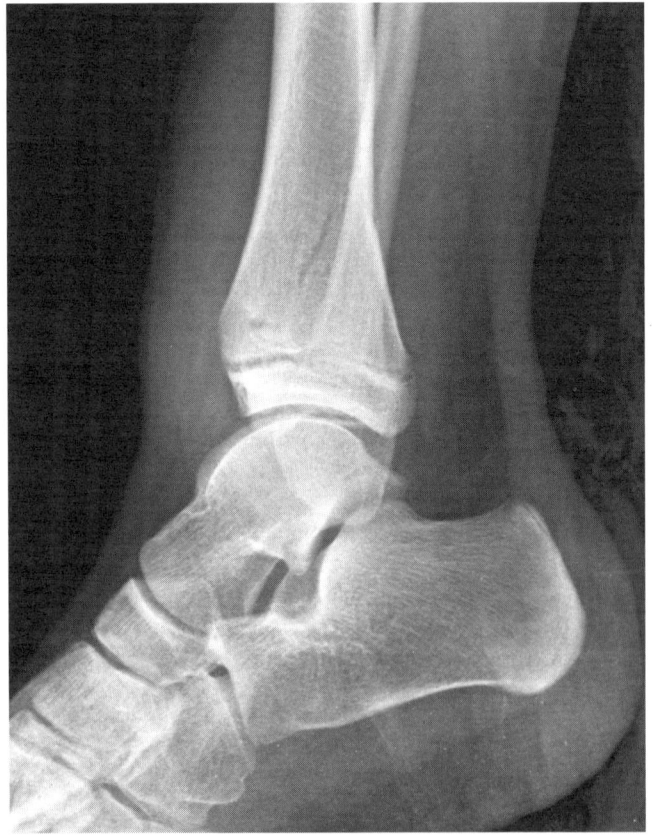

A. Juvenile rheumatoid arthritis

B. Lyme disease

C. Septic arthritis

D. Toxic synovitis

E. Uremia

308. A 34-year-old man with known HIV infection presents to his primary care physician with complaints of dyspnea, dry cough, and fever of 6 days' duration. The patient appears fatigued and is having difficulty breathing. Physical examination reveals that the skin is warm and moist without lesions. Cardiovascular examination findings are unremarkable. Blood work demonstrates a CD4 count of less than 200/mm^3 and increased lactate dehydrogenase. PaO$_2$ is 70 mm Hg. Chest x-ray demonstrates a mild right pneumothorax and two small cavitations on the left. What is the most appropriate treatment for this patient?

A. Amphotericin B

B. Isoniazid and rifampin

C. Prednisolone

D. Prednisone

E. Trimethoprim-sulfamethoxazole

309. A 23-year-old woman presents to the student health clinic with complaints of vaginal irritation and discharge. She admits to being sexually active and occasionally uses condoms. Physical examination reveals a "fishy" malodorous discharge, and mild erythema is noted. A wet preparation of a vaginal swab has a pH of 5 to 6 and reveals clue cells. What is the most appropriate treatment for this patient?

A. Bacitracin

B. Doxycycline

C. Metronidazole

D. Ketoconazole

E. Penicillin

310. A 32-year-old male custodian comes to see his primary care physician for a routine visit. He lives alone and has never been involved in a serious relationship. When asked why, he states, "I've just never really been interested. I'm just sort of a hermit I guess." Today he is wearing a purple cloak, a bright green sweatshirt, and dark sunglasses. When you ask him how he is feeling today, he replies, "Not too good. My bill for lunch today came to $13.13, so I just know something terrible is going to happen. Plus, it's a full moon tonight, so you know what that means . . ." You ask him if he has any concerns and he says, "Well, I have a feeling that the other guys at work are talking about me behind my back, and telling my boss stuff to try to get me fired." His speech is difficult to follow, as it takes him awhile to get to the point. What is the most likely diagnosis?

A. Avoidant personality disorder

B. Borderline personality disorder

C. Paranoid personality disorder

D. Schizoid personality disorder

E. Schizotypal personality disorder

311. A 63-year-old man with a 60 pack/year history of smoking complains of gross hematuria. Physical examination findings of the heart, lungs, and abdomen are within normal limits. The prostate is approximately 40 g and is symmetric. Intravenous pyelography reveals normal kidneys and ureters bilaterally. A small filling defect is noted within the floor of the urinary bladder. Cystoscopy is performed, and a sessile, papillary growth of approximately 2 × 4 cm is noted proximal to the left ureteral orifice. What is the most likely diagnosis based on biopsies taken of this lesion?

A. Adenocarcinoma

B. Carcinoid tumor

C. Sarcoma

D. Squamous cell carcinoma

E. Transitional cell carcinoma

312. A 40-year-old Asian woman with a history of perineal warts presents to her primary care physician for annual follow-up. She does not report any melena or hematochezia. She has a history of diet-controlled diabetes mellitus and hypertension. Her current medications include glyburide. Physical examination findings of the head/neck, heart, lungs, and abdomen are within normal limits. Rectal examination reveals stool in the vault, but her Hemoccult test is positive after 50 seconds. Results of laboratory studies are shown below:

Electrolytes, serum

Na, serum	144 mEq/L
Cl, serum	99 mEq/L
K, serum	3.9 mEq/L
Bicarbonate, serum	26 mEq/L
Magnesium, serum	1.8 mEq/L
Creatinine, serum	1.1 mg/dL

Leukocyte count and differential

Leukocyte count	8500/mm^3

What is the next most appropriate step in the evaluation of this patient?

A. No further steps necessary; her Hemoccult was negative 20 seconds after the developer was applied

B. Send her home with three Hemoccult cards she can use herself, then mail the cards to her physician

C. Barium enema

D. Endoscopy (upper gastrointestinal tract)

E. Endoscopy (lower gastrointestinal tract)

313. A 47-year-old woman complains of 4 hours of severe generalized abdominal pain and intermittent vaginal bleeding that has increased over the past 2 days. She presents to her primary care physician for evaluation. Her prior obstetric history is notable for abruptio placentae with her only pregnancy at age 33, which resulted in a stillborn product. Presently she complains of dizziness, nausea, and constipation. Her last menstrual period was 40 days ago, and her menstrual periods typically occur every 26 days. Blood pressure is 96/70 mm Hg, pulse 110 beats/min, and respirations 18 breaths/min, and she demonstrates lower abdominal tenderness to deep palpation. Pelvic examination reveals a slightly open cervix with no evidence of blood in the vaginal vault. What is the most appropriate next step in the workup and treatment of this patient?

- **A.** Blood work: CBC, serum electrolytes, and liver function test
- **B.** Diagnostic culdocentesis
- **C.** Ultrasonography (abdominal, pelvic, and renal)
- **D.** Ultrasonography (transvaginal)
- **E.** Urine pregnancy test

314. Parents bring their 4-year-old daughter to the pediatric clinic because they have concerns about her development. Upon interacting with the child, you notice that she has a long face, and is in the fifth percentile for height. Her left eye is medially deviated. She does interact with you, but she seems easily distractible and her mother says her activity at home is as if her daughter "were being driven by a motor." Her language skills are mildly lacking for her age. On physical examination, you detect a late systolic murmur on cardiac auscultation. What is true about this child's condition?

- **A.** It is the result of a chromosomal trisomy
- **B.** It can be caused by abnormal CGG repeats in the patient's affected chromosome
- **C.** It is caused by a partial deletion in chromosome 5
- **D.** This patient may exhibit compulsive eating behavior
- **E.** It is inherited in an autosomal-dominant fashion

315. A 41-year-old man who is a known alcoholic complains of epigastric pain that radiates to the back, nausea, and vomiting for 7 days. Physical examination reveals a poorly nourished male whose vital signs are blood pressure 90/60 mm Hg, pulse 110 beats/min, repirations 17 breaths/min. Cardiac auscultation reveals tachycardia. Pulmonary examination is notable for bibasilar rales. Abdominal examination reveals hypoactive bowel sounds and a palpable mass in the midepigastrium. Blue discoloration of the periumbilical area is noted. Results of laboratory studies are presented below:

Amylase, serum	400 U/L
Bilirubin, serum	1.0 mg/dL
Calcium, serum	11.5 mg/dL
Na, serum	136 mEq/L
Cl, serum	99 mEq/L
K, serum	3.3 mEq/L
Bicarbonate, serum	22 mEq/L
Magnesium, serum	1.4 mEq/L
Creatinine, serum	1.6 mg/dL
Osmolality, serum	288 mOsmol/kg
Albumin, serum	3.3 g/dL
Urea nitrogen, serum (BUN)	17 mg/dL
Hematocrit	34%
Hemoglobin, blood	11.2 g/dL
Leukocyte count	10,000/mm^3
Platelet count	177,000/mm^3
Alanine aminotransferase, serum	30 U/L
Aspartate aminotransferase, serum	35 U/L

Which of the following is the most specific laboratory study test for this condition?

- **A.** Serum amylase
- **B.** Serum calcium
- **C.** Serum glucose
- **D.** Serum hepatic transaminase
- **E.** Serum lipase

316. A 2-month-old girl presents to the pediatric clinic for evaluation. Her parents state that she has been in good health without any difficulties feeding. The parents have noticed that the infant has a long, narrowed face and they are concerned this may be permanent. Physical examination reveals that vital signs are normal and the infant is greater than fiftieth percentile for both weight and height. Primitive reflexes are present, but sagittal cranial sutures are not palpated. What is the most appropriate treatment for this patient?

- **A.** Molding the head via a helmet
- **B.** Observation only
- **C.** Radiation followed with surgical reopening of the cranial sutures
- **D.** Surgically reopening the cranial sutures followed by chemotherapy
- **E.** Surgically reopening the cranial sutures

317. A 20-year-old woman was diagnosed with a major depressive episode 1 month ago. She did not start on any medications, but began receiving counseling. Before this, she has had no psychiatric problems or depression. The past 4 days, however, she has felt great. Her mood has been fabulous. She feels her self-esteem has turned completely around and she feels great about herself. She has been sleeping 3 hours a night and feels well rested. She has been very talkative, and has enjoyed going out nightly again with her friends, driving home drunk most weeknights from the bar. She returns for her counseling appointment and explains to her psychiatrist how she feels. What is the most likely explanation of these findings?

A. Bipolar I disorder
B. Bipolar II disorder
C. Cyclothymic disorder
D. Manic episode
E. Recovery from depression

318. A 25-year-old woman who is 30 weeks pregnant presents to the emergency department with complaints of vaginal bleeding and severe abdominal pain. She has experienced some irregular contractions. Physical examination reveals a heart rate of 95 beats/min, blood pressure of 134/80 mm Hg, and respirations of 18 breaths/min. A fetal monitoring strip shows variable decelerations with occasional late decelerations. What is the most likely substance abused by this patient?

A. Alcohol
B. Caffeine
C. Cocaine
D. Marijuana
E. Opioids

319. A 37-year-old woman comes to the emergency department after breaking her tibia in a motor vehicle accident. She has caused a disturbance in the waiting room. She refuses to be seen by a resident and is demanding to be seen by "only the best physician at the hospital." You come to talk with her and she tells you that she is a "wildly successful" lawyer, and describes multiple awards she has received for outstanding achievement. She complains about the wait, and tells you that she should have been your top priority. When you explain that there are many other patients who are also in need of attention, she replies, "Other patients do not concern me, I deserve medical attention immediately!" What is the most likely diagnosis?

A. Borderline personality disorder
B. Histrionic personality disorder
C. Narcissistic personality disorder
D. Obsessive-compulsive personality disorder
E. Schizotypal personality disorder

320. A 60-year-old man presents to the ambulatory care clinic with a 2-month history of progressive, watery diarrhea. He claims to have four to eight loose stools a day. "The diarrhea seems to be worse when I get excited or upset," the patient says. "And when I get nervous or excited, my whole face and neck turns beet red, and I can't breathe air in or out for several minutes." Physical examination reveals that the abdomen is nondistended and has no scars. Auscultation yields hyperactive bowel sounds. Percussion is mostly dull with a few patch areas of resonance. With deep palpation, there is no hepatomegaly or splenomegaly but a small mass at the McBurney point is palpable. What is the most likely diagnosis?

A. Carcinoid syndrome secondary to appendiceal carcinoid
B. Carcinoid syndrome secondary to liver metastases of carcinoid tumor
C. Carcinoid syndrome secondary to rectal carcinoid tumor; incidental finding of mass in the right lower quadrant of the abdomen
D. Diverticulitis
E. Partial bowel obstruction secondary to fecal impaction in cecum

The response options for items 321 and 322 are the same. You will be required to select one answer for each item in the set.

A. Angelman syndrome
B. Fragile X syndrome
C. Prader-Willi syndrome
D. Rett syndrome
E. Turcotte syndrome
F. Turner syndrome

For each patient with mental retardation, select the most appropriate diagnosis.

321. A 19-year-old institutionalized obese man is evaluated for an insatiable appetite. He is mentally retarded. He is also loquatious and emotionally labile. Physical examination reveals a man who appears 6 years his junior. His height is 4 feet 11 inches. Physical examination of the heart, lungs, and abdomen are unremarkable. Musculoskeletal examination reveals decreased tone in all extremities.

322. A 24 year old institutionalized mentally retarded man presents for a follow-up examination. He has a history of abnormal gait and seizures. He speaks in a poorly intelligible fashion but laughs, smiles, and is very excitable. Physical examination findings of the heart, lungs, and abdomen are unremarkable.

The response options for items 323 and 324 are the same. You will be required to select one answer for each item in the set.

A. Broca aphasia
B. Conduction aphasia
C. Global aphasia
D. Subcortical aphasia
E. Transcortical motor aphasia
F. Transcortical sensory aphasia

323. A 73-year-old man with a history of diabetes mellitus, hypertension, and atrial fibrillation has a stroke. He is evaluated by the medical team on day 8. His speech is nonfluent and his attempted speech output is characterized by hesitations. He states that he "wants go store" and substitutes the word "spool" for "spoon." Comprehension is preserved. CT scan reveals infarct of the distribution of the right middle cerebral artery.

324. A 69-year-old man with a history of hypertension, prostate cancer, and colon cancer has a stroke. He is evaluated by the medical team on day 10. He is asked to repeat the sentence "The boy in the car is eating popcorn." However, he makes paraphrasic errors which he cannot correct. He does have intact comprehension. CT scan reveals atrophy of the arcuate fasciculus.

325. A 29-year-old homeless man with a 3-week history of fevers, rigors, and myalgias presents to the ambulatory care clinic for evaluation. He is a homosexual. He has a 10 pack/year history of smoking and is a former intravenous drug user. Physical examination reveals no evidence of cervical or axillary nodes, but inguinal adenopathy is noted bilaterally. Pharyngeal examination reveals erythema bilaterally. Cardiac examination reveals a regular rate and rhythm. Pulmonary examination does not demonstrate wheeze, rhonchi, or rales. Gastrointestinal examination reveals no evidence of peritoneal signs. Which of the following is an appropriate test to order next in the evaluation of this patient?

A. Enzyme immunoassay test
B. Erythrocyte sedimentation rate
C. HIV p24 antigen
D. Plasma p24 antigen
E. Western blot test

326. A 58-year-old woman presents to her primary care physician with complaints of labial itching and pain. She states that she has been seen by several other physicians who have told her she has a yeast infection. She believes that the antifungal medications and steroid creams have not helped. Pelvic examination reveals a grade I cystocele and diffuse raised brown lesions on the labia. What is the most likely diagnosis?

A. Candidiasis refractory to treatment
B. Paget disease
C. Syphilis
D. *Trichomonas vaginalis* infection
E. Vulvar intraepithelial neoplasia (VIN)

327. An 18-month-old boy is brought to the pediatric clinic for routine evaluation. The mother states that her child has been in good health, other than suffering from three otitis media infections. Physical examination reveals that the child is below the fifth percentile for both weight and height. Retinal and vitreous hemorrhages are identified in both eyes. Heart and lungs are normal. What is the most likely explanation for these findings?

A. Acute bacterial conjunctivitis
B. Cataract
C. Child abuse
D. Hyphema
E. Increased intraocular pressure

328. A 25-year-old man presents to his primary care physician with the complaint of excessive daytime sleepiness. After further questioning you find out that he has extreme difficulty falling asleep at night. He tells you that this has lasted approximately 3 months. About 2 months ago, he started falling asleep on the job and because of this, his boss has threatened to fire him. The patient denies any other medical or psychological problems. He does not use alcohol or any recreational drugs. A nighttime polysomnogram is obtained and results are shown in Table 328. What is the most likely diagnosis?

Table 328

Monitoring time	450 min
Sleep time	300 min
Sleep latency	75 min
REM latency	70 min
Apnea index	0
Nocturnal myoclonus index	0

A. Breathing-related sleep disorder
B. Dyssomnia not otherwise specified
C. Narcolepsy
D. Primary hypersomnia
E. Primary insomnia

329. A 19-year-old man who was a participant in a robbery attempt was struck by police with a club in an effort to apprehend him. The individual sustained injury to his right hand and complained of diminished sensation over the fourth and fifth digits. He is an alcoholic and uses marijuana frequently. Three weeks after the incident, wasting of the small hand muscles of the fourth and fifth digits are noted. There is no evidence of healed laceration or other physical deformity. Which of the following is the most likely injured structure?

A. Axillary nerve
B. Musculocutaneous nerve
C. Palmar interosseus nerve
D. Radial nerve
E. Ulnar nerve

330. A newborn baby boy was taken to the neonatal intensive care unit for jaundice that was so severe that he required an exchange transfusion. Laboratory studies revealed normocytic anemia, reticulocytosis, an indirect hyperbilirubinemia. Osmotic fragility test was positive. What protein in the RBC membrane is mostly likely responsible for this patient's condition?

A. Dystrophin
B. Dyein
C. Elastin
D. Spectrin
E. Thrombin

331. A 43-year-old woman presents to her primary care physician complaining of 2 weeks of generalized itching. She cannot think of any causes for the itching, including skin contact or new medications. She denies having pain, fevers, headaches, vision problems, palpitations, cough, dyspnea, nausea, vomiting, constipation, or voiding problems. She has noticed increased fatigue over the past 2 weeks, as well as gradual loosening of stools, which are now foul smelling and tend to float. Physical examination reveals an uncomfortable-appearing woman in acute distress. Integument appears to be excoriated diffusely, but there is no evidence of underlying irritation, including urticaria or rash. The pupils are equally round and reactive to light, and there is no conjunctival injection bilaterally. However, there is a faint yellowing of both sclera. The oropharynx is nonerythematous. No lymphadenopathy is palpable in the cervical region. The abdomen is soft and nontender. The liver span is 8 cm in the midclavicular line. Laboratory and radiographic studies obtained are shown below:

Alanine aminotransferase (ALT)	20 U/L
Aspartate aminotransferase (AST)	33 U/L
Alkaline phosphatase	364 U/L
Bilirubin, serum (total, direct)	2 mg/dL, 0.3 mg/dL
Antimitochondrial antibody	Positive
Ultrasonography	No dilated bile ducts
Liver biopsy	Intralobar bile duct destruction

What is the most appropriate treatment for this patient?

A. Liver transplantation
B. 5-fluorouracil and levamisole
C. Cholestyramine
D. Ursodeoxycholic acid
E. Endoscopic retrograde pancreatic cholangiography with stent placement

332. A 29-year-old woman has just recently given birth to a healthy baby boy. During her pregnancy, she had developed gestational diabetes, which was well controlled with an insulin regimen. On follow-up, the patient inquires about her postnatal diabetic care. What is the most appropriate statements to make to this patient?

A. She can manage her diabetes on a restricted, diabetic diet
B. She no longer requires any diabetic management postpartum
C. She will be changed to an oral hypoglycemic postpartum
D. She will need to be given an oral glucose tolerance test approximately 6 weeks postpartum to determine if continued treatment will be necessary
E. She will need to continue an insulin regimen which should be much lower postpartum

333. At the end of a visit with a patient whom you are seeing for diabetes control, the patient tells you that he has been experiencing vivid, frightening dreams. He states that these have been going on for as long as he can remember and they seem to happen about once a week. He seems to be worried about the distress these dreams cause him and asks you to tell him a little bit about what he is experiencing. What would be appropriate to tell this patient about these dreams?

A. "You are experiencing night terrors, which occur during deep, or slow-wave, sleep. Benzodiazepines can be used in treatment because they reduce the amount of time spent in slow-wave sleep."
B. "You are experiencing night terrors, which occur in REM sleep. Benzodiazepines can be used in treatment because they reduce the amount of time spent in REM sleep."
C. "You are experiencing nightmares, which occur in REM sleep. Tricyclic antidepressants can be used for treatment because they reduce the time spent in REM sleep."
D. "You are experiencing nightmares, which occur in slow-wave sleep. Benzodiazepines can be used for treatment because they reduce the time spent in slow-wave sleep."
E. "You are experiencing nightmares, which occur in slow-wave sleep. Tricyclic antidepressants can be used for treatment because they reduce the time spent in slow-wave sleep."

334. A 38-year-old man has a 2-year history of dysphagia and regurgitation of nonacidic material. He achieves minimal relief of symptoms with oral over-the-counter antacid therapy. He presents to his primary care physician for evaluation. Physical examination reveals a palpable thyroid gland without masses. Cardiac examination reveals no evidence of rubs, murmurs, or gallops. Pulmonary auscultation reveals no evidence or wheeze or rhonchi. Gastrointestinal examination reveals mild tenderness in the midepigastric region without focal peritoneal signs. Rectal examination reveals a normal size prostate, and the patient is guaiac negative with stool in the vault. Esophagography reveals a fluid-filled, dilated esophagus with a distal stricture. What is the most likely diagnosis?

A. Achalasia
B. Esophagitis (viral)
C. Esophageal carcinoma
D. Pill-related esophagitis
E. Scleroderma

335. A 74-year-old man with a history of diabetes mellitus and hypothyroidism presents for evaluation of intermittent gross hematuria with small clots noted upon urination. He complains of nocturia three times per night and decreased force of urinary stream with hesitancy. He is a nonsmoker but admits to drinking one beer per week for the past 20 years. His medications include an oral hypoglycemic agent and a synthethic thyroid hormone preparation. Physical examination reveals no evidence of rubs, murmurs, or gallops. Pulmonary auscultation reveals decreased breath sounds at the bases bilaterally. Gastrointestinal examination reveals some tenderness along the sigmoid colon without evidence of guarding or rebound tenderness. Rectal examination is guaiac positive with stool in the vault. A small internal hemorrhoid is noted in the left lateral position. Urinalysis reveals +2 hematuria with no evidence of leukocytes or nitrates. Kidney and bladder sonography reveal no evidence of hydronephrosis. The bladder is smooth walled with few trabeculations. Results of laboratory studies are shown below:

Na, serum	133 mEq/L
Cl, serum	100 mEq/L
K, serum	4.9 mEq/L
Bicarbonate, serum	23 mEq/L
Magnesium, serum	1.5 mEq/L
Creatinine, serum	1.4 mg/dL
Albumin, serum	4.2 g/dL
Urea nitrogen, serum	12 mg/dL
Hematocrit	33%
Hemoglobin, blood	11.2 g/dL
Leukocyte count	9200/mm^3
Platelet count	330,000/mm^3

What is the most likely diagnosis?

A. Acute prostatisis
B. Bladder carcinoma
C. Prostate hyperplasia
D. Renal calculi
E. Urinary tract infection

336. A 30-year-old woman who is taking fertility drugs, because of a strong desire to conceive experiences some unusual and troubling side effects. She feels suddenly hot for no reason, she has severe mood swings, and is feeling depressed about her visual changes. She is most likely taking which of the following?

A. Clomiphene citrate
B. Danocrine
C. Human chorionic gonadotropin
D. Pulsatile gonadotropin-releasing hormone
E. Pergonal (human gonadotropins)

337. A 33-year-old woman presents to her primary care physician because of slurred speech and a 1 year history of generalized weakness, which gets worse when she climbs stairs, combs her hair, or repeatedly lifts objects. For the past 6 months she has also noticed that she has been choking on her food. Physical examination reveals bilateral ptosis that worsens with upward gaze, a smile that resembles a snarl. After administration of 2 g of intravenous edrophonium the patient's ptosis disappears. MRI of her chest reveals an anterior mediastinal mass. What is the next best step in the treatment of this patient?

A. Azathioprine
B. Lifelong plasmapheresis
C. Mechanical ventilation for possible respiratory paralysis
D. Radiation therapy
E. Thoracotomy

338. A full-term, 3200-g neonate is delivered vaginally in an occiput-anterior fashion after a prolonged labor. Physical examination reveals the newborn to have diffuse, edematous swelling of the scalp, which extends across suture lines and the midline of the scalp. What is the most likely diagnosis?

A. Caput succedaneum
B. Cephalohematoma
C. Hydrocephalus
D. Hydrops fetalis
E. Hydronephrosis

339. A 15-year-old girl was 5 feet 8 inches tall and weighed 130 pounds at the beginning of her soccer season last fall. She presents to her primary care physician for an annual checkup. She got on the scale and was elated when it read 85 pounds. Over the winter she became very obsessed with her weight and began exercising 3 hours a day. She became very picky about food, and decreased her calories to less than 700 per day. She would cut her food into small pieces, and eat only a few bites at every meal. She would also weigh everything she consumed. Every morning when she awoke, she would weigh herself, and if she had not lost weight, she would become very scared that she was going to become fat. All of her thoughts most of the day were on food and her weight, and she would go home from class crying many days because she was upset about her weight. She had not had her period for 4 months and is not sexually active. What is the best treatment of this patient?

A. Begin fluoxetine immediately
B. Begin intensive psychotherapy
C. Begin the patient on a 3000 calorie per day diet
D. Diet education in clinic and then follow-up in clinic in 1 month
E. Hospitalize and closely monitor

The response options for items 340–342 are the same. You will be required to select one answer for each item in the set.

A. Atenolol
B. Captopril
C. Furosemide
D. Hydrochlorthiazide
E. Sodium nitroprusside
F. Terazosin
G. Valproic acid
H. Valium
I. Valtrex
J. Verapamil

For each patient with hypertension, select the most appropriate therapeutic agent.

340. A 47-year-old man with non-insulin-dependent diabetes mellitus and asthma has hypertension. He has been on medical therapy for some time now. Physical examination findings are unremarkable. Results of laboratory studies are shown below:

Electrolytes, serum

Na, serum	143 mEq/L
Cl, serum	100 mEq/L
K, serum	3.1 mEq/L
Creatinine, serum	1.0 mg/dL
Monocytes	4%

Blood, plasma, serum

Alanine aminotransferase (ALT)	10 U/L
Amylase, serum	50 U/L
Aspartate aminotransferase (AST)	10 U/L
Hematocrit	43%
Triglycerides, serum	375 mg/dL
Urea nitrogen, serum (BUN)	10 mg/dL

341. A 69-year-old man with a history of hypertension has a recent history of urinary frequency, nocturia, and decreased force of stream. Pressure/flow voiding study reveals a flow rate of 9 mL/sec with high pressures and a straining pattern. His post void residual is significant.

342. A 64-year-old man with a history of asthma and chronic bronchitis is hospitalized for an exacerbation of his asthma. Pulmonary auscultation reveals bilateral scattered wheezes with decreased breath sounds at the lung bases.

343. A 6-year-old boy is brought to his primary care physician. His mother says that she is fed up with him and cannot control his behavior. She cannot get him to go to sleep, and once he gets to sleep, he is usually up very early. During the day, he has an endless reserve of energy. If she asks him something he often forgets. She gives the example of asking him to get her book out of her bedroom, but he got sidetracked on the way and never finished the task. He is in the first grade, but his teacher feels he may have to repeat. You suspect that he may have attention deficit hyperactivity disorder. What is the most likely side effect of the medication used for this condition?

A. Alopecia
B. Bradycardia
C. Decreased appetite
D. Growth inhibition
E. Hypotension

344. A 33-year-old hirsute bachelor presents to his primary care physician with diffuse pustules over his body, but particularly in areas more covered with hair. They are growing out of his hair follicles. They do not have any pigmentation and have no central umbilication. He denies any immunologic disorders, skin allergies, or eczema. The pustules are itchy. He does not take any medications. Social history is negative for alcohol and smoking. He denies switching detergents, clothing materials, or using incense in the past few months. He says a few

of his girlfriends also have some of these pustules on random spots near hair follicles as well. He has sexual relations with all of them and has especially enjoyed doing so in his hot tub. What is the most likely explanation of these findings?

A. *Pseudomonas aeruginosa* that has been growing in his hot tub has infected his follicles
B. *Staphylococcus aureus* that has been growing in his hot tub has infected his follicles
C. *Streptococcus pyogenes* that has been growing in his hot tub has infected his follicles
D. Type I neurofibromatosis that the patient had and passed on to his girlfriends
E. Molluscum contagiosum that the patient had and passed on to his girlfriends

345. A 31-year-old woman who is 32 weeks pregnant presents to the emergency department with severe abdominal pain and vaginal bleeding. The father of the baby is unknown. Reviewing her records reveals that she is hepatitis B (anti–hepatitis B surface antigen) positive and has a positive history for herpes simplex virus. She is rubella immune, HIV negative, and Rh negative. After examination, the mother and fetus appear to be stable. What is the next most appropriate step in treating this patient?

A. Check fetal scalp pH
B. Give mother hepatitis immunoglubulin and vaccine
C. Give mother RhoGam to prevent isoimmunization
D. Induce labor since the patient is in her third trimester
E. Start acyclovir to prevent transmission to the fetus

346. A 58-year-old woman is brought into the emergency department with a history of abdominal pain followed by nausea and vomiting since earlier that morning. The patient has not passed any stools for the past 2 days and reports no flatus since the night before. Past medical history is significant for numerous abdominal surgeries, including appendectomy and three cesarean sections. On examination, the abdomen is mildly distended and the patient reports diffuse tenderness over her entire abdomen. There is no generalized rebound or involuntary guarding. Bowel sounds are high pitched. Upright abdominal x-rays show no free air under the diaphragm and multiple air-fluid levels in a stepladder orientation in the small bowel. What is the most likely diagnosis?

A. Adynamic ileus
B. Large bowel obstruction
C. Perforated large bowel
D. Small bowel obstruction (mechanical)
E. Small bowel obstruction (strangulated)

347. A 57-year-old man presents to his primary care physician because of a long history of progressive right-sided hearing loss. He is now unable to pick up the telephone and place the receiver to his right ear. He also complains of tinnitus and difficulty maintaining his balance. He has a prior medical history of benign prostatic hyperplasia. His current medications include an alpha blocker. Physical examination findings of the heart, lungs, and abdomen are unremarkable. Results of otoscopic examination are normal bilaterally. MRI of the head is performed and is shown below (Figure 347). What is the most likely diagnosis?

Figure 347

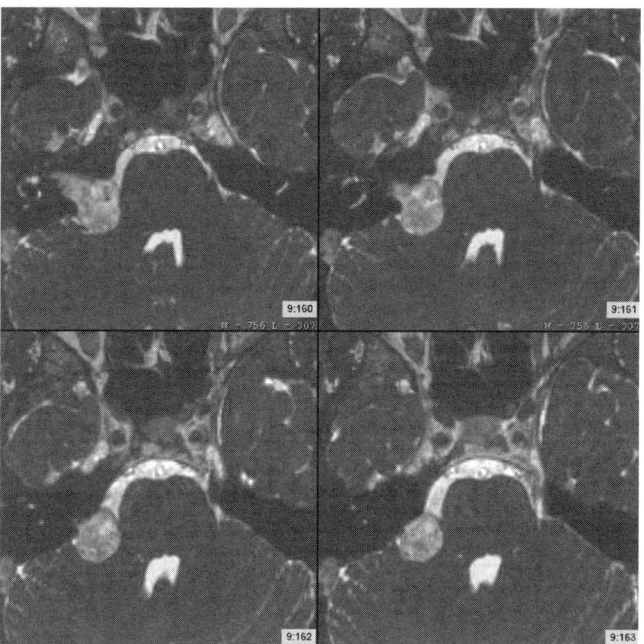

A. Acoustic neuroma
B. Brain abscess
C. Cerebellar atrophy
D. Ménière disease
E. Meningioma of the frontal lobe

348. A 3-month-old girl is brought to the pediatric clinic for evaluation of jerking movements over the past 2 days. The parents describe the movements as repetitive mixed flexor-extensor spasms. The patient has a history of herpes encephalitis, which was successfully treated. Physical examination reveals spasms of the lower extremities. Electroencephalography (EEG) reveals hypsarrhythmia. What is the most likely diagnosis?

A. Cerebral palsy
B. Grand mal seizures
C. Infantile spasms
D. Myoclonic seizures
E. Petit mal seizures

349. A two-year-old boy is brought to the pediatric clinic by his mother. She notes that the patient has been having frequent nosebleeds and gingival bleeding with brushing his teeth. Laboratory testing reveals a normal prothrombin time, prolonged activated partial thromboplastin time (APPT), and prolonged bleeding time. Von Willebrand factor antigen (vWF:Ag) and vWF actinomycin (vWF:Act) are low

and there is normal platelet aggregation. What is the genetic mode of inheritance for this patient's condition?

A. X-linked
B. Autosomal dominant
C. Autosomal recessive
D. Mitochondrial inheritance
E. Ribosomal inheritance

350. A 34-year-old nulliparous female with a 5-year history of dysmenorrhea presents to her gynecologist with increasing complaints of pelvic pain. She describes the pain as being associated with deep penetration during intercourse as well as intermittent pain with passing stool. Physical examination findings of the heart, lungs, and abdomen are within normal limits. Pelvic examination reveals a grade I cystocele, grade I rectocele, and nodularity of the uterosacral ligaments. Significant pain in the adenexa is noted on bimanual examination. Results of laboratory studies are shown below:

Electrolytes, serum

Na, serum	143 mEq/L
Cl, serum	100 mEq/L
K, serum	3.7 mEq/L
Bicarbonate, serum	24 mEq/L
Magnesium, serum	2.0 mEq/L
Creatinine, serum	1.0 mg/dL

Leukocyte count and differential

Leukocyte count	12,000/mm^3
Segmented neutrophils	75%
Bands	7%
Eosinophils	3%
Basophils	1%
Lymphocytes	27%
Monocytes	4%

Blood, plasma, serum

Alanine aminotransferase (ALT)	10 U/L
Amylase, serum	50 U/L
Aspartate aminotransferase (AST)	10 U/L
Calcium, serum	9 mg/dL
Glucose, serum	100 mg/dL
Hematocrit	33%
Urea nitrogen, serum (BUN)	10 mg/dL

Urinalysis

Urine pH	6.0
RBC count	2/HPF
WBC count	2/HPF
Nitrates	Negative
Bacteria	Negative

This patient is at increased risk for:

A. Breast cancer
B. Infertility
C. Pelvic inflammatory disease
D. Urinary tract infections
E. Uterine cancer

351. A 3-year-old girl presents to the pediatric clinic with a weeping rash consisting of many erythematous papules. She has moderate edema and the rash is severely pruritic. Her mother tells you she was diagnosed with atopic dermatitis (eczema) last year. She is being treated with topical steroids and antipruritics. What phase of eczema does this child have?

A. Phase I
B. Phase II
C. Phase III
D. Phase IV
E. Phase V

352. A 14-year-old boy is seen in the emergency department after he sustained deep second-degree burns to his hands when he fell on some hot coals during a camping trip. After evaluation, he is deemed to be at high risk for infection. Which of the following medications can be used to decrease the likelihood of infection in this patient?

A. Amoxicillin
B. Ciprofloxacin
C. Penicillin
D. Topical silver sulfadiazine
E. Topical steroid creams

353. A 24-year-old male chemistry student finally comes in to the clinic after canceling his appointment on four previous occasions. He admits that he was anxious about coming to see you because he was afraid of what you might tell him. He has a few friends, but has never been involved in an intimate relationship. He is slow to make new friends. He avoids interaction with his co-workers, and never eats lunch with them, despite repeated invitations. He tells you that he wants to join them, but is afraid that they would not like him. He tells you that last week someone mentioned that his "shoes were looking a little worn out." This really bothered him, and he immediately bought new shoes and disposed of the others. When speaking with you, he makes poor eye contact, and offers very little information on his own. What is the most likely diagnosis?

A. Avoidant personality disorder
B. Dependent personality disorder
C. Panic disorder with agoraphobia
D. Paranoid personality disorder
E. Schizoid personality disorder

354. A 38-year-old obese female from rural West Virginia presents to her primary care physician with complaints of constant fatigue, poor quality of sleep, and decrease in exercise intolerance. She reports no changes in her life recently with regard to medications, stress, and illnesses. Her husband says that she snores loudly and has done so for years. She is 5 feet 2 inches tall and weighs 350 pounds. Her temperature is 97.5°F, blood pressure 160/100 mm Hg, pulse 88 beats/min, and respirations 18 breaths/min. She has no audible wheezes or stridor. Physical examination of the heart and abdomen are within normal limits. Results of laboratory studies are shown below:

Alanine aminotransferase, serum (ALT)	15 U/L
Amylase, serum	50 U/L
Calcium, serum	9 mg/dL
Creatinine, serum	1.2 mg/dL
Na, serum	138 mEq/L
Cl, serum	95 mEq/L
K, serum	5.1 mEq/L
Hematocrit	65%

What is the most likely diagnosis?

A. Dysthymic disorder
B. Hypertension
C. Hypoventilation syndrome
D. Polycythemia vera
E. Seasonal allergies

355. A 48-year-old woman presents to her primary care physician with symptoms of menopause. She is concerned about the risk for bone loss and breast cancer. She has a family history of osteoporosis and breast cancer in a mother and sister. Physical examination findings of the heart, lung, abdomen, and pelvic area are normal. Her serum follicle-stimulating hormone and luteinizing hormone levels are elevated. What is the most appropriate therapy for this patient?

A. Calcium
B. Calcium and premarin
C. Calcium and raloxifene
D. Calcium, raloxifene, and vitamin D
E. Premarin

356. A 12-year-old girl presents to the pediatric clinic with complaints of 2 months of intermittent joint pain, swelling, and limitation of range of motion in her elbows, knees, ankles, and wrists bilaterally. She reports that her symptoms are worse in the morning. She has an intermittent low-grade fever associated with her joint pain. She denies having traveled recently outside her hometown in Florida and denies getting any recent insect bites. She admits to feeling fatigue over the past couple of months. Her erythrocyte sedimentation rate is elevated, and synovial fluid from joint space reveals a WBC count of 15,000/mm³, elevated protein, and low glucose and complement. What is the most appropriate treatment for this patient?

A. Acetaminophen
B. Inflammatory-suppression drugs and physical therapy
C. Narcotics
D. Physical therapy
E. Surgery

357. A 19-year-old woman presents to the emergency department by ambulance accompanied by her parents. She had been feeling depressed since her boyfriend sexually assaulted her 2 weeks ago, but then her mood improved abruptly 2 days ago. However, her parents found her unconscious in the bathtub with her mother's empty alprazolam prescription bottle on the floor. Physical examination reveals that she is nonresponsive. What is the most appropriate first step in the treatment of this patient?

A. Administer flumazenil

B. Administer activated charcoal

C. Obtain serum toxicology

D. Obtain intravenous access and establish airway

E. Straight catheterize bladder for urine for a urine drug screen

358. A 7-year-old boy presents to the emergency department with a history of passing a large, bloody bowel movement. Vital signs are stable. Further workup using a technetium scan localizes ectopic gastric mucosa in the lower abdomen. Failure to obliterate which structure in the developing fetus gives rise to this anomaly?

A. Cardinal veins

B. Ductus venosus

C. Omphalomesenteric duct

D. Stenson duct

E. Vitelline duct

359. A 13-year-old boy presents to the emergency department with right wrist pain after falling off his skateboard. On examination, he has multiple abrasions of the right palm, medial forearm, and elbow. An anteroposterior radiograph of the right wrist is ordered and is shown below (Figure 359). What is the most likely diagnosis?

A. Colle fracture

B. Greenstick fracture

C. Smith fracture

D. Torus fracture

E. Type IV fracture (Salter-Harris) of the right distal radius

Figure 359

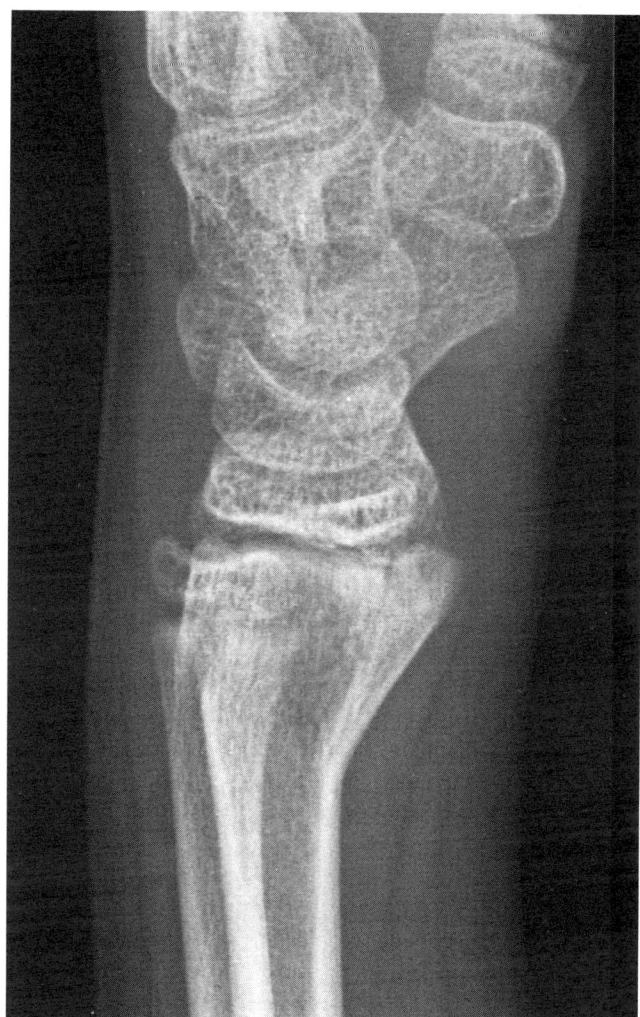

360. A 25-year-old woman presents to her primary care physician because of fear of colon cancer after reading an article in a local newspaper. The article described a prominent individual who died suddenly of metastatic colorectal cancer. She reports that she has had no rectal bleeding, abdominal fullness, or tenderness, and has never had any testing performed thus far. She does report a father who died of familial polyposis coli at age 52. What is the appropriate screening regimen for this patient?

A. Colonoscopy every year from age 25 to 35

B. Digital rectal examination yearly starting at age 40, occult blood test of stool yearly starting at age 50, and sigmoidoscopy every 3 to 5 years starting at age 50

C. Occult blood testing of the stool every year

D. Sigmoidoscopy every year from age 25 to 35

E. Total colectomy before the age of 30

361. A 26-year-old G1P0 woman at 38 weeks' gestation is found to have a blood pressure of 146/92 mmHg on a routine office visit. Her baseline pressure over the course of her prenatal care has been approximately 110/80 mmHg. The patient's urine dipstick reveals 3+ protein and repeat blood pressure was 142/94 mmHg. A 24-hour urine collection showed 356 mg protein. What is the most appropriate course of action?

A. Bed rest for the remainder of the pregnancy

B. Immediate delivery via cesarean section

C. Induction of labor for anticipated vaginal delivery

D. Start antihypertensives and magnesium sulfate immediately

E. Start seizure prophylaxis with magnesium sulfate immediately

362. A 34-year-old construction worker presents to his primary care physician because his wife is worried about his drinking. Social history reveals that he started drinking 4 or 5 years ago, and has noticed that he needs to drink much more than he used to in order to feel drunk. On occasion, he goes out with his friends, intending to have only a few drinks, but ends up drinking so much that he vomits. He wants to quit, and has tried to cut back several times, but has been unsuccessful. He has a history of gastroesophageal reflux disease, and knows that the alcohol makes his reflux worse, but he still cannot seem to cut back. For the past few months, often when he gets drunk, he gets into arguments with his wife over his drinking and the effects it has on their relationship. Which of the following scenarios would suggest a diagnosis of alcohol abuse rather than dependence?

A. An increasing alcohol tolerance

B. Continued drinking despite recurrent arguments with spouse

C. Continued drinking despite knowledge that his reflux is made worse by it

D. Recurrent instances of drinking more than intended

E. Unsuccessful efforts to cut back

363. A 6-year-old boy is brought to his pediatrician because of fatigue. He states he only gets 4 to 5 hours of sleep per night and often awakes with a headache. His father also notes that the patient snores very loudly. He denies having any fever, chills, night sweats, or abdominal pain. Physical examination of the oropharynx reveals obstructing tonsils bilaterally. The lungs are clear to auscultation, and no murmurs are heard. What is the most appropriate treatment for this patient?

A. Antibiotics

B. Observation

C. Nightime continuous positive airway pressure (CPAP)

D. Sleep with the head of the bed in an elevated position

E. Tonsillectomy

364. A 51-year-old man with a history of hyperplastic colon polyps discovered 3 years ago undergoes a follow-up colonoscopy. He has a prior medical history of hypertension and laryngeal carcinoma. His current medications include a calcium channel blocker. Physical examination reveals a well-developed man who appears his stated age. There is pigmentation of the buccal mucosa. Cardiac, pulmonary, and gastrointestinal examination findings are within normal limits. Colonoscopy reveals the presence of numerous hamartomatous polyps throughout the descending and transverse colon. Results of laboratory studies are shown below:

Leukocyte count and differential

Leukocyte count	7000/mm³
Segmented neutrophils	60%
Bands	5%
Eosinophils	4%

The most appropriate treatment is which of the following?

A. Chemotherapy (multiagent), 6-week course

B. Radiotherapy (template focused), 6-week course

C. Subtotal colectomy and external beam radiation therapy

D. Subtotal colectomy with proctectomy

E. Surveillance colonoscopy

365. A 28-year-old man presents to the ambulatory care clinic complaining of fever and a productive cough. He states that he has always been sick, particularly with fevers with productive coughs. He does not appear to be in any acute distress. Head and neck examination is remarkable for mild erythema of the pharynx. Cardiac examination has a regular rate and rhythm without murmurs, rubs, or gallops. Pulmonary examination reveals bilateral rales more prominent on the left side. Chest x-ray demonstrates bilateral cystic lesions with fluid levels in the middle and lower lung zones. What is the most likely diagnosis?

A. Bronchiectasis
B. Cystic fibrosis
C. Foreign body obstruction
D. Pneumonia
E. Sarcoidosis

366. A 28-year-old woman complains of painful menses since the inception of her periods at age 12. She has a prior medical history of recurrent urinary tract infections. She has a past surgical history of septorhinoplasty and tonsillectomy. Physical examination findings of the heart, lungs, and abdomen are within normal limits. What is the most likely explanation for these findings?

A. Elevated prostaglandins
B. Endometriosis
C. Luteinizing hormone:follicle-stimulating hormone (LH:FSH) ratio greater than 2.5
D. Ovulatory pain on the third or fourth day of menstruation
E. Pelvic adhesions

367. A 28-year-old man presents to the emergency department with rapid onset of hoarseness, difficulty swallowing, sore throat, and cough. Physical examination reveals a temperature of 38.9°C, cervical lymphadenopathy, drooling, and stridor. Physical examination findings of the heart, lungs, and abdomen are within normal limits. What is the most likely diagnosis?

A. Acute epiglottitis
B. Asthma
C. Bronchitis
D. Foreign body aspiration
E. Mononucleosis
F. Pneumonia

368. A 47-year-old man who has been the night watchman for a car dealership for the past 15 years presents to his primary care physician. His hygiene is very poor. He has had many jobs involving a trade, such as carpentry and auto mechanics, but was let go because he never seems to finish a project. His aunt raised him after his family was killed by a tornado when he was 9 years old. He was helping his father construct a storm shelter before the tornado struck. He often dreams about making the shelter but never can seem to finish it. His only friends are his aunt and uncle, even though his uncle was physically abusive to him and his aunt. He has never had a sexual relationship, and does not seem to want one. What is the highest Erickson stage of development that this patient has mastered?

A. Autonomy versus shame
B. Initiative versus guilt
C. Industry versus inferiority
D. Identity versus role confusion
E. Intimacy versus isolation

369. A 13-year-old girl moved to a new town and went to her physician to get a physical before starting school. She has no medical problems and her parents are healthy and very supportive. She denies use of medications or any substances and has no thoughts of suicide. Her affect is very restricted, and upon questioning, her physician learns that she quit school in her old town. She states that a little over a year ago she felt like her energy became really low and she did not feel like doing anything. She felt down nearly every day and she was always tired. She stopped going to school because she found herself sleeping over 12 hours every day and had a lot of trouble getting out of bed in the morning. She also stated that she has not felt very good about herself or very happy and therefore has trouble making friends. She has not had any episodes where she has felt that her mood was good. What is the most likely diagnosis?

A. Cyclothymic disorder
B. Depression (major)
C. Dysthymic disorder
D. Minor depressive disorder
E. Recurrent brief depressive disorder

370. A 22-year-old female presents to the student health clinic for a follow up examination. She was started on oral contraceptive pills (estrogen/progesterone) and complains of increasing acne. She states that she has tried using topical benzoyl peroxide without improvement. Physical examination is unremarkable except for facial acne. What is the most appropriate course of action to take?

A. Change the pill to one with less androgenic activity
B. Change the pill to one with less estrogenic activity
C. Change the pill to one with less progestin activity
D. Maintain the current dosage and reevaluate in 3 months
E. Suggest that the patient use another form of birth control

BLOCK 1	BLOCK 2	BLOCK 3	BLOCK 4
1. **A**	47. **C**	93. **D**	140. **C**
2. **A**	48. **B**	94. **C**	141. **E**
3. **E**	49. **E**	95. **D**	142. **A**
4. **C**	50. **E**	96. **E**	143. **B**
5. **C**	51. **A**	97. **E**	144. **C**
6. **A**	52. **B**	98. **B**	145. **A**
7. **C**	53. **A**	99. **A**	146. **E**
8. **D**	54. **B**	100. **D**	147. **C**
9. **A**	55. **C**	101. **C**	148. **B**
10. **I**	56. **E**	102. **D**	149. **B**
11. **G**	57. **B**	103. **E**	150. **D**
12. **D**	58. **C**	104. **C**	151. **B**
13. **E**	59. **B**	105. **D**	152. **A**
14. **A**	60. **A**	106. **B**	153. **B**
15. **C**	61. **A**	107. **E**	154. **C**
16. **A**	62. **B**	108. **D**	155. **D**
17. **E**	63. **B**	109. **C**	156. **A**
18. **B**	64. **A**	110. **D**	157. **A**
19. **B**	65. **D**	111. **B**	158. **D**
20. **B**	66. **C**	112. **D**	159. **A**
21. **B**	67. **D**	113. **E**	160. **A**
22. **C**	68. **B**	114. **J**	161. **C**
23. **D**	69. **B**	115. **A**	162. **H**
24. **C**	70. **B**	116. **F**	163. **D**
25. **E**	71. **A**	117. **G**	164. **A**
26. **D**	72. **F**	118. **E**	165. **D**
27. **E**	73. **E**	119. **B**	166. **D**
28. **B**	74. **B**	120. **C**	167. **A**
29. **D**	75. **F**	121. **A**	168. **C**
30. **D**	76. **E**	122. **D**	169. **C**
31. **C**	77. **C**	123. **C**	170. **E**
32. **D**	78. **A**	124. **A**	171. **C**
33. **A**	79. **D**	125. **D**	172. **B**
34. **A**	80. **C**	126. **A**	173. **C**
35. **E**	81. **A**	127. **D**	174. **C**
36. **A**	82. **E**	128. **A**	175. **C**
37. **D**	83. **B**	129. **B**	176. **C**
38. **A**	84. **E**	130. **D**	177. **B**
39. **E**	85. **B**	131. **B**	178. **A**
40. **A**	86. **A**	132. **A**	179. **C**
41. **C**	87. **E**	133. **A**	180. **C**
42. **D**	88. **B**	134. **B**	181. **A**
43. **E**	89. **D**	135. **E**	182. **D**
44. **B**	90. **B**	136. **A**	183. **A**
45. **C**	91. **B**	137. **E**	184. **B**
46. **E**	92. **E**	138. **B**	185. **B**
		139. **C**	

BLOCK 5	BLOCK 6	BLOCK 7	BLOCK 8
186. **B**	233. **C**	279. **C**	325. **A**
187. **E**	234. **D**	280. **C**	326. **E**
188. **D**	235. **B**	281. **A**	327. **C**
189. **A**	236. **C**	282. **D**	328. **E**
190. **C**	237. **B**	283. **B**	329. **E**
191. **F**	238. **E**	284. **D**	330. **D**
192. **H**	239. **D**	285. **A**	331. **D**
193. **C**	240. **A**	286. **B**	332. **D**
194. **B**	241. **C**	287. **B**	333. **C**
195. **E**	242. **A**	288. **E**	334. **A**
196. **E**	243. **B**	289. **B**	335. **C**
197. **A**	244. **B**	290. **D**	336. **A**
198. **D**	245. **B**	291. **B**	337. **E**
199. **E**	246. **B**	292. **E**	338. **A**
200. **A**	247. **C**	293. **D**	339. **E**
201. **A**	248. **A**	294. **C**	340. **C**
202. **A**	249. **A**	295. **A**	341. **F**
203. **C**	250. **B**	296. **B**	342. **J**
204. **A**	251. **G**	297. **C**	343. **D**
205. **E**	252. **D**	298. **C**	344. **A**
206. **A**	253. **A**	299. **A**	345. **C**
207. **A**	254. **E**	300. **B**	346. **D**
208. **A**	255. **A**	301. **C**	347. **A**
209. **B**	256. **B**	302. **C**	348. **C**
210. **B**	257. **B**	303. **A**	349. **B**
211. **C**	258. **D**	304. **E**	350. **B**
212. **C**	259. **B**	305. **B**	351. **B**
213. **E**	260. **B**	306. **A**	352. **D**
214. **D**	261. **E**	307. **A**	353. **A**
215. **C**	262. **A**	308. **E**	354. **C**
216. **B**	263. **D**	309. **C**	355. **D**
217. **E**	264. **C**	310. **E**	356. **B**
218. **A**	265. **D**	311. **E**	357. **D**
219. **C**	266. **D**	312. **B**	358. **E**
220. **C**	267. **C**	313. **E**	359. **C**
221. **A**	268. **D**	314. **B**	360. **D**
222. **A**	269. **D**	315. **E**	361. **C**
223. **D**	270. **B**	316. **E**	362. **B**
224. **B**	271. **E**	317. **B**	363. **E**
225. **B**	272. **A**	318. **C**	364. **E**
226. **A**	273. **A**	319. **C**	365. **A**
227. **C**	274. **A**	320. **B**	366. **A**
228. **D**	275. **B**	321. **C**	367. **A**
229. **E**	276. **A**	322. **A**	368. **B**
230. **C**	277. **C**	323. **A**	369. **C**
231. **A**	278. **A**	324. **B**	370. **A**
232. **C**			

1. **A.** Modern views of the pathogenesis indicate that there is a major role for *Helicobacter pylori* in the pathophysiology of peptic ulcer disease. This urease-producing organism colonizes the gastric antral mucosa in 100% of patients with duodenal ulcer and 70% of patients with gastric ulcer. Eradication of this organism is that mainstay of therapy for ulcer disease.

B. Classic teaching regarding the pathogenesis of peptic ulcer disease considers impaired blood flow as a key contributor to this condition. Modern views of peptic ulcer disease dispute this finding.

C. Impaired gastric epithelial cell turnover is not felt to contribute to the current pathogenesis of ulcer disease.

D. Prostaglandin inhibition, while accounting for salicylate and nonsteroidal antiinflammatory agent ulcer disease, actually contributes to less than 30% of cases of gastric ulcer.

E. Thinning of the mucous layer may occur as a result of toxic effects of *H. pylori* on the duodenal mucosa; however, on its own it is a small contributor to the pathophysiology of peptic ulcer disease.

2. **A.** In addition to antibiotics and drainage, improving the clearance of secretions by using bronchodilators and chest physiotherapy may be beneficial.

B. Bronchoscopy and any surgery are inappropriate at this stage.

C. Lung transplantation is not appropriate at this stage.

D. Respiratory isolation is unlikely to be of benefit for this patient.

E. Surgical resection is not indicated at this stage.

3. **E.** This patient has symptoms of ulcerative colitis. Typical symptoms include bloody and watery diarrhea. Pregnancy does not exacerbate this disease. Inflammatory bowel disease can be associated with anal fissure disease. The fissures are typically lateral in location, in contrast to idiopathic anal fissures, which are in the midline. Severe disease is associated with an increased risk for spontaneous abortion and premature labor. Treatment consists of a low-residue diet, antidiarrheals, and sulfasalazine.

A. Appendicitis is typically associated with the acute onset of periumbilical pain, nausea, and vomiting.

B. Gastroesophageal reflux occurs postprandially and is associated with midepigastric pain.

C. Hepatitis is associated with right upper quadrant pain and elevation of liver function tests (transaminases).

D. Hyperemesis gravidarum is associated with protracted nausea and vomiting with pregnancy.

4. **C.** The patient described has meconium ileus and must be evaluated for cystic fibrosis. Either a sweat chloride level should be determined or the patient can undergo genetic testing for diagnosis.

A. A child that has not passed meconium within the first 24 hours needs further evaluation.

B. Transrectal biopsy is indicated if there is evidence of Hirschsprung disease, which would present similarly but with a dilated proximal bowel on abdominal radiograph.

D. A repeat abdominal radiograph is unlikely to reveal any new information. This procedure is not indicated.

E. This neonate is stable and does not require laparotomy. This procedure is not indicated.

5. **C.** This patient likely has testicular carcinoma. The peak incidence is between the ages of 20 and 40 years. Cryptorchid testes are at increased risk. Early orchiopexy may protect against testis cancer but not always. Seminoma accounts for 50% of cases and is the most common pathology seen. Seminoma often presents with painless enlargement of the testis. It is radiosensitive and has a high cure rate.

A. Embryonal cell carcinoma (20%) is a nonseminomatous germ cell tumor of the testis. Such tumors often present with pain in the testis or metastasis. Serum human chorionic gonadotropin levels are often increased in these individuals.

B. Endodermal sinus tumor (5%) is a common testis tumor in newborn males. It is extremely rare in adults.

D. Teratocarcinoma (20%) is a nonseminomatous germ cell tumor of the testis. It is a combination of teratoma and embryonal carcinoma.

E. Teratoma (15%) is a malignant nonseminomatous germ cell tumor of the testis.

6. **A.** Fibroadenoma is a lobular, firm, well-circumscribed solitary mass that is common in young females. Surgical excision is the treatment of choice in women over the age of 25. Younger patients may be treated with needle cytology and surveillance.

B. Fibrocystic change is associated with breast tenderness and swelling premenstrually. Patients with severe atypia or hyperplasia on biopsy are at risk for breast carcinoma.

C. Sarcoma of the breast represents a small percentage of breast cancers and is more common in women over the age of 40.

D. Infiltrating ductal cell carcinoma is the most common form of breast cancer. Lesions are typically hard, scirrhous, and infiltrating.

E. Intraductal papilloma is the most common cause of bloody nipple discharge (90% of the time) and is a benign condition. The papilloma arises from an isolated mammary duct, which should be excised.

7. **C.** This patient is likely a drug abuser. Such patients often complain of chronic pain, often related to previous trauma. Chronic back pain or other orthopedic pain related to an old injury and chronic headache are the two most common complaints. This patient only has pain relief to his analgesics of choice (pentazocine and meperidine).

A. This patient does not display features of chronic lumbar pain syndrome.

B. Physical examination reveals no evidence of deformity of the lumbar spine.

D. There is no history of or physical examination findings of prior lumbar spine fractures.

E. This patient does not have a somatiform pain disorder.

8. **D.** *Staphylococcus aureus* respiratory infections are characterized by chest pain, systemic toxicity, and dyspnea. It is typical in tracheally intubated hospitalized patients. A lobar infiltrate and gram-positive cocci in clusters is found on imaging and sputum studies, respectively.

A. Aspiration pneumonia is usually anaerobic, more common in alcoholics, and shows organisms with mixed morphology on Gram stain.

B. *Haemophilus influenzae* is common within the first 5 days of hospitalization. This organism is more common in smokers and those with chronic obstructive pulmonary disorder. Typically a lobar pneumonia will result, and pleomorphic gram-negative rods can be seen on Gram stain.

C. *Mycobacterium tuberculosis* infection will show white blood cells but no organisms on Gram stain.

E. *Streptococcus pneumoniae* will also cause a lobar pneumonia. Gram stain shows gram-positive diplococci. It is more likely to present within the first 5 days of hospitalization.

9. **A.** Alport syndrome is an X-linked-dominant condition with associated abnormalities of the basement membrane of the eye, cochlea, and glomerulus. Affected individuals have nephritis and high-frequency sensorineural hearing loss. Progression to end-stage renal disease occurs after childhood.

10. **I.** This newborn has evidence of posterior urethral valves. This is the most common obstructive urethral lesion in newborns and is found at the distal prostatic urethra. Treatment consists of valve ablation.

11. **G.** This newborn has congenital nephrotic syndrome. This condition appears within the first 6 months of life and is common in persons of Scandinavian descent. Placentomegaly is common. Proteinuria and elevated serum creatinine are typical. Unfortunately, most children die due to infection or renal failure by age 5.

12. **D.** The clinical scenario reveals a history of a patient presumably with Guillain-Barré syndrome. Even though the natural history of the disease is self-limiting in nature, plasmapheresis is the only treatment shown to both decrease the likelihood of persistent neurologic deficits and hasten recovery in the acute setting. Albumin-cytologic dissociation is the classic finding from cerebrospinal fluid analysis.

A. Although intravenous immunoglobulin is sometimes substituted for plasmapheresis, specifically in children and adults with cardiovascular problems, this treatment has been shown to be associated with higher rates of recurrence.

B. Although this disease is associated with antecedent infection with *Clostridium jejuni*, it is believed to be immunologic in nature and not associated with active infection.

C. Although fluids, pressors, and heparin may be needed in the acute setting, they do not affect the course of future neurologic deficits. Intravenous immunoglobulin can decrease the duration of the acute phase.

E. This patient would benefit most from plasmapheresis.

13. **E.** Anal fissure is a split in the midline of the posterior anoderm 90% of the time. This is the most common location of anal fissures. Symptoms of acute fissures include tearing pain on defecation and blood in the stool or on the toilet paper. Surgical therapy is reserved for chronic, nonhealing fissures, and the procedure of choice is lateral sphincterotomy.

A. There is no role for intravenous antibiotic therapy in the management of acute anal fissures.

B. There is no role for oral antibiotic therapy in the management of acute anal fissures.

C. Rubber band ligation is an appropriate treatment for hemorrhoids.

D. Treatment of choice for acute fissures includes stool softeners, sitz baths, and dietary bulking agents.

14. **A.** The natural response to a fall is to extend a hand in order to decrease the impact to the rest of the body. When the outstretched limb strikes the ground, however, the distal radius is commonly fractured. This is called a Colles fracture. Radiographic assessment of this type of fracture commonly shows fracture of the distal radius with or without a fracture line and dorsal angulation.

Figure 14

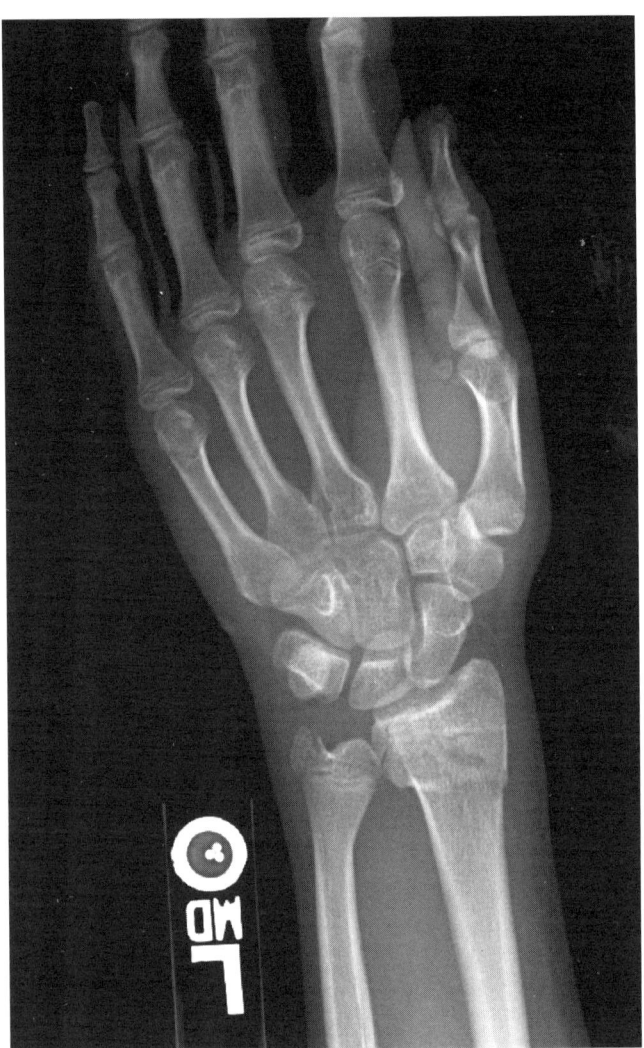

B. Like a torus fracture, a greenstick fracture is found in children and also is an incomplete break. In this case, the long bone resembles an immature branch that has been broken and is subsequently bowed. One surface will have displacement while the other will have a curved appearance.

C. A Smith fracture is also a fracture of the distal radius but with volar angulation of the distal fragment. This fracture also occurs after a fall onto an outstretched hand.

D. A torus fracture can be easily differentiated from other fractures of the distal radius. You will find a curve in the straight edge of the distal radius as you trace its edge. Indeed, this curved disruption is the buckle that results from a bending force. In the upper extremity, this can result from a fall on an outstretched hand; in the lower extremity, this can result from jumping or falling from greater than 6 feet above the ground. These fractures are frequently found in children.

E. The Salter-Harris Classification defines five types of epiphyseal fractures. Salter-Harris type IV is an epiphyseal break in which the fracture line runs from the joint surface through the epiphyseal plate, epiphysis, and metastasis. There is no involvement of the epiphysis in our patient's radiograph.

15. **C.** Sensitivity and specificity of a test do not change. They are fixed regardless of the population's disease status. This makes them much less useful clinically because they assume you already know whether the patient has the disease. Positive and negative predictive values are much more useful clinically because they change according to the prevalence of disease in a population. A good clinician uses this to his or her advantage. For example, it is not a good idea to get a stress test on someone in their twenties or thirties without many risk factors because the number of false positives in this age group is high due to the low prevalence of disease.

A. Sensitivity stays the same.

B. Positive predictive value increases.

D. Sensitivity stays the same and positive predictive value increases.

E. Sensitivity stays the same and positive predictive value increases.

16. **A.** Mastitis can be treated with oral antibiotics, commonly dicloxacillin; patients should continue to breast-feed to prevent intraductal accumulation of infected material.
    The condition is generally unilateral. The usual cause is *Staphylococcus aureus*. There are two forms: sporadic and epidemic.

B and **C.** Patients are encouraged to continue breast-feeding.

D. Antibiotics are the treatment of choice for mastitis.

E. Antibiotics are warranted for mastitis as well as the continuance of breast-feeding.

17. **E.** Wegener granulomatosis is a systemic vasculitis that involves the upper and lower respiratory tracts and kidneys. A presentation dominated by pulmonary findings is not unusual. Some patients are asymptomatic. Other typical symptoms include polyarthralgias or myalgias, oral or nasal ulcerations, and palpable purpura or petechiae.

A. Alveolar hemorrhage often presents acutely with significant hemoptysis.

B. Anti–glomerular basement membrane disease is found in younger male patients and is a rapidly progressive glomerulonephritis.

C. The significant morbidity of Churg-Strauss syndrome is caused by coronary arteritis and myocarditis. Other associations include eosinophilia and asthma.

D. Pulmonary abscess typically presents with fever and night sweats. Associated abnormalities on chest x-ray range from lobular consolidation with air bronchograms to diffuse patchy interstitial infiltrates.

18. B. Acute onset of perirectal pain associated with straining and blood on the toilet tissue suggests the diagnosis of fissure-in-ano. Risk factors for the development of this condition include straining during bowel movements, constipation, and anal intercourse. Ninety percent of cases occur in the posterior midline, while the remainder occur in the anterior midline. Medical treatment includes stool softeners, dietary bulk, and sitz baths. Surgical treatment is reserved for chronic, nonhealing fissures.

A. External hemorrhoids are abnormally dilated anal veins below the dentate line. They may show a skin tag and occasionally erode through the skin.

C. Fistula-in-ano describes perianal pain and a mass in the perianal skin associated with discharge of liquid from the perianal area.

D. Internal hemorrhoids are veins with mucosa above the dentate line. They are prone to prolapse and bleeding.

E. Proctitis may be either inflammatory or caused by radiation exposure. Inflammatory diseases might include ulcerative colitis, whereas radiation proctitis is noted following radiotherapy. Treatment for both conditions might involve steroids and steroid enemas.

19. B. Hyperglycemia will cause a hypertonic hyponatremia due to an excess of osmotically active particles in serum. When blood glucose becomes acutely elevated, water is drawn from the cells to the extracellular space, diluting the serum Na and increasing serum osmolality. Infusion of hypertonic solutions containing osmotically active osmoles (e.g., mannitol) may also cause this. This patient gives no history of taking any medicines, drugs, or radiocontrast agents, so the onset of diabetes mellitus with hyperglycemia.

A. Dehydration is a hypovolemic hypotonic hyponatremia. Urine Na will be less than 10 mEq/L and the patient will show signs of fluid deprivation.

C. Hyperlipidemia (or hyperproteinemia) will cause an isotonic hyponatremia because plasma osmolality is unaffected by lipids or proteins. A decreased volume of water results, so that the Na concentration in total plasma volume is decreased. Because the Na concentration in the plasma water is actually normal, this situation is usually called a pseudohyponatremia.

D. Nephrotic syndrome is a hypervolemic hypotonic hyponatremia. The kidneys are working ineffectively and Na and water are retained, producing edema and a urine Na of less than 10 mEq/L.

E. SIADH will cause a hypotonic hyponatremia. This is usually a euvolemia and in such a situation, determinations of urine osmolality and urine Na can be useful to help determine a diagnosis. SIADH is usually a disease of the CNS that results in increased production of ADH and resulting hyponatremia, decreased serum osmolality, inappropriately increased urine osmolality, and urine Na greater than 20 mEq/L.

20. B. The key to this scenario is bullae that rupture almost immediately after they appear. This is indicative of staphylococcal scalded skin caused by *Staphylococcus aureus*. This rash begins with diffuse erythema followed 12 to 24 hours later by bullae that enclose sterile fluid. After rupturing, the lesions leave a red, weeping surface. A positive Nikolsky sign (epidermal separation upon light rubbing) is also an associated feature. This microbe can also cause bullous impetigo, but this rash begins as macules that lead to bullae with an erythematous base. *Staphylococcus aureus* can be cultured from fluid within the lesions. Bullous impetigo can unfortunately be confused with child abuse because it may resemble cigarette burns.

A. This presentation is not typical for *Haemophilus influenzae*.

C. This presentation is not typical for beta-hemolytic streptococcus. This agent is a common cause of pharyngitis.

D. This presentation is not typical for *Sarcoptes*. Scabies is an infection of the skin by a contagious mite and results in pruritus.

E. This presentation is not typical for *Strongyloides*. These infections are uncommon in the United States.

21. B. This patient has an imperforate hymen. She has never had a menarche/menses because the imperforate hymen has not allowed her menses to egress. She should have started menarche well within the past four years because thelarche occurred at age 9 (breast bud formation), and indeed she did, but her menses did not pass on account of the imperforate hymen blocking its path. This would be a case of primary amenorrhea. Hematocolpos is an accumulation of menstrual blood because of an obstruction of the introitus.

A. A Bartholin gland cyst would be on one side of the introitus and exquisitely painful.

C. Rectocele is unlikely because she is so young. This would be distention of the rectum through the vagina.

D. Child sexual abuse must always be suspected and is to be reported to the correct authorities when it is suspected. This is not the most likely choice from this history and presentation.

E. Uterine prolapse typically occurs after multiple childbirths.

22. **C.** This is a rare but significant side effect of thioridazine. It is important to periodically monitor blood pressure in patients taking this medication.

A. Agranulocytosis is a side effect of another antipsychotic, clozapine.

B. Delayed ejaculation is a side effect of some of the selective serotonin reuptake inhibitors, such as Zoloft.

D. Pigmented retinopathy is not an adverse reaction of thioridazine.

E. Weight gain can also be a problem with some of the selective serotonin reuptake inhibitors, such as paroxetine.

23. **D.** All patients with an indwelling catheter will eventually develop bacteriuria. After the catheter has been in place for approximately 10 days, nearly all patients will have asymptomatic bacteriuria. This patient should not receive antibiotic therapy unless he becomes symptomatic and develops fever or chills. Treatment of patients with bacteriuria without symptoms will lead to development of resistant organisms, which will ultimately become a problem when the patient develops a true urinary tract infection.

A. This patient should not receive antibiotic therapy when the catheter is removed unless there is clinical evidence of infection.

B. Gross hematuria in the absence of a positive urinalysis or urine culture result and should not be treated with antibiotics.

C. As mentioned above, pyuria in the absence of clinical evidence of infection should not be treated with antibiotics.

E. Patients with indwelling Foley catheters who receive a urine culture may grow two organisms. These individuals should not receive antibiotic therapy unless they have clinical evidence of infection.

24. **C.** This patient has Reiter syndrome, which is a special type of reactive arthritis characterized by arthritis, urethritis, and conjunctivitis. Reactive arthritis seems to be precipitated by infectious diarrhea (due to *Salmonella, Shigella, Campylobacter,* or *Yersinia*) or genitourinary infection (*Chlamydia*) and usually occurs within 3 weeks after infection. Keratoderma blenorrhagica, as described in the question, is the classic skin lesion of Reiter syndrome and mimics pustular psoriasis. In addition, balanitis circinata, which manifests as shallow painless ulcers on the penis, is also seen in Reiter syndrome.

A. Bamboo spine is not a common feature of Reiter syndrome.

B. *Chlamydia* infection on Gram stain is not a common feature of Reiter syndrome.

D. Mitral valve stenosis is not a common feature of Reiter syndrome.

E. Pleural effusion is not a common feature of Reiter syndrome.

25. **E.** In well-controlled diabetics without complaints, induction of labor is undertaken at 38 to 40 weeks given the increased risk for fetal death after 40 weeks. This is possible because of maternal glucose instability (with possible acidosis) and placental insufficiency.

A. Given the increased risk for fetal death, this is not an appropriate selection.

B. The patient is a well-controlled diabetic—no need to check hemoglobin A1C levels at this time. In addition, serial ultrasonography is performed every 4 to 6 weeks after 30 weeks.

C. Given the increased risk for fetal death, this is not an appropriate selection.

D. There is no indication for cesarean section.

26. **D.** Sickle cell anemia is the most common cause of hemolytic anemia in the African-American population. It is also the most common autosomal-recessive disorder in African Americans. Sickle cell anemia results from a valine for a glutamine substitution in the sixth amino acid position of the beta globin chain. Under deoxygenation, RBCs distort to a sickled shape, resulting in chronic hemolytic anemia. These sickled cells can also cause microvascular obstruction, which leads to tissue ischemia and infarction. Sickling of cells can be exacerbated by hypoxia, acidosis, and increased or decreased temperature and dehydration. Common manifestations include pallor, jaundice, splenomegaly, systolic ejection murmur in the pulmonic region, and dactylitis in infants.

A. Anemia of chronic disease is hypochromic and microcytic.

B. There is no reason to suspect a ferritin deficiency in this case.

C. This child has no evidence of hereditary spherocytosis.

E. This child has no evidence of transient erythroblastopenia.

27. **E.** Thiamine should always be given to alcohol-dependent patients before they are given fluids and electrolytes. Glucose depletes thiamine stores. Alcoholics usually have poor caloric intake, which leads to a depletion of thiamine and predisposes the patient to developing Wernicke-Korsakoff disease.

A. Carbamazepine has been used successfully to treat alcohol withdrawal, but usually only in mild to moderate withdrawal. This patient may have had a seizure earlier that day and is having auditory hallucinations. This indicates that it is a more severe withdrawal episode. Lorazepam would be a better choice.

B. Folic acid is necessary for an alcoholic, but it is not the first thing that should be given.

C. This may help for the patient's hallucinations, but is not the first thing that should be done.

D. Sodium bicarbonate is usually only given in severe cases of metabolic alkalosis. It is not necessary in this patient.

28. **B.** This patient likely has bulimia nervosa. Bulimia is characterized by recurrent episodes of binge eating followed by attempts to prevent any weight gain. The symptoms must occur at least twice a week for 3 months, and the individual's self image is influenced by his or her body shape and weight.

A. Anorexic individuals would not have a normal BMI.

C. This patient has findings consistent with bulimia nervosa.

D. Kluver-Bucy syndrome is also characterized by hyperphagia, but this individual does not meet any other criteria for this particular syndrome.

E. This patient has findings consistent with bulimia nervosa.

29. **D.** The most likely diagnosis is an unconjugated hyperbilirubinemia from hemolysis secondary to a hemoglobinopathy such as sickle cell disease. Bilirubin levels greater than 5 mg/dL are considered abnormal in the neonate, and a conjugated, or direct, bilirubin level of greater than 2 mg/dL or 15% of the total bilirubin is consistent with conjugated hyperbilirubinemia. In addition, the child's history, presentation, and laboratory studies reveal a picture of hemolysis and anemia.

A. ABO incompatibility is another cause of unconjugated hyperbilirubinemia; however, one would expect a positive Coombs test result in this scenario.

B. Biliary atresia is a cause of conjugated hyperbilirubinemia.

C. Dubin-Johnson syndrome is a cause of conjugated hyperbilirubinemia.

E. There is no evidence to suggest an underlying malignancy in this patient.

30. **D.** Animal bites on the hand should be left open because closed wound infections of the hand may result in loss of function. Amoxicillin/clavulonate or ampicillin/sulbactam are the preferred antibiotics. The duration of therapy is 10 to 14 days.

A. Ampicillin/sulbactam is the antibiotic of choice for cat bites.

B. The wound should not be closed. It should be left open with wet to dry dressings to be changed daily as needed.

C. Thirty percent to 50% of cat bites become infected and should be treated with prophylactic antibiotics.

E. Penicillin is the antibiotic of choice for human bites.

31. **C.** On subsequent pregnancies, there is a 25% to 30% increased risk for developing preeclampsia given her prior history. Aspirin has been shown to decrease this risk. Antihypertensives and magnesium sulfate are not usually given for prophylaxis, and there is no reason that this patient would be at increased risk for delivery by cesarean section.

A. This patient is at risk for developing preeclampsia because of her prior obstetric history.

B. Antihypertensives and magnesium sulfate are not given prophylactically to prevent preeclampsia.

D. This patient is at no increased risk for delivery by cesarean section.

E. This patient is at increased risk for the development of preeclampsia.

32. **D.** The patient has a suspected diagnosis of coronary artery disease, which can be confirmed with an exercise stress test. Symptoms include angina associated with activity or emotional upset, relieved quickly by rest or nitroglycerine.

A. Cardiac echocardiography is indicated if ECG and cardiac enzymes shows the possibility of a myocardial infarction (MI).

B. Chest radiography will help diagnose a pneumonia, but physical examination of this patient's lungs showed that they were normal, ruling out this diagnosis.

C. Coronary angiography is also indicated if an MI is suspected and can be used to identify the precise location of a thrombus. It is usually performed in the setting of an acute MI with the goal of mechanical revascularization.

E. The patient did not have any right upper quadrant pain or tenderness, and the patient's pain is not associated with meals or colic. It is unlikely to be gallstones.

33. **A.** Status epilepticus is a medical emergency and is associated with a 20% mortality rate. It is defined as a seizure that lasts greater than 15 to 30 minutes or recurrent seizures between which the patient does not return to consciousness. Immediate management consists of assessing the airway, assuring that the patient is breathing and has a heartbeat (ABCs). Next, intravenous benzodiazepines and a loading dose of phenytoin are administered for treatment.

B. Phenobarbital is preferred in neonates and young infants who experience status epilepticus.

C. Ethosuximide has no role in the treatment of status epilepticus.

D. Valproic acid is not indicated for this condition.

Figure 34

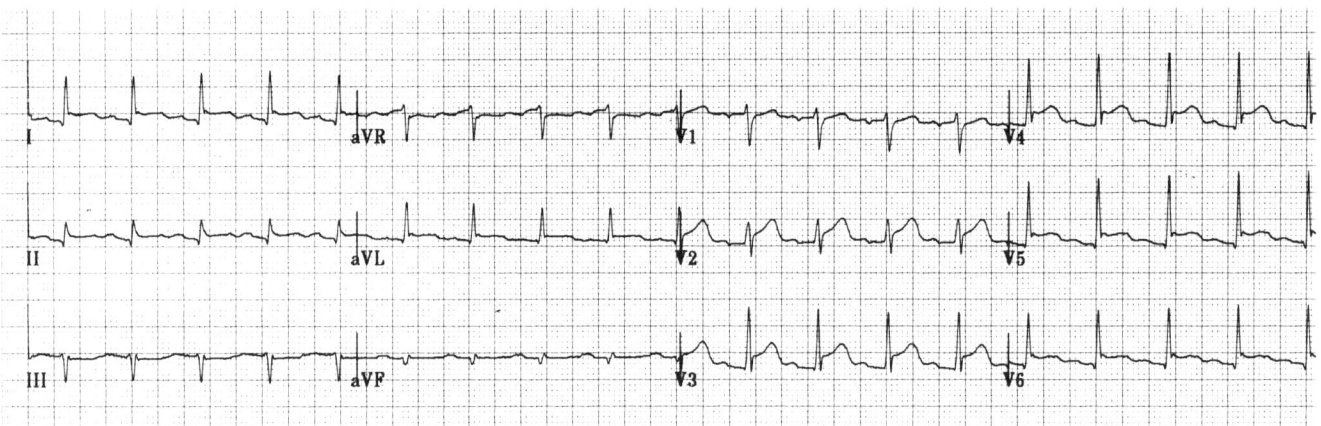

E. Although continuous monitoring is appropriate, intravenous medication is required to prevent recurrence of seizures.

34. **A.** This is the presentation of acute pericarditis. The chest pain is usually pleuritic, although it can present as anginal pain. Two key features of the disease is chest pain that gets worse when the patient leans forward and a pericardial friction rub. The rub is present in 85% of patients with acute pericarditis. The ECG is characterized by diffuse ST segment elevation, as is present with our patient. The first step in the management of this patient involves reducing pericardial inflammation. This can be achieved by the use of aspirin or nonsteroidal antiinflammatory drugs (NSAIDs).

B. Although a chest x-ray is not the best next step in the management of this patient, it does play a significant role in these patients. An important finding is new cardiomegaly. If this is present in a patient with acute pericarditis, then follow-up echocardiography should be performed to rule out pericardial effusion.

C. A potential life-threatening sequela of pericarditis is cardiac tamponade due to pericardial effusion. In this scenario, inflammation of the pericardium causes fluid exudation around the heart into the pericardial sac. This increased fluid compresses the heart and thus impairs its filling. In all patients with acute pericarditis, pericardial effusion or tamponade must be ruled out. Although tamponade is a clinical diagnosis, echocardiography can reveal the presence of fluid in the pericardial sac, which indicates effusion.

D. If there is evidence of effusion or tamponade, then pericardiocentesis is indicated. This will relieve the pressure around the heart and restore cardiac filling.

E. This management option delves into finding a cause for the pericarditis. Viral and idiopathic pericarditis are by far the most common diagnoses made. Both are successfully treated with salicylates or NSAIDs and pericardiocentesis for effusion or tamponade. If the etiology is unknown and the disease persists, then a pericardial biopsy can be helpful in establishing the etiology.

35. **E.** Toxic shock syndrome (TSS) is usually caused by staphylococci but may also be caused by *Streptococcus*. It is more common in women of menstruating age due to use of superabsorbant tampons. TSS is characterized by high fever (above 102°F), vomiting, watery diarrhea, myalgias, confusion, and headache. An erythematous macular rash may be present with desquamation 1 to 2 weeks later. The rash begins on the trunk and spreads to the arms and legs, involving palms and soles.

A. Botulism would be uncommon to present with sore throat, myalgias, or rash.

B. Kawasaki disease occurs in children and consists of at least 5 days of fever with desquamation, conjunctivitis, rash, lymphadenopathy, and oral changes.

C. This patient does not have Lyme disease. There is no mention of the characteristic bulls-eye rash. Not usually associated with desquamation.

D. There is no history of camping or tick bites. Vomiting and diarrhea are not usually associated with Rocky Mountain spotted fever.

36. **A.** Because of this patient's age and smoking, the use of a combined oral contraceptive pill (due to the estrogen component) is contraindicated. Such pills have been shown to increase the risk for cardiovascular disease, and the dose-related hypercoagulability caused by oral contraceptives has been associated with increased risk for heart attack, stroke, and deep venous thrombosis.

B. There is no contraindication to condom use in this case.

C. There is no contraindication for use of a diaphragm in this case.

D. An intrauterine device would be an appropriate choice of contraception.

E. There is no contraindication for progestin-only pill in this case.

37. D. Multiple myeloma is a malignancy of monoclonal proliferation of plasma cells of the bone marrow. It is characterized by lytic bone lesions that commonly cause rib and back pain. The lesions are created from accelerated osteoclast activity that leads to hypercalcemia and subsequent renal failure. Light chains from increased antibody production can be detected in the urine; however, dipstick evaluation is commonly negative for protein. Pancytopenia often leads to increased susceptibility to pneumonias and pyelonephritis.

A. Chronic myelogenous leukemia does produce thrombocytopenia and anemia, but a characteristic blast crisis usually creates a leukocytosis.

B. Hyperparathyroidism is a cause of hypercalcemia, but it would not explain the pancytopenia.

C. Lymphoma is characterized by lymphadenopathy and nonspecific symptoms of fever, night sweats, and lethargy.

E. Waldenström macroglobulinemia is a malignancy of lymphoplasmacytoid cells of the bone marrow that secrete IgM. The disease is characterized by hepatosplemomegaly, lymphadenopathy, pancytopenia, and absence of the bone lesions and hypercalcemia seen in multiple myeloma.

38. A. This patient has acute stress disorder, which occurs when an individual has been exposed to a traumatic event, and the person experienced, witnessed, or was confronted with an event or events that involved actual or threatened or serious injury, or a threat to the physical integrity of self or others. In addition, the person's response involved intense fear, helplessness, or horror. Other associated symptoms often include depersonalization, derealization, dissociative amnesia, detachment, flashbacks, and nightmares. The individual avoids stimuli that bring about recollections of the trauma. Symptoms of anxiety or increased arousal are also present, and the symptoms cause impairment in functioning. Symptoms of acute stress disorder occur within 4 weeks of the event and last for a minimum of 2 days and a maximum of 4 weeks.

B. Generalized anxiety disorder is characterized by excessive anxiety or worry over numerous events or activities occurring more days than not for at least 6 months.

C. Major depressive episode would not be the diagnosis if symptoms of hyperarousal, efforts to avoid recollection of the trauma, and reexperience of the trauma were the most prominent symptoms.

D. Panic disorder consists of recurrent or unexpected panic attacks that occur suddenly and reach a peak within 10 minutes, unlike this individual's symptoms.

E. Posttraumatic stress disorder consists of nearly identical symptoms but must last for more than 1 month.

39. E. In treating myoglobinemia-myoglobinuria, intravenous hydration, mannitol, and alkalinization of the urine with sodium bicarbonate are the standards of therapy. Mannitol is an osmotic diuretic that will help the kidney diurese. Sodium bicarbonate will serve to alkalinize the urine to a pH of greater than 6; as a result, the myoglobin will remain soluble and not crystallize within the renal tubules and thus be excreted. An elevated potassium level is also a concern in crush injuries, but there was no mention of electrocardiogram changes due to hyperkalemia that would warrant the use of calcium gluconate. There is no evidence of pre-existing renal failure; therefore, hemodialysis is most likely not necessary.

A. Removal of the urinary catheter will not treat the underlying condition.

B. This patient needs mannitol and sodium bicarbonate in addition to the intravenous fluids.

C. This patient needs administration of sodium bicarbonate, mannitol, and intravenous fluids.

D. This patient also needs administration of sodium bicarbonate.

40. A. Certain forms of amyloidosis commonly involve the kidney and specifically affect the glomeruli. This creates nephrotic range proteinuria and an impaired glomerular filtration rate. Hypertension is sometimes present in these patients. Renal size is normal or slightly enlarged. Rectal biopsy or abdominal fat pad biopsy may obviate the need for renal biopsy. The glomerular basement membrane is thickened, and large nodular eosinophilic masses eventually develop. There is apple-green birefringence with Congo red stain, and immunofluorescence is only weakly positive due to the expression of the variable region of immunoglobulin expression rather than the constant region.

B. Hypersensitivity nephropathy usually develops after several weeks of drug exposure before evidence of renal injury appears. Hematura, pyuria, or proteinuria may all be present. The glomeruli appear normal histologically, and the interstitium shows lymphocytic infiltration. Immunofluorescence studies may show linear deposition of complement or immunoglobulins. Light chains would not be elevated specifically, and the sample would not stain with Congo red.

C. Multiple myeloma can cause a light chain deposition disease of the kidney due to proliferation of plasma cells within bone marrow. Nephrotic range proteinuria and renal impairment usually occur. Immunofluorescence studies are strongly positive for monoclonal light chains, in contrast to amyloidosis, because the constant region rather than the variable region of the chains are deposited. The deposits do not stain with Congo red.

D. Renal ultrasonography revealed no stenosis to suggest a decrease in perfusion to the kidneys. This disease could produce proteinuria but would not elevate immunoglobulin light chain specifically. Renal biopsy would not stain with Congo red.

E. Waldenström macroglobulinemia is characterized by an IgM-secreting clone of plasma cells. The abnormally high levels of the IgM paraprotein can cause hyperviscosity of the blood and compromise renal blood flow and glomerular filtration rate. Large amorphous deposits of eosinophilic material can develop in glomerular capillaries. Laboratory results would show a large increase in light chains due to expression of the constant region on immunofluorescence and would not show apple-green birefringence. Although this disease can lead to amyloidosis, it would not itself show the characteristic findings mentioned above.

41. **C.** This elderly patient needs constant supervision because he is at risk for foreign body obstruction most likely to occur during meals. A complete obstruction would likely have presented acutely; however, a partial obstruction allows air to enter the lung on inspiration, causing a hyperinflation of the affected side. This is termed a ball-valve obstruction.

A. Atelectasis involves the risk for a complete obstruction, which would present acutely.

B. This patient's symptoms are not suggestive of an infectious pathology. He is afebrile and has no findings consistent with a pneumonia.

D. The mediastinum would shift right or away from the lung with the blockage.

E. An inspiratory film may be normal, but after 1 week, hyperinflation is likely to be seen on inspiration as well as expiration.

42. **D.** Kallmann syndrome is the congenital absence of gonadotropin-releasing hormone (GnRH) and often it is associated with anosmia. It is a cause of infertility. Normally the anterior pituitary releases follicle-stimulating hormone and luteinizing hormone in response to GnRH released from the hypothalamus. These patients do not ovulate.

A. Anorexia nervosa can present with low body fat, but one should also look for lanugo (wispy body hair) and thinning brittle hair with a history that should alert you to an eating disorder (not eating in front of other people, being a very picky eater, etc.). Anorexia is not associated with anosmia.

B. Brain tumors could compress the pituitary stalk or the arcuate nucleus and simulate infertility similar to that seen in this patient, although such tumors are not likely to be associated with isolated anosmia.

C. Constitutionally delayed puberty is unlikely to be associated with anosmia.

E. Swyer syndrome, also called gonadal agenesis, in a genotype of 46 XY. When the testes do not develop, müllerian inhibiting factor despite a male genotype is not released, so internal and external genitalia remain female.

43. **E.** This child has diabetic ketoacidosis (DKA). Immediate objectives for treating this condition include fluid and electrolyte replacement. Initial fluid replacement should be a 20 mL/kg intravenous bolus of normal saline or lactated Ringer solution. Half the fluid deficit and maintenance should then be given over the first 8 hours, followed by the remainder of the deficit and maintenance over the next 16 hours.

A. Acidosis is usually corrected by rehydration and insulin therapy. Bicarbonate is administered only when the pH falls below 7.10.

B and **C.** Although carbohydrates and glucagons can be given in a state of hypoglycemia, this case clearly depicts DKA. In DKA the greatest concern should be volume replacement.

D. In DKA, insulin replacement to reverse the catabolic state is imperative. However, replacing insulin too quickly can lead to cerebral edema. Insulin therapy should begin with a 0.1 unit/kg bolus followed by 0.1 U/kg/h in order to decrease glucose levels by 100 mg/dL/h.

44. **B.** The patient described above can be diagnosed with periodic limb movement syndrome (PLMS) or nocturnal myoclonus. This is distinct from, although typically confused with, restless leg syndrome (RLS). Patients affected by RLS are aware of their excessive movements, whereas those with PLMS are often not aware, and thus a nighttime polysomnogram is needed for diagnosis. Many behavioral and pharmacologic treatments are available, but dopamine agonists remain the preferred treatment.

A. Acetylcholine has not been implicated as a major factor in PLMS. The loss of acetylcholinergic neurons, such as that which occurs in Alzheimer dementia, results in decreased slow-wave sleep and REM sleep.

C. GABA is not the target system affected by first-line medical treatment for PLMS.

D. Glutamate is not the target system affected by first-line medical treatment for PLMS.

E. Norepinephrine is not the target system affected by first-line medical treatment for PLMS.

45. **C.** This patient has multiple endocrine neoplasia type I. Everything on the problem list can also be explained by hyperparathyroidism (i.e., the disease of "bones, stones, and abdominal groans"), including psychological manifestations. Hyperparathyroidism causes an increase in blood calcium levels, which can lead to calcium deposition in the kidneys, causing stones. In order to increase calcium levels, the parathyroid hormone activates osteoclastic bone resorption. If neurologic, vascular, and psychogenic causes of impotence are unlikely, is there an endocrine cause of impotence associated with hyperparathyroidism? In this patient, prolactinoma (a pituitary tumor) as part of multiple endocrine neoplasia type I is the likely diagnosis.

A. This patient does not have any of the classic features of factitious disorder. In addition, the history of three kidney stones suggests a metabolic cause.

B. This patient more likely has organic impotence because his nocturnal penile tumescence test does not reveal nocturnal erections.

D. This patient does not manifest classic findings of multiple sclerosis. Multiple sclerosis is a demyelinating disease confined to the central nervous system characterized by the depletion of myelin-producing oligodendrocytes, which manifests clinically with exacerbations followed by remissions. Typical symptoms include weakness of lower extremities, visual disturbances, retrobulbar pain, and loss of bladder control (incontinence). It is often associated with the Charcot triad, which consists of nystagmus, intention tremors, and scanning speech.

E. This patient does not have any of the classic features of somatization disorder. In addition, the history of three kidney stones suggests a metabolic cause.

46. **E.** Squamous cell carcinoma is the second most common skin cancer, it is most likely to present on people who have had a significant history of sun exposure (UVB and UVC waves cause skin cancer) and those who are fair skinned. Ulcers and crusts will be seen when presenting as a significantly advanced lesion.

A. Actinic keratosis appears as the many rough spots on the patient's sun-exposed skin. When these are not frozen off or treated with 5-fluorouracil cream, they can become squamous cell carcinomas.

B. Even though basal cell carcinomas are the most common skin cancer and will also present as papules on sun-exposed areas of light-skinned individuals, they will appear to be more and have small vessels seen growing on them.

C. Melanomas typically present as A (**a**symmetric), B (with irregular **b**orders), C (very dark in **c**olor with many different shades), D (with a **d**iameter >6 mm). These kill more people than either basal cell or squamous cell carcinomas.

D. Rosacea typically presents on middle-aged men as small vessel growth in normal skin around the nose and can progress to a stereotypically large and deformed cystic nose.

47. C. *Trichomonas vaginalis* is a protozoan organism that lives in the urethra and vagina. This organism can be freely transmitted during sexual intercourse. Symptoms of infection include vulvar itching, burning, copious discharge with rancid odor, dysuria, and dyspareunia. Examination may reveal edema and erythema of the vulva and petechiae of the upper vagina and cervix. The secretions are often yellow-green with a pH of greater than 6.5. Wet smear will reveal the *Trichomonas* organism. Treatment is by oral metronidazole, and 1-day therapy regimens will result in a 90% cure rate.

A and B. Amoxicillin and ampicillin are not appropriate treatment choices for *Trichomonas vaginalis*.

D and E. Miconazole and terconazole are topical synthetic imidazoles for the treatment of vaginal candidiasis.

48. B. Osteogenesis imperfecta is a group of related genetic disorders that result from abnormal synthesis of type I collagen. Clinical characteristics include a history of multiple fractures, blue sclera of the eyes, conductive hearing loss, and short stature.

A. An abnormal FGF receptor is the cause of achondroplasia, which manifests as dwarfism.

C. Child abuse must be considered in this case, but no information in the history or physical examination suggests abuse.

D. Deficiency in vitamin D causes rickets in children, and would manifest with characteristic bowing of the legs.

E. There is no evidence that the patient has an underlying bone tumor.

49. E. The etiology of syndrome X is unknown. It is a variant angina that is a diagnosis of exclusion. A clue is the normal angiogram with ergonovine, which induces vasospasm. The etiology may relate to microvascular angina and a hypersensitivity to pain. Treatment may include calcium channel blockers, beta blockers, or angiotensin-converting enzyme inhibitors.

A. This patient lacks significant risk factors and symptoms typical for myocardial infarction (MI). Electrocardiogram findings do not reveal the typical ST, T, and Q wave changes that might be expected in MI.

B. Costochondritis is associated with chest pain produced during chest palpation. ECG is normal.

C. Esophageal dysmotility would not be expected to cause ST segment depression.

D. Mitral valve prolapse is characterized by chest pain, palpitations, dizziness, and anxiety secondary to neuroendocrine or autonomic dysfunction.

50. E. Patients who are not stressed will have a resting energy expenditure of 10% more than their basal energy expenditure. Various situations can alter the resting energy expenditure such as starvation, trauma, sepsis and burns. Burns will change the energy expenditure by 50 to 100%. Thus, this patient requires 3600 kcal/day of energy.

51. A. Axis I consists of the clinical disorders that may be a focus of clinical attention. In this category, medical conditions such as diabetes mellitus, hypertension, thyroid disorders, and parathyroid disorders should be included. The multiaxial evaluation allows for categorization of physical, social, and psychological disorders to be characterized to allow for maximization of patient diagnosis and subsequent care.

B. Axis II consists of personality disorders and mental retardation.

C. Axis III represents any physical disorder or general medical condition that is present in addition to the mental disorder.

D. Axis IV is used to code the psychosocial and environmental problems that can contribute to an individual's current psychosocial disorder. Stressors can affect the individual in a positive or negative fashion, and such information may be important in formulating a therapeutic plan for an individual that will maximize removal of the psychosocial stressor.

E. Axis V represents the global assessment of functioning (GAF) scale. This scale judges the psychological, social, and occupational functioning based on a continuum of mental health and mental illness.

52. B. Treatment of cytomegalovirus (CMV) retinitis involves ganciclovir, foscarnet, and cidofovir. These agents have produced response rates of 70% to 90% for CMV retinitis. The drugs are given as an initial induction phase and then a later life-long phase. Neutropenia is the major toxic effect and occurs in 15% to 30% of patients. Ganciclovir can also be given in an intraocular implantable form.

A. Erythromycin is not indicated in the treatment of CMV retinitis.

C. Penicillin VK is not useful in the management of CMV retinitis.

D. Oral corticosteroids are unproven in the treatment of CMV retinitis.

E. Oral prednisolone is unlikely to be of benefit in the treatment of CMV retinitis.

53. **A.** This patient has signs and symptoms of acute appendicitis. The diagnosis is suspected when nausea and vomiting is preceded by anorexia and periumbilical or right lower quadrant pain. The gravid uterus may mask the diagnosis by altering the position of the appendix and inflammatory exudate. Appendectomy with or without antibiotic therapy is necessary.

B. Gastroesophageal reflux occurs postprandially and is associated with midepigastric pain.

C. Hepatitis is associated with right upper quadrant pain and elevation of liver function tests (transaminases).

D. Hyperemesis gravidarum is associated with protracted nausea and vomiting with pregnancy.

E. Perforated tuboovarian abscess would require demonstration of fluid collection around the fallopian tube and ovary with an imaging study such as a CT scan or ultrasonography. Neither study was provided in this case.

54. **B.** Surgical resection of the terminal ileum has significant consequences to intestinal homeostasis. Fat malabsorption results in a deficiency of fat-soluble vitamins A, D, E, and K.

A. Constipation results due to resection of the ileocecal valve and often due to electrolyte/fat malabsorption.

C. Bile salts are minimally reabsorbed after ileal resection and can contribute to the diarrhea.

D. Vitamin B_{12} absorption will decrease, not increase. Vitamin B_{12} is mainly absorbed in the terminal ileum.

E. Vitamin D absorption is decreased with terminal ileum resection.

55. **C.** *Streptococcus pneumoniae* was isolated in middle ear aspirates (35% of the time). *Haemophilus influenzae* and *Moraxella cateralis* were isolated in 25% and 15% of the cases, respectively.

A. *Haemophilus influenzae* (25%) is the second most common organism isolated in patients with acute otitis media.

B. *Moraxella cateralis* (14%) is a common isolate from middle ear exudates and is poorly eradicated with amoxicillin due to increasing incidence of resistance.

D. *Streptococcus pyogenes* (3%) contributes to a minority of cases of otitis media.

E. It is important to remember that 15% of middle ear exudates cultured will show no growth. Treatment with antibiotics should still be completed despite lack of growth.

56. **E.** Foreign bodies must be removed from the airway to prevent further aggravation of symptoms. The lung tissue can be damaged from obstruction and ischemia; thus, removal is indicated as soon as possible after diagnosis.

A. Definitive management needs to be instituted. The object needs to be removed.

B. Blind finger sweeps are no longer indicated in any situation, especially where the oropharynx looks clear. If the foreign body is not into the bronchus, a finger sweep could push it into the bronchus.

C. This patient is not unstable, and respiratory distress will subside after removal of the object.

D. This scenario will not correct on its own and needs proper management.

57. **B.** This patient has evidence of gonococcal urethritis. Such patients need to be treated with agents that cover both *Neisseria gonorrhoeae* and *Chlamydia trachomatis*. The differential diagnosis of urethritis in men should also include *Trichomonas vaginalis, Mycoplasma genitalum, Ureaplasma urealyticum*, and herpes simplex virus. The treatment for *Neisseria gonorrhoeae* is a third-generation cephalosporin. Doxycycline should also be given.

A. Ceftriaxone will only eradicate *Neisseria gonorrhoeae*.

C. Ciprofloxacin is a treatment for *Chlamydia trachomatis*.

D. Doxycycline is a treatment for *Chlamydia trachomatis*.

E. This combination is ineffective for either *Neisseria gonorrhoeae* or *Chlamydia trachomatis* infections.

58. **C.** This patient is 46XY. Testicular feminization is an androgen insensitivity caused by a dysfunctional or completely absent testosterone receptor. This results in a phenotypically female patient. Because müllerian inhibiting factor was secreted, such individuals have an absence of all the structures derived from the müllerian duct. Estrogen is often produced, and they grow breasts and are very feminine and attractive. The vagina is reconstructed for sex, but no reproduction is possible.

A. Imperforate hymen is a cause for primary amenorrhea but is not in itself a cause for infertility because it can be perforated surgically.

B. Phenotypically she is female, although she is genotypically male and she is infertile.

D. 47XXY is Klinefelter syndrome, in which the affected individual presents as a phenotypic male.

E. 45X0 is Turner syndrome. In this syndrome the ovaries undergo rapid atresia. Often these patients have a webbed neck and short stature.

59. **B.** This clinical scenario is classic for Duchenne muscular dystrophy (DMD). DMD is an X-linked recessive disorder and is caused by an abnormality in a protein named dystrophin. Patients are likely to present at age 5 and display delayed achievement of motor developmental milestones. Patients are typically wheelchair bound before their teens and are likely to die from respiratory insufficiency, respiratory infection, and decompensation of the heart.

A. Women are not susceptible to DMD because it is X-linked recessive.

C. Since the disease is X-linked recessive, the gene was inherited from the mother, and the father would not have been likely to display similar symptoms.

D. Anticipation is a phenomenon where symptoms tend to become more severe from generation to generation while also displaying an earlier age of onset. Anticipation is a characteristic of myotonic dystrophy, an autosomal-dominant disease.

E. Defects also occur in the heart in DMD and can result in arrhythmias or even heart failure.

60. **A.** The extrapyramidal reaction that the patient is experiencing is from decreased dopamine availability caused by the antipsychotic's mechanism of action, which includes a dopamine receptor blockade. Antiparkisonian medications such as benztropine and amantidine may help, which work by correcting the imbalance between dopamine (decreased) and acetylcholine (increased).

B. Betamethasone is a corticosteroid useful for decreasing inflammation.

C. Cannabis is useful for treating glaucoma and nausea.

D. Lorazepam is a benzodiazepine that works by stimulating the GABA receptor, leading to increased inhibition in the central nervous system, and is useful for anxiety.

E. Propranolol is a nonselective beta blocker useful for treatment of hypertension and social phobias.

61. **A.** This patient has developed magnesium sulfate toxicity; consequently, she has developed early signs of respiratory depression and absent deep tendon reflexes. Intravenous calcium gluconate is the treatment of choice.

B. Magnesium sulfate toxicity is best managed by intravenous calcium gluconate therapy. Supplemental oxygen therapy and monitoring are important adjuncts to this treatment.

C. Immediate cesarean section is not indicated for this patient.

D. Intubation may be required if the respiratory rate and oxygen saturation continue to decline.

E. Oral calcium gluconate will take time to be absorbed. Intravenous calcium gluconate is preferred.

62. **B.** These symptoms of upper and lower respiratory symptoms is classic for *Mycoplasma* pneumonia. The laboratory values and chest x-ray also correlate. Treatment is doxycycline or erythromycin.

A. The symptoms of *Chlamydia* pneumonia are similar to those of *Mycoplasma* pneumonia, but the prodromal phase lasts longer.

C. *Pneumocystis* pneumonia is more common in immuno-suppressed patients.

D. Rubeola consists of fever, coryza, cough, and conjunctivitis. Affected patients may also have Koplik spots. The rash begins on the face and moves downward.

E. *Streptococcus* pneumonia usually presents with high fever, productive cough, and sometimes hemoptysis. This would not explain the upper respiratory symptoms.

63. **B.** This patient has diverticulitis. The radiographic features of diverticulitis include nonspecific ileus or obstruction. CT scan of the abdomen may reveal thickening of the sigmoid colon with inflammation of the adjacent fat. Extraluminal gas may also be present.

Figure 63

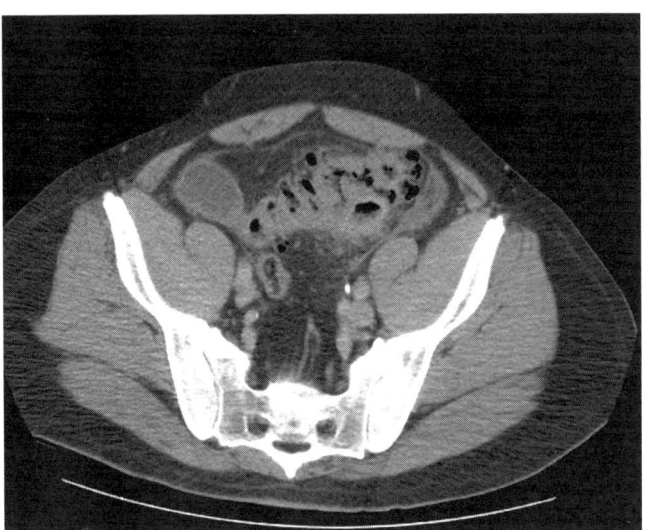

A. There is no evidence of abscess on this CT scan.

C. Crohn disease is more likely to occur in the terminal ileum and right colon.

D. Ulcerative colitis is unlikely given the normal colonoscopic findings.

E. Ulcerative proctitis is unlikely given the normal colonoscopic findings.

64. **A.** The urinary tract stone as described is likely to pass with conservative measures (analgesics and hydration). Aggressive hydration remains somewhat controversial. The other selections are incorrect but could be considerations if the stone is large (>5 mm) and the patient has intractable pain or hydronephrosis. In this latter situation, placement of a ureteral stent would be most appropriate.

B. A large stone (2 cm or larger) with associated hydronephrosis may require a percutaneous nephrostomy to unobstruct the kidney.

C. Shock-wave lithotripsy may be indicated for a larger (1–2 cm) nonobstructing renal stone.

D. Ureteroscopic stone extraction may be indicated for larger distal ureteral stones.

E. Although stenting is a reasonable option for this patient, the small stone size and lack of hydronephrosis suggests a more conservative approach. However, should pain persist despite analgesics and hydration, placement of a ureteral stent is indicated.

65. **D.** This patient has vitamin B_{12} deficiency, which is needed for DNA synthesis. This condition is rare in developed countries because stores are large. It is found in meat, fish, eggs, and cheese. Clinical manifestations include glossitis, diarrhea, and weight loss. Neurologic sequelae include paresthesias, peripheral neuropathies, dementia, ataxia, and posterior column degeneration. Vitiligo is the main dermatologic manifestation. This patient should be treated with vitamin B_{12} injections (50–100 μg) intramuscularly once a month. Response is usually rapid, and anemia may resolve within 1 to 2 months.

A. Corticosteroid therapy is not indicated for vitamin B_{12} deficiency.

B. Folate supplementation is not the treatment for vitamin B_{12} deficiency.

C. Iron supplementation is the treatment for iron deficiency anemia.

E. Watchful waiting is not the recommended treatment for vitamin B_{12} deficiency.

66. **C.** Irritable bowel syndrome (IBS) presents with similar symptoms as those of inflammatory bowel disease (ulcerative colitis and Crohn disease). IBS is not autoimmune related and usually occurs during times of stress. Presenting symptoms are abdominal pain with an urge to defecate, pain relieved with defecation, bloating, and diarrhea. Weight loss is uncommon with IBS.

A. Crohn disease is chronic. Patients will often have diarrhea, fevers, and weight loss.

B. Gastroenteritis is usually more severe in nature and is the result of an infectious process by bacteria, viruses, or parasites, all of which are usually ingested. The patient will have fever, diarrhea, or vomiting, but would also experience signs of dehydration if the diarrhea were to persist for any more than a day or two. Other findings include orthostatic hypotension, tachycardia, poor capillary refill, dry mucous membranes, and decreased skin turgor.

D. Although stress is a risk factor for developing peptic ulcers, and patients will present with abdominal pain, diarrhea will not be present. Patients with peptic ulcers may also present with melena, vomiting, or hematemesis. Pain is relieved by food or antacids. More than 90% of peptic ulcer disease is associated with *Helicobacter pylori* infections.

E. Although ulcerative colitis will cause abdominal pain with diarrhea, a sense of urgency, and waxing and waning symptoms, the diarrhea is usually bloody.

67. **D.** A chest x-ray and bronchoscopy together will elaborate the source of bleeding in the vast majority of cases. With moderate amounts of hemoptysis, it is crucial to find the source of bleeding; therefore, bronchoscopy is mandatory.

A. Watchful waiting is not an appropriate option for a patient with hemoptysis.

B. It is important to visualize the source of bleeding with bronchoscopy, not merely find a "shapshot" of blood-filled lungs with x-ray or CT alone.

C. The source of bleeding should be visualized.

E. It is far more important to localize the bleeding than it is to determine whether or not an infectious cause exists.

68. **B.** The scenario describes a patient with narcolepsy. Narcolepsy is a disorder typically composed of excessive daytime sleepiness and cataplexy. Cataplexy is loss of muscle tone typically resulting from emotionally charged situations. Patients will often complain of sleep paralysis, which is thought to occur when awakening out of REM sleep. First-line treatment of narcolepsy is with stimulants, which is the same as for attention deficit hyperactivity disorder. Cataplexy, one feature of the disorder, can be treated with clomipramine.

A. Treatment for amyotrophic lateral sclerosis is mainly supportive. Glutamate inhibitors have been shown to prolong life but have no effect on quality of life.

C. First-line therapy for major depression is psychotherapy and/or antidepressant therapy with a selective serotonin reuptake inhibitor.

D. Restless leg syndrome is treated either with dopamine agonists or benzodiazepines.

E. Benzodiazepines and baclofen can by used to treat spasticity in stiff man syndrome.

69. **B.** The caloric requirements for a healthy, growing, preterm neonate is approximately 120 kcal/kg/day. Based on this need, the child's weight, and the caloric contents of the formula, the mother should feed her child 30 ounces of formula per day.
(120 kcal/kg/day) × (5 kg)/(20 kcal/ounce of formula) = 30 ounces of formula/day.

70. **B.** This patient has a fever of unknown origin (FUO). This is defined as a fever of 101°F or greater for at least 3 weeks. Most cases of FUO are due to infection, neoplasm, or collagen vascular disease. Chest x-ray is an important first step in the evaluation of these patients to rule out pneumonia or other pulmonary process.

A. A barium enema should be performed if symptoms suggest a lower gastrointestinal cause.

C. Echocardiogram should be performed if endocarditis or myxoma is suspected.

D. Lumbar puncture may be useful if the patient complains of a headache, photophobia, stiff neck, neurologic abnormalities, or if the patient seizes.

E. PET scans are expensive and should not be administered as a first-line method of evaluation of FUO.

71. **A.** The first stage of thelarche, the development of breast buds, is usually the first phenotypical change to occur in girls. This usually occurs at around 11 years of age. In order of average age of onset, breast bud development is first.

B. An increase in sebaceous gland secretion is not a hallmark phenotypical sign of pubertal development.

C. The onset of pubic hair growth occurs around 12 years of age.

D. Menarche usually occurs around 12 to 13 years of age.

E. Peak height velocity occurs around 12 to 13 years of age.

72. **F.** This patient has a prolactinoma, the most common functioning pituitary adenoma. Prolactinomas are characterized by hypogonadism and galactorrhea. The most confirming laboratory study in the diagnosis of this patient would be prolactin levels elevated above 150 mg/L.

A. Dopamine can mediate suppression of serum prolactin levels.

B. Decreased Na is unlikely to assist with the diagnosis of prolactinoma.

C. CEA protein levels may be elevated in colorectal carcinoma but are unlikely to assist with the diagnosis of prolactinoma.

D. Growth hormone levels are unchanged with prolactinoma.

E. Leutinizing hormone levels are unchanged with prolactinoma.

73. **E.** In hypovolemic shock there can be a decline in cardiac output and systemic vascular resistance due to fluid loss. This condition can result from loss of blood (hemorrhage), loss of plasma fluids (burn patients), and loss of fluid and electrolytes (third spacing seen in pancreatitis).

74. **B.** Cardiogenic shock can result from cardiac pump failure or valvular failure. As described by the scenario in this question, rupture of the intraventricular septum can also occur with immediate decline in cardiac output and systemic vascular resistance.

75. **F.** Etiologies of obstructive shock include tension pneumothorax, pericardial diseases, disease of the pulmonary blood vessels, cardiac tumor (left atrial myxoma), mural thrombus, and valvular obstructive diseases. In this condition, there is a decrease in cardiac output and an increase in systemic vascular resistance.

76. **E.** This patient has hypovolemic shock. Loss of electrolytes and fluid, known as third spacing, is a major contributor to shock in patients with acute pancreatitis. There can be a decline in cardiac output and systemic vascular resistance due to fluid loss.

77. **C.** This patient is described as having a pneumopericardium, or air within the pericardial sac. This can occur after a closed chest trauma and may develop into a cardiac tamponade. Radiography with pneumopericardium demonstrates the shifting of pericardial air when comparing supine films to erect films.

A. Although heart failure and other causes of right-sided heart failure are in the differential diagnosis, they are less likely given this patient's presentation.

B. A pericardial rub would indicate pericarditis, which would not be heard after the development of an effusion.

D. Although heart failure and other causes of right-sided heart failure are in the differential diagnosis, they are less likely given this patient's presentation.

E. Pneumomediastinum as opposed to pneumopericardium is associated with subcutaneous emphysema in the suprasternal notch in as many as half of patients.

78. **A.** Young patients with diabetes mellitus should undergo an initial ocular examination within 5 years of diagnosis. However, this patient with gestational diabetes should be examined as soon as the diagnosis of diabetes is established.

B–E. Young nonpregnant patients with DM should have an ocular examination within 5 years of the diagnosis.

79. **D.** Duchenne muscular dystrophy (DMD) is an X-linked disorder that results from a deficiency of dystrophin. Muscle weakness is most pronounced in the proximal muscle groups. Examination reveals calf pseudohypertrophy and a positive Gower sign. Definitive diagnosis is made by muscle biopsy. Treatment is supportive, but most children become wheelchair bound in the early second decade of life and die by age 30.

A. DNA analysis will demonstrate the dystrophin mutation, but one would not be able to differentiate DMD from Becker-type muscular dystrophy.

B. EMG would show polyphasic potentials and increased recruitment, but would not confirm the diagnosis.

C. Creatinine kinase is consistently elevated, but is nonspecific and does not confirm the diagnosis.

E. The diagnosis of DMD is not a clinical one. Muscle biopsy is necessary.

80. **C.** Fever and sore throat accompanied with malaise and cervical lymphadenopathy suggest mononucleosis. Heterophile antibody and monospot test results should be positive within 4 days.

A. Mononucleosis does not require inpatient therapy.

B. Chest x-ray is not indicated in this patient.

D. With lack of exudate on the patient's throat streptococcal pharyngitis is unlikely.

E. The Weil-Felix titer screens for rickettsial disease and is not indicated in this patient.

81. **A.** Alcoholic hallucinosis is the presence of unpleasant auditory hallucinations with a clear sensorium. These are the only two essential findings. Once the sensorium is altered, the patient is moving toward delirium tremens.

B. Flat affect is not an essential finding for alcoholic hallucinosis.

C. Flight of ideas is not an essential finding for alcoholic hallucinosis.

D. Inability to write is not an essential finding for alcoholic hallucinosis.

E. Loss of abstract thought is not an essential finding for alcoholic hallucinosis.

82. **E.** An occluded left anterior descending branch (LAD) of the left coronary artery produces an anterior myocardial infarction. This manifests on ECG as Q waves in leads V_1, V_2, V_3, and V_4. Some researchers also describe a septal infarct. This is when only the first two precordial chest leads are involved, since these leads most accurately reflect the electric potential of the intraventricular septum. By this definition, the patient has a septal infarct of undetermined age most likely produced by occlusion of the LAD.

A. Occlusion of a branch of the right coronary artery (RCA) produces a posterior infarction of the left ventricle. This shows up on ECG as a large R wave in V_1 and V_2 with or without a Q wave in V_6. For an acute posterior infarction, look for ST depression in V_1 or V_2 (and occasionally V_3).

B. Usually, the inferior portion of the left ventricle is supplied by the RCA; however, the left coronary artery (LCA) supplies this area in a small portion of the population. So in a patient with the RCA as the supplier, occlusion of this artery would produce an inferior myocardial infarction (MI). Conversely, a patient with the LCA as the supplier would sustain an inferior MI with subsequent occlusion of this artery. In either case, this will show up on ECG as appropriate changes in the inferior leads II, III, and AVF.

C. The circumflex branch supplies blood to the lateral portion of the left ventricle; hence, occlusion of this artery produces a lateral MI. On ECG, one will see signs of infarction in leads I and AVL, which are the lateral leads.

D. A patient with the LCA as the supplier would sustain an inferior MI with subsequent occlusion of this artery. In either case, this will show up on ECG as appropriate changes in the inferior leads II, III, and AVF.

Figure 82

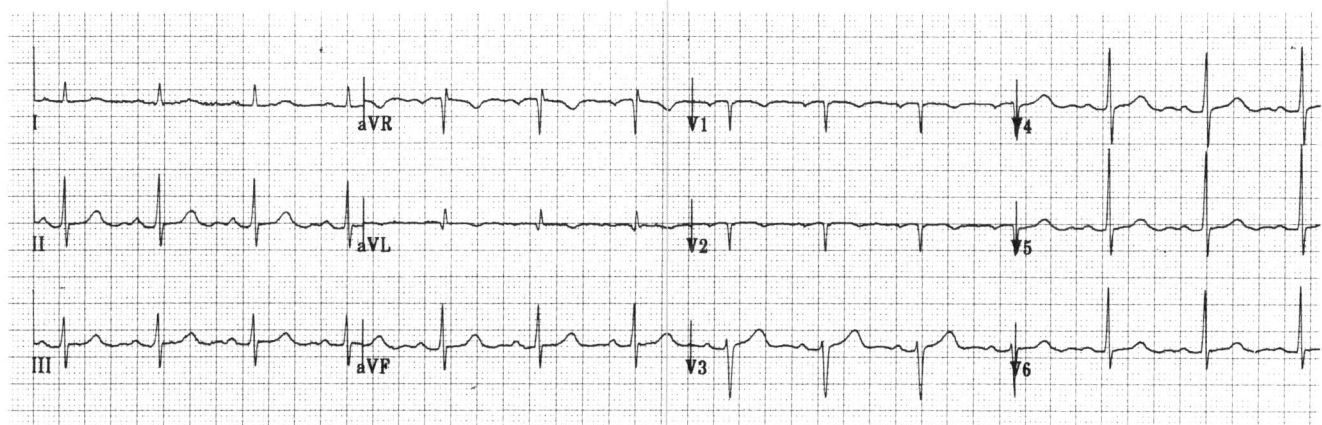

83. **B.** Children with constitutional delay have family members of average height but usually one or more relatives have a history of short stature in childhood and delayed puberty. These children develop at or below the fifth percentile but at normal growth velocities. In addition, they usually have delayed bone age.

A. Achondroplasia is an autosomal-dominant disorder leading to disproportionate short stature.

C. Cushing disease is a rare cause of diminished growth, and those affected would have other symptoms of the syndrome.

D. Children with familial short stature usually have at least one parent with short stature, and puberty is not delayed. Those affected grow at or below the fifth percentile and have normal bone age.

E. Growth hormone deficiency is a rare cause of short stature. It accounts for less than 5% of cases. Children grow at a decreased growth velocity (<5 cm/yr) and may have a history of birth asphyxia, neonatal hypoglycemia, or microphallus.

84. **E.** It is important to rule out pregnancy before restarting the patient's oral contraceptive pills. It is reasonable to allow her to take the oral contraceptives for another month before altering her regimen.

A–D. If the pregnancy test is negative, it is reasonable to allow her to resume her current regimen for another month.

85. **B.** The patient is suffering from paranoid personality disorder (axis II). This disorder is characterized by a pattern of pervasive distrust and suspiciousness of others, and the interpretation that their motives are malevolent. They are often reluctant to confide in others for fear that the information will be used against them, and they tend to read hidden demeaning or threatening meaning into benign remarks. They may be very unforgiving of personal slights, and are quick to counterattack. They may also have recurrent suspicions regarding the fidelity of their sexual partner. Personality disorders and mental retardation are classified under axis II.

A. Axis I refers to the clinical syndrome.

C. Axis III refers to the physical disorder present.

D. Axis IV refers to the degree of psychosocial stress present during the past year.

E. Axis V refers to the Global Assessment Scale of Functioning and evaluates the current level of functioning and the highest level attained throughout the prior year.

86. **A.** Crohn disease is an inflammatory disease of the small or large bowel with spontaneous remissions and acute exacerbations. This condition typically occurs in young adults who present with intermittent abdominal pain, diarrhea, weight loss, and extraintestinal manifestations such as perianal fistulas, fissures, and abscesses. Small bowel series in these individuals may reveal a nodular contour, luminal narrowing, linear ulcers, sinuses, and clefts.

B. Small bowel leiomyoma is the most common benign tumor of the small bowel. These lesions are often asymptomatic or present with occult bleeding.

C. Small bowel lipoma represents the second most common benign tumor of the small bowel. Often asymptomatic, these lesions can cause obstruction by intussusception.

D. Tuberculous enteritis occurs as a secondary infection in a patient with pulmonary tuberculosis. This condition can involve the iliocecal region.

E. Villous adenomas are benign small bowel tumors that have a 35% to 55% malignant potential. The majority of these patients are asymptomatic.

87. **E.** This patient has a disorder of humoral immunity known as X-linked (Bruton) agammaglobulinemia. A history of recurrent infections with organisms such as *Haemophilus influenzae* and *Streptococcus pneumoniae* (encapsulated organisms) and failure to respond to antibiotic therapy is suspicious for a primary B-cell deficiency.

A. Chronic granulomatous disease is a disorder of phagocytic immunity resulting in recurrent skin infections.

B. Common variable immunodeficiency is distributed equally among genders and infections are less severe.

C. DiGeorge syndrome is a disorder of cell-mediated immunity.

D. Selective IgA deficiency is the mildest as well as the most common immunodeficiency. Serum levels of other antibodies are normal and patients react normally to viral infections.

88. **B.** This patient has the CREST variant of scleroderma, which is characterized by calcinosis, Raynaud phenomenon, esophageal dysmotility, sclerodactyly, and telangiectasia. Elevated erythrocyte sedimentation rate would be expected in all forms of connective tissue disease, and thus would be present but is not specific to CREST syndrome. Likewise, anticentromere antibody is detected in only 60% of individuals with CREST syndrome, but is considered specific for this syndrome.

A. Antinuclear antibody is the most common autoantibody in connective tissue disease and is also not specific.

C. Anti-dsDNA is seen in systemic lupus erythematosus.

D. Anti-Jo immunoglobulin is associated with polymyositis/dermatomyositis.

E. Anti-Smith antibody is seen in systemic lupus erythematosus.

89. **D.** The appropriate management of this patient, who is presenting with tardive dyskinesia, is benztropine. Tardive dyskinesia is the result of chronic antipsychotic treatment.

A. Benztropine is the treatment for this condition.

B. Clozapine will cause tardive dyskinesia.

C. Haloperidol is associated as a causative agent of tardive dyskinesia.

E. Tardive dyskinesia is by definition caused by medicines, and therefore not a primary symptom of her schizophrenia.

90. **B.** Endomyometritis is a polymicrobial infection of the uterine lining. Endomyometritis commonly occurs 5 to 10 days after delivery. The infection usually begins at the placental site and is common in the puerperium. Premature rupture of membranes, a long labor, and a cesarean delivery increase the risk for uterine infection.

A. There is no evidence of atelectasis; usually fever occurs sooner.

C. There is no evidence of kidney stones with the patient's symptoms.

D. There is no evidence of a urinary tract infection on urinalysis.

E. There is no evidence of wound infection in this patient.

91. **B.** This patient has Kawasaki disease, which is a systemic vasculitis. Fever, lymphadenopathy, and mucocutaneous lesions characterize it. It occurs mostly in infants and young children and more often in boys. The most serious complication is coronary vasculitis. Prognosis of this disease is associated with severity of cardiac involvement.

A. Aseptic meningitis is not a typical complication of Kawasaki disease.

C. Gastroenteritis is not a typical sequela of systemic vasculitis.

D. Testicular torsion is not a typical complication of Kawasaki disease.

E. Uveitis is not a typical complication of Kawasaki disease.

92. **E.** The electroencephalogram (EEG) helps to rule in or out a variety of conditions and can differentiate between organic and functional conditions. Patients with degenerative dementia of the Alzheimer type will have a normal EEG greater than 50% of the time. However, reversible forms of dementia often produce abnormal EEG findings.

A. Diffuse EEG slowing can be seen in patients with delirium.

B. Drugs can alter the EEG tracing. For example, sedative-hypnotics increase fast activity.

C. Intermittent rapid and slow activity on the EEG are not typical of primary degenerative dementia.

D. Partial slowing of activity on the EEG is not typical of Alzheimer disease.

93. **D.** A solitary pulmonary nodule is defined as an abnormal round density up to 4 cm in diameter surrounded by a rim of normal lung tissue that is free from cavitation. In nonsmokers under the age of 35, there is a small chance for malignancy; therefore, diagnosis with bronchial brush biopsy and observation are appropriate. Eighty percent of solitary pulmonary nodules are benign, and of these, almost 90% are granulomas.

A. Adenocarcinoma is rare in patients under the age of 45, especially among those patients who are nonsmokers.

B. Arteriovenous malformation is difficult to assess on a routine chest x-ray and therefore is not a likely answer to this question.

C. Bronchogenic tumors include cylandroma and mucoepidermoid type. Their location is usually central, and treatment involves en bloc surgical resection.

E. Hamartoma is a disorganized pulmonary tumor that is composed of muscle, fibrous, and fatty tissue.

94. **C.** By history, this patient appears to have carotid sinus syncope. Symptoms are provoked by wearing tight-fitting neck collars. The next step to further evaluate this entity is gently compressing the carotid artery with simultaneous electrocardiographic monitoring.

A. Cardiac catheterization is not the appropriate next step in evaluating carotid sinus syncope.

B. Carotid massage is not indicated because it may dislodge an embolus.

D. Observation as an inpatient is not appropriate for a patient with impending carotid sinus syncope. This patient needs more immediate intervention.

E. This patient needs more intensive evaluation and treatment rather than routine follow-up outpatient reevaluation.

95. **D.** The heart becomes infarcted (i.e., necrotic) when an area of the myocardium is deprived of blood. Using ECG technology it is possible to determine when this happens and which area of the heart muscle is involved in a myocardial infarction (MI). There are three cardinal signs of infarction: significant Q waves (see below), ST segment elevation, and T wave inversion. These correspond to three different associations for the hemodynamic state of the myocardium, which are necrosis, injury, and ischemia, respectively. Note that by definition, an infarction indicates necrosis of a tissue. So the presence of significant Q waves indicates MI; however, if there is just ST segment elevation, then the diagnosis of non–Q wave infarction may be made.

Depending on the leads that these three markers show up in, we can infer which area of the myocardium is involved. When describing the location for an MI, it is important to note that we are not talking about the entire heart. The changes on ECG specifically refer to areas of the left ventricle. The diagnosis of inferior MI is made by finding significant Q waves in leads II, III, and AVF, which are the inferior leads. Significant Q waves are those greater than 1 mm (0.04 sec) or more than one third of QRS amplitude. By convention we refer to a "Q" wave to mean a significant Q wave and a "q" wave to be not significant. Our patient most likely sustained an infarction during his episode of chest pain 2 to 3 months ago since there are no indications of acute injury such as ST elevation; however, without ST segment elevation to indicate acute infarction, the exact age of the MI cannot be determined by ECG. Some researchers would call this an old inferior MI, which is also an acceptable diagnosis.

▌ **Figure 95**

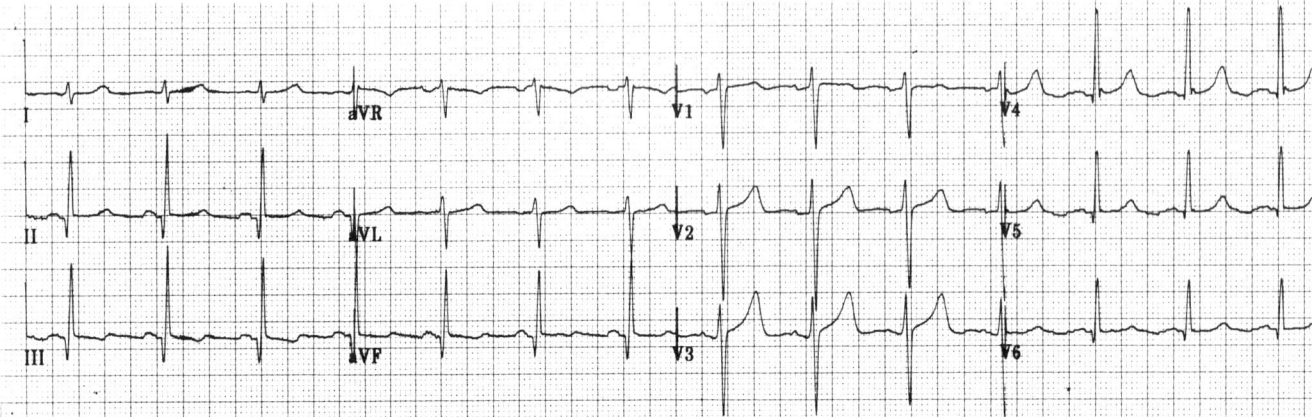

A. This electrocardiogram is not normal if it has Q waves present in one or more of the leads.

B and **E.** There is no ST segment elevation in the inferior leads that would suggest acute injury to the inferior portion of the left ventricle and, thus, an inferior MI.

C. A lateral MI is an infarction of the lateral wall of the left ventricle. This would show up on ECG as Q waves in the lateral leads I and AVL.

96. **E.** This patient has symptoms of pica. Pica is a craving for nonfoodstuffs such as laundry starch, ice, dirt, or clay and is common in pregnancy. Its true incidence is underestimated due to denial. This condition can be serious when ingestion of materials interferes with needed food and mineral intake. Poor nutrition can result. Treatment consists of detection, counseling, and encouragement to control pica.

A. Hyperemesis gravidarum is associated with protracted nausea and vomiting.

B. Manic depression is associated with a manic component and a depressive component.

C. This patient does not display typical features of obsessive-compulsive disorder.

D. Oral contraceptive use during pregnancy is contraindicated.

97. **E.** The Global Assessment of Functioning (GAF) scale judges the psychological, social, and occupational functioning based on a continuum of mental health and mental illness. The scale is coded on axis V and is a 100-point scale, where 100 represents the highest level of functioning in areas mentioned above.

A. Axis I consists of the clinical disorders that may be a focus of clinical attention.

B. Axis II consists of personality disorders and mental retardation.

C. Axis III represents any physical disorder or general medical condition that is present in addition to the mental disorder.

D. Axis IV is used to code the psychosocial and environmental problems that can contribute to an individual's current psychosocial disorder. Stressors can affect the individual in a positive or negative fashion, and such information may be important in formulating a therapeutic plan for an individual that will maximize removal of the psychosocial stressor.

98. **B.** Developmental dysplasia of the hip (DDH) results when contact between the acetabulum and the femoral head is lost during intrauterine development. It is diagnosed by the Barlow and Ortolani maneuvers. Treatment includes the use of the Pavlik harness, which maintains hip flexion and abduction.

A. Hip adduction is not therapeutic for DDH.

C. Observation is contraindicated due to the possible complications of untreated DDH.

D. Avascular necrosis of the femoral head is the most common complication. Surgery is not indicated for DDH.

E. Intravenous antibiotics are not a treatment for DDH.

99. **A.** In this individual with chronic constipation and a normal physical examination for rectal pathology, one must consider a secondary cause for constipation. Hypercalcemia is an endocrine cause of constipation and might be related to hypercalcemia of malignancy in this patient with known metastatic renal cell carcinoma.

B. Hypokalemia is associated with constipation. Hyperkalemia may be associated with diarrhea.

C. Hyperglycemia of diabetes mellitus may be an endocrine cause of constipation.

D. Hyperparathyroidism is associated with hypercalcemia, which can cause constipation.

E. Hypopituitarism, not thyrotoxicosis, is a metabolic cause of chronic constipation.

100. **D.** Typically, scirrhous adenocarcinoma of the breast begins in the upper outer quadrant of the breast. It takes approximately 5 to 8 years for the typical breast cancer to become palpable (>1 cm in size). With enlargement of the mass, fibrosis will shorten Cooper ligaments and cause dimpling of the skin. Systemic spread of this cancer is to the lung (65%), bone (56%), and liver (56%).

A. Fibroadenoma is a lobular, firm, well-circumscribed solitary mass that is common in young females. Surgical excision is the treatment of choice in women over the age of 25. Younger patients may be treated with needle cytology and surveillance.

B. Fibrocystic change is associated with breast tenderness and swelling premenstrually. Patients with severe atypia or hyperplasia on biopsy are at risk for breast carcinoma.

C. Sarcoma of the breast represents a small percentage of breast cancers and is more common in women over the age of 40.

E. Intraductal papilloma is the most common cause of bloody nipple discharge (90% of the time). It is a benign condition. The papilloma arises from an isolated mammary duct, which should be excised.

101. **C.** Mallory-Weiss tears occur in the mucosa near the gastroesophageal junction. Patients are usually alcoholics and give a history of vomiting that precedes emesis of a large amount of blood. Physical examination is often unremarkable. Diagnosis is made by endoscopy, and treatment strategies include H2 receptor blockade.

A. Esophagitis is typically an inflammatory condition in response to acid reflux from an incompetent lower esophageal sphincter. It is not a fungal or viral infection.

B. As mentioned above, esophagitis is typically an inflammatory condition in response to acid reflux from an incompetent lower esophageal sphincter. It is not a fungal or viral infection.

D. Peptic ulcer disease may be associated with upper gastrointestinal bleeding.

E. Tuberculosis is more likely to be associated with respiratory complaints such as chest pain, dyspnea, and hemoptysis. Hematemesis is uncommon with tuberculosis.

102. **D.** This patient either may have a vaginal foreign body or may have been a victim of sexual abuse. Diagnosis usually depends on the graphic history, often offered by the child, mother, or friend. Physical examination may be helpful. However, it is also important to be alert to verbal and nonverbal clues to possible abuse when consulting with young patients and their family members. These observations may prove more fruitful than further examinations.

A. There is no role for the use of diagnostic hysteroscopy in the evaluation of a child.

B. There is no role for the use of vaginal speculum examination. It is often difficult in a prepubertal child and may be both traumatic and unyielding.

C. There is no role for the use of diagnostic culposcopy in the evaluation of a young child of suspected rape.

E. CBC and serum electrolytes will probably add little to the diagnosis of sexual abuse.

103. **E.** Vulvar carcinoma accounts for 4% of gynecologic malignancies. The typical clinical profile is a female patient over the age of 65 who complains of vulvar pruritus. Physical examination often reveals an ulcerative or exophytic lesion on the labia majus. The etiology of this carcinoma is thought to be prior intraepithelial lesions and human papilloma virus.

A. Melanoma is a raised pruritic and pigmented lesion of the vulva.

B. Paget disease is often associated with underlying disease of the colon and breast and is an intraepithelial disease.

C. Squamous hyperplasia is a hyperplastic lesion associated with skin thickening with excoriation.

D. Vaginal neoplasia is often multifocal and associated with other lower genital tract intraepithelial or invasive lesions.

104. **C.** Intestinal secretion is indicative of *Clostridium perfringens* food poisoning. This is the second or third most common cause of food poisoning in the United States. Primary sources are recooked meats, meat products, and poultry.

A. Impulses sent to the medullary center are indicative of *Staphylococcus* food poisoning.

B. Epithelial necrosis of the colon is indicative of *Clostridium difficile* colitis.

D. A superficial gut infection with little invasion is indicative of *Salmonella* food poisoning.

E. Blockade of acetylcholine receptors at the neuromuscular junction is indicative of *Clostridium botulinum* food poisoning.

105. **D.** The neonate described in the question has congenital toxoplasmosis. Felines are the definitive host of the parasite, and the mother's history is suspicious for exposure to cats. Intrauterine meningoencephalitis is common among infants infected early in pregnancy. At birth, these children present with microcephaly, chorioretinitis, microphthalmia, intracranial calcifications, and seizures. Mental retardation and learning disabilities are unfortunate long-term sequelae. Toxoplasmosis is treated with the synergistic combination of pyrimethamine and sulfadiazine. Because these antibiotics inhibit folic acid, it must be given in conjunction with the drugs.

A. Herpes simplex type II viral infections are treated with acyclovir.

B. Intravenous immunoglobulin is an appropriate pharmacotherapy for congenital HIV infection.

C. Penicillin is used to treat congenital syphilis.

E. Intravenous immunoglobulin and trimethoprim are appropriate pharmacotherapies for congenital HIV infection.

106. **B.** Small, noninfected decubitus ulcers (pressure sores) can be managed by positional changes, wet-to-dry dressings, foam padding, and other supportive measures, but signs of infection and tissue ischemia require drainage and débridement. In order for the wound to heal, prolonged pressure on the area must be avoided and the wound must have ample blood supply. Primary closure and skin grafting are not good choices for two fundamental reasons: (1) cutaneous tissue will not survive in absence of an underlying blood supply, which is usually compromised by pressure necrosis and débridement, and (2) either type of skin graft fails to "pad" the area to reduce pressure. Note that most decubitus ulcers form over bony prominences such as the sacrum, ischium, and greater trochanter.

A. Healing by secondary intention is a poor choice for this patient.

C. This option is not the first choice for this patient.

D. This option is not the first choice for this patient.

E. Débridement is usually significant, because subcutaneous damage is frequently more extensive than the superficial wound would suggest.

107. **E.** This patient has equal volume periods occurring less than 21 days apart that include less than 80 mL of blood loss each time. This is polymenorrhea because it is regular, only on an abnormally shortened time frame.

A. Menorrhagia is the condition of heavy blood loss and is defined as blood loss of 80 mL with each period. Patients describe their periods as "pouring out" or "gushing." These patients must be evaluated for vaginal cervical and rectal bleeding as well. Quantity of blood is determined by weighing of pads or a history of more than 24 pads per day during their periods.

B. Menometrorrhagia is heavy bleeding (>80 g).

C. Metrorrhagia is the condition when there is bleeding between periods normally less than or equal to normal period flow.

D. Oligomenorrhea is having periods that are more than 35 days apart.

108. **D.** Two doses of tetanus 1 to 2 months apart with a booster 6 to 12 months later is the recommended regimen for patients with no prior tetanus vaccine. This should be given to this patient at this office visit.

A. A tetanus booster will not provide adequate immunity for this patient. Two doses followed by a booster is more appropriate.

B and **C.** Although adults should not receive pertussis vaccines, a tetanus-diphtheria vaccine is appropriate.

E. Tetanus immune globulin is the treatment for tetanus, but there is no clinical suspicion of tetanus in this patient.

109. **C.** Aortic stenosis commonly can present later in life without the patient having preexisting heart problems in the past. A systolic ejection murmur is commonly heard with it.

A. Aortic dissection presents with abrupt, excruciating onset of pain. No murmur is associated with it.

B. Aortic regurgitation has a crescendo-decrescendo diastolic murmur.

D. Mitral regurgition is associated with a pansystolic murmur.

E. Mitral stenosis is associated with a low-pitched, rumbling diastolic murmur with an opening snap.

110. **D.** Neuroblastoma is the most common neoplasm of infancy, and can present as a nontender abdominal mass. CT or MRI will usually reveal an adrenal mass. Urine studies often shows elevated levels of vanilmandelic acid and homovanillic acid levels. Treatment may involve surgical excision with postoperative chemotherapy.

A. Autosomal-dominant polycystic kidney disease presents in patients over 20 years of age. Typical findings include flank pain and hematuria.

B. Autosomal-recessive polycystic kidney disease presents in infants with bilateral large cystic kidneys and renal failure.

C. Wilms tumor often presents as a nontender abdominal mass, but may also cause elevated blood pressure and microscopic hematuria.

E. A Meckel diverticulum normally presents with painless rectal bleeding in infants.

111. **B.** This patient exhibits features of exhibitionism. Patients are typically timid males who become sexually aroused by exposing their genitals to unsuspecting females (adults or children). They are only rarely aggressive. They may masturbate during the exposure and need a shock reaction from the female for satisfaction.

112. **D.** The young male has evidence of frotteurism. This condition involves arousal from touching or fondling a nonconsenting person, usually in a crowded place where escape is possible. Usually involves teenage or young adult males.

113. **E.** This patient has evidence of hypoactive sexual desire disorder. Affecting approximately 20% of the population, this condition is more common in women and may present as inhibited excitement or inhibited orgasm. Depression, anxiety, and stresses of the relationship may also play a role.

114. **J.** Vaginismus is an involuntary spasm during coitus of the muscles surrounding the outer third of the vagina, which prevents penile entrance. It may be related to physical causes producing pain-dyspareunia. However, in this patient with a normal examination and a history of past sexual trauma, vaginismus is the most likely diagnosis.

115. **A.** This patient has evidence of dyspareunia. It is often related to a physical condition (50%), cervical or vaginal infection, or anatomic abnormality. Anxiety about sexual activity can produce pelvic muscle tightening and pain. However, pain from organic causes can also produce anxiety, which exacerbates the pain.

116. **F.** This patient has evidence of retrograde ejaculation into the bladder. This is often due to organic factors such as anticholinergic drugs and can occur after transurethral prostate surgery. Psychotherapy is rarely helpful for these patients. Medical therapy with an alpha agonist to contract the bladder neck may be helpful in some patients.

117. **G.** This patient has evidence of paraphilia. These patients become sexually excited only by unusual or bizarre stimuli (practices or fantasies). Orgasmic release occurs by masturbation during or following the event. Etiology is uncertain but may relate to biologic, learned, and/or dynamic instincts. These conditions frequently coexist with personality disorders.

118. **E.** Fifty percent of patients with primary amyloidosis have cardiac involvement, and if infiltrative is usually dominated by right-sided heart failure. The narrowed pulse pressure results from the low stroke volume. This diagnosis should be suspected in any patient with an otherwise unexplained cardiomegaly, heart failure, heavy proteinuria, or hepatomegaly. Treatment is supportive.

A. Air in the vasculature may have dire consequences and present with a sudden onset of cardiopulmonary and neurologic decompensation. Dyspnea is almost a universal finding.

B. Budd-Chiari syndrome presents with hepatomegaly and ascites in nearly 100% of patients and may demonstrate right-sided heart failure secondary to impaired outflow.

C. Congestive heart failure is not the best explanation for the constellation of signs and symptoms.

D. Cor pulmonale is an alteration of right ventricular structure due to pulmonary hypertension caused by diseases affecting the lung.

119. **B.** Fabry disease is a hereditary condition that is the result of accumulation of glycosphingolipids with terminal alpha galactosyl moieties in lysosomes of glomerular, tubular, vascular, and interstitial cells, which can be observed with renal biopsy. Renal disease manifests in the late teens to early twenties with lipiduria, proteinuria with minimal hematuria, nephrotic syndrome, hypertension, and progressive renal insufficiency. Diagnosis can be made by physical examination of the above findings. Measurement of urinary glycosphingolipids and estimation of peripheral leukocyte alpha-galactosidase levels help confirm the diagnosis.

A. Alport syndrome is an X-linked disease resulting in abnormal production of type IV collagen. Males develop microscopic hematuria, proteinuria, and progressive renal insufficiency. Light microscopy on renal biopsy reveals mesangial hypercellularity, focal and segmental glomerulosclerosis, chronic tubulointerstitial fibrosis, atrophy, and

accumulation of foam cells. Sensorineural hearing loss is also common. Glycosphingolipids and elevated alpha-galactosidase levels are not characteristic.

C. Lecithin-cholesterol acyltransferase deficiency has renal manifestations of proteinuria, microscopic hematuria, and progressive renal insufficiency. Renal biopsy reveals focal and segmental glomerulosclerosis. Glycosphingolipids and elevated alpha-galactosidase levels are not characteristic.

D. Lipodystrophy may be acquired or congenital as an autosomal-recessive trait. The disease causes metabolic abnormalities and loss of body fat. Painful nodular swellings of adipose tissue can occur. Renal manifestations common occur in girls between the ages of 5 and 14 years. Nephrotic range proteinuria and progressive renal insufficiency are common. Low C3 levels are also common.

E. Nail-patella syndrome is an autosomal-dominant disease. It is characterized by bony abnormalities, usually of the elbows and knees, and nail dysplasia. About half of patients have nephropathy. Light microscopy findings from renal biopsy reveal local glomerular basement membrane thickening, tubular atrophy, interstitial fibrosis, and varying degrees of glomerular sclerosis. The disease usually manifests as asymptomatic hematuria and proteinuria. Progression to end-stage renal disease is rare. Glycosphingolipids and elevated alpha-galactosidase levels are not characteristic.

120. **C.** Between 20 and 36 weeks' gestation, fundal height, measured from the symphysis pubis, corresponds to the weeks of gestation to within 2 weeks.

121. **A.** Acute lymphocytic lymphoma (ALL) has a peak incidence at 3 to 5 years of age, and is the most common pediatric neoplasm. Common presenting symptoms include fever, pallor, lethargy, malaise, and bone pain. Diagnosis is by bone marrow aspiration.

B. A radiograph of the chest would be performed to rule out mediastinal involvement.

C. A CT scan may be performed, but would not be diagnostic of ALL.

D. The presence of the Philadelphia chromosome, which indicates a 9,22 translocation, is diagnostic of chronic myelogenous leukemia.

E. A peripheral blood smear frequently reveals "blast cells," but this may not reflect the true bone marrow morphology.

122. **D.** Guillain-Barré syndrome (GBS) is a progressive, ascending weakness caused by peripheral nerve demyelination. It has an acute onset, and normally develops 7 to 21 days after viral infection or *Campylobacter jejuni* infection. A lumbar puncture reveals an albuminocytologic dissociation. Treatment is intravenous immune globulin or plasmapheresis.

A. Acyclovir is used for herpes encephalitis.

B. Antibiotics would not be used for GBS, but would be indicated for bacterial meningitis.

C. Anticholinesterase therapy is used in myasthenia gravis, but has no role for GBS.

E. Intubation is often used for GBS if there are signs of respiratory failure, but the presented patient is breathing comfortably.

123. **C.** A patient with a pulmonary embolism classically presents with sudden onset of chest pain, cough, dyspnea, and tachypnea. Patients with a pulmonary embolism have usually developed a clot in the deep veins that can be related to the Virchow triad of endothelial injury, stasis, and hypercoagulable status. In this case we suspect an active pulmonary embolism, and the only way to definitively rule out this diagnosis is pulmonary arteriography.

A. Chest x-ray is not specific enough to detect the presence of a pulmonary embolism.

B. Spiral CT is fast becoming a measure used to detect emboli, but unfortunately has not found its way into standardized testing.

D. Ventilation/perfusion scanning is a less invasive method, but when given the choice, the gold standard (pulmonary arteriogram) should always be done first.

E. Vascular studies are appropriate to screen for deep venous thrombosis in the presence of obvious clinical findings (unilateral lower extremity swelling and erythema).

124. **A.** Menopause marks the termination of the reproductive phase in a woman's life through the resultant loss and atresia of oocytes. During this period, luteinizing hormone and follicle-stimulating hormone (FSH) levels gradually increase in response to decreased negative feedback from diminished estrogen production secondary to this primary ovarian failure.

B. Blood serum FSH levels will not establish a diagnosis of menopause.

C. Blood serum testosterone levels will not establish a diagnosis of menopause.

D. Ovarian tissue biopsy cannot establish the diagnosis of menopause.

E. Papanicolaou smear will identify cervical dysplasia or neoplasia.

125. **D.** This patient has clinical and radiologic evidence of a renal stone. The kidney, ureter, and bladder (KUB) image demonstrates a large right renal calcification. The CT scan shows that the large stone is in the renal pelvis. Approximately 80% to 90% of urinary tract calculi will appear radiodense on plain x-rays.

Figure 125a

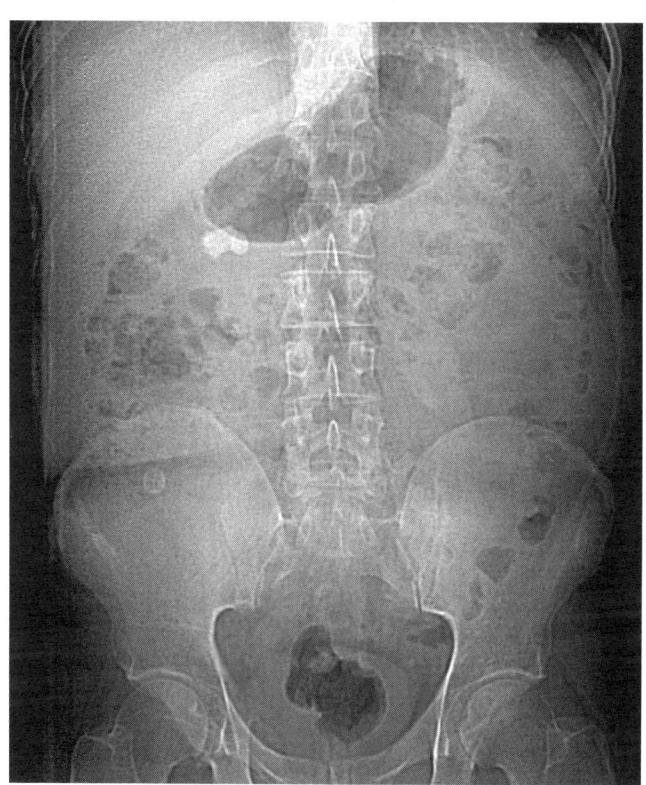

Figure 125b

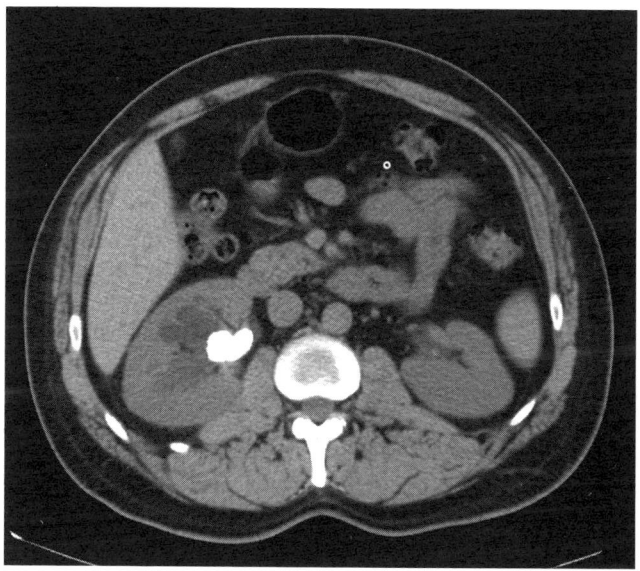

A and **B.** Although one might be confused that this is a gallstone on the KUB image, the CT scan clearly shows that this stone is in the kidney.

C. A phlebolith is a pelvic vein stone. This stone is neither in the pelvis nor in a vein.

E. Transitional cell carcinoma of the renal pelvis would appear dark on CT scan.

126. **A.** This patient may have suffered a ruptured berry aneurysm (saccular aneurysm). This is possible based on the history of hypertension, smoking history, and the classic clinical picture. If the patient's diagnosis is in question and the patient is stable, it may be prudent to consider a lumbar puncture. However, with a good suspicion of ruptured berry aneurysm, a lumbar puncture is not necessary. CT scan is a fairly sensitive and noninvasive method to diagnose berry aneurysm.

B and **C.** Withdrawal of cerebral spinal fluid only contributes to morbidity by risking herniation and/or further bleeding.

D. Angiography performed within 6 to 8 hours after presentation may increase the risk for rebleeding. Second, although an angiogram is essential in the preoperative evaluation, the patient is not a surgical candidate until he stabilizes.

E. Watchful waiting is not a prudent option for a patient with a suspected ruptured berry aneurysm because it can result in death secondary to brain ischemia caused by loss of adequate blood flow to the brain.

127. **D.** This child's presentation is consistent with diabetes insipidus (DI). Common symptoms of this disease include polyuria, polydipsia, and increased thirst. This leads to hypernatremic dehydration. However, differentiating nephrogenic from central DI cannot be determined by symptomatology alone. Both conditions are characterized by a normal blood glucose and elevated serum osmolality. In nephrogenic DI, antidiuretic hormone (ADH) levels are normal but the nephron tubules are unresponsive to ADH. Therefore, when DDAVP is given in a test dose to patients with DI, urine output is unchanged in those with nephrogenic DI but is significantly decreased in those with central DI.

A. In central DI, the posterior pituitary does not release adequate amounts of ADH.

B. Diabetes mellitus would be characterized by an increased blood glucose.

C. Glomerulonephritis presents with hematuria, azotemia, and oliguria.

E. Renal tubular acidosis is characterized by a hyperchloremic metabolic acidosis.

128. **A.** Adenocarcinoma of the esophagus accounts for over 40% of esophageal cancer in some Western countries. The most common etiologic factor in the development of this condition is Barrett esophagus, which is a metaplastic change in the lower esophageal lining from squamous to columnar. There is no evidence that medical therapy or an antireflux procedure removes the risk for neoplastic transformation in the distal esophagus.

B. Leiomyoma comprises 50% of benign esophageal tumors, and most are located in the distal two thirds of the esophagus.

C. Lymphoma is an uncommon tumor of the esophagus.

D. Sarcomas are rare esophageal neoplasms that often present with dysphagia. The masses can expand intraluminally.

E. Squamous cell carcinoma accounts for the majority of esophageal cancers and can be linked to environmental factors such as food additives (nitrous compounds) and deficiencies of zinc and molybdenum not to reflux.

129. **B.** This is a pregnant patient who has a urinary tract infection. Initial treatment with trimethoprim/sulfamethoxazole for urinary tract infections is appropriate in this patient. Treatment for 7 days or more yields a better cure than treatment for less than 7 days regardless of the drug used.

A. Ordering an intravenous pyelogram would not be the next step in the treatment given the findings on physical examination.

C. Intravenous ampicillin and gentamicin would be appropriate treatment for pyelonephritis.

D. Ciprofloxacin is contraindicated in pregnancy.

E. Tetracycline is contraindicated in pregnancy.

130. **D.** This is a classic presentation of adult respiratory distress syndrome (ARDS) with the acute onset of dyspnea, wheezing, cough, and tachypnea. Most commonly ARDS occurs 12 to 24 hours after sepsis. Other causes include (but are not limited to) aspiration, severe pneumonia, drug effects, or shock. ARDS is a neutrophil-mediated event where damage to the lung tissue occurs through the release of enzymes (protease) and free radicals and other inflammatory mediators. This in turn causes capillary damage, allowing protein-rich fluid to seep into the alveoli—hence the alveolar pattern on the film. Edematous change decreases compliance and elasticity and results in a ventilation/perfusion (V/Q) mismatch.

A. Depression of the respiratory center produces a respiratory acidosis also, but without a V/Q mismatch.

B. The type II pneumocyte is damaged, which decreases surfactant production. Subsequent alveolar collapse ensues.

C. The A-a gradient in ARDS is increased (>30 mm Hg), further indicating V/Q mismatch. The intrapulmonary shunting resulting from the alveolar collapse causes this increase in gradient.

E. A blood gas for ARDS would show a respiratory acidosis.

131. **B.** The current therapy for Alzheimer disease, which is this patient's most likely diagnosis, is a cholinesterase inhibitor. This condition represents 50% of all dementias (5% of people over age 65). It is usually a diagnosis of exclusion. Onset is insidious and can progress to death within 10 years.

A. Anticholinergic agents would have the opposite the desired effect in Alzheimer dementia, since there actually is a decrease in cholinergic activity in this condition.

C. Electroconvulsive therapy is not effective treatment for Alzheimer disease.

D. Reassurance is not appropriate because the course of Alzheimer dementia is progressive.

E. Selective serotonin reuptake inhibition is not an effective treatment for Alzheimer disease.

132. **A.** Cervicofacial actinomycosis is a slowly developing disease. Abscesses drain to the surface for a long time, and masses of filamentous organisms or sulfur granules may be seen in the pus. Pain is usually minimal. Bony involvement may be seen on x-ray.

B. *Listeria* causes five types of infection: infection during pregnancy, granulomatosis infantisepticum, bacteremia, meningitis, and focal infections.

C. *Haemophilus influenzae* would not explain these symptoms.

D. *Providencia stuartii* is a common cause of urinary tract infections in hospitalized patients.

E. *Streptococcus viridans* causes subacute bacterial endocarditis.

133. **A.** Asherman syndrome. Multiple dilation and curettages, cesarean section, and endometritis are all risk factors for Asherman syndrome, which is characterized by adhesions in the endometrial cavity. These adhesions show up on ultrasonography in classic "bridging" patterns.

B. An LH:FSH ratio of greater than 2.5 is associated with polycystic ovarian disease and not with this patient's clinical picture.

C. Premature ovarian failure would be suspected in elevated LH and FSH values (not the case in this question) and would not be likely with this presentation.

D. Stein-Leventhal syndrome is one end of the spectrum of presentations of polycystic ovarian disease syndrome. It is characterized by anovulation, diminished or absent menses, hirsutism, obesity, and enlarged ovaries, with multiple cysts appearing on ultrasonography as the classic "string of pearls."

E. Swyer syndrome is not associated with this patient's history, in fact it is the name for gonadal agenesis in a genotypical male who subsequently presents phenotypically as a female.

134. **B.** This patient has true sciatica (pain radiating below the knee in L4–S3 distribution) as indicated by positive straight leg test. Most cases of sciatica resolve after 2 to 3 weeks with a brief period of bed rest (not more than 3 days), nonsteroidal antiinflammatory agents, physical therapy, and local heat. Extended periods of bed rest have been shown to worsen back pain. Current recommendations are that bed rest should not be extended for longer than 3 days.

A. Bed rest should not be extended for longer than 3 days. In addition, referral to the pain clinic is unnecessary at this time.

C. Long-term disability is unnecessary at this time.

D. This patient does not have any signs or symptoms that would indicate immediate surgical intervention (bowel or bladder incontinence or motor/sensory deficits).

E. Surgical removal of a herniated disk may be considered for patients with persistent or disabling symptoms, but a period of conservative treatment should be instituted first.

135. **A.** Protein levels are not significant to diagnose preeclampsia, and patient blood pressure not exceedingly high (usually expect >140/90 mm Hg on at least two recordings to consider preeclampsia). Bed rest would be appropriate for a stable, preterm mother with mild preeclampsia.

B. Bed rest would be appropriate for a stable, preterm mother with mild preeclampsia.

C. Cervical examination may be important to determine cervical effacement and dilation but is not a treatment for preeclampsia.

D. This patient does not require immediate induction of labor. She does not meet criteria for preeclampsia.

E. This patient should not be treated with hydralazine because she does not meet criteria for preeclampsia or eclampsia.

136. **A.** Estrogen is increased in polycystic ovarian syndrome because of chronic anovulation that results in increased levels of androgens and estrogens. These increased androgens and estrogens are then converted in the body's fat to estrone.

B. The combination of being hyperandrogenic and obese often leads to insulin resistance and eventually hyperinsulinemia. One can understand, then, the increased incidence of associated type II diabetes mellitus.

C. This state of excess estrogen may be reflected in an LH:FSH ratio above 2.5, but, although less likely, there may also be a normal LH:FSH ratio.

D. The high levels of androgens result in lowered levels of sex hormone–binding globulin, which then, naturally, results in even higher levels of free estrogen and androgens.

E. This state of excess estrogen may be reflected in an LH:FSH ratio above 2.5, but, although less likely, there may also be a normal LH:FSH ratio.

137. **E.** This patient has experienced deep venous thrombosis (DVT), thrombus formation from the deep veins of the leg or pelvis. DVTs are most often seen in postoperative patients (especially hip and prostate surgery), pregnant women, obese or bedridden patients, females using oral contraceptives, or occurring after fractures of long bones. Local swelling or tenderness to deep palpation may be present over the affected vein.

A. Tachycardia rather than bradycardia is the most common symptom seen after embolization of DVT to the pulmonary circulation.

B. Although cellulitis after fracture of long bones is part of the differential diagnosis, DVT is more likely given the sudden onset of the condition.

C. A positive Homan sign may be associated with DVT. Pain is elicited by dorsiflexing the foot on the affected side.

D. The Virchow triad indicates increased risk for thrombus formation. It includes stasis, endothelial trauma, and hypercoagulability. Hypercoagulable states include protein C deficiency, nephrotic syndrome, high estrogen states, and cancer.

138. **B.** This child has a history of recurrent pyogenic infections. The appropriate treatment of this patient would be antibiotic therapy against the offending organisms and periodic gammaglobulin administration.

A. Antibiotic therapy alone will not improve morbidity and mortality in this patient.

C. Bone marrow transplantation is suggested for patients with DiGeorge syndrome.

D. Daily prophylactic trimethoprim would be indicated for chronic granulomatous disease.

E. Watchful waiting is not appropriate in patients with recurrent pyogenic infections. These should be treated with antibiotic therapy and immune system bolstering with gammaglobulin.

139. **C.** This patient has Takayasu arteritis, which is a vasculitis seen most often in adolescent females. Almost all forms of vasculitis are associated with erythrocyte sedimentation rates of greater than 100 mm/hr and other nonspecific signs of inflammation, including fever, malaise, weight loss, and normochromic, normocytic anemia. Hypertension is seen in forms of vasculitis that affect the renal vasculature, including polyarteritis nodosa, Wegener granulomatosis, Henoch-Schonlein purpura, and Takayasu arteritis. Takayasu arteritis, or "pulseless disease," affects large arteries (aorta, subclavian) and leads to diminished peripheral pulses. A chest x-ray should always be obtained and may display a widened aorta. Takayasu arteritis may also affect the carotid arteries, leading to syncope and stroke.

A. Antineutrophil cytoplasmic antibody, specifically the cytoplasmic type (c-ANCA) is diagnostic for Wegener granulomatosis but is not seen in Takayasu arteritis.

B. Blood cultures could reasonably be ordered, but a vasculitis rather than infection should be suspected based on all the given information.

D. There is no indication at this time for head CT. Takayasu arteritis should be treated with steroids in all cases, methotrexate in severe cases, and aggressive surgical repair of the affected arteries.

E. There is no indication at this time for joint aspirate analysis.

F. Temporal artery biopsy would be necessary when temporal arteritis is suspected, but this would be seen in older individuals with complaints of headache, temporal pain, and vision changes.

140. C. Although most chest radiographs will be unremarkable, some, like the one given, will show peribronchial cuffing and hyperinflated lungs. Hyperinflation is indicated by more than 10 posterior ribs seen above the diaphragm. Peribronchial cuffing is simply the radiographic appearance of edema around the bronchial tree. The diagnosis of asthma is supported with the evidence of decreased oxygenation, wheezes auscultated on examination, and history of onset in an allergen-abundant environment. The history of past difficulty breathing suggests that this disease process has been going on for quite some time even though it had yet to be diagnosed.

Figure 140

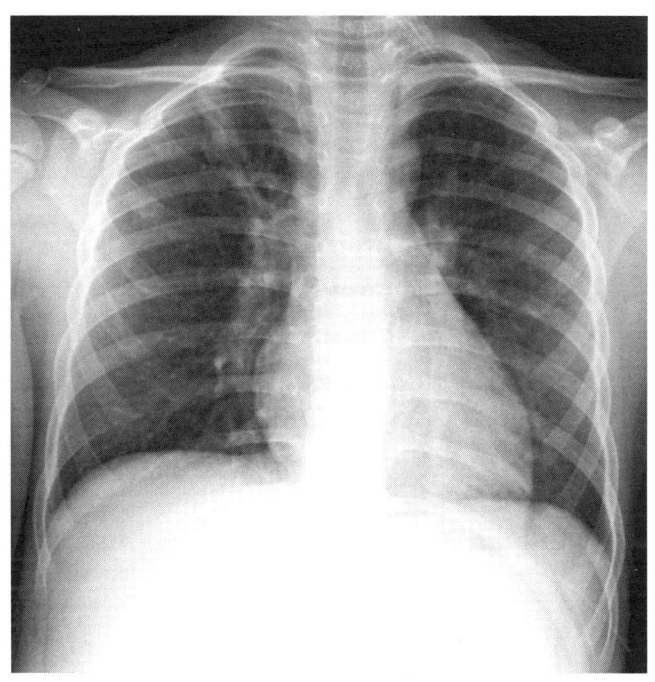

A and E. Although the patient's age puts him well out of range for cancer to be the most likely etiology, there are no history or physical examination findings that support these two diagnoses. Also, the radiographic appearance shows no pulmonary nodules.

B and D. Despite the symptoms of cough and rhinitis, it is unlikely to see these kinds of severe respiratory compromise in patients with the common cold (rhinovirus infection) or allergic rhinitis. Also, the radiographic findings do not support these diagnoses.

141. E. This patient has symptoms of ptyalism. Ptyalism, or excess salivation, can be quite bothersome to patients. Affected individuals can produce up to 1 liter of saliva per day. Treatment strategies include atropine, which produces a small decrease in secretions. Patients should be reassured that this condition will remit as the pregnancy progresses and is not dangerous.

A. The diagnosis of acute appendicitis is suspected when nausea and vomiting is preceded by anorexia and periumbilical or right lower quadrant pain.

B. Gastroesophageal reflux occurs postprandially and is associated with midepigastric pain.

C. Hepatitis is associated with right upper quadrant pain and elevation of liver function test results (transaminases).

D. Hyperemesis gravidarum is associated with protracted nausea and vomiting with pregnancy.

142. A. Adjustment disorder is a common psychiatric condition. This patient is suffering from normal grief secondary to the loss of a loved one. This is a traumatic event and the symptoms that this patient has are typical of an adjustment disorder.

B. Brief reactive psychosis is unlikely given this patient's symptoms and duration.

C. Atypical depression is more common in females with a history of psychiatric disorders.

D. Major depression is a possible sequela if adjustment disorder does not resolve in this patient.

E. Schizoaffective disorder is unlikely given this patient's symptoms and and their duration.

143. B. Fragile X is an X-linked disorder characterized by moderate mental retardation, macrosomia, macroorchidism, macrognathia, large head circumference, and large ears. It occurs with a frequency of 1 out of every 1000 males.

A. Down syndrome is an autosomal chromosomal abnormality that occurs once in every 700 live births. Those affected may have the following: upslanted palpebral fissures, small ears, microcephaly, micrognathia, a flat occiput, a flat nasal bridge, a short sternum, excess skin on the back of the neck, brachydactyly, clinodactyly, duodenal atresia, hypotonia, septal defects, hypothyroidism, and moderate mental retardation.

C. Klinefelter syndrome is an abnormality of sex chromosomes that occurs in 1 out of every 1000 males. This disorder is due to a sex chromosome abnormality. The most common karyotype is 47 XXY. Pubertal males have a female body habitus, decreased body hair, microorchidism, a small phallus, and hyposermia, and tend to be taller than average.

D. Trisomies 13 and 18 are examples of autosomal trisomies. These conditions are associated with craniofacial abnormalities, congenital heart abnormalities, abnormalities of the extremities, as well as developmental delays. Unlike Down syndrome and fragile X syndrome, Klinefelter syndrome usually results in mild mental retardation.

E. This disorder is not Y-linked.

144. | **C.** Chondrosarcoma is a malignant tumor of cartilage, most commonly seen in the metaphyses of long bones and in the pelvis. The typical patient is 30 to 60 years of age. Treatment involves wide surgical resection or amputation. Chemotherapy and radiation are of limited success and often used in palliative efforts.

A. Adamantinoma is a tumor that arises in the diaphyses or metaphyses of long bones such as the tibia.

B. Aneurysmal bone cyst is a vascular lesion in the metaphysis of young children and may respond to radiation therapy.

D. Tumors that are metastatic to bone include breast, prostate, lung, thyroid, and kidney. Pathologic fractures are the usual presenting symptom.

E. Unicameral bone cyst is an expansile, benign bone lesion of childhood. Usually affecting the femur or humerus, this fluid-filled cavity can be associated with pathologic fractures. The lesion often resolves spontaneously after bone maturity occurs.

145. | **A.** This patient likely has Huntington chorea. Pathology is located in the caudate nucleus. This is a subcortical dementia with symptoms that range from neurotic to psychotic (including dementia). It is important to remember to check other family members for this disease, which is inherited in an autosomal-dominant fashion.

B. The cerebellar cortex is not involved in Huntington disease.

C. The corpus callosum is not involved in Huntington disease.

D. Diffuse cortical involvement is not typical with Huntington disease.

E. Parkinson disease is a disease of the substantia nigra.

146. | **E.** Because this man has no symptoms of end organ damage, he is presenting with hypertensive urgency. Any systolic blood pressure measurement greater than 210 mm Hg or diastolic pressure greater than 120 mm Hg is considered a medical emergency and must be treated with a fast-acting antihypertensive such as nitroprusside, diazoxide, or labetolol. Had symptoms of end organ damage (e.g., encephalopathy, left ventricular failure, or acute renal failure) been present with or without a drastically elevated blood pressure, he would have been in a hypertensive emergency.

A. If he had been symptom-free with a diastolic blood pressure less than 120 mm Hg, it would have been appropriate to correctly diagnose hypertension by obtaining three separate measurements. Stage I hypertension is either a systolic pressure greater than 140 mm Hg or a diastolic pressure greater than 90 mm Hg on three separate measurements. Prehypertension is defined as systolic pressure greater than 120 mm Hg or diastolic pressure greater than 80 mm Hg on three separate measurements, and should be treated with lifestyle modifications.

B and **C.** Although lifestyle modifications are acceptable to recommend to any patient with an unhealthy lifestyle, they cannot be recommended for the purpose of lowering blood pressure until the official diagnosis of hypertension has been made.

D. Although angiotensin-converting enzyme (ACE) inhibitors are very effective for reducing blood pressure (but less so in blacks) and have the additional benefit of reducing the risk for stroke and heart attack, they do not work immediately enough to lower the dangerously elevated pressure in this case. Sodium nitroprusside is more appropriate. ACE inhibitors should also be used in all type II diabetics, whether or not they have hypertension, due to the reduced risk for diabetic nephropathy and retinopathy when a patient is on an ACE inhibitor. Such is not the case if they cannot tolerate the side effects.

147. | **C.** The management of adult respiratory distress syndrome (ARDS) involves treating any underlying causes, intubation, and beginning oxygen therapy with mechanical ventilation to correct the hypoxia and ventilation/perfusion mismatch.

A. There is no proven benefit to steroids in ARDS.

B. This patient needs adequate treatment to prevent the progression. The most frequent cause of mortality in ARDS is multisystem organ failure.

D. PEEP increases intrathoracic pressure and would therefore not be the best answer. Increasing intrathoracic pressure could worsen the condition by worsening pulmonary edema.

E. If permissible, airway intubation is the option for treatment of this patient.

148. **B.** Osteoporosis is the progressive reduction and weakening of bone as a result of the aging process. Several important risk factors for osteoporosis have been identified: female gender, white or Asian race, smoking, early menopause, family history of osteoporosis, and low body weight. Other factors associated with increased risk for osteoporosis may include excessive alcohol intake, low calcium intake, nulliparity, and lack of exercise. The most likely individual to develop osteoporosis is the 47-year-old Asian woman who has a history of thyroid disease and weighs 95 pounds. She has 3 risk factors: female gender, Asian race, and low body weight.

A. This individual possess none of the above-mentioned risk factors for osteoporosis development.

C. This individual has one risk factor (female gender) for osteoporosis development.

D. This individual has one risk factor (female gender) for osteoporosis development.

E. This individual has one to two risk factors (female gender, overweight, and possibly inactive) for osteoporosis development.

149. **B.** Patients with solitary pulmonary nodules should receive follow-up chest x-rays to evaluate progression of the lesion. Solitary pulmonary nodules are usually surrounded by normal lung and without satellite lesions. Lesions are well circumscribed with smooth contours. A solitary nodule that does not change in size or shape in 2 years is most likely to be benign.

A. The most common location of an aspirated foreign body is the right middle lobe. The x-ray findings note that the lesion is in the right lower lobe.

C. The progression of malignant melanoma is rapid, and this patient would have exhibited signs of metastasis and progression of the chest x-ray findings by this time.

D. Bronchogenic carcinoma is exceedingly rare in this age group. The progression of such carcinoma is rapid, and this patient would have exhibited signs of metastasis and progression of the chest x-ray findings by this time.

E. Primary bronchogenic carcinoma is rare before the age of 45 and is often associated with cough and blood-tinged sputum production.

150. **D.** A 15-mm induration is needed for a healthy patient in a low-risk population. A 10-mm induration is considered positive in health-care workers, intravenous drug users, patients with medical illnesses, and children under 4 years of age. A 5-mm induration is considered positive in HIV-infected patients, patients with recent contact to active TB, and patients with fibrotic chest radiographs.

A–C. This patient does not need to be treated for TB. He is considered low risk on the basis of his medical history.

E. This patient has no medical reason for termination from the workplace. He is considered low risk to acquire TB on the basis of his medical history.

151. **B.** The dermatologic problem described in the question is consistent with erythema toxicum neonatorum, a rash found on 50% of full-term babies. This rash typically presents 24 to 72 hours after birth and is most commonly found on the trunk, face, and extremities. Microscopic examination of the vesicular contents characteristically reveals eosinophilic leukocytes. The rash is transient and usually resolves without treatment in 3 to 5 days.

A. Cutis marmorata is a pink, marble-like mottling of the skin in neonates. It is a normal and physiologic phenomenon.

C. Milia are benign subepidermal keratin cysts commonly found on the chins, noses, and foreheads of neonates. They are also transient and require no treatment.

D. Mongolian spots are found in over 90% of African-American, Asian, and Indian infants. They are transient, darkly pigmented macules most often found over the lower back and buttocks.

E. Seborrheic dermatitis, or "cradle cap," is found in areas dense with sebaceous glands, such as the scalp, face, postauricular, and intertriginous areas. The lesions are dry, scaly, erythematous, and can be pruritic. It typically presents later than erythema toxicum neonatorum, between 2 and 10 weeks of life.

152. **A.** The history and physical findings are consistent with compartment syndrome, which can be caused by muscle contusions, hemorrhage, prolonged compression, or reperfusion injury after revascularization (i.e., after arterial embolism or trauma). Classically the signs and symptoms of decreased perfusion are the "six P's": pallor, paresthesia, pulselessness, pain, paralysis, and poikilothermy (cold). Swelling or hemorrhage causes increased interstitial pressure in the unyielding compartments of the leg to the point that it exceeds capillary perfusion pressure. *Warning:* Do not rule out compartment syndrome if distal pulses are palpable; systolic pressures are much higher than the pressure needed to make the muscles and nerves ischemic. Compartment syndrome is predominantly a clinical diagnosis, and the patient should undergo an immediate fasciotomy because it only takes 6 to 8 hours for irreversible muscle and nerve damage.

B. The clinical picture suggests the diagnosis of compartment syndrome.

C. The Thompson test results in an intact Achilles tendon.

D. Because the clinical picture already confirms compartment syndrome, fasciotomy must be performed immediately.

E. The clinical picture already shows compartment syndrome, so these physical examinations are not needed.

153. **B.** A CD4 count of greater than 500/mm³ implies early HIV disease for which the most common finding is lymphadenopathy. This finding is considered to be a part of the group III classification of HIV infection. Group I and II classifications include acute HIV syndrome and asymptomatic infection, respectively. Group IV disease consists of infectious, neoplastic, and neurologic complications of HIV.

A. Herpes zoster infection typically occurs in patients with CD4 counts of 200 to 500/mm³.

C. As with herpes zoster infection, Kaposi sarcoma will occur in patients with CD4 counts of less that 500/mm³.

D. Non-Hodgkin lymphoma is a neurologic opportunistic infection that occurs with CD4 counts of 200 to 400/mm³.

E. Oral thrush is an infectious (group IV) complication of HIV disease that typically occurs in patients with CD4 counts of less than 500/mm³.

154. **C.** Panic disorder is defined as recurrent unexpected panic attacks. A panic attack is a period of intense fear or discomfort that develops suddenly and peaks within 10 minutes. Four of the classic thirteen symptoms of panic attacks must be present to diagnose panic disorder. In addition, for at least 1 month following one of the attacks, one of the following must be present: persistent concern about having additional attacks, worry about the implications or consequences of an attack, or a significant change in behavior related to the attack. Panic disorder can occur with or without agoraphobia. This individual does not have agoraphobia.

A. Agoraphobia is an intense fear of places or situations in which escape might be difficult. Conditions that are feared are avoided or are endured with much distress.

B. Obsessive-compulsive disorder is characterized by recurrent obsessions and compulsions that cause significant distress and occupy a significant portion of the individual's life. From the information given, this patient does not have obsessions about anything, nor does she display compulsive behavior.

D. Social phobia is an anxiety disorder where individuals have a great fear of being scrutinized in public places. This woman clearly fits criteria for a panic attack, and has persistent worry about having another panic attack. Her desire for social interaction is displayed by her working at a bar to support herself before she finds another job. Therefore, her anxiety is not due to fear of social situations or being scrutinized.

E. This patient had normal cardiac enzymes, a normal ECG, and a normal chest x-ray. In addition, this patient is a healthy young woman who is a nonsmoker and therefore has none of the risk factors for coronary artery disease.

This patient's symptoms occurred only when she was interviewing, peaked within 10 minutes, and fit all of the criteria for panic disorder. Therefore, unstable angina would not be the most likely diagnosis.

155. **D.** Progestin therapy is considered helpful in patients with hirsutism (due to increased levels of LH) who have a contraindication to estrogen therapy. This woman is a smoker, which is a contraindication due to a hypercoagulable state associated with estrogen. Progesterone decreases levels of LH, which results in less androgen production, and the relative decrease of androgen levels allows for increased catabolism of testosterone. This then results in lowered levels of testosterone. This woman likely has polycystic ovarian syndrome with the LH:FSH ratio of 3 and the association of diabetes with this syndrome. She therefore has an ovarian cause for her hirsutism.

A. Combined oral contraceptive pill preparations can be used to suppress LH and FSH and increases sex hormone–binding globulin. Because it contains estrogen, this is contraindicated in this patient, since she is a smoker.

B. Gonadotropin-releasing hormone agonists like leuprolide acetate (Lupron depot), nafarelin acetate (Synarel) and goserelin (Zoladex) work by suppressing LH and FSH. This treatment also results in a hypoestrogenic state, and the patient would need estrogen supplementation along with this treatment. This is contraindicated in this patient because she is a smoker and obese.

C. Prednisone is the treatment for adrenal nonneoplastic conditions, not ovarian conditions.

E. Spironolactone has antiandrogen effects that have been useful in androgen suppression due to an adrenal nonneoplastic origin. It has a temporary effect and so is not ideal.

156. **A.** Cocaine may adversely affect any organ system and is associated with significant morbidity and mortality. Typical cardiovascular effects include left ventricular dysfunction, hypertension, aortic rupture, angina pectoris, cardiac arrhythmia (any type is possible), and coronary artery disease.

B. The autonomic effects of cocaine use include tachycardia and hypertension.

C. Mitral valve rupture is a possible cardiac sequela of cocaine use. Mitral valve prolapse is more common in young females.

D. Pulmonary valvular dysfunction and pulmonary hypertension can result from cocaine use.

E. Left ventricular dysfunction is a possible cardiac sequela of cocaine use.

157. A. Subdural hematoma is seen frequently after automobile accidents with head trauma. The CT results are pathognomonic for acute subdural hematoma.

B. Chronic subdural hematoma is typically seen in the elderly or alcoholics, and over a couple of weeks mental function deteriorates. This was a sudden loss of consciousness.

C. Diffuse axonal injury shows diffuse blurring of the gray and white matter and multiple small hemorrhages.

D. Epidural hematoma would show a lens-shaped hematoma on CT scan. Also, epidural hematoma is associated with a lucid interval followed by a progressive deterioration in level of consciousness.

E. Subarachnoid hematomas are not usually associated with trauma. They present with sudden onset of a severe headache described as the worst headache of my life. They are associated with ruptured berry aneurysms.

158. D. The patient described has slipped capital femoral epiphysis (SCFE). The disorder is most common in adolescent males. The cause is unknown, and it is not associated with trauma. Patients may present with either hip or knee pain, and diagnosis is made with frog-leg radiographs. Treatment consists of surgical fixation of the slipped femoral head into correct position.

Figure 158

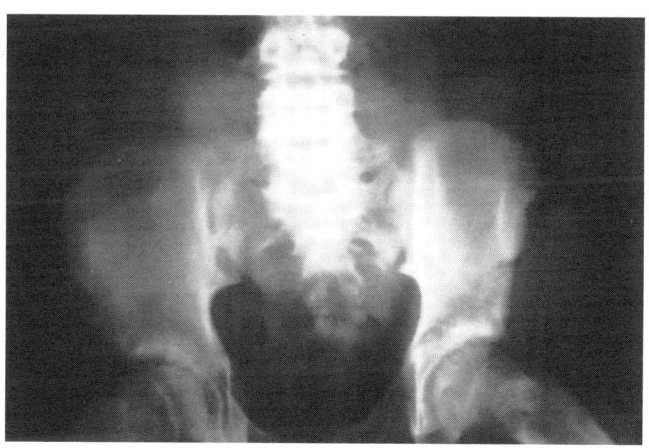

A. Physical therapy is not indicated for SCFE. These patients should be advised to not bear weight on the affected limb until stabilized.

B. Rest and pharmacotherapy is not appropriate for these patients.

C. Observation is not appropriate for these patients.

E. Arthroscopy has no benefit for patients diagnosed with SCFE.

159. A. The combination of delayed social development and vocabulary make autism a likely diagnosis. This condition can begin in childhood and progress into adulthood. It is considered a psychosis.

B. Attention deficit hyperactivity disorder is unlikely in a patient with delayed social development.

C. Congenital deafness is unlikely in this patient.

D. This patient has no evidence to suggest fragile X syndrome.

E. Mental retardation is not a likely possibility in this case.

160. A. Analgesics such as acetaminophen, ibuprofen, and codeine are considered safe during pregnancy. Antibiotics such as penicillins, erythromycin, and cephalosporins are also considered safe in pregnancy. These medications usually do not require dose adjustments.

B–E. Ciprofloxacin, methotrexate, valproic acid, and warfarin are contraindicated during pregnancy.

161. C. This patient most likely has infective endocarditis. Blood cultures are an important diagnostic test, and three sets of blood cultures should be drawn prior to starting antibiotics. Positive blood cultures are considered a major criterion for the diagnosis of infective endocarditis.

A. Nafcillin, penicillin, and gentamycin are an appropriate regimen to start until cultures and sensitivities are known, but blood cultures should be drawn prior to starting antibiotics.

B. The chest x-ray may show evidence of a cardiac abnormality but is not as important as blood culture results.

D. Transfusion of fresh frozen plasma is not indicated in the evaluation of infective endocarditis.

E. Valve replacement is not part of the initial workup for endocarditis.

162. H. This newborn has 18p- syndrome. This condition is characterized by mild growth deficiency. In addition, ptosis, hypertelorism, micrognathia, large ears, small hands, and small feet can be present.

163. D. This newborn has triploidy 69 XXX. This condition is characterized by a placenta with hydatiform changes. Stillborn or early neonatal death is possible. Other findings on physical examination include hypospadias and cryptorchidism.

164. A. This newborn has trisomy 8. This syndrome is characterized by thick lips, deep-set eyes, prominent ears, and camptodactyly (permanent flexion of the interphalangeal joints).

165. **D.** This patient presents 5 days after her operation complaining of constipation that can be attributed to her use of narcotic medications. Unfortunately, some patients will misuse or abuse pain medication, particularly narcotics. It is crucial to first rule out surgical causes before assuming medication abuse. In this vignette, the patient admits to using medication excessively, and since constipation is a side effect of narcotics that does not yield to tolerance, we would expect a certain level of persistent bowel discomfort.

A. Adhesions become evident months after the surgical procedure and are less likely after laparoscopic surgeries.

B. Iatrogenic bowel injury would manifest with peritoneal signs on physical examination.

C. Ileus is defined as nonmechanical obstruction of the bowel that prevents normal functioning. The small bowel does not manifest ileus postoperatively, gastric ileus can persist from 24 to 48 hours, and colonic ileus may last from 3 to 5 days. Ileus can be made worse by inflammation or blood in the peritoneal cavity. Narcotics also delay the return of bowel function.

E. Postoperative inflammatory bowel disease is more likely to cause chronic diarrhea than constipation.

166. **D.** This patient likely has a pancreatic insulinoma. His history of headaches, diaphoresis, nausea/vomiting, tachycardia, loss of consciousness, and relief of symptoms with food or intravenous dextrose corresponds with hypoglycemic states. The markedly elevated levels of insulin and protein C indicate that the extra insulin is coming from his own body (protein C is cleaved from preinsulin when insulin is made). Pancreatic insulinomas fit in the category of carcinoid tumors, which include tumors that secrete other hormonal and bioactive agents, including gastrin, serotonin, somatostatin, histamine, bradykinin, and kallikrein.

A. The patient's symptoms would be closer to those of volume depletion and hyperthermia, the insulin and protein C levels would be normal, and glucose would not relieve his symptoms.

B. Even though his symptoms would be identical with self-injection of insulin, his protein C levels would be normal or decreased.

C. This individual does not have evidence of exogenous ingestion of thyroid hormone. His symptoms would resemble hyperthyroidism, his thyroid-stimulating hormone would be decreased, and his insulin and protein C would be normal.

E. This patient does not have diabetes mellitus. His symptoms would not be relieved with eating. Exercise is recommended with type II diabetes in order to lower glucose levels to within normal limits and improve insulin sensitivity.

167. **A.** According to the definition, a person is dependent on a drug if he or she exhibits three of the following signs: tolerance; withdrawal; repeated and unintended use; persistent failed efforts to cut down; excessive time spent trying to obtain the drug; reduction in social, occupation, or recreational activities; and continued use despite awareness that the drug can cause psychological or physical problems. Due to the fat-soluble properties of marijuana, it is almost unheard of to have withdrawal symptoms. It is slowly released from the fat in the body. However, you can have enough symptoms to still be considered dependent without withdrawal.

B. Addiction to a drug is more of a quantitative description of how the drug affects a person's life, rather than a physical condition. This means that the person may psychologically be seeking a drug constantly but does not physically need it.

C. It is possible to be addicted without being physically dependent. It is also possible to be dependent and tolerant to a drug without being addicted, such as narcotic use in terminally ill patients.

D. It is possible to be addicted without being physically dependent. It is also possible to be dependent and tolerant to a drug without being addicted, such as narcotic use in terminally ill patients.

E. This patient is both addicted to and dependent on the drug in question.

168. **C.** This patient has symptoms consistent with Wolff-Parkinson-White syndrome. Pertinent findings include tachycardia and preexcitation on ECG as well as the slurred upstroke, or delta wave. The appropriate cure for reentrant circuits is radiofrequency ablation.

A. Beta blockers cannot control an accessory cardiac pathway. Radiofrequency ablation is a better alternative.

B. Calcium channel blockers are ineffective in controlling an accessory pathway. They may be indicated when there is associated atrial fibrillation with a very rapid (>250/min) ventricular rate and hemodynamic compromise.

D. Digoxin may be useful in the treatment of narrow QRS complex tachycardia. One must take note of side effects such as nausea, atrioventricular block, and ventricular or supraventricular arrhythmias.

E. This patient is not experiencing tachycardia from dehydration. Thus, rehydration with saline is unlikely to be of benefit for this patient as a primary therapeutic intervention.

169. **C.** Stress incontinence is characterized by loss of urine with straining (coughing, sneezing, laughing) or exertion. It is commonly associated with pelvic relaxation and displacement of the urethrovesical junction. Urge incontinence or detrusor instability is loss of urine associated with uninhibited and involuntary bladder contractions.

A. This describes an areflexic bladder.

B. Neurogenic bladder results from injury, congenital abnormality, or disease process involving the central or peripheral nervous system supply to the bladder.

D. This describes an unstable bladder with loss of urine from uninhibited contractions.

E. Total incontinence is the continuous leakage of urine resulting from fistula formation occurring secondary to pelvic surgery or pelvic radiation.

170. **E.** Prostate cancer incidence increases with age and has been found to be most common in African-American men. Adenocarcinoma of the prostate typically arises at the periphery of the gland; therefore, digital rectal examination is one of the best screening tests for prostate cancer. Upon palpation of a mass, transrectal needle biopsy should be used to confirm the diagnosis. Spread of prostate cancer is by local extension, with the most common location of metastasis being the axial skeleton. Widespread bone metastases may respond to several therapies, including androgen ablation, orchiectomy, luteinizing hormone–releasing hormone agonists, or antiandrogens such as flutamide.

A. Flutamide is an antiandrogen used to treat advanced prostate cancer.

B. Nilutamide is an antiandrogen used to treat advanced prostate cancer.

C. This patient should have a prostate needle biopsy based on abnormal findings during digital rectal examination. Prostate-specific antigen (PSA) levels are not diagnostic for prostate cancer, but are considered to be a screening tool. Increased PSA can indicate adenocarcinoma or benign prostatic hyperplasia (BPH). Free PSA must then be assessed, and if low, adenocarcinoma of the prostate is more likely than BPH.

D. Radical prostatectomy is the gold standard treatment for organ-confined prostate cancer in patients with at least a 10-year life expectancy. However, in the above scenario, the patient has not yet been diagnosed with prostate cancer.

171. **C.** This patient suffers from schizoid personality disorder. Patients with this disorder show a pervasive pattern of social detachment and a restricted range of emotions and expression in interpersonal settings. They must meet four of the following criteria: (1) lack a desire for intimacy, (2) choose solitary activities. (3) have little interest in sexual experiences, (4) take pleasure in few, if any, activities, (5) lack close friends, (6) appear indifferent to praise or criticism, and (7) show emotional coldness or detachment.

A. Autistic disorder is distinguished by more severe social impairment, as well as stereotyped behaviors and interests.

B. In avoidant personality disorder this isolation is due to fear of being embarrassed or found inadequate, and there is excessive anticipation of rejection.

D. Schizoid personality disorder may be distinguished from schizophrenia by a lack of psychotic symptoms.

E. Schizotypal personality disorder tends to be characterized by more cognitive and perceptual distortions. Although schizoid and avoidant personality disorder are both marked by social isolation.

172. **B.** This patient has clinical and radiographic evidence of Crohn disease. CT scan shows thickening of the terminal ileum. Inflammation of the adjacent mesenteric fat, abscesses, and fistulas can also be seen in severe cases. This condition typically occurs in the terminal ileum but can arise from any portion of the gastrointestinal tract from mouth to anus.

Figure 172

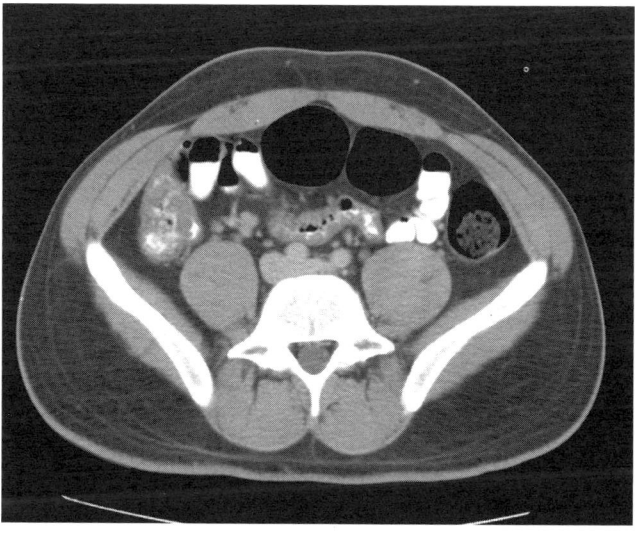

A. Adenocarcinoma of the small bowel is an uncommon lesion, especially in young people.

C. Meckel diverticulitis typically occurs in 2% of the population and is 2 feet from the iliocecal valve.

D. Mesenteric ischemia is associated with poor blood flow to the small bowel. It typically occurs in elderly patients who have pain out of proportion to their physical examination findings.

E. Ulcerative colitis occurs in the colon and is associated with bloody diarrhea.

173. **C.** Uterine atony is the leading cause of postpartum hemorrhage. Patients are at higher risk secondary to chorioamnionitis, multiple gestation, macrosomic fetus, use of anesthesia, use of oxytocin, and prolonged labor.

A. Cervical laceration is most often associated with rapid cervical dilatation.

B. Placenta acceta is the abnormal adherence of part or all of the placenta to the uterine wall. May be associated with a normally implanted placenta or a placenta previa. It is often asymptomatic in the antepartum period but can cause profuse hemorrhage and shock with substantial maternal morbidity and mortality. This is due to the inability of the placenta to separate from the uterine wall after delivery.

D. Uterine rupture is associated with previous uterine surgery (i.e., prior cesarean section or myomectomy) or if fetal parts are palpable abdominally.

E. The clinical picture suggests uterine atony, but vaginal lacerations are also a common cause of postpartum hemorrhage. They are generally ruled out by careful physical examination.

174. **C.** Wilms tumor can present as a painless flank mass during the first 5 years of life. Associated signs may include hypertension, fever, and hematuria. Risk factors include genitourinary anomalies, sporadic aniridia, hemihypertrophy, and a positive family history. Initial tests should include a CBC, urinalysis, and renal function tests. He will then need an abdominal imaging study such as ultrasonography, CT, or MRI.

A. Abdominal CT would be used later in the workup to evaluate extension of the tumor.

B. Abdominal ultrasonography would follow the initial blood work to define the origin of the tumor within the kidney.

D. MRI would be used later to evaluate possible extension of the tumor.

E. Percutaneous biopsy is not indicated for management of Wilms tumor.

175. **C.** This patient has signs and symptoms of anal carcinoma. This condition is associated with chronic rectal irritation from hemorrhoids, perineal fistula, leukoplakia, and trauma from anal intercourse. Women are more commonly affected than men, and typical presenting features include bleeding, pain, and a perineal mass. Radiotherapy and chemotherapy together lead to a complete response in 80% of patients when the lesion is smaller than 3 cm.

A. Chemotherapy alone is less effective than combination therapy for anal carcinoma.

B. Radiotherapy alone is less effective than combination therapy for anal carcinoma.

D. Subtotal proctocolectomy may be indicated for patients with large or recurrent lesions.

E. Surgical resection of the polyp is less effective than combination therapy for anal carcinoma because polyps are likely to recur.

176. **C.** This patient has rubeola. A 3- to 4-day history of fever, coryza, conjunctivitis, and cough followed by a maculopapular rash starting at the head and neck and spreading downward is characteristic. The rash becomes brown and desquamating in 5 to 6 days.

A. Erythema infectiosum is caused by parvovirus B19 and has a characteristic slapped cheek appearance. The rash consists of maculopapules on the extremities.

B. Infective mononucleosis has a maculopapular rash similar to rubella preceded by fever, adenopathy, and sore throat.

D. Rubella has little or no prodrome and a maculopapular rash that begins on the head and neck spreading downward. It fades in 3 days.

E. Varicella is characterized by a fever followed in 1 to 2 days by a macular to papular rash that becomes vesicular and crusts.

177. **B.** Discontinue clozapine. Agranulocytosis is a known side effect of clozapine; it happens in 1% of patients on this drug. Increasing the dose is inappropriate management. This patient is leukopenic, and decreasing the dose is not appropriate to prevent agranulocytosis.

A, C, and **D.** Clonidine is not effective against leukopenia induced by clozapine.

E. Electroconvulsive therapy is not effective management of the negative symptoms of schizophrenia.

178. **A.** The most likely reason for amenorrhea in a woman of reproductive age is pregnancy. Analysis of beta human chorionic gonadotropin must be performed to rule out pregnancy as the cause for amenorrhea in this patient, who has established fertility (G2P2002).

B. CA 125 is a tumor marker for ovarian cancer that can also be elevated by liver disease and peritoneal irritation, not the first choice for determining the most likely cause of amenorrhea in this patient.

C. Luteinizing hormone and follicle-stimulating hormone levels in this patient would be normal for values drawn early in pregnancy but would not be a confirmatory test for pregnancy. These levels would be assessed if an anovulatory cause were suspected, as in polycystic ovary syndrome.

D. Percentage body fat would be low in an anorexic patient, who could have cessation of menses secondary to low body fat. Extreme athleticism could also result in amenorrhea.

E. Thyroid-stimulating hormone would be an important level to check in the workup of amenorrhea (positive for abnormal bleeding) because hypothyroidism can result in oligomenorrhea and hyperthyroidism can result in menorrhagia.

179. **C.** When malignant cells are killed by chemotherapy, intracellular components are released from within the cells. A triad of hyperkalemia, hyperphosphatemia, and hyperuricemia occurs, known as tumor lysis syndrome. Both before and during chemotherapy, metabolic support for this is essential.

A. Granulocyte infusion is controversial and rarely used.

B. Intravenous antibiotics are given if the leukemic patient becomes febrile.

D. RBC transfusions are given once the hematocrit level is less than 20%.

E. Platelets are transfused if the count becomes less than 20,000/mm^3.

180. **C.** Ovarian failure presents with elevated FSH and LH because the ovaries have stopped producing estrogen, which normally acts in a negative feedback loop to suppress FSH and LH.

A. GnRH overstimulation would result in increased levels of FSH and LH but not amenorrhea.

B. Hypothalamic disorder presenting with decreased FSH and LH (not increased) would result in amenorrhea.

D. Pituitary disorder resulting in amenorrhea would more likely have decreased FSH and LH as well.

E. Sheehan syndrome would present with amenorrhea caused by destruction of the pituitary secondary to postpartum hemorrhage.

181. **A.** Chédiak-Higashi disease is an autosomal-recessive disease characterized by impaired chemotaxis and phagolysosome fusion in neutrophils and monocytes. Patients get recurrent infections and the above symptoms. Presentation can occur in adolescence.

B. Chronic granulomatous disease reflects a group of disorders of granulocyte and monocyte oxidative metabolism. The disease shows an X-linked recessive pattern. Hydrogen peroxide production is diminished, and infection with catalase-positive bacteria is common. Aphthous ulcers and chronic inflammation of the nares are usually present. Granulomas are frequent and can cause obstruction. Excessive inflammatory reactions probably reflect abnormal turnoff of inflammation by failure to degrade chemoattractants and failure to degrade antigens that cause persistent neutrophil accumulation. Impaired killing of intracellular microorganisms by macrophages may lead to persistent cell-mediated immunity and granuloma formation.

C. Drug-induced neutropenia reflects a lack in production of neutrophils rather than impaired chemotaxis.

D. Felty syndrome is a disease of immunoglobulins directed toward neutrophils. A triad of rheumatoid arthritis, splenomegaly, and neutropenia are usually present. Patients may respond to splenectomy.

E. Myeloperoxidase deficiency is an autosomal-recessive trait and is the most common neutrophil defect. Microbicidal activity of neutrophils is delayed but not absent. However, if another defect, such as poorly controlled diabetes mellitus, is present, then host defenses may be significantly reduced.

182. **D.** Osteoid osteoma affects children and young adults 10 to 20 years of age and has a male predominance. It usually arises in the femur and tibia. The cardinal feature is pain, which is more severe at night. Signs of inflammation are unusual. X-ray reveals a sharply demarcated radiolucent nidus of osteoid tissue surrounded by sclerotic bone.

A. Aneurysmal bone cyst is a vascular lesion in the metaphysis of young children and may respond to radiation therapy. MRI may reveal blood-filled cystic spaces in affected areas. Treatment can also involve curettage or resection, except when the lesion is inaccessible.

B. Chordoma is a tumor of notochord origin that is slow growing and occurs in middle-aged adults.

C. Histiocytic lymphoma occurs in the diaphyses of long bones in patients over the age of 20.

E. Unicameral bone cyst is an expansile, benign bone lesion of childhood. Usually affecting the femur or humerus, this fluid-filled cavity can be associated with pathologic fractures. The lesion often resolves spontaneously after bone maturity occurs.

183. **A.** Delirium is a rapidly developing disorder of disturbed attention that fluctuates with time. Individuals often have clouding of the consciousness, attention deficits, perceptual disturbances, and sleep-wake alteration. Disorientation, memory impairment, incoherence, and altered psychomotor activity may also be noted. It is often difficult to distinguish a delirium from an acute functional psychosis. Electroencephalograms in this condition often reveal diffuse slowing. Treatment is usually supportive, with an active search for the underlying cause of the delirium.

B. Dementia is a loss of cognitive and intellectual functions sufficiently severe to interfere with social or occupational functioning. The most common cause of dementia is Alzheimer disease.

C. Depression in the elderly may coexist with dementia. Many patients with dementia become depressed as they understand the severity of their dementia. However, this patient does not exhibit classical signs of depression.

D. Normal aging is associated with a decreased ability to learn new material and a slowing of thought processes. Occupational and social functioning are normal in these individuals.

E. The history in this question gives no indication that the patient has suffered any recent loss of a loved one. Although he is experiencing difficulties on the job, his behavior is not typical of a grief reaction.

184. **B.** Erythematous, swollen, monoarticular joint pain of acute onset should lead the physician to initially evaluate for infection and gout. Gout is a condition resulting from intraarticular deposition of monosodium urate crystals and most commonly occurs in men (90%). It most commonly affects the first metatarsophalangeal joint, knees, ankles, and wrists, sparing the hips and shoulders. It is diagnosed by joint aspirate containing needle-shaped, negatively birefringent crystals and an elevated WBC count. Patients with long-standing gout may develop tophi leading to deformed joints and "bite" lesions of cortical bone. Allopurinol and probenecid are appropriate treatments for gout.

A. Initial treatment should be with colchicines, indomethacin, or steroids. Allopurinol and probenecid can be used prophylactically in patients with recurrent episodes. Allopurinol is contraindicated in acute attacks because it may precipitate an acute gouty attack.

C. Cephalexin is not likely to be effective in the management of gout.

D. Antibiotic is not recommended for this patient because laboratory studies clearly indicate gout rather than infection.

E. Loop and thiazide diuretics may also worsen hyperuricemia and are not appropriate treatments for gout.

185. **B.** Asherman syndrome is caused by adhesions in the endometrial cavity secondary to multiple dilation and curettage procedures, cesarean section, and/or endometritis. The progestin challenge is performed in the evaluation of patients who present with secondary amenorrhea to determine if enough endogenous estrogen is present and if the outflow tract is intact.

A. Anorexia is a condition that can present with secondary amenorrhea and have the above criteria in common.

C. Hyperthyroidism is a condition that can present with secondary amenorrhea and have the above criteria in common.

D. Hypothyroidism is a condition that can present with secondary amenorrhea and have the above criteria in common.

E. Polycystic ovarian syndrome is a condition that can present with secondary amenorrhea and have the above criteria in common.

186. **B.** Legg-Calve-Perthes disease is defined as avascular necrosis of the femoral epiphysis. It is most common in boys 4 to 8 years of age, and occasionally is bilateral. There is no association with trauma. Pain may be present, either in the hip or radiating to the knee. Bracing or surgery may be necessary to prevent collapse of the femoral head.

A. Developmental dysplasia of the hip, if untreated, will lead to avascular necrosis of the femoral head. However, symptoms would present much earlier.

C. Oscood-Schlatter disease occurs in adolescents and presents with pain over the tibial tuberosity.

D. Rickets is due to vitamin D deficiency and causes bowing of the legs.

E. Slipped capital femoral epiphysis is associated with limping and pain. Radiographs demonstrate epiphyseal displacement.

187. **E.** Several drugs can cause a syndrome resembling systemic lupus erythematosus (SLE). The syndrome is most common with procainamide, which induces the presence of antinuclear antibodies in up to 75% of individuals within a few months. There is a genetic predisposition to drug-induced SLE determined by drug acetylation rates. Typical symptoms include systemic complaints and arthralgias. The initial therapeutic approach is withdrawal of the offending drug.

A. Erythromycin is not implicated in causing drug-induced SLE.

B. Ferrous sulfate is not implicated in causing drug-induced SLE.

C. Hydralazine is the second most common cause of drug-induced SLE and induces antinuclear antigen positivity in up to 30% of patients taking this medication.

D. Penicillin has not been shown in clinical studies to cause a lupuslike reaction.

188. **D.** This patient's most likely diagnosis by her physical findings is iron deficiency anemia. It is the most common cause of anemia during childhood and is usually seen between 6 and 24 months of age. It may result from a nutritional iron deficiency, usually with rapid growth or from blood loss (i.e., microscopic intestinal hemorrhage). Mild iron deficiency is relatively asymptomatic. With moderate to severe iron deficiency, infants may develop anorexia, irritability, apathy, and fatigability. On physical examination patients may appear pale and sallow and have glossitis, angular stomatitis, spoon nails, and tachycardia with a systolic ejection murmur at the left sternal border. Very severe anemia may result in signs of congestive heart failure. If this is high on the differential, a serum iron level, TIBC, and ferritin level are needed for analysis. Other helpful tests include a CBC with differential and RBC indices, reticulocyte count, and blood smear.

A. Serum hematocrit determination will not aid in the diagnosis of iron deficiency anemia.

B. Serum lead level is important to determine but will not aid in the diagnosis of iron deficiency anemia.

C. Thyroid-stimulating hormone level is unlikely to aid in the diagnosis of iron deficiency anemia.

E. Urinalysis is unlikely to be of benefit in the diagnosis of iron deficiency anemia.

189. **A.** Bereavement occurs in the first 2 months following the death of a loved one. Therefore, the initial symptoms of this patient can be accounted for by bereavement. This patient's current symptoms meet criteria for major depressive disorder. Major depressive disorder is classified after a single episode of major depression. Five out of nine symptoms must be present to diagnose major depressive disorder. It is necessary that one symptom be either depressed mood or loss of interest or pleasure. This patient displays anhedonia. Other symptoms used in the diagnosis of this patient include change in sleep patterns, guilt, decreased energy, and change in appetite.

B. One episode of mania is required to meet the criteria for this disorder. This patient does not meet criteria for a manic episode.

C. Cyclothymia consists of recurrent mood disturbances changing between hypomania and dysthymia. It cannot be diagnosed if the patient has had a manic or major depressive episode.

D. Dysthymia is diagnosed by a minimum of 2 years of chronically depressed mood most of the time.

E. The diagnosis of hypothyroidism cannot be made on the symptoms found in this patient alone.

190. **C.** Hyperemesis gravidarum is intractable emesis during pregnancy. It occurs in 4 of 1000 pregnancies and is associated with severe gastrointestinal symptoms, weight loss, dehydration, ketosis, and electrolyte abnormalities. Hospitalization for fluid and electrolyte repletion is required. Diet can be reinstituted slowly and progressively.

A. Pyelonephritis is associated with fever, chills, flank pain, and a urinary tract infection.

B. Endometriosis is associated with the physical findings of uterosacral nodularity and pain on pelvic examination.

D. Peptic ulcer disease is associated with burning and gnawing pain in the midepigastric region after meals.

E. This patient does not display any features of psychosis.

191. **F.** Psoriasis is a chronic, recurrent disorder characterized by well-circumscribed erythematous plaques with silvery surfaces. These lesions are distributed on the extensor surfaces such as the knees, elbows, and buttocks. Onycholysis, pitting or thickening of the nail plate with subungual debris, may also be noted. Treatment strategies involve topical corticosteroids, coal tar ointment, ultraviolet light therapy, and methotrexate.

192. **H.** Seborrheic dermatitis is a chronic noninfectious process with erythematous patches and associated greasy yellowish scale. Lesions are often located on the scalp, eyebrows, nasolabial folds, axillae, chest, and posterior auricular areas. Treatment involves shampoos that contain coal tar, salicyclic acid, or selenium sulfide.

193. **C.** Erythema multiforme is a skin reaction composed of erythematous papules and bullae. Target lesions may also be noted and consist of erythema and normal flesh-colored skin with a central vesicle. Lesions may appear on the palms and soles of the feet. Drug reactions to penicillins and sulfonamides represent a common cause of this reaction.

194. **B.** Basal cell carcinoma is the most common form of skin cancer and occurs frequently on sun-exposed areas. Predisposing factors include fair complexion and exposure to inorganic arsenic. The clinical appearance is a pearly, translucent smooth papule with rolled edges and surface telangiectases. Treatment is surgical removal.

195. **E.** Pityriasis rosea is a self-limiting condition that lasts approximately 8 weeks. Lesions include oval erythematous patches with a peripheral rim of scale. These lesions begin as herald patches and later progress. Lesions are found along the trunk and proximal extremities. Treatment consists of oral antihistamines for pruritus as well as topical glucocorticoids. Most cases are self-limiting.

196. **E.** Omphalocele results from a failure of migration of the bowel from the umbilical coelom. It is characterized by herniation of the abdominal viscera, including the liver and spleen in large defects, through the umbilical and supraumbilical portions of the abdominal wall. The herniation is contained within a sac consisting of peritoneum and amniotic membrane. Omphalocele is associated with polyhydramnios in utero, and 10% of infants with this condition are born prematurely.

A. There is no evidence to suggest congenital diaphragmatic hernia.

B. Duodenal atresia is complete obstruction of the duodenum owing to failure of the normal recanalization process during the eighth to tenth weeks of gestation. Infants with this condition present with bilious emesis shortly after their first feeding.

C. Congenital hypothyroidism causes profound mental retardation if left untreated, but it is not associated with abdominal malformations.

D. Gastroschisis is differentiated from omphalocele by the absence of a sac, such that the herniated viscera is uncovered and adherent. Unlike omphalocele, gastroschisis is a surgical emergency. The herniation in gastroschisis occurs two centimeters lateral to the umbilicus.

197. **A.** This patient has a pleural effusion. Aspiration of the pleural fluid by thoracentesis indicates that this fluid is a transudate. Congestive heart failure is known to cause a transudative effusion, usually right sided. Other potential causes of transudates include nephrotic syndrome, cirrhosis, hypothyroidism, fluid overload, and constrictive pericarditis.

B. Mesotheliomas typically produce bloody effusions.

C. It is unlikely that this patient has pneumonia because there are no complaints of a fever or productive cough. Signs of effusion are dictated by gravity, not by lobar anatomy, as with the consolidation of pneumonia.

D. Sarcoidosis would be associated with bilateral hilar lymphadenopathy on chest x-ray. In addition, other systemic symptoms may be expected with this disease.

E. Tuberculosis causes an exudative lymphocytic effusion. Lymphocytes predominate on smear. Closed biopsy is required for diagnosis.

198. **D.** This patient is suffering from delirium. Elderly people are more prone to delirium, especially in nursing home settings. These patients may seem bizarre, confused, or even wild. On the other hand, some patients with delirium may appear somnolent or normal during the day and then decompensate dramatically at night. An electroencephalogram has a characteristic pattern of diffuse slowing.

A. This patient has no evidence to suggest acetaminophen overdose.

B. This patient has no evidence to suggest alcohol overdose. Intoxication can mimic mania, depression, or schizophrenia symptoms.

C. This patient does not display features of Alzheimer disease.

E. Stroke is unlikely because there are no signs of focal neurologic deficits.

199. **E.** A young woman with pathologic nipple discharge requires further evaluation by the physician. The most common cause of bloody nipple discharge (90% of the time) is intraductal papilloma, a benign condition. The papilloma arises from an isolated mammary duct, which should be excised.

A. Fibroadenoma is a lobular, firm, well-circumscribed solitary mass that is common in young women. Surgical excision is the treatment of choice in women over the age of 25. Younger patients may be treated with needle cytology and surveillance.

B. Fibrocystic change is associated with premenstrual breast tenderness and swelling. Patients with severe atypia or hyperplasia on biopsy are at risk for breast carcinoma.

C. Sarcoma of the breast represents a small percentage of breast cancers and is more common in women over the age of 40.

D. Infiltrating ductal cell carcinoma is the most common form of breast cancer. Lesions are typically hard, scirrhous, and infiltrating.

200. **A.** Given this patient's recent history of embolic strokes, bowel infarction is the most likely explanation for her weight loss. The slow course of her weight loss and lack of abdominal pain leads one to believe that the embolus lodged in her mesenteric artery was nonocclusive in nature. The finding of thumbprinting on x-ray is characteristic of the formless loops of bowel or intestine after atrophy from the decreased flow of nutrients.

B. Cholecystitis is not likely based on the presentation and findings of this case. She does not complain of right upper quadrant pain. There are no ultrasound findings of thickening of the gall bladder wall with inflammation.

C. Colon cancer is not likely based on the presentation and findings of this case. No laboratory values suggest anemia and there are no changes in bowel habits.

D. Depression can cause weight loss and is more prevalent in the elderly; however, it is not as likely given the past medical history.

E. Hyperthyroidism can cause weight loss but is also associated with other somatic findings not present in this patient.

201. **A.** This patient has classic symptoms of iron deficiency anemia, including microcytosis, hypochromia, low ferritin levels, and high iron-binding capacity. Such patients also have a low MCV and a lack of stored iron. For this disorder, it is important to find the cause of blood loss.

B. Anemia of chronic disease is associated with normal/high ferritin levels, low serum iron levels, and normal/increased iron-binding capacity.

C. Hemolytic anemia is associated with macrocytic anemia with an increased reticulocyte count.

D. Folate deficiency is associated with macrocytosis.

E. Sideroblastic anemia is associated with high ferritin levels, high serum iron levels, and low iron-binding capacity. This is typically caused from lead and medications like isoniazid or chloramphenicol.

202. **A.** Adenomatous polyps are benign glandular proliferations. They may be pedunculated or sessile. Approximately 80% have tubular histology, 10% villous histology, and 10% tubulovillous histology. These polyps are carcinoma precursors. Treatment is colonoscopic polypectomy.

B. Hyperplastic polyps are more common than adenomatous polyps and occur with increased incidence in the elderly.

C. Juvenile polyps are associated with intestinal bleeding, obstruction, and intussusception. This represents the most common cause of pediatric gastrointestinal bleeding.

D. Peutz-Jegher syndrome involves hamartomatous polyps that occur throughout the gastrointestinal tract. Mucocutaneous pigmentation is also associated with this condition.

E. Turcot polyps are familial adenomatous polyps and are associated with concurrent cerebral tumors.

203. **C.** This patient has clinical and radiologic evidence of small bowel obstruction. The KUB images demonstrate dilated air-filled loops of small bowel (supine film) and air-fluid levels (upright film). One of the most common causes of small bowel obstruction is adhesions that form scarlike bands around the small bowel.

A. There are no images of the lungs on this abdominal x-ray.

B. There is no radiographic evidence of foreign body.

D. There is no evidence of renal calculus on this x-ray.

E. Tumor thrombus is better assessed via CT, MRI, or venacavography.

Figure 203a

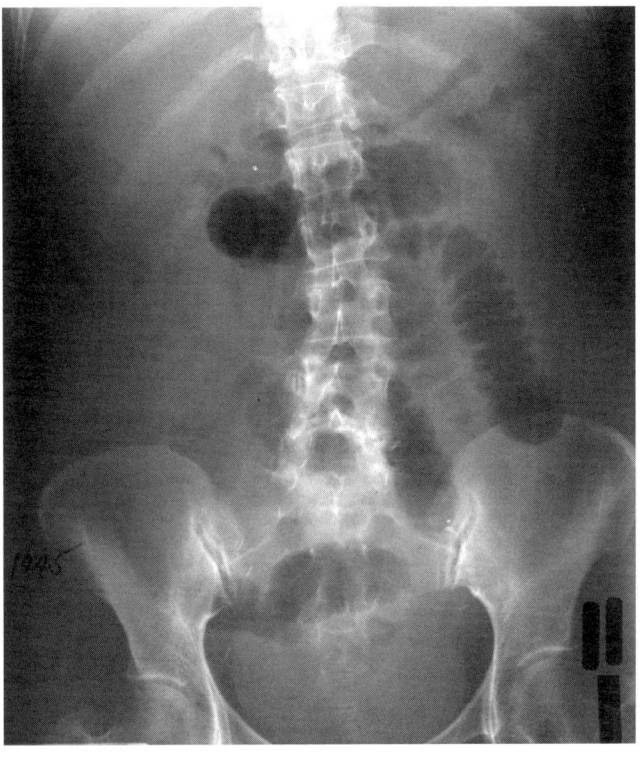

Figure 203b

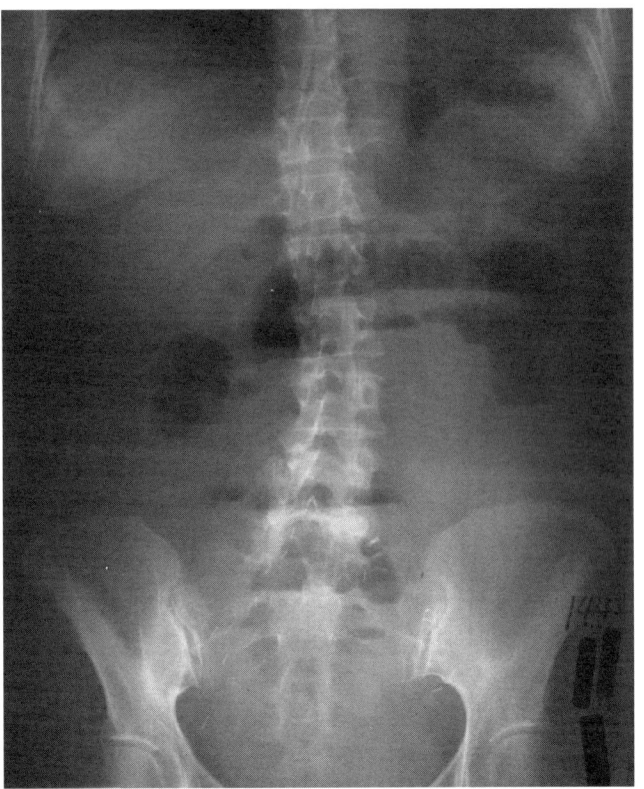

204. **A.** This patient likely developed renal insufficiency secondary to dye toxicity from cardiac catheterization. This causes acute tubular necrosis (ATN), which reveals a fractional excretion of Na (FeNa) of greater than 1 and granular or tubular epithelial casts on urinalysis.

B. Glomerulonephritis is not as likely as ATN given the timing and the events. Chronic hypertension can increase the risk for unstable angina or myocardial infarction (MI) and renal failure, but usually takes years to develop.

C. Malignant hypertension is not as likely as ATN given the timing and the events. Chronic hypertension can increase the risk for unstable angina/MI and renal failure, but usually takes years to develop.

D. Pyelonephritis is not as likely as ATN given the timing and the events. Chronic hypertension can increase the risk for unstable angina/MI and renal failure, but usually takes years to develop.

E. Renal artery stenosis is not as likely as ATN given the timing and the events. Chronic hypertension can increase the risk for unstable angina/MI and renal failure, but usually takes years to develop.

205. **E.** This patient is experiencing posttraumatic stress disorder (PTSD). PTSD is characterized by an extreme traumatic stressor followed by persistent reexperience of the trauma, efforts to avoid recollecting the trauma, and hyperarousal. Symptoms often include anxiety, agitation, flashbacks, and nightmares. The symptoms must be present for longer than a month, and must significantly affect daily life.

A. Acute stress disorder is similar to PTSD, but the symptoms must occur within 4 weeks of the event, and last from 2 days to 4 weeks.

B. Borderline personality disorder should also be considered in the differential diagnosis of a patient with PTSD, but it is characterized by unstable relationships, reactive and angry affect, impulsiveness, brief paranoia, and dissociative symptoms. A key in the history is the traumatic event that precedes PTSD.

C. Generalized anxiety disorder is characterized by intense worry over every aspect of life and is associated with physical manifestations of anxiety such as restlessness, irritability, sleep disturbance, difficulty concentrating, fatigue, and muscle tension.

D. Although malingering should be considered in the differential diagnosis, this patient clearly had a preceding trauma to his symptoms, which are very characteristic of PTSD.

206. A. Ewing sarcoma occurs primarily in adolescents and is 1.5 times more likely in males than females. It normally involves the diaphysis of long bones. Radiographs reveal a lytic bone lesion with calcified periosteal elevation ("onion-skinning"). Treatment consists of radiation, chemotherapy, and surgery.

B. Osteochondromas are slow-growing benign lesions that normally occur in the metaphysis of long bones.

C. Osteomyelitis presents with fever, bone pain, erythema, and edema. It needs bone aspiration for definitive diagnosis.

D. Osteogenic sarcoma shows the characteristic "sunburst" pattern on radiographs.

E. Rheumatoid arthritis normally causes bilateral disease of smaller joints, and normally presents with morning stiffness of joints.

207. A. The liver lies in the right upper quadrant of the body and is divided into a right and left lobe by the falciform ligament anteriorly. This ligament attaches directly to the peritoneum. The ligamentum venosum divides the right and left liver lobes posteriorly. The ligamentum venosum is formed from the degradation of the fetal ductus venosus.

B. The gallbladder serves to further subdivide the right lobe of the liver.

C. Neither the gallbladder fundus nor the gallbladder body serve to divide the right and left lobes of the liver.

D. The left hepatic artery is a branch of the common hepatic artery, which is a branch of the celiac artery. The vessel traverses both right and left hepatic lobes.

E. The right hepatic artery is also a branch of the common hepatic artery and traverses both right and left hepatic lobes.

208. A. 3-beta-hydroxysteroid dehydrogenase induces the inability to convert pregnenolone to progerone and the inability to convert dehydroepiandrosterone (DHEA) farther down the androgen synthesis pathway. The result is an accumulation of DHEA and its sulfate DHEAS. Both of these have a mild androgenic quality that results in too much androgen in females and not enough androgen in males, resulting in the condition described in this question stem.

B. Patients with 11-beta-hydroxylase deficiency present with similar symptoms of androgen excess because precursors are shunted toward androgen production.

C. Patients with 17-alpha-hydroxylase deficiency would not be able to make androgens.

D. Patients with 21-alpha-hydroxylase deficiency do not make 17-alpha-hydroxyprogesterone and present with salt wasting and adrenal insufficiency at the time of birth. The pathway is shifted then to make more androgens than normal. Female infants present with ambiguous genitalia from excess androgens.

E. Patients who have used anabolic steroids present with masculinization, although men may present with gynecomastia and shrunken testicles after he has stopped using steroids.

209. B. The patient is afflicted by sleep terrors. This parasomnia occurs in slow-wave sleep as opposed to nightmares, which occur in REM sleep. Understanding this, it is easy to see that treatment can be directed at reducing the duration of slow-wave sleep. Benzodiazepines (diazepam) are useful for this.

A. Amitriptyline is a tricyclic antidepressant. It has not been shown to be effective in treating sleep terrors.

C. Diphenhydramine is an antihistamine that induces drowsiness and is available over the counter. It has not been shown to be effective in treating sleep terrors.

D. Paroxetine is a selective serotonin reuptake inhibitor. It has not been shown to be effective in treating sleep terrors.

E. Zolpidem belongs to the sedative/hypnotic class of drugs and is frequently used as a sleep aid. It has not been shown to be effective in treating sleep terrors.

210. B. Congestive heart failure is a cause of prerenal azotemia. Through calculating the fractional excretion of Na (FENa), the value is determined as less than 1, indicating prerenal azotemia. The BUN to creatinine ratio is greater than 20, which also indicates prerenal azotemia. The presence of hyaline casts raises the suspicion of prerenal azotemia because they are found in no other cause of acute renal failure.

A. Acute tubular necrosis is a cause of intrinsic renal azotemia and would show an FENa of greater than 1 and granular or tubular epithelial cell casts.

C. Pyelonephritis usually presents with costovertebral angle tenderness, fever, and a urinalysis showing leukocytes, proteinuria, RBCs, and bacteria.

D. Renal artery thrombosis is also a cause of intrinsic renal azotemia and is associated with atrial fibrillation. The FENa would be less than 1, and the patient may have mild proteinuria or occasional red cells on microscopy.

E. Urinary tract obstruction might be present in a patient with trouble voiding, a palpable bladder, or abdominal/flank pain.

211. **C.** Idiopathic thrombocytopenic purpura has no apparent cause. It results from antiplatelet antibodies that adhere to platelets. Clinical manifestations typically present 1 to 4 weeks after a viral illness or immunization. Manifestations include abrupt onset of petechiae and ecchymoses of the skin and bleeding of mucosal membranes. CBC is normal, other than some thrombocytopenia. Peripheral blood smear may reveal large platelets, and antiplatelet antibodies are noted on serology. Bone marrow aspirate is not needed for diagnosis, but if done, it often reveals normal myeloid and erythroid elements with an increased number of megakaryocytes.

A. This patient has no history of any recent drug use.

B. This patient's spleen is not enlarged. CBC is normal, with the exception of decreased platelets.

D. If this patient had leukemia, one would expect an increase in the WBC count.

E. There is nothing on this patient's physical examination or in her history to suggest that she is septic.

212. **C.** This patient may have a deep venous thrombosis (DVT). The risk factors for this condition include venous stasis, endothelial injury and hypercoagulable stage. This particular patient requires Doppler ultrasonography to rule out DVT. Pregnancy is considered a hypercoagulable state.

A and **D.** This patient requires a duplex Doppler study to rule out DVT.

B. Physical therapy may be helpful to reduce peripheral edema once DVT has been diagnosed.

E. Analgesics, warm compresses, and bed rest are appropriate adjunct therapies for DVT.

213. **E.** This patient has mucormycosis. Diabetic ketoacidosis, steroids, and chronic renal failure are predisposing factors. Biopsy is usually required for diagnosis. Sinuses, lungs, and orbits can be affected. Black necrotic lesions and new cranial nerve abnormalities should raise suspicion of this disease.

A. *Aspergillus fumigatus* may affect sinuses or lungs of immunocompromised patients.

B. Blastomycosis usually occurs in men who acquire the illness during outdoor activities. Most common is pulmonary infection. Lesions of skin, bones, and urogenital systems can be seen with dissemination.

C. *Cryptococcus* often affects the central nervous system but may affect any organ.

D. Most cases of histoplasmosis are asymptomatic or subclinical. Symptomatic infections last 1 to 4 days with an influenza-like infection.

F. Sporotrichosis occurs after contact with soil or decaying wood and is caused by *Sporothrix schenckii*. It often begins with a hard, nontender, subcutaneous nodule and later ulcerates.

214. **D.** Schizophreniform disorder is essentially schizophrenia that fails to last for 6 months and does not involve social withdrawal. It is, by definition, self-limited. The time frame includes prodromal, active, and residual phases. Diagnosis changes to schizophrenia if symptoms last more than 6 months, even if in the residual phase.

A. This has been going on too long to be a brief psychotic disorder (<1 month) and too short to be schizophrenia (>6 months).

B. Delusional disorder is characterized by nonbizarre delusions. Most people would consider an alien takeover bizarre.

C. Schizophrenia requires that the symptoms be present for greater than 6 months.

E. This patient has evidence and meets criteria for a schizophreniform disorder.

215. **C.** This patient likely has bronchopneumonia. Radiography shows the characteristic pattern of patchy alveolar opacification. This pattern is shown in the right middle lobe. This diagnosis is supported by the fever and the physical examination findings. The sputum culture grew normal flora, indicating a poorly attained specimen; however, this should not cause you to disregard the prominent radiographic features of the bronchopneumonia.

Figure 215

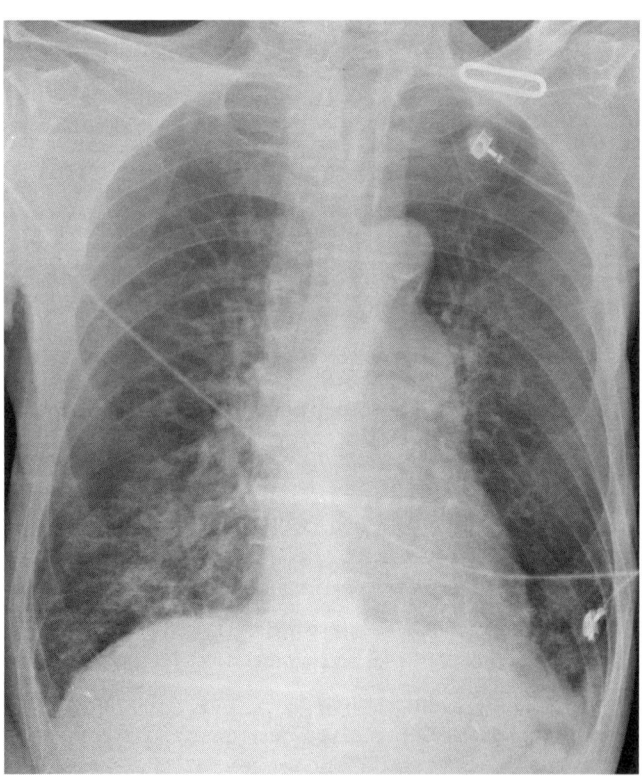

A. The radiographic picture of adult respiratory distress syndrome is one of diffuse, bilateral alveolar infiltrates.

B. The chest radiograph of a patient with asthma will usually be unremarkable; however, some will show peribronchial cuffing and hyperinflated lungs.

D. There is no opacification in a lobar distribution.

E. The classic picture of sarcoidosis on chest x-ray is that of bilateral, hilar lymphadenopathy. This is clearly not present in the provided figure.

216. **B.** Hyperchloremic, non–anion gap metabolic acidosis is characteristic of renal tubular acidosis (RTA). However, the information in this question is most consistent with a diagnosis of type 4, distal RTA. This is the most common RTA in both children and adults. It is characterized by aldosterone resistance or deficiency, which results in hyperkalemia. Urine anion gap is positive. The urine pH is usually less than 5.5.

A. Types 1 and 2 RTA, which are due to inability to secrete hydrogen ions into the distal tubule and impaired reabsorption of bicarbonate in the proximal tubule, respectively, result in either hypo- or normokalemia.

C. Lactic acidosis and uremia both result in an increased serum anion gap.

D. In type 2 RTA, pH is also less than 5.5, but the urine anion gap is negative. The urine pH is typically greater than 5.5 with type 1 RTA.

E. There is no evidence to suggest uremia.

217. **E.** Although exogenous estrogen replacement has been found to promote breast cancer growth, it has not been found to induce breast cancer. Estrogen is important in maintaining the integrity of urethral, vaginal, and uterine tissues by preventing tissue atrophy. It is also important in the maintenance of bone mineral content.

A. Estrogen has been found to aid in the maintenance of bone mineral content by preventing the relative loss via reabsorption through excessive osteoblastic activity. Osteoclasts are the cellular component responsible for laying bone down.

B. Exogenous estrogen has been linked to an increased incidence of endometrial hyperplasia and endometrial cancer; however, it has been shown to reduce the incidence of ovarian cancer.

C. Exogenous estrogen replacement has been found to pose an additional risk in the development of endometrial cancer.

D. Exogenous estrogen replacement has been found to pose an additional risk in the induction of breast cancer.

218. **A.** This patient has brucellosis, a zoonosis caused by four species of aerobic gram-negative bacilli. Combination therapy is needed due to a relapse rate as high as 50% with monotherapy.

B. Penicillin is not effective in the treatment of brucellosis.

C. This is not an appropriate regimen to treat brucellosis.

D. Streptomycin can replace gentamycin in the above combination or when used with trimethoprim-sulfamethoxazole as an effective regimen but is ineffective when used alone.

E. Therapy is needed to help prevent complications such as spondylitis and endocarditis.

219. **C.** Back pain is the most common neurologic symptom in patients with systemic cancer. Metastatic carcinoma, multiple myeloma, and lymphoma can involve the spine. Pain is often unrelieved with rest. MRI reveals metastasis with sparing of the disc space. Lytic bone lesions associated with multiple myeloma occur mainly in the skull and axial skeleton. They appear as "punched out" lesions that are caused by an osteoclast-activating factor secreted by the neoplastic plasma cells, which can also result in hypercalcemia. These lesions often cause severe "bone pain."

A. Without a history of trauma, low back strain is not a likely diagnosis.

B. Lumbar arachnoiditis may follow an inflammatory response to local tissue injury in the subarachnoid space.

D. Spondylolisthesis is slippage of the anterior spine while leaving the posterior elements behind. Lumbar radiculopathy can result.

E. Vertebral osteomyelitis is associated with low back pain that is unrelieved by rest, focal spine tenderness, and an elevated erythrocyte sedimentation rate.

220. **C.** There is a decreased incidence of ectopic pregnancy. This risk is not lowered as far as it is by oral contraceptives, but it is lower than no contraception at all. Disadvantages of this device include cramping, expulsion during menses, and ectopic pregnancy.

A. Intrauterine devices (IUDs) do not affect ovulation. A proposed mechanism of action for all IUDs is an induction of a sterile inflammatory response that engulfs and destroys sperm.

B. Progesterone-containing IUDs increase cervical mucus viscosity and thin the endometrial lining. The copper-containing IUD has a supposed mechanism of reducing sperm motility and capitation.

D. The rate of spontaneous abortions is raised to 40% to 50% in women who conceive with an IUD in place. If pregnancy is realized, the IUD must be removed by continuous gentle traction. No birth defects are associated with pregnancies started while using an IUD.

E. Absolute contraindications to IUD use are a history of pelvic inflammatory disease, undiagnosed abnormal uterine bleeding, suspected uterine or other gynecologic cancers, presence of any infection from the cervix and above, or a current pregnancy.

221. **A.** This patient likely has seasonal allergic rhinitis, which is a type I hypersensitivity immune response to environmental allergens, including airborne pollens. The allergen binds IgE on mast cells and inflammatory mediators are subsequently released in the upper respiratory tract.

B. Type II reactions are cytotoxic, causing cell lysis or phagocytosis commonly seen in Rh disease or Goodpasture syndrome.

C. Type III reactions are immune complex reactions. This type of reaction is seen in serum sickness.

D. Type IV reactions are delayed (cell-mediated) reactions. Examples include contact dermatitis or transplant rejection.

E. This patient is having a type I hypersensitivity reaction.

222. **A.** This patient likely has the antisocial personality disorder. This diagnosis is made when three or more of the following criteria are met: (1) failure to conform to social norms with respect to lawful behaviors, (2) deceitfulness, (3) impulsivity, (4) irritability and aggressiveness, (5) disregard for safety of self or others, (6) consistent irresponsibility, and (7) lack of remorse for harmful actions. The individual must also be at least 18 years old, and there must be evidence of a conduct disorder with onset before age 15.

B. People with borderline personality disorder are manipulative to gain attention or empathy. However, patients with antisocial personality disorder are manipulative to gain profit, power, or material gratification. They also tend to be less emotionally unstable and more aggressive.

C. Conduct disorder is a diagnosis usually made in childhood, and is excluded if the individual meets criteria for antisocial personality disorder.

D. Patients with histrionic personality disorder tend to be more exaggerated in their emotions, and do not characteristically demonstrate antisocial behaviors.

E. Patients with narcissistic personality disorder do not have the characteristics of impulsivity, aggression or deceit, and usually lack a history of conduct disorder or criminal behavior.

223. **D.** Dysfunctional uterine bleeding (DUB) is often caused by disorders of the hypothalamic-pituitary axis that result in a continuous supply of estrogen to the endometrium. The endometrium proliferates until it outgrows its blood supply and sloughs off, revealing exposed, torn blood vessels. Estrogen should be given to a hemodynamically unstable woman with DUB.

A. In hemodynamically stable patients, nonsteroidal anti-inflammatory agents have been found to be useful in ovulatory DUB. They reduce menstrual flow by 20% to 50% and may be used in coordination with estrogen and progesterone management.

B. Dilation and curettage is for those patients whose disorder does not respond to medical management. This is diagnostic and often therapeutic.

C. Further surgical methods of management include endometrial ablation and hysterectomy. One must be absolutely sure there is no cancer when deciding to use endometrial ablation because it may mask the symptoms of a growing cancer later.

E. Progesterone can then be used to cycle the patient once the bleeding has been controlled and stopped.

224. **B.** Aplastic anemia is characterized by pancytopenia and a low reticulocyte count. Most cases are acquired, but some are inherited, such as Fanconi anemia. Some common acquired causes include drugs, radiation, benzene/insecticides, and pregnancy. Chronic exposure at low-dose radiation increases incidence. For instance, patients receiving radiation treatments for ankylosing spondylitis are at increased risk.

A. Acute myeloid leukemia is characterized by an elevated WBC count and platelet count. Weight loss, fever, and bone and joint pain are some of the common characteristics.

C. Hereditary spherocytosis is an RBC membrane disorder that impairs correct formation of the cytoskeleton of the cell membrane. The disease is genetic and is transmitted as an autosomal-dominant trait. The clinical features are anemia, splenomegaly, and jaundice.

D. Myelodysplastic syndrome is a group of acquired blood disorders characterized by pancytopenia and a low reticulocyte count. In addition, this disease can be created secondary to an aplastic anemia. However, the transition from aplastic anemia to this disease takes many years to develop instead of the 2 weeks mentioned above. This disease often progresses to acute leukemia. The exact cause is unknown, but certain factors have been found to be contributors. These include radiation, genetic disorders such as Down syndrome and Fanconi anemia, drugs and chemicals, and aplastic anemia.

E. Polycythemia vera is a clonal disorder involving a multipotent hematopoietic progenitor cell in which there is overproduction of phenotypically normal red cells, granulocytes, and platelets. The disease shows an erythrocytosis in the absence of high or normal erythropoietin.

225. **B.** The patient in this question has neuroleptic malignant syndrome, which can be caused by antipsychotic pharmacotherapy. The elevated temperature, blood pressure, leukocytosis, elevated CPK, and delirium are characteristic of neuroleptic malignant syndrome. Bromocriptine is the treatment of choice.

A. Acetaminophen is not appropriate treatment for neuroleptic malignant syndrome.

C. Infection is not likely, so blood cultures will not help determine the treatment plan of this patient.

D. Sodium bicarbonate is used in tricyclic antidepressant overdose, another psychiatric emergency.

E. Dantrium is used in malignant hyperthermia, not neuroleptic malignant syndrome.

226. **A.** Medulloblastoma is the second most common brain tumor in children. It occurs most often between 3 and 5 years of age and arises from the floor of the fourth ventricle. The tumor may metastasize; thus, examination of the cerebrospinal fluid (CSF) is crucial. Treatment is surgical excision and radiation with adjuvant chemotherapy.

B. A chest radiograph may be beneficial if metastatic disease is suspected.

C. Preoperative chemotherapy is a treatment option. However, CSF examination is needed prior to starting any treatment.

D. Preoperative radiation is a treatment option. However, CSF examination is needed prior to starting any treatment.

E. The complete extent of tumor should be determined before any treatment is initiated.

227. **C.** Dubin-Johnson and Rotor syndrome both cause conjugated hyperbilirubinemia. They are also autosomal recessive and have mostly asymptomatic courses besides the jaundice. Dubin-Johnson syndrome is more common than Rotor syndrome and is therefore more likely. Dubin-Johnson syndrome results from impaired transport of the intracellular conjugated bilirubin into the extracellular bile canaliculi.

A. Crigler-Najjar syndrome type I causes unconjugated hyperbilirubinemia due to the complete inactivity of UDP-glucuronosyl transferase and is fatal in neonates.

B. Crigler-Najjar syndrome type II causes unconjugated hyperbilirubinemia. It is autosomal dominant and has a mostly mild course and normal life span, but the skin is markedly jaundiced and there is a risk for kernicterus.

D. Gilbert syndrome causes unconjugated hyperbilirubinemia. It is the most common cause of jaundice in the adult and is usually very mild.

E. Even though Rotor syndrome causes conjugated jaundice and has a mild course, it is less common than Dubin-Johnson and therefore less likely for causing this patient's jaundice.

228. **D.** The progesterone-only pill or Depo-Provera injections are indicated if the woman is breast-feeding. The breast-feeding woman can remain amenorrheic for several months. Ovulation may not begin for approximately 3 months.

A and **E.** These selections will not provide adequate birth control.

B. Combined oral contraceptive pills have been shown to decrease milk production.

C. Use of an intrauterine device involves a higher rate of extrusion in the immediate postpartum period.

229. **E.** Plummer-Vinson syndrome consists of postcricoid dysphagia, upper esophageal webs, and iron deficiency anemia. Improvement in dysphagia after iron therapy provides evidence for an association between the two. The iron deficiency leads to symptoms such as angular cheilitis (cracks at the corners of the mouth), glossitis (smooth red tongue), and koilonychia (spoon nails).

A. Achalasia is defined by aperistalsis. Dysphagia is often present, but patients often do not present with lethargy, glossitis, cheilitis, and koilonychias. Barium studies show aperistaltic contractions in a segment of the esophagus with dilatation of the esophagus proximal to the effected segment. The lower esophageal sphincter also fails to completely relax with swallowing.

B. Cytomegalovirus (CMV) infections are known to cause many problems, such as retinitis and meningitis; however, the symptoms mentioned in this vignette do not in any way suggest a CMV infection.

C. Esophageal adenocarcinoma can present with dysphagia and weight loss. However, patients often do not present with glossitis, cheilitis, and koilonychias.

D. Mallory-Weiss syndrome includes longitudinal lacerations in the esophagus at the esophagogastric junction caused by severe wretching and vomiting in the setting of toxic gastritis with failure of the lower esophageal sphincter. This causes severe bleeding/hematemesis, enough so that the patient may lose consciousness. These symptoms are most often associated with alcoholics.

230. **C.** This patient has panic disorder with agoraphobia. These attacks tend to occur several times per week. This condition is chronic, with exacerbations and remissions, and has an excellent prognosis with therapy. Medication is essential for panic disorder. Tricyclic antidepressants such as imipramine are good choices for these patients and often produce a response within 2 to 3 weeks.

A. Alprazolam is a medication used in the treatment of panic disorder but is associated with depression, addiction, and the need for frequent dosing.

B. Clonazepam, not clonidine, is useful in the management of panic disorder with agoraphobia.

D. Propranolol is also a possible treatment for panic disorder but is not as effective as imipramine.

E. Trazodone is a serotonin reuptake inhibitor that has unproven benefits in the management of panic disorder.

231. **A.** Gestational diabetes is suspected in patients with several risk factors, such as prior birth history of infants weighing greater than 4000 g, a history of repeated spontaneous abortions, a history of unexplained stillbirths, or a strong history of diabetes mellitus, obesity, and glucosuria. This mother has several risk factors for gestational diabetes and should be given a 1-hour glucola screening at the onset of prenatal care.

B and **C.** In patients lacking risk factors, the 1-hour glucola screening is usually performed between 24 and 28 weeks' gestation.

D and **E.** The 3-hour glucose tolerance test should be administered to patients whose glucose value on the 1-hour glucola test exceeds 140 mg/100 mL.

232. **C.** The Minnesota multiphasic personality inventory is a self-administered personality test that produces a general description of the patient's personality characteristics. Although this test is useful for a global description of the patient, its uses diagnostically are somewhat limited.

A. The Bender-Gestalt test involves having the patient draw nine specific geometric figures on a blank sheet of paper to detect visual motor impairment and organic defects.

B. The draw-a-person test asks the patient to draw the picture of a person and then a picture of a person of the opposite sex.

D. The Rorschach test is an unstructured projective test that asks a patient to describe what he sees in a series of ten standardized ink blots. It can be used diagnostically to help identify psychoses and personality disorders.

E. The thematic apperception test is a projective test similar to the Rorschach which draws conclusions from the patient's responses to a series of suggestive and ambiguous drawings.

233. **C.** This patient has Rocky Mountain spotted fever, which is caused by infection with *Rickettsia rickettsii* after begin bitten by the *Ixodes* tick. The rash usually appears on the third day in 50% of cases, beginning as pink macules on the wrists and ankles. Lesions spread centripetally, convert to maculopapules that branch on compression, and can become petechial.

A. Lyme disease is also contracted by a tick bite. It is caused by *Borrelia burgdorferi* and the rash is called erythema chronicum migrans and does not involve the palms or soles.

B. Coxsackie A causes hand foot and mouth disease with a rash on the palms and soles but is most common in children and infants.

D. *Rickettsia typhi* is the cause of endemic typhus.

E. *Treponema pallidum*, the causative agent of syphilis, can cause a palm and sole rash in tertiary syphilis but does not fit this clinical picture.

234. **D.** This patient has irritable bowel syndrome, which is a motor disorder characterized by altered bowel habits, and abdominal pain in the absence of detectable organic disease. This entity represents the most common gastrointestinal disease seen by physicians in clinical practice. Treatment involves reassurance and a supportive physician-patient relationship, avoidance of stress, and dietary bulking agents.

A. Amitriptyline is an experimental agent that may have promise in the treatment of this condition in the future.

B. Leuprolide acetate is a gonadotropin-releasing hormone analogue that has shown some use in the treatment of irritable bowel syndrome. However, this is not considered a first-line therapy.

C. Rowasa (corticosteroid) enemas are indicated in the treatment of inflammatory bowel disease, not irritable bowel syndrome.

E. Oral tetracycline is useful in the treatment of intestinal pseudoobstruction when bacterial overgrowth contributes to this condition.

235. **B.** A common complication of vagotomies (especially those with partial gastrectomies) is dumping syndrome, which is the result of too rapid an emptying of the stomach, and is characterized by abdominal pain, postprandial diarrhea, palpitations, nausea, and bloating. Treatment is usually with octreotide.

A. Anesthetic side effects relating to gastrointestinal motility would be problematic early on after surgery.

C. Duodenal ulcers usually present with epigastric pain described as gnawing, aching, or burning. Someone with a vagotomy would be much more prone to diarrhea than an obstruction, unless he or she was chronically abusing narcotics or taking another drug that is known to constipate.

D. Mechanical obstruction by postoperative adhesions usually occur months after surgery.

E. Short gut syndrome is the result of resection of large amounts of small bowel intestine, especially in conditions such as inflammatory bowel disease.

236. **C.** Idiopathic scoliosis is often found in healthy children, and is more common in females. It is normally not associated with pain. If curves are less than 25 degrees, the patient can be observed with close follow-up. Curves greater than 25 degrees require bracing, and curves greater than 45 degrees generally require spinal fusion surgery. Thus, this patient can be observed with interval follow-up visits.

A. Bracing is recommended if the curve is greater than 25 degrees.

B. Antiinflammatory medication has not been shown to manage scoliosis.

D. Physical therapy may help strengthen the back musculature, but it has not been shown to prevent scoliosis.

E. Spinal fusion is recommended if the curve is greater than 45 degrees.

237. **B.** Grief is a normal process following the death of a loved one. Regarding the management of grief, having a small group of people who knew the deceased talk about the person in the presence of the grieving person may help in the dissipation of grief.

A. Encourage the ventilation of feelings and allow the person to talk about their loved one.

C. Frequent short visits with the physician are better than fewer long ones.

D. Do not prescribe antianxiety medications on a regular basis. If the person becomes acutely agitated it is important to talk to the patient about his or her feelings before prescribing medication.

E. Do not prescribe antidepressant medications on a regular basis. If the person becomes acutely depressed, talk to the patient about his or her feelings before prescribing medication.

238. **E.** This patient fits the criteria for a manic episode and would be diagnosed with bipolar I disorder. However, her mania developed directly after treatment with an antidepressant, so it appears that this is the likely cause. When this occurs, the patient is diagnosed with substance-induced mood disorder, not bipolar disorder. Her antidepressant medication should be discontinued initially.

A. This patient fits the criteria for a manic episode and would be diagnosed with bipolar I disorder. However, her mania developed directly after treatment with an antidepressant, so it appears that this is the likely cause.

B. This patient does not meet the criteria for bipolar II disorder.

C. Although borderline personality disorder is characterized by impulsiveness and risk-taking behavior, unstable relationships, unstable self-image, and unstable affect are other characteristics of this disorder.

D. This patient does not display characteristics of histrionic personality disorder, which include attention-seeking and theatrical behavior, as well as excessive emotionality.

239. **D.** This patient exhibits signs and symptoms of Tourette disorder. Multiple motor and vocal tics occur several times daily. Simple motor tics can include eye blinking and facial grimacing. Simple vocal tics include coughing and grunting. Complex motor tics include hitting oneself and jumping, whereas complex vocal tics include repeating one's own words and the repeating others' words. Excessive swearing can also be noted. Eighty-five percent of patients improve with haloperidol and its associated sedative properties.

A. Elective mutism is the persistent refusal to talk in school in a child who both speaks and comprehends.

B. This rare disorder of childhood relies on the adult criteria for depression for the diagnosis.

C. Schizophrenia of childhood requires the presence of delusions and hallucinations. This condition is diagnosed using the adult criteria.

E. Undifferentiated attention deficit disorder describes very inattentive children who are not hyperactive.

240. **A.** This patient has evidence of acute cholecystitis. Symptoms include right upper quadrant pain, fever, nausea, and vomiting. Pain can be referred to the scapula and the gallbladder may be palpable. Murphy sign may be positive in acute cholecystitis (tenderness with inspiratory arrest during right upper quadrant palpation).

B. Ascending cholangitis is an uncommon cause of right upper quadrant pain.

C. Ultrasonographic findings do not reveal evidence of gallstones.

D. Pancreatitis is uncommon given that no laboratory values are given (one would expect elevated amylase and lipase levels).

E. Peptic ulcer disease is unlikely given the lack of findings associated with meals. No evidence of endoscopic abnormalities of gastric or duodenal ulcerations were presented to further suggest this diagnosis.

241. **C.** Hodgkin lymphoma typically presents with nontender adenopathy in the neck, supraclavicular, or mediastinal areas. Mediastinal adenopathy is also possible, and such patients will present with cough. Spread of disease tends to be in contiguous node groups.

A. Acute myelogenous leukemia is unlikely in this patient. This is a clonal malignancy of myeloid bone marrow precursors in which poorly differentiated cells accumulate in the bone marrow and circulation.

B. Mononucleosis typically presents with pharyngitis and lymphadenopathy that is more generalized or confined to the posterior cervical lymph nodes.

D. Asymmetric lymphadenopathy associated with systemic symptoms in this age group raises concerns of Hodgkin lymphoma over non-Hodgkin lymphoma.

E. Sarcoidosis is associated with bilateral hilar adenopathy and/or interstitial changes in the lungs.

242. **A.** Antihypertensive therapy is indicated if the diastolic blood pressure is repeatedly above 110 mm Hg. Hydralazine is the initial antihypertensive of choice and is given in 5-mg increments until blood pressure reduction is achieved. This agent will have no effect on cardiac output or renal blood flow but can cause lethargy, fever, headache, and lupuslike syndrome.

B. Labetalol is an alpha- and beta-adrenergic blocker that causes a decrease in cardiac output and renal blood flow. This agent is also associated with a possible decrease in placental perfusion, which can manifest as decreased fetal movements.

C. Methyldopa is a beta blocker and can decrease cardiac output and renal blood flow.

D. Prazosin is a direct vasodilator with cardiac effects. This agent can increase cardiac output without change in renal blood flow.

E. This agent is a first-line therapy for hypertensive emergencies. It is important to remember that this agent can only be given intravenously and has an ultrashort duration of action.

243. **B.** This CT scan and the clinical history suggest an intracerebral hematoma. This can occur following trauma but can also be seen with tumors, arteriovenous malformations, and amyloidosis. The CT image demonstrates blood within the left frontal lobe, which originated from an arteriovenous malformation.

Figure 243

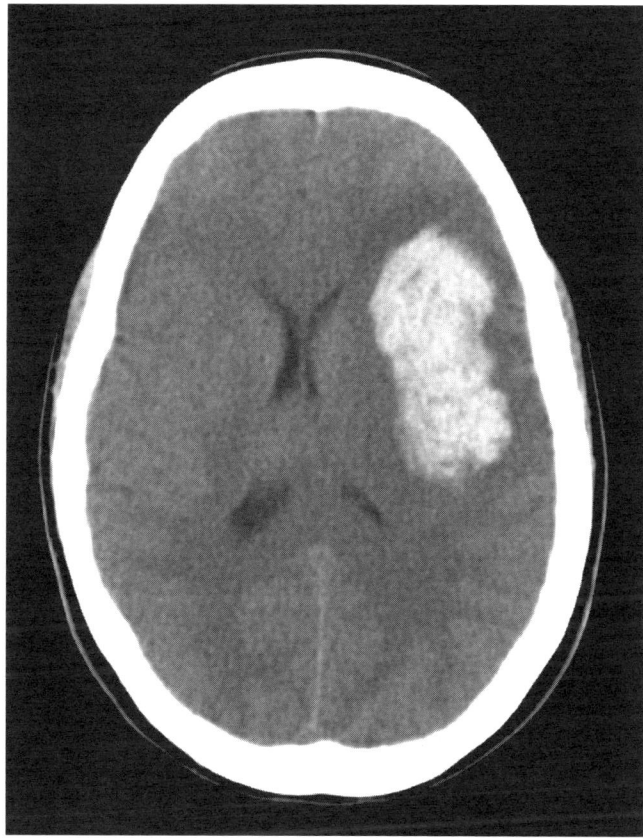

A. There is no evidence to suggest brain abscess in this patient. This lesion is focal.

C. There is no other history given to suggest metastatic tumor to brain.

D. There is no evidence of multiinfarct dementia.

E. There is no evidence of subdural hematoma. There is no crescent hematoma below the dura.

244. **B.** Mild to moderate iron deficiency anemia without evidence of congestive heart failure should be treated with 3 to 6 mg/kg/day of iron for a minimum of 3 months for hematocrit normalization and replenishment of iron stores. In severe cases infants must be transfused slowly with 3 to 5 mL/kg of packed RBCs every 4 hours until stabilized.

A. Folate supplementation is unlikely to benefit this patient.

C. Splenectomy is not indicated in this patient.

D. Thyroid hormone replacement is not indicated in this patient.

E. Iron supplementation is the most appropriate option for this patient.

245. **B.** This patient has delusional disorder. The patient's delusions are nonbizarre (involving situations that occur in real life) and have lasted at least 1 month, and there is no marked impairment of function apart from the impact of the delusions. Other criteria that must be met for delusional disorder include (1) not meeting criteria for schizophrenia; (2) mood disturbances, if present, have been brief compared with the delusional episodes; and (3) the disturbance is not due to the effects of a substance or medical condition. Tactile or olfactory hallucinations may be present as long as they are associated with the delusion.

A. In brief psychotic disorder, the symptoms must last no longer than 1 month.

C. Paranoid personality behavior tends to be a more generalized, enduring pattern of behavior rather than one specific delusion.

D. In schizophrenia, the symptoms must persist for at least 6 months.

E. In schizophreniform disorder, one would see more active symptoms (e.g., prominent auditory or visual hallucinations, bizarre delusions, disorganized speech, grossly disorganized or catatonic behavior, negative symptoms). Delusional disorder usually produces less impairment in occupational or social functioning than does schizophreniform disorder. In paranoid personality disorder, there must be no clear-cut or persisting delusional beliefs.

246. **B.** Conn syndrome (primary hyperaldosteronism) is a rare cause of hypertension associated with metabolic alkalosis, hypernatremia, and hypokalemia. This refers to an adrenal cause and can be due to either an adrenal adenoma or bilateral adrenal hyperplasia.

A. Addison's disease is an adrenal insufficiency and presents with hypotension and hyponatremia.

C. Pulmonary edema typically presents with shortness of breath and crackles on lung examination. Metabolic alkalosis is uncommon.

D. Pheochromocytoma is a secondary cause of hypertension, but is not usually associated with hypokalemia, hypernatremia, and metabolic alkalosis.

E. Acute renal tubular injury of the kidney secondary to dehydration or toxins can be associated with abnormal renal function.

247. **C.** Paget disease is characterized by long-standing vulvo-dynia and vulvar itching, and velvety red lesions that become eczematous and form white plaques. Lesions can be on the labia perineum or perianal regions. It is CEA positive, S-100 antigen negative, and melanoma antigen negative. Definitive diagnosis is made by biopsy.

A. Herpes genitalis is characterized by clear vesicles that rupture into shallow, painful ulcers.

B. Although melanoma is similar to Paget disease, it is CEA negative, S-100 negative, and melanoma antigen positive. Melanoma accounts for 5% to 10% of vulvar cancers.

D. Vulvar intraepithelial neoplasia is similar to Paget disease, but it is CEA negative, S-100 positive, and melanoma antigen negative.

E. This patient does not have evidence of vulvovaginal carcinoma.

248. **A.** This patient has obsessive-compulsive disorder (OCD). It is characterized by recurrent obsessions that cause much distress, and compulsions that are performed to neutralize the obsessions. The best treatment for OCD is clomipramine, selective serotonin reuptake inhibitors, or behavior therapy.

B. Clonazepam is less well studied, but can be used in refractory patients.

C. Lithium may be added to augment clomipramine if the initial treatment is unsuccessful.

D. Phenelzine is not a first-line agent for OCD.

E. Venlafaxine has also shown success as a second-line agent for OCD.

249. **A.** Always perform a physical examination. In closed head injuries, all of the imaging studies have a role in evaluating the patient and should be chosen based on type of injury, clinical presentation, etc. On the other hand, lumbar puncture will not provide much information after a head injury. A "normal" lumbar puncture can easily miss an intracranial hematoma. And positive findings (blood, increased cerebrospinal fluid pressures) cannot localize the injury.

B. CT scan may miss findings of closed head injury.

C. Lumbar puncture can miss intracranial bleeding.

D. MRI can miss findings of closed head injury.

E. Skull x-ray is difficult to interpret.

250. **B.** Cardiovascular complications, increased gallbladder disease, and benign hepatic tumor are all disadvantages to the pill in addition to the requirement of having to take a medication every day. There is a decreased risk for ectopic pregnancy in patients who are taking oral contraceptives.

A, C, D, and **E.** The risk for developing colorectal carcinoma, malignant breast cancer, thyroid carcinoma, and uterine teratoma is not decreased with the use of oral contraceptives.

251. **G.** This patient has an overdose of isoniazid. The key from the case is the history of tuberculosis in the patient's mother. Isoniazid is part of the treatment regimen and is a likely medicine of abuse in this case. Clinical findings include nausea, vomiting, slurred speech, dizziness, seizures, and coma.

252. **D.** This patient has had an overdose of digoxin. Clinical features of this overdose include vomiting, diarrhea, visual disturbances, confusion, bradycardia, cardiac block, and hyperkalemia.

253. **A.** The patient has signs of hyperkalemia due to overdose of trimethoprim. The possibility of dangerous arrhythmias requires prompt treatment with the following agents: furosemide, bicarbonate, dextrose (glucose), insulin, fludrocortisone, albuterol, sodium polystyrene sulfonate (kayexalate), calcium gluconate, and dialysis in severe cases. Calcium gluconate helps to stabilize membranes and prevents the effects of excess potassium.

B. Hydrochlorothiazide is a moderate-acting diuretic and would not be indicated in this case.

C. An increased dosage of bicarbonate would not be necessary since the underlying acid base disorder was already corrected.

D. Potassium chloride would only exacerbate the problem.

E. Spironolactone is a potassium-sparing diuretic and would exacerbate the patient's condition.

254. **E.** Testicular torsion is the most likely diagnosis. It is a uro-logic emergency. A high riding testicle in a horizontal lie in which elevation of the testicle provides relief is the classic presentation of testicular torsion. The critical time of ischemia for testicular torsion is 4 hours, and if a gangrenous testicle is missed, the patient will be at a high risk for sterility due to his body mounting an autoimmune response to his own sperm. Appropriate management is immediate bilateral orchiopexy because the contralateral testicle is also at an increased risk for torsion.

A. Epididymitis is unlikely in this scenario due to the lack of fever or systemic illness in this patient. Epididymitis is not a urologic emergency and can be treated with intravenous antibiotics. If this patient presented with epididymitis, a sonogram would still be of value to rule out testicular torsion. When raised, the testicle would actually cause more pain to occur rather than relieve the pain.

B. Prostatitis is unlikely given the clinical presentation and the lack of urinary symptoms.

C. Henoch-Schonlein purpura is associated with a purpuric rash on the scrotum and fever.

D. Testicular cancer is most commonly found in young men, but the usual presentation is a painless testicular mass.

255. **A.** The patient is diagnosed with somnambulism, also known as sleepwalking. These episodes, like sleep terrors, occur during slow-wave, or delta, sleep. Since patients have been known to hurt themselves unknowingly during episodes, treatment should consist of taking precautions to prevent injury if future episodes occur. Medications that reduce time spent in slow-wave sleep can also be used.

B–E. Somnambulism only occurs in delta sleep.

256. **B.** Treatment of deep venous thrombosis during pregnancy involves the use of heparin. Initially, the treatment is with intravenous heparin, which may be continued with subcutaneous heparin for the remainder of pregnancy and postpartum.

A and **D.** Coumadin is contraindicated in pregnancy.

C. This would be appropriate treatment for superficial vein thrombosis.

E. Treatment of deep venous thrombosis during pregnancy involves heparin.

257. **B.** Herpes virus 6 or roseola infantum is a common illness of young children characterized by a maculopapular rash that begins on the trunk and then spreads to the extremities. Those infected usually report acute onset of fever (102–106°F) lasting up to 5 days. Leukopenia is noted 1 to 2 days after fever begins.

A. Fifth disease or erythema infectiosum is caused by DNA parvovirus B19. Like rubella, fever is usually limited and there is no prodrome. The rash begins with erythematous cheeks followed by a maculopapular rash originating on the arms that migrates to the trunk and legs.

C. Rubella (German measles) is caused by an RNA togavirus that has an incubation period of 14 to 21 days. There is no prodrome, and the maculopapular rash tends to be discrete. If it does occur, fever is usually limited.

D. Rubeola (measles) is a paramyxovirus that exists with a prodrome of flulike symptoms. Two to three days after the onset of symptoms Koplik spots appear on the oral mucosa and 2 days later a maculopapular rash appears. The rash tends to appear first on the head and then spreads to the feet. Rubeola has an incubation period of 8 to 12 days. Diagnosis of rubella as well as rubeola may be confirmed by a fourfold increase in hemagglutination inhibition antibodies or viral isolation.

E. Syphilis is associated with a chancre in the primary stage and a maculopapular rash in the secondary stage.

258. **D.** *Pneumocystis carinii* is the most common form of respiratory failure in HIV/AIDS patients. It has a clinical picture similar to adult respiratory distress syndrome. It typically presents with a CD4 count of less than 200/mm³ and increased lactate dehydrogenase.

A. Cytomegalovirus and fungal infections typically present when the CD4 count is less than 100/mm³.

B. Although presenting with cough, dyspnea, and fever, Kaposi sarcoma also may involve hemoptysis and oral/skin lesions.

C. *Mycobacterium avium-intracellulare* and fungal infections typically present when the CD4 count is less than 100/mm³.

E. Tuberculosis lymphadenitis occurs in greater than 25% of cases of extrapulmonary tuberculosis and is particularly common among HIV-infected patients.

259. **B.** This is a classic vignette describing flail chest. Flail chest occurs when four or more ribs are fractured in at least two locations, leading to paradoxic movement of the chest wall during respiration. This commonly occurs after trauma such as a motor vehicle accident. The true danger in patients with flail chest is the frequent underlying pulmonary contusion. In this patient the blood gas indicates a decreased respiratory effort, suggesting that he is not properly respiring. The ABCDE's of trauma must be adhered to in any trauma situation, particularly flail chest. Intubation of this patient and mechanical ventilation are important in the management of this patient.

A. The maintenance of the airway takes priority in the management of this patient.

C. Observation may precipitate respiratory distress in this patient.

D. The respiratory distress of this patient with flail chest requires more oxygen support than can be given by nasal cannula.

E. Sand bags will decrease respiratory effort in a patient with already compromised respiratory ability due to flail chest.

260. **B.** Fresh frozen plasma is the treatment of choice for patients suffering from disseminated intravascular coagulation (DIC) subsequent to bleeding. This solution is appropriate to replenish the spent clotting factors and platelet concentrates characteristic of DIC. This will correct the thrombocytopenia.

A. Antibiotics would be appropriate in a patient who is septic and subsequently developed DIC. However, we have no evidence to suspect that the patient has an active infection.

C. Heparin is an appropriate prophylactic treatment in patients with mild-onset DIC to prevent progression in certain populations, such as patients with acute promyelocytic leukemia. The drug would not be a good choice for acute DIC following trauma.

D. Packed RBCs would be an appropriate consideration had hemoglobin and hematocrit been diminished. However, the most important next step in this patient is replenishment of platelets and spent clotting factors with fresh frozen plasma.

E. Warfarin seems like a logical consideration for treatment of chronic DIC. Unfortunately, DIC does not respond well to oral warfarin. The drug would not be a good choice for acute DIC following trauma.

261. **E.** This child has the classic presentation of pyloric stenosis. The typical history is that of nonbilious vomiting, classically projectile in an otherwise well child between 2 and 8 weeks of age. Depending on the severity of vomiting, weight loss, dehydration, and lethargy may be present. The palpable "olive" in the epigastric region represents the enlarged pylorus and is best appreciated after the infant has vomited. The hypochloremic, hypokalemic metabolic alkalosis is typical of extended periods of vomiting.

A. Gastric ulcers are uncommon in infants.

B. Gastroenteritis is uncommon in a 3-week-old infant.

C. The clinical history is not consistent with meconium ileus.

D. Necrotizing enterocolitis presents commonly at birth and is associated with gut ischemia.

262. **A.** This patient needs to be further evaluated. She likely has adenomyosis. In patients over 35 years of age with menorrhagia, endometrial cancer should be ruled out by endometrial biopsy of fractional dilation and curettage specimens and/or by hysteroscopy.

B. If severe symptoms of adenomyosis are refractory to medicinal management, hysterectomy may be indicated.

C. Although the patient should be followed closely, this patient needs a diagnostic hysteroscopy to evaluate any uterine pathology.

D. If menorrhagia is severe or if the dysmenorrhea is disabling, the use of mifepristone may provide relief.

E. If menorrhagia is severe or if the dysmenorrhea is disabling, the use of a GnRH agonist may provide relief.

263. **D.** The radiograph shows a bacterial lobar pneumonia with the classic appearance of alveolar opacification in a lobar distribution. This diagnosis is supported by the signs of bacterial infection, high fever, and high WBC count. In the setting of a nosocomial (i.e., hospital-acquired) pneumonia, many factors must be taken into account in order to determine the most likely cause. In this case, the patient's history of diabetes puts him at significant risk for *Staphylococcus aureus* causing the pneumonia.

Figure 263

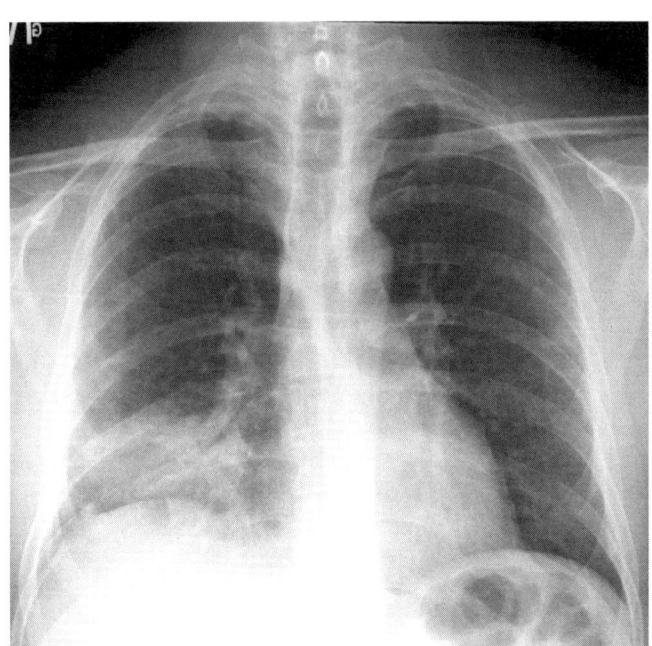

A. In a patient with recent abdominal surgery or a witnessed aspiration, anaerobes are a significant source of nosocomial pneumonia; however, since none of these risk factors are present, we do not consider this to be the most likely cause in this patient.

B and **E.** Although *Streptococcus pneumoniae* and *Haemophilus influenzae* are common causes of nosocomial pneumonias in patients that are fewer than 5 days into their hospital stay, you must consider *S. aureus* as the most likely etiologic agent in a patient with diabetes.

C. In patients on high-dose steroids, *Legionella* species are considered a significant source of nosocomial pneumonia. This patient, however, is taking no medications.

264. **C.** It is acceptable to observe this man for 12 months because he has no risk factors for coronary artery disease (CAD). He is under 45 years of age, he does not have a history of cigarette smoking, he has no significant family history of premature heart attacks, he does not have hypertension or diabetes, and his HDL is level is over 35 mg/dL.

A. Had his total fasting cholesterol level been greater than 239 mg/dL, it would have been appropriate to check LDL to look for levels greater than 159 mg/dL. If the LDL level had been 160 to 180 mg/dL in this patient, diet modification would be appropriate.

B. Triglyceride levels alone have not been shown to be a risk factor for developing CAD. However, elevated triglycerides along with elevated LDL cholesterol confer a higher risk for developing CAD than does elevated LDL alone.

D. Had his total fasting cholesterol level been greater than 239 mg/dL, it would have been appropriate to check LDL to look for levels greater than 159 mg/dL. If the LDL level had been 160 to 180 mg/dL in this patient, diet modification would be appropriate. If the LDL level had been greater than 180 mg/dL in this patient, a medication such as lovastatin should have been prescribed.

E. Had his total fasting cholesterol level been greater than 239 mg/dL, it would have been appropriate to check his LDL to look for levels greater than 159 mg/dL. If his LDL level had been 160 to 180 mg/dL, diet modification would be appropriate. If the LDL level had been greater than 180 mg/dL in this patient, medications should have been prescribed. Niacin is an appropriate agent.

265. **D.** The patient would at this time have a diagnosis of residual schizophrenia. This means he met the criteria for schizophrenia at one time, but now has residual negative symptoms, and attenuated delusions, hallucinations, or thought disorders.

A. He may, at one time, have had a diagnosis of catatonic type, which includes motoric immobility or excessive, purposeless motor activity, and maintenance of a rigid echolalia.

B. He does not have a diagnosis of paranoid type, which includes paranoid delusions, frequent auditory hallucinations, and not a flat affect.

C. He probably, at one time, also had a diagnosis of undifferentiated type, which means that criteria are not met for the paranoid, catatonic, disorganized, or residual types.

E. This type of schizophrenia does not exist in DSM-IV.

266. **D.** This patient has what is referred to as prehypertension. In three recordings of his blood pressure, he did not have one value equal to or below 120/80 mm Hg, but he did have a value less than 140/90 mm Hg. This has been shown to be a risk factor for developing stage I hypertension and consequently arteriosclerosis. This is best treated with lifestyle modifications and diet control (although it should be noted that reducing salt intake has not shown to benefit blood pressure in otherwise healthy individuals).

A. This patient has prehypertension and does not require oral therapy at this time.

B. This is not an appropriate choice for this patient with prehypertension.

C. Black patients tend to respond better to calcium channel blockers and diuretics than beta blockers.

E. This choice would only be appropriate if one of his three recordings had been below or equal to 120/80 mm Hg.

267. **C.** A defect in 17,20-desmolase. This woman has gonadal agenesis and is 46XY. This enzyme is involved in testicular steroid production, so this patient will not produce testosterone. Müllerian inhibiting factor (MIF) will still be produced in these patients, so there will be absence of all internal female organs.

A. Absence of MIF would result in the müllerian-derived structures not being inhibited and thus, there would be a uterus and ovaries and fallopian tubes present.

B. A 17-beta-hydroxylase does not exist. It is 17-alpha-hydroxylase that is involved in testosterone production, so the above reason applies to this one as well.

D. An elevated 17-alpha-hydroxyprogesterone level would result from the defect of 21-alpha-hydroxylase, which would result in a build-up of testosterone and virilization in women.

E. The question stem states she has had no surgeries.

268. **D.** This patient has histrionic personality disorder. Individuals with this disorder show pervasive and excessive emotionality and attention-seeking behavior. They are uncomfortable when they are not the center of attention. They are often sexually provocative or seductive, and use their physical appearance to draw attention to themselves. Emotional expression may be rapidly shifting, and they are characterized by theatrical and exaggerated expression of emotion.

A. People with histrionic personality disorder generally do not engage in antisocial behaviors.

B. Borderline personality disorder is not the best choice because these individuals tend to show self-destructiveness, angry relationship disruptions, and chronic feelings of deep emptiness and identity disturbance.

C. In dependent personality disorder, the patient lacks excessive flamboyant and exaggerated emotional features.

E. People with narcissistic personality disorder tend to praise their superiority.

269. **D.** Osteogenic sarcoma is the most common primary malignant tumor of bone. It occurs more commonly in adolescents, and is two times more common in males than females. Bone pain and edema are the most common presentations, and 10% to 15% may have lung metastases. Radiographs reveal a "sunburst" pattern, indicating new bone formation. Treatment consists of surgical resection and chemotherapy.

A. Observation has no role in the treatment of osteogenic sarcoma.

B. Osteogenic sarcoma is not radiosensitive at conventional doses.

C. Surgical resection alone is associated with a 20% survival rate, whereas surgical resection plus chemotherapy has a greater than 50% survival rate.

E. Osteogenic sarcoma is not radiosensitive at conventional doses.

270. **B.** This patient is suspicious for having *Legionella* pneumonia. He has a history of immunosuppression and upper respiratory symptoms. Several other guests have similar symptoms, suggesting aerosol spread of this organism. Culture on charcoal-yeast agar has an 80% to 90% sensitivity and should be the next test ordered.

A. Sputum and transtracheal aspirate are nearly 100% specific for *Legionella*.

C. This is not a sensitive test for *Legionella*.

D. Pulmonary function tests are not an appropriate next step in the workup.

E. Legionnaires disease is a pneumonia caused by *Legionella pneumophila*. Treatment is with erythromycin.

271. **E.** *Trichomonas vaginalis* is a protozoan organism that lives in the urethra and vagina. This organism can be freely transmitted during sexual intercourse. Symptoms of infection include vulvar itching, burning, copious discharge with rancid odor, dysuria, and dyspareunia. Examination may reveal edema and erythema of the vulva and petechiae of the upper vagina and cervix. The secretions are often yellow-green with a pH of greater than 6.5. Wet smear will reveal the *Trichomonas* organism. Treatment is by oral metronidazole, and 1-day therapy regimens will result in a 90% cure rate.

A. Candidiasis is associated with variable amounts of white discharge, a vaginal pH of 4 to 5, and the presence of mycelia on potassium hydroxide microscopic preparations.

B. *Gardnerella* infections are associated with a gray-white discharge, a foul smelling odor, and a vaginal pH of 5 to 5.5. Clue cells are present on microscopic examination.

C. Hidradenitis suppurativa is a chronic, unrelenting skin infection that causes deep, painful scars and a foul-smelling discharge. Treatment involves local antibiotics and steroids.

D. Physiologic vaginal secretions are yellow-white in color, with a pH of 3.5 to 4.5. The patient is asymptomatic, and physical examination will reveal no evidence of erythema. Microscopy will reveal few WBCs.

272. **A.** This patient has mild preeclampsia, which is defined as the development of hypertension in pregnancy with proteinuria or edema or both, usually in the second half of pregnancy. This patient has mild preeclampsia because her blood pressure is less than 160/110 mm Hg and proteinuria is less than 2+. Management of mild preeclampsia is bed rest in the lateral decubitus position to maximize uterine blood flow while normalizing maternal blood pressures.

B. Antihypertensive therapy is indicated if the diastolic blood pressure is repeatedly above 110 mm Hg. Hydralazine is the agent of choice.

C. Antihypertensive therapy is indicated if the diastolic blood pressure is repeatedly above 110 mm Hg. Hydralazine is the agent of choice. This agent can be given intravenously to hospitalized patients.

D. Prazosin is a direct vasodilator that can be used in the treatment of moderate or severe preeclampsia.

E. Thiazides cause a decrease in cardiac output and plasma volume and can be used in the treatment of moderate preeclampsia.

273. **A.** Churg-Strauss syndrome is a vasculitis affecting blood vessels of all different sizes leading to fever, malaise, and weight loss. Eosinophilia is the hallmark of this disease and leads to new-onset recurrent asthma symptoms. Pulmonary infiltrates may be seen in both Wegener granulomatosis and Churg-Strauss syndrome. Palpable purpura (as described in the question stem) can be seen in any of the vasculitides, but is most common in Churg-Strauss syndrome. Prednisone (1 mg/kg/day) until symptomatic improvement occurs, with tapering to avoid long-term side effects, is the recommended treatment for this condition.

B. These features are not typical for polyarteritis nodosa.

C. These features are not typical for rheumatoid arthritis.

D. These features are not typical for Takayasu arteritis.

E. These features are not typical for temporal arteritis.

274. **A.** This patient meets criteria for attention deficit hyperactivity disorder (ADHD), and as such, treatment with an amphetamine is indicated. Such patients can be easily distracted, impulsive, unable to tolerate stress, and can be restless.

B. Cognitive therapy is not effective by itself in treatment of this condition.

C. The patient is old enough to have his behavior at school addressed.

D. ADHD typically resolves by adolescence; most children do not have symptoms in adulthood.

E. ADHD children have a higher risk for developing adult antisocial personality disorder.

275. **B.** For all stages of seminoma, treatment first involves inguinal orchiectomy for histopathologic diagnosis and staging. For higher stage disease, retroperitoneal lymph node dissection is undertaken. When positive lymph nodes are found, radiotherapy and chemotherapy are instituted.

A. Chemotherapy is not the primary therapy for seminoma.

C. External beam radiotherapy, not interstitial radiotherapy, is a treatment for seminoma.

D. Chemotherapy and radiotherapy may be required for the treatment of advanced seminoma following orchiectomy.

E. Transcrotal orchiectomy is not indicated in the treatment of testis cancer. It is possible that during removal of the tumor by this approach that lymphatic seeding of tumor cells can occur, making the situation gravely worse.

276. **A.** Hemophilia A is caused by a deficiency of factor VIII and occurs in 1:5000 males. This disorder is X-linked recessive. The deficiency in factor VIII results in a delay in production of thrombin. Thus, the primary fibrin clot cannot form. There are three forms: severe, moderate, and mild. These correlate with the amount of factor VIII the patient has. Children with severe hemophilia may have spontaneous bleeding and will bleed with minor trauma. Patients with moderate hemophilia require moderate trauma to bleed, and those with mild hemophilia may go undiagnosed for years because significant trauma is required to induce bleeding and spontaneous bleeding does not occur.

B. Hemophilia B has a similar presentation, but factor IX is deficient in this type of hemophilia.

C. Vitamin B_{12} deficiency is associated with pernicious anemia.

D. Vitamin K deficiency is associated with deficient coagulation factors II, VII, IX, and X and proteins C and S.

E. Von Willebrand disease is associated with low von Willebrand factor (vWF) antigen and vWF actinomycin and normal factor VIII and IX.

277. **C.** The black widow spider is the most common biting spider in the United States. The venom is neurotoxic and centers around the spinal cord. Symptoms include muscular pain, nausea, vomiting, and headache. Treatment consists of narcotics for pain relief and a muscle relaxant. Antivenin therapy is rarely required.

A. Although antibiotics are part of the treatment plan, they are secondary to pain control and relief of muscle spasm.

B. Corticosteroids are not required in the treatment of black widow spider bites.

D. Plasmapheresis is not required in the treatment of black widow spider bites.

E. Although an antivenin is available, it is rarely required for the treatment of black widow spider bites.

278. **A.** This individual has brief reactive psychosis. This condition is defined by a symptom constellation of less that 1 month's duration and follows an obvious stress on the patient's life. Patients exhibit an increase in volatility and lability, confusion, disorientation, and affective symptoms. This condition is highly associated with individuals who have a preexisting personality disorder and those who have experienced a major life stressor such as a natural disaster.

B. Posttraumatic stress disorder occurs following a severe loss or stress such as rape, car accident, or natural disaster and is notable for marked anxiety, personality change, insomnia, and nightmares.

C. This patient has symptoms that are clearly identifiable with a psychiatric disorder.

D. Schizoaffective disorder is a vague and poorly defined disorder meant for people with evidence of both schizophrenia and major depression.

E. Schizophrenia is the most common psychotic disorder, with varying degrees of severity. Affected individuals have an impaired sense of reality and may be confused and disoriented.

279. **C.** The primary treatment for vaginal carcinoma is by radiotherapy, which will shrink large tumors rather well. Following radiotherapy, it is possible that chemotherapy or surgical excision will be viable options. This cancer typically occurs in women over 40 with classical symptoms of vaginal bleeding and urinary symptoms from compression on the bladder.

A. Chemotherapy provides poor results for patients with vaginal carcinoma.

B. Intravesicular chemotherapy is appropriate for carcinoma in situ of the bladder.

D. Surgical excision, although an appropriate additional therapy for this condition, should be attempted after radiotherapy.

E. Watchful waiting is an inappropriate strategy for the management of vaginal carcinoma.

280. **C.** This patient has evidence of *Clostridium difficile* enterocolitis infection, which is caused by antibiotic use, especially ampicillin and clindamycin. The treatment is metronidazole or vancomycin. If the patient initially fails metronidazole, it is reasonable to switch to vancomycin. Relapses are much more common than treatment failures.

A. Ampicillin is not effective against *C. difficile*.

B. Ceftriaxone only covers gram-negative organisms and some gram-positive organisms.

D. Trimethoprim is not effective against *C. difficile*.

E. Watchful waiting will likely be associated with a worsening of symptoms. Therefore, this patient should be treated promptly.

281. **A.** Valproate levels should be monitored regularly until stable blood levels occur. However, liver function tests should be measured at baseline and then frequently during the first 6 months. Serious idiosyncratic side effects of valproate include fatal hepatotoxicity, fulminant pancreatitis, and agranulocytosis. Fatal hepatotoxicity is most common during the first 6 months of therapy.

B. This medication has hepatic effects. Thus, liver function tests should be ordered.

C. This medication has hepatic effects. Thus, liver function tests should be monitored.

D. Valproate levels should be monitored at regular intervals.

E. There is no indication to obtain an abdominal CT scan in this patient.

282. **D.** Anal fissure is a split in the midline of the posterior anoderm 90% of the time. This is the most common location of anal fissures. Symptoms of acute fissures include tearing pain on defecation and blood in the stool or on the toilet paper. Treatment of choice for acute fissures includes stool softeners, sitz baths, and dietary bulking agents.

A. There is no role for intravenous antibiotic therapy in the management of acute anal fissures.

B. There is no role for oral antibiotic therapy in the management of acute anal fissures.

C. Rubber band ligation is an appropriate treatment for hemorrhoids.

E. Surgical therapy is reserved for chronic nonhealing fissures, and the procedure of choice is lateral sphincterotomy.

283. **B.** Gestational diabetes is carbohydrate intolerance of varying severity, with onset or first recognition during pregnancy. It is characterized by insulin resistance as well as impaired insulin secretion. The GLT is a screening test for gestational diabetes. If the result is greater than 140 mg/dL, then it is positive and a GTT is necessary.

A. The 1-hour GLT is only a screening test, not diagnostic.

C. Betamethasone followed by cesarean section would not be an appropriate next step.

D. Insulin regimens are generally not used during pregnancy because they cross the placenta and are potentially teratogenic.

E. The GLT is a screening test, not diagnostic for diabetes mellitus.

284. **D.** Septic arthritis is most commonly caused by *Staphylococcus aureus*, and the hip is the most common joint involved in this age group. Diagnosis is made by aspiration of the synovial fluid, which shows greater than 25,000 WBCs/mm³. Treatment includes intravenous antibiotics.

A. Avascular necrosis of the femoral head is not associated with fever or other signs of infection.

B. There is no history that would suggest a fracture of the femoral neck.

C. There is no history that would suggest a pelvic fracture.

E. Toxic synovitis causes joint pain in children, and most often occurs after a viral infection. It is not commonly associated with fever and other signs of infection. Treatment consists of analgesics and rest.

285. **A.** AFP is most likely to be elevated in hepatomas and hepatocellular cancers. Thus, in a patient with palpable liver nodules, AFP is likely to be elevated.

B. CA-125 is a marker for colon and breast cancer.

C. CEA is a marker for colorectal cancer.

D. HCG is a marker for testicular cancer.

E. PSA is a marker for prostate cancer.

286. **B.** Beta-thalassemia can be divided into homozygous (major) and heterozygous (minor) forms. Beta-thalassemia major is characterized by severe hemolytic anemia with marked splenomegaly during the first year of life. Without treatment the child can develop bone marrow hyperplasia and extramedullary hematopoiesis that produces tower skull, frontal bossing, maxillary hypertrophy, and overbite along with failure to thrive. Death may occur in the first few years of life if not treated with blood transfusions. Death is usually by progressive CHF. In beta-thalassemia major, reticulocytopenia is present and peripheral blood smears exhibit hypochromia, microcytosis, anisocytosis, and poikilocytosis. On electrophoresis, hemoglobin A is markedly decreased or totally absent and hemoglobin F accounts for up to 95% in the B0/B0 genotype and 20% to 80% in B+/B+ genotype.

A. This patient has no evidence to suggest alpha-thalassemia. This condition is a hereditary microcytic anemia resulting from decreased production of the hemoglobin alpha chain.

C. Beta-thalassemia can be divided into homozygous (major) and heterozygous (minor) forms. This patient has evidence of beta-thalassemia major.

D. This patient has no evidence to suggest fragile X syndrome.

E. This patient has no evidence to suggest hemoglobin Bart disease.

287. **B.** The positive predictive value (PPV) measures the distribution of people who receive a positive test result. PPV = true positives/(true positive + false positive).

Table 287	Diabetes	
SCREENING TEST RESULT	**PRESENT**	**ABSENT**
Positive	250	450
Negative	50	50

288. **E.** A clue to this diagnosis is the onset of severe back (flank) pain that radiates to the ipsilateral abdomen. Although 85% to 90% of urinary tract calculi are seen with x-ray, uric acid stones are radiolucent. (Hint: the patient has a history of gout.) For obscure reasons, colicky pain of renal origin results in ipsilateral rectus spasm. Thus, the correct answer is ureteral calculi.

A. The film is also consistent with ileus, not obstruction (where you might see distal gasless bowel of smaller caliber).

B. This patient has no evidence to suggest the diagnosis of diverticulitis.

C. The patient does not have peritoneal signs consistent with pancreatitis (she is thrashing around and has no rebound tenderness).

D. This patient has clear-cut evidence of a ureteral calculi.

289. **B.** The presence of antibodies against the surface antigen (HBsAg) is indicative of resolved hepatitis B infections (or immunity if the vaccine was given), and no further treatment is needed. These levels are usually detectable approximately 4 months after infection and will last throughout the patient's lifetime assuming he or she maintains a healthy immune system. This patient should also be tested for the presence of hepatitis D as well because it can coincide with and only with hepatitis B, and the presence of a superimposed hepatitis D virus infection gives a poorer prognosis to the patient in terms of developing either fulminant acute hepatitis or chronic hepatitis.

A. Administration of the hepatitis B vaccine has not been shown to help give immunity to those already infected.

C. Patients can have detectable levels of IgG antibodies against the core antigen, yet still progress to chronic hepatitis in the absence of the surface antigen antibodies.

D. Patients can have detectable levels of IgG antibodies against the viral envelope antigen, yet still progress to chronic hepatitis in the absence of the surface antigen antibodies.

E. Interferon-alpha is the treatment of choice for chronic hepatitis B. It will induce immunity (anti-HBsAg IgG) in 50%.

290. **D.** The Apgar scoring system is used to assess the need for neonatal resuscitation and is determined by evaluating five physiologic parameters at 1 and 5 minutes after birth: heart rate, respiration, muscle tone, reflex irritability, and body color. All parameters are scored as either 0, 1, or 2. Heart rate is scored as 0 beats/min (0), less than 100 beats/min (1), or greater than 100 beats/min (2). Respiration is scored as none (0), weak cry (1), or vigorous cry (2). Muscle tone is assessed as none (0), some extremity flexion (1), or arms and legs well flexed (2). Reflex irritability is measured as none (0), some motion (1), or cry and withdrawal (2). Body color is either blue (0), pink body with blue extremities (1), or pink all over (2). According to this scoring system, the child in the question should have an Apgar score of 9 at 1 minute. Weight is not a parameter used is assessing the Apgar score.

291. **B.** This patient has radiographic and clinical evidence of an epidural hematoma. The CT scan shows a lens-shaped, high-attenuation collection in the frontal region. Occasionally, the hematoma can cross the midline. Nearly all patients with an epidural hematoma have a skull fracture.

Figure 291

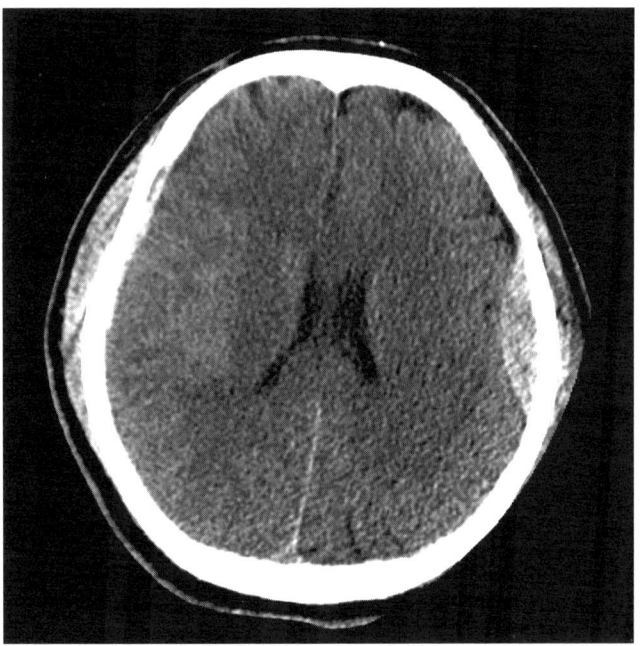

A. There is no evidence of brain abscess in this patient given the history of trauma.

C. There is no evidence of a space-occupying mass lesion on the CT scan.

D. Subarachnoid hemorrhage is unlikely given the CT findings presented in this case.

E. Subdural hematoma is a collection of blood within the potential space between the dura mater and the pia mater.

292. **E.** Propranolol is a nonselective beta blocker that is very useful for social phobic situations such as giving speeches. It crosses the blood-brain barrier and diminishes central arousal, as well as acting peripherally by decreasing tachycardia, tremor, and sweating. It may not be a good choice for someone with asthma, since it can exacerbate asthma symptoms.

A. Atenolol is also a beta blocker, but it does not cross the blood-brain barrier, making it less effective at altering mood.

B. Clonidine is a central nervous system alpha 2 adrenoreceptor agonist that is useful for decreasing autonomic symptoms in opiate withdrawal and it is also an antihypertensive.

C. Diphenhydramine is an anticholinergic that can be used for sedation, congestion, and even neuroleptic movement disorders.

D. Methylphenidate is a psychostimulant used to treat narcolepsy and attention deficit disorder.

293. **D.** Wide local excision of Paget lesions should be curative, but because there is often microscopic disease beyond the gross lesion, the margins should be examined to be sure they are clear of disease. Adenocarcinoma is found underlying the skin changes in 20% of Paget disease. Thus, careful pathologic examination of margins is important.

A. Without adenocarcinoma, Paget disease rarely metastasizes. Thus, radiation is unnecessary. Metastasis is common with adenocarcinoma, and once the disease spreads to the nodes it is often fatal.

B. Antifungal agents would be the treatment for candidiasis or other fungal infections.

C. Antibiotics would be the treatment for an infectious disease.

E. Paget disease should be treated in a proactive fashion. Watchful waiting is not appropriate in this case.

294. **C.** This patient, who was suffering from chronic low back pain, has experienced a herniated nucleus pulposus at the level of L4–L5. A history of sudden movement yielding "shooting pain" into his big toe as well as a positive straight leg raise test and pain elicited by the Valsalva maneuver support this diagnosis. The Valsalva maneuver causes an increase in venous pressure in the venous plexus of the spinal cord that will exacerbate the pain caused by a herniated lumbar disc.

A. There is no evidence to suggest a lumbar vertebral fracture.

B. This patient has evidence of a herniated disc at L4–L5.

D. If the pain was shooting into his little toe, then the most likely level for herniation would be L5–S1. An MRI is the diagnostic modality of choice to detect herniated discs. The presence of numbness or weakness in the lower extremities would necessitate referral to a neurosurgeon for surgical treatment.

E. This patient has evidence of a herniated disc at L4–L5. Also, at this level, there are no "discs" because the bone (sacrum) is fused.

295. **A.** The spleen is one of the most commonly injured abdominal organs in blunt trauma. A history of a motor vehicle accident and the findings of bruised ribs in the left upper quadrant increase our suspicion for splenic injury. This patient may need to be taken to the operating room eventually but first he must be stabilized. The ABCDE's of trauma must be cleared. This patient is hemodynamically unstable and may need blood and fluids before surgery. If splenectomy is performed for hemostasis, it is critical to administer vaccinations against encapsulated organisms because these patients lose their ability to filter such organisms.

B. Administration of pain medications delays the ultimate need of this patient, which is stabilization with intravenous fluids and blood.

C. Although splenectomy may ultimately be needed for this patient, administration of fluids and blood should be undertaken first.

D. Transesophageal echocardiogram will not provide useful information about abdominal injuries in this patient.

E. Obtaining a blood alcohol level is important, but not in the setting of acute abdominal bleeding.

296. **B.** Absence (petit mal) seizures occur only in children and are described as "staring spells." The child has a brief staring episode associated with an alteration of consciousness. Electroencephalography demonstrates the classic 3-per-second spike-and-wave pattern. First-line treatment is ethosuximide.

A. Carbamazepine is used for partial seizures and tonic-clonic seizures.

C. Methylphenidate is used for the treatment of attention deficit syndrome.

D. A child who is having active seizures must be medically treated.

E. Phenytoin is used for the treatment of tonic-clonic seizures and partial seizures.

297. **C.** IgA nephropathy is a nephritic glomerulopathy that typically occurs in association with infection or systemic disease. Hematuria is present, and urinary protein is elevated but is below the nephrotic range. It is the most common cause of asymptomatic hematuria in adults.

A. Focal segmental glomerular sclerosis is associated with hypertension and hematuria. The primary form is similar to minimal change disease of nephritic syndrome.

B. Goodpasture syndrome is a nephritic syndrome, and respiratory symptoms such as hemoptysis and infiltrates on chest x-ray are typically seen in conjunction with renal abnormalities.

D. Membranous glomerulonephritis and focal segmental glomerulosclerosis are generally nephrotic syndromes characterized by massive proteinuria, edema, hypoalbuminemia, and hyperlipidemia.

E. Poststreptococcal glomerulonephritis is most common in childhood. Nephritis develops 1 to 3 weeks after pharyngeal or cutaneous infection with nephritogenic strains of group A beta-hemolytic streptococci.

298. **C.** This patient has clinical features of preeclampsia. She should be further evaluated with measurement of blood pressure and a urinalysis. This condition is characterized by hypertension plus generalized edema and/or proteinuria occurring after the 20th week of gestation. This condition can be further divided into mild and severe based on blood pressure and laboratory findings.

A. Adnexal and cervical examinations are unlikely to provide further information about preeclampsia.

B. Echocardiography is not indicated in the evaluation of preeclampsia.

D. Renal ultrasonography is likely to reveal hydronephrosis, which is a normal finding in the third trimester of pregnancy.

E. Watchful waiting is not indicated because this patient likely has preeclampsia.

299. **A.** Continuous positive airway pressure (CPAP) is the desired treatment for obstructive sleep apnea. CPAP helps keep the upper airway open during sleep. Uvulopalatopharyngoplasty is a second-line treatment for this condition.

B. Nasal surgery is not a first-line therapy for sleep apnea.

C. Sedative medications are not considered first-line therapy for sleep apnea. These should be discontinued if they are being used as they may be increasing the severity of the disturbance.

D. Uvulopalatopharyngoplasty is not a first-line treatment for sleep apnea.

E. Weight loss may be helpful in the treatment of sleep apnea as an adjunct to a first-line treatment.

300. **B.** Leukoplakia is a precancerous lesion seen in tobacco users. The lesion should be examined via biopsy to rule out neoplastic processes. The description given is consistent with this lesion and is especially worrisome when the lesion does not rub off. Pathology will be able to distinguish different types of leukoplakia. Some types of leukoplakia are more prone to undergo malignant transformation.

A. The patient does not likely have thrush, caused by *Candida albicans* because there is no mention of corticosteroid usage, broad-spectrum antibiotic usage, or evidence of an immunosuppressed state such as HIV infection.

C. Although lung cancer should always be suspected in patients who smoke, there is no symptomatic evidence of a lung mass. A screening chest x-ray is not proper usage of a screening test in asymptomatic smokers.

D. Although hairy leukoplakia is a concern in patient with HIV, these lesions are rarely located outside the lateral aspect of the tongue.

E. The patient should not be reassured that this is a normal hyperkeratosis because only pathology can distinguish which lesions possess more risk.

301. **C.** This patient has disseminated intravascular coagulation (DIC). In this condition, normal homeostasis between hemorrhage and thrombosis is altered by severe illness. There is activation of both coagulation and fibrinolysis. Platelets, fibrinogen, and factors II, V, and VIII are consumed, as are anticoagulant proteins. The diagnosis is clinical and is supported with laboratory results. Bleeding diathesis is diffuse. Thrombotic lesions are also possible. Both ischemic and hemorrhagic stroke can occur. Laboratory tests often reveal thrombocytopenia, prolonged prothrombin time, partial thromboplastin time, and thrombin time. Levels of fibrinogen and factors V and VIII are low, and those of fibrin split products and D-dimers are elevated.

A. Aplastic anemia is associated with pancytopenia.

B. Diamond-Blackfan syndrome is an autosomal-recessive red cell aplasia of unknown etiology.

D. Hemophilia B is associated with decreased factor IX.

E. Idiopathic thrombocytopenia purpura (ITP) is a thrombocytopenia with abrupt onset of petechiae and ecchymoses.

302. **C.** Fibroids may be seen to be associated with recurrent pregnancy failure, heavy periods, and pain. These are discrete, rounded, firm, benign tumors of the myometrium composed mostly of smooth muscle and connective tissue. Approximately 95% arise from the uterine corpus, whereas 5% arise from the cervix.

A. Endometriosis is associated with cyclic pelvic pain.

B. Endometritis cases present commonly with an elevated temperature and pelvic pain.

D. The presence of an intrauterine device is a risk factor for uterine and total infertility. However, it is less likely to be associated with the triad of pregnancy failure, heavy periods, and pain.

E. The presence of pelvic inflammatory disease raises concern for ectopic pregnancy if the infection caused enough damage to the fallopian tubes to hinder the passage of the egg. However, it is less likely to be associated with the triad of pregnancy failure, heavy periods, and pain.

303. **A.** This patient has acute angle-closure glaucoma. Acute glaucoma comes on rapidly. The most common symptom is severe pain in one eye. Vomiting often occurs. Patients complain of impaired vision and halos around lights. Treatment involves reduction of intraocular pressure. Intravenous acetazolamide should be given.

B. Acute episcleritis is a localized inflammation of the eye which is usually tender and sore.

C. Acute iridocyclitis is an inflammation of the iris and ciliary body.

D. Bacterial conjunctivitis is associated with purulent discharge and conjunctival irritation.

E. Viral conjunctivitis can be due to adenovirus. Discharge is watery.

304. **E.** The child in this question presents with classic findings of glomerulonephritis: hematuria, azootemia, hypertension, and edema. Hematuria can be microscopic or gross, and parents often report findings of urine discoloration. A renal biopsy is the gold standard for determining the specific etiology. Crescent formation is pathognomonic for rapidly progressive glomerulonephritis, a description given to a number of glomerulonephropathies that frequently cause deterioration over a period of weeks with renal failure, uremia, and encephalopathy.

A. Acute poststreptococcal glomerulonephritis is the most common glomerulonephritis in childhood and marked by granular deposits of IgG and C3 below the glomerular basement membrane.

B. Alport syndrome is a hereditary nephropathy characterized by defective, thickened bands of glomerular basement membrane.

C. Focal segmental glomerulosclerosis is considered a nephritic, not a nephrotic, disorder.

D. IgA nephropathy is characterized by mesangial IgA deposits in the glomeruli.

305. **B.** The Salter-Harris classification system defines five types of epiphyseal fractures. Our radiographs demonstrate a type II of the distal tibia. This involves extension of the fracture through the epiphyseal plate, resulting epiphyseal displacement, and a fractured, triangular segment of metaphysis. Despite the numerous changes, the epiphysis remains intact. This results in a good prognosis for a patient with this type of injury, but growth disturbances can occur with any of the five types of epiphyseal fractures.

A. A Salter-Harris I fracture only involves extension of the fracture through the epiphyseal plate, with resulting epiphyseal displacement. Like a type II fracture, this fracture spares the epiphysis and thereby results in a good prognosis for the patient.

C. A Salter-Harris III fracture runs from the joint surface through the epiphyseal plate and epiphysis. The higher the grade, the worse the prognosis, with growth disturbances being the main concern. Still, this type of fracture has a similar prognosis to that of types I and II, even though the epiphysis is fractured.

D. A Salter-Harris IV fracture involves an epiphyseal break in which the fracture line runs from the joint surface through epiphyseal plate, epiphysis, and metastasis. This type of epiphyseal fracture has a worse prognosis than the preceding types and is at high risk for growth disturbances.

E. A Salter-Harris V fracture is a crush injury to the epiphyseal plate. Because of this, such fractures may be difficult to identify on radiographs. Of course, this type is also associated with a high risk for growth disturbances.

Figure 305a

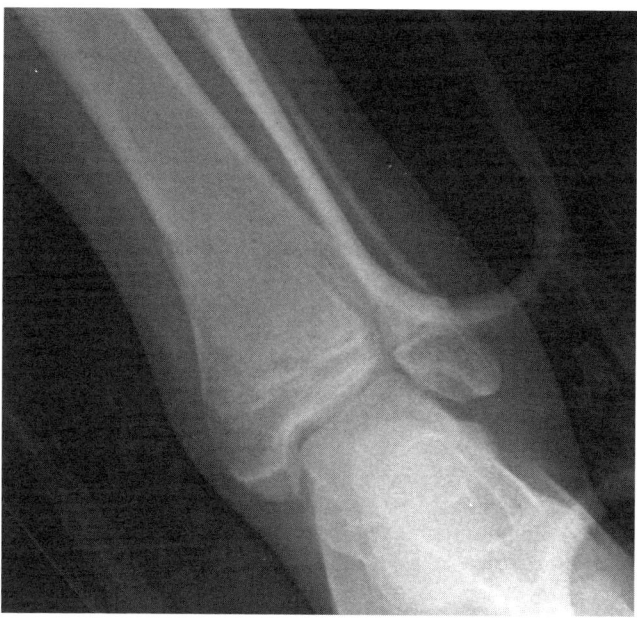

Figure 305b

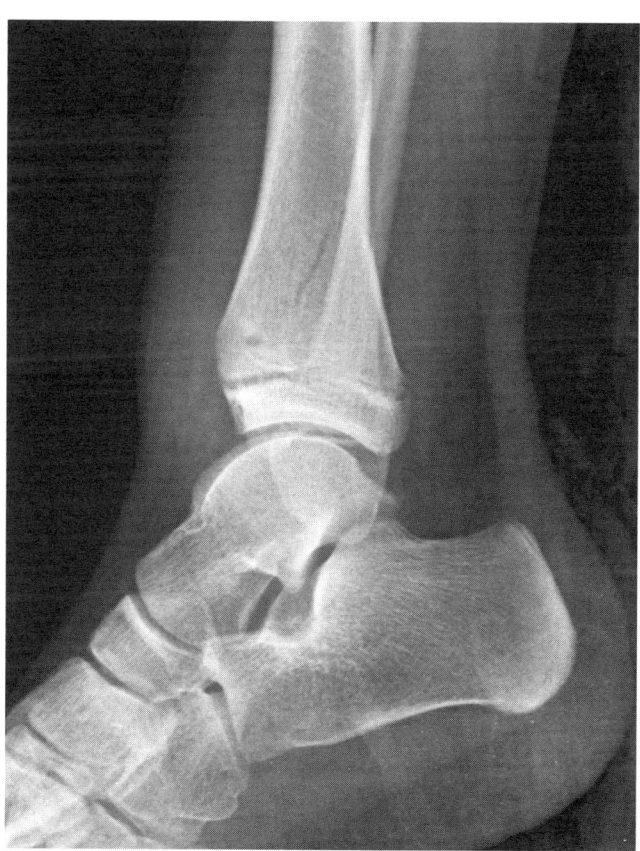

306. **A.** Mayer-Rokitansky-Kuster-Hauser syndrome is a condition where patients have müllerian agenesis or dysgenesis. Patients can either have vaginal agenesis and absence of a uterus, or a partial vaginal agenesis with a partially developed uterus combined with a distal vagina.

B. Savage syndrome is a case of the ovaries failing to respond to follicle-stimulating hormone and luteinizing hormone. This is thought to be because of a defective receptor.

C. Swyer syndrome, or gonadal agenesis, in a 46XY individual presents similarly to ovarian agenesis. Because testes do not develop, there is never a release of müllerian inhibiting factor (MIF), and these patients present phenotypically as female. These patients do not develop breasts.

D. Testicular feminization is a defect of the testosterone receptor such that a phenotypic female presents with chromosomes 46XY. MIF is secreted in these patients, so there are no müllerian-derived structures. These patients can develop breasts but cannot reproduce. Patients with testicular feminization would not have pubic hair, so would not achieve Tanner stage IV.

E. In vaginal atresia the müllerian system develops and the distal portion of the vagina is made up of tissue that is fibrotic. These patients will be 46XX and have ovaries and a uterus.

307. **A.** This patient has signs and symptoms of juvenile rheumatoid arthritis. This condition is more common in girls. Diagnostic criteria include age of onset less than 16 years; arthritis in more than one joint; duration greater than or equal to 6 weeks; type of onset may be polyarticular, oligoarthritic, or systemic; and exclusion of other forms of juvenile arthritis should be ruled out.

B. Lyme disease is unlikely in this patient because she has no history of travel to endemic areas.

C. Septic arthritis is a purulent infection of joint space, and incidence is highest among infants and young children. The most likely pathogen is *Staphylococcus aureus*. Joints most affected are the hip and knee. It is not common for septic arthritis to involve multiple bilateral joints.

D. Toxic synovitis often follows a viral infection. The hip joint is most commonly involved. Range of motion is minimally limited. WBC count, sedimentation rate, and temperature are normal or only minimally elevated.

E. This patient has no evidence of uremia.

308. **E.** Trimethoprim-sulfamethoxazole is the treatment of choice for *Pneumocystis carinii* pneumonia (PCP) and is given for 2 to 3 weeks. It can be used as lifelong prophylaxis when the CD4 count is less than 200/mm^3, as in this patient. PCP responds well to treatment but must be recognized early. It can progress to respiratory failure and is associated with a high mortality rate.

A. Amphotericin B is appropriate for a disseminated fungal infection.

B. Isoniazid and rifampin are treatments for tuberculosis.

C. Systemic corticosteroids are appropriate treatment for *Pneumocystis carinii* pneumonia in states of hypoxia or interstitial pneumonitis.

D. Systemic corticosteroids are appropriate treatment for *Pneumocystis carinii* pneumonia in states of hypoxia or interstitial pneumonitis.

309. **C.** Metronidazole is first-line treatment for bacterial vaginosis. This condition is a clinical diagnosis describing an overgrowth of certain facultative and obligate anaerobic bacteria. These organisms are derived from the patient's endogenous flora.

A. Bacitrarin is appropriate treatment for skin infections.

B. Doxycycline is appropriate treatment for *Chlamydia trachomatis*.

D. Fluconazole is appropriate treatment for candidiasis. Ketoconazole is a treatment for systemic fungal infections.

E. Penicillin is not appropriate treatment for bacterial vaginosis.

310. **E.** This patient has schizotypal personality disorder. Patients with this disorder tend to have odd, eccentric, or magical beliefs. They are often suspicious or paranoid, and may have circumstantial speech. There is usually a pervasive pattern of social and interpersonal deficits. Although borderline personality disorder may have transient psychotic symptoms, they are usually more closely associated with affective shifts in response to stress, and are more dissociative than cognitive.

A. In avoidant personality disorder, an active desire for relationships is constrained by fear of rejection, whereas in schizotypal personality disorder, there is a lack of desire for intimate relationships, as well as more persistent detachment.

B. The psychotic-like symptoms in schizotypal personality disorder are more pervasive. Patients with borderline personality disorder also tend to demonstrate more impulsive or manipulative behaviors.

C. This patient does not display features of paranoid personality disorder. Paranoid personality behavior tends to be a more generalized, enduring pattern of behavior rather than one specific delusion.

D. This patient does not display features of schizoid personality disorder. These are seclusive people who have little wish or capacity to form interpersonal relationships. Treatment involves psychotherapy.

311. **E.** The incidence of bladder cancer in the United States is approximately 60,000 cases per year, with a median age at detection of 65 years. Smoking accounts for 50% of the risk. Greater than 90% of tumors are derived from transitional epithelium. Hematuria is the initial sign in approximately 90% of patients. Superficial tumors can be removed at cystoscopy.

A. Adenocarcinoma represents 2% of all bladder carcinomas.

B. Carcinoid tumors represent less than 1% of all bladder carcinomas.

C. Sarcoma represents less than 1% of all bladder carcinomas.

D. Squamous cell carcinoma represents approximately 3% of all bladder cancers.

312. **B.** Hemoccult cards are sensitive for gastrointestinal bleeding, but not very specific. Many foods can cause the cards to show false-positive results. As long as the patient's vitals signs are stable, they do not appear anemic, and they do not report any gross bleeding, melena, or hematochezia, it is reasonable to send them home to use three cards with three subsequent bowel movements to test at home themselves. As long as one of the three cards is negative, nothing else is necessary except for further follow-up with their primary care physician.

A. Hemoccult cards that show a positive result are considered positive, no matter how long it takes once the developer is applied. Hence, it is a good idea for the examiner not to throw away the card 10 seconds after the developer is applied just because it is not immediately positive.

C. Barium enema is not as sensitive as colonoscopy at detecting polyps or other sources of gastrointestinal bleeding. In addition, they are not able to inspect any part of the tract proximal to the ileocecal junction.

D. Although direct visualization of the gastrointestinal tract is sensitive at detecting sources of bleeding, this is invasive and unnecessary to determine the etiology of a single positive Hemoccult result.

E. Lower gastrointestinal endoscopy is an invasive measure for determining the etiology of a single positive Hemoccult result.

313. **E.** Ectopic pregnancy should be considered in the differential diagnosis of any sexually active female in the reproductive age group who presents with pain, menstrual bleeding, and/or amenorrhea. The initial step in the treatment of this patient should include a urine pregnancy test, which can detect human chorionic gonadotropin (hCG) as early as 14 days after conception and is positive in greater than 90% of cases of ectopic pregnancy.

A. This test is unlikely to aid in the diagnosis of pregnancy.

B. Culdocentesis can aid in the identification of hemoperitoneum, which might indicate the presence of ectopic pregnancy. Although aspiration of blood suggests a ruptured ectopic pregnancy, a negative culdocentesis result does not rule out this condition.

C. Transabdominal sonography is a useful adjunct to quantification of hCG levels and cannot rule out a pregnancy outside the uterine cavity. It can, however, confirm the intrauterine presence of a gestational sac.

D. Transvaginal sonography is more sensitive than transabdominal sonography and can detect pregnancy when the hCG level is 1500 mIU/mL or greater.

314. **B.** This patient most likely has fragile X syndrome. This syndrome can be caused by abnormal CGG repeats in the X chromosome. The murmur of mitral valve prolapse (MVP), along with the physical characteristics, point to fragile X. MVP is not typical of Down syndrome; those patients are more likely to have cardiac malformations.

A. This condition is not related to a chromosomal trisomy.

C. A deletion in chromosome 5 causes cri-du-chat syndrome, not fragile X syndrome.

D. Patients with cri-du-chat syndrome are more likely to have compulsive eating behavior.

E. Fragile X syndrome is not inherited in an autosomal-dominant fashion.

315. **E.** The serum lipase level is very specific for pancreatic disease and remains elevated for 10 to 14 days. This is important in this patient, whose symptoms began 1 week ago.

A. Serum amylase levels may suggest the diagnosis of acute pancreatitis, but normal serum levels do not exclude this diagnosis, and the degree of elevation does not predict the severity of the disease.

B. Serum calcium is lowered in 25% of patients with acute pancreatitis but is not a specific marker.

C. Hyperglycemia is a common finding in patients with acute pancreatitis, but this test is nonspecific.

D. Serum bilirubin, alkaline phosphatase, and aspartate aminotransferase levels are commonly elevated in acute pancreatitis. However, these markers are not specific for this disease.

316. **E.** Premature closure of one or more cranial sutures, craniosynostosis, may be idiopathic or occur as part of a syndrome. If the sagittal suture is involved, a long and narrowed face (dolichocephaly) may result. Most defects are treated surgically before age 2 years for cosmetic reasons.

A. There is no evidence that molding the head by using a helmet corrects craniosynostosis.

B. Observation may be adequate, but for cosmetic purposes, surgery is the best choice.

C. Radiation is not indicated for craniosynostosis.

D. Chemotherapy is not beneficial for craniosynostosis.

317. **B.** Bipolar II disorder is similar to bipolar I disorder but less severe. These patients experience at least one major depressive episode and one hypomanic episode. Hypomania is a period of elevated, expansive, or irritable mood lasting at least 4 days with three to four of the following symptoms during the same time period: inflated self-esteem or grandiosity, decreased need for sleep, pressured speech, flight of ideas, distractibility, increase in goal-directed activity or psychomotor agitation, and excessive involvement in pleasurable activities that could have painful consequences. This patient's symptoms meet criteria for bipolar II disorder.

A. Bipolar I disorder is characterized by one manic and one major depressive episode.

C. Cyclothymic disorder is a chronic form of bipolar disorder in which the mood alternates between a dysthymic mood and hypomania.

D. A manic episode must last for at least 1 week.

E. This patient meets the criteria for bipolar II disorder.

318. **C.** Cocaine abuse has been correlated with abruptio placentae and central nervous system effects. Studies also reveal an increased incidence of prematurity.

A. Alcohol has a high correlation with teratogenic effects, most importantly, fetal alcohol syndrome.

B. Caffeine has been correlated with an increased risk for spontaneous abortions.

D. Marijuana has not been proven to be teratogenic or cause placenta abruption.

E. Opioids have not been correlated with abruptio placentae.

319. **C.** This patient has narcissistic personality disorder. This disorder is characterized by a pattern of grandiosity, need for admiration, and lack of empathy. Patients often are preoccupied with fantasies of power or success and believe that they are "special" or unique, and should only associate with high-status people. They may have a sense of entitlement (i.e., unreasonable expectations of favorable treatment). They are often manipulative of others and show arrogant or haughty behaviors or attitudes. They are frequently envious of others, or believe that others are envious of them.

A. This patient does not meet criteria of borderline personality disorder.

B. The most useful characteristic in discriminating narcissistic personality disorder from histrionic and borderline personality disorders is the grandiosity characteristic of narcissistic personality disorder. Although patients with all three of these disorders often need attention, those with narcissistic personality disorder need that attention to be admiring.

D. Although patients with obsessive-compulsive disorder may also profess a commitment to perfectionism and believe that others cannot do things as well, they tend to express self-criticism, which is absent in narcissistic personality disorder.

E. Traits that distinguish schizotypal personality disorder are suspiciousness and social withdrawal.

320. **B.** The history is consistent with carcinoid syndrome. Approximately half of carcinoid tumors originate in the appendix. Occasionally they can be found in the small bowel, the rectum, the bronchi, and even the stomach, ovary, or testicle. Carcinoid tumors are often asymptomatic. Alternatively, they can cause small bowel obstruction, bleeding, weight loss, dermatitis, and diarrhea. Carcinoid syndrome, on the other hand, is the constellation of bronchospasm, diarrhea, flushing, and right-sided congestive heart failure due to valve problems. Carcinoid syndrome occurs in the minority of carcinoid tumors, and its presence depends entirely on the location of the tumor. When the tumor is drained by the portal venous system, the liver detoxifies the released substances, and carcinoid syndrome is not present. When the tumor gains access to systemic (caval) circulation, the products cause the unique effects of the syndrome.

A. Appendiceal carcinoids cannot cause carcinoid syndrome (without metastasis). Both rectal carcinoids and liver metastases of carcinoids can cause carcinoid syndrome. Statistically, liver metastases are a more likely cause (especially if you were able to palpate the primary tumor in the appendix).

C. Carcinoid syndrome due to rectal carcinoid is less common than that secondary to liver metastasis.

D. Diverticulitis typically occurs on the left side associated with crampy abdominal pain and bright red blood per rectum. Patients with diverticulitis also usually present with fever.

E. Fecal impaction is more common in the rectum than the cecum and is not a common cause of diarrhea.

321. **C.** This patient has Prader-Willi syndrome. This uncommon inherited disorder is associated with absence of segment 11–13 on the long arm of paternally derived chromosome 15. Features include mental retardation, decreased muscle tone, short stature, emotional lability, and insatiable appetite.

322. **A.** This patient has Angelman syndrome. This is an uncommon neurogenetic disorder associated with deletion of segment 11–13 on the maternally derived chromosome 15. Features include mental retardation, abnormal gait, seizures, and inappropriate social behavior (laughing, smiling, and excitability). This syndrome is sometimes referred to as the happy puppet syndrome.

323. **A.** This patient has evidence of Broca aphasia. This is a problem of language production. Comprehension is preserved. Fluency and repetition are impaired. Commonly associated signs include right hemiparesis. This stroke can involve the distribution of the middle cerebral artery.

324. **B.** This patient has a conduction aphasia. This condition is characterized by an inability to repeat what is said, with preserved fluency and comprehension. The lesion is in the arcuate fasciculus, which is the white matter connections between the Broca and Wernicke areas. Paraphrasic errors are common in this condition.

325. **A.** The initial diagnostic test for HIV infection is the enzyme immunoassay. This test is highly sensitive (>99%) and is quite specific. The results of this test must be confirmed with the results of the Western blot test and detects antibodies to HIV antigens of specific molecular weights.

B. Erythrocyte sedimentation rate is not a specific test for HIV but may be elevated due to acute inflammation.

C. HIV p24 antigen can be measured by a capture assay. This is not a first-line test for HIV infection.

D. Plasma p24 antigen levels increase during the first few weeks after HIV infection, prior to the appearance of anti-HIV antibodies.

E. Western blot is the most commonly used confirmatory test and detects antibodies to HIV antigens of specific molecular weights.

326. **E.** Vulvar intraepithelial neoplasia (VIN) presents with vulvar pruritus and vulvodynia and patients have often been seen several times and diagnosed with candidiasis with no relief of symptoms with treatment. Lesions may be diffuse or focal, raised or flat, or white, red, brown, or black. Diagnosis is made by biopsy.

A. It is uncommon for candidiasis to not respond to multiple treatments with no improvement, and the characteristic "cottage cheese" like, thick white discharge is not present. Also, lesions are not usually associated with candidiasis.

B. Paget disease is characterized by velvety red or white plaquelike lesions.

C. The vulvar lesion of syphilis is a firm, painless chancre.

D. This patient does not have any of the features of *Trichomonas* infection.

327. **C.** Retinal and vitreous hemorrhages indicate shaken-baby syndrome, a form of child abuse. This may be the only verifiable sign of abuse. If not treated, permanent vision loss may occur.

A. Acute bacterial conjunctivitis would cause purulent discharge, and is not associated with retinal or vitreous hemorrhages.

B. Cataracts are the most common cause of leukocoria in an infant or child.

D. Hyphema is blood in the anterior chamber of the eye, and is caused by trauma.

E. Increased intraocular pressure causes glaucoma, and is not associated with retinal or vitreous hemorrhages.

328. **E.** In the DSM-IV, the criteria for diagnosis of primary insomnia include a difficulty of initiating sleep for at least 1 month; the disturbance causes distress in social, occupational, or other areas of functioning; the disturbance cannot be accounted for by certain other sleep disorders or occur during the course of another psychological illness; and it is not due to the effects of a substance. This patient meets all of these criteria.

Table 328	
Monitoring time	450 min
Sleep time	300 min
Sleep latency	75 min
REM latency	70 min
Apnea index	0
Nocturnal myoclonus index	0

A. A breathing-related sleep disorder would present with a significant increase in the apnea index. Examples of such disturbances include obstructive sleep apnea, central sleep apnea, and central alveolar hypoventilation syndrome.

B. This patient meets the criteria for primary insomnia.

C. A patient with narcolepsy would have a distinctly different history. In addition, the REM latency would be reduced. Diagnosis would require a multiple sleep latency test.

D. The diagnosis of primary hypersomnia requires demonstration of an adequate amount of sleep. This patient does not show this.

329. **E.** This individual has claw hand deformity, which results in hyperextension of the fingers at the metacarpophalangeal joints, flexion at the interphalangeal joints, and wasting of the small hand muscles. Sensation along the fourth and fifth digits is also diminished in this condition, which involves damage to the ulnar nerve.

A. The axillary nerve innervates the deltoid muscle and functions to abduct the upper arm.

B. The musculocutaneous nerve innervates the biceps muscle and functions to flex the supinated arm.

C. The palmar interosseous nerve extends and adducts the hand at the wrist, extends the metacarpophalangeal joints, and supinates the extended forearm.

D. The radial nerve extends the forearm and extends and abducts the hand at the wrist.

330. **D.** This patient has hereditary spherocytosis, which is an autosomal-dominant hemolytic anemia caused by a defect in the protein spectrin. Spectrin is the major supporting protein of RBCs. This defect results in a loss of membrane fragments and the formation of microspherocytes. These rigid microspherocytes become trapped in microvasculature of the spleen and are hemolyzed. Clinical manifestations vary greatly from severe hemolytic anemia with growth failure, splenomegaly, and chronic transfusion requirements requiring a splenectomy to asymptomatic mild hemolytic anemia that may be discovered incidentally.

A. Dystrophin is a component of skeletal muscle.

B. Dyenin is not a supporting component of RBCs.

C. Elastin is a supporting component of collagen.

E. Thrombin is a component of the coagulation cascade.

331. **D.** This patient has primary biliary cirrhosis. Most patients present with near normal levels of AST/ALT, but have elevated alkaline phosphatase levels, gamma-glutamyl transferase and conjugated bilirubin. Primary biliary cirrhosis, some drug reactions, and primary sclerosing cholangitis are examples of intrahepatic bile duct obstructions. These do not show dilated bile ducts on ultrasonography (although primary sclerosing cholangitis can show a narrow-beaded appearance of the intrahepatic and extrahepatic ducts on endoscopic retrograde pancreatic cholangiography). Antimitochondrial antibody titers have a 95% sensitivity in cases of primary biliary cirrhosis, but are not elevated in primary sclerosing cholangitis. Ursodeoxycholic acid is the treatment of choice in early cases of primary biliary cirrhosis. It is thought to decrease the accumulation of bile salts in the body, thereby relieving the pruritus. It also delays the need for liver transplantation.

A. This patient's symptoms are not nearly severe enough to warrant transplantation, although it might be necessary if complications of cirrhosis or cholestasis develop, such as recurrent ascites, bleeding from varices, encephalopathy, or malnutrition due to decreased absorption of fat-soluble vitamins.

B. 5-Fluorouracil and levamisole are chemotherapeutic agents used in the treatment of colon cancer.

C. Cholestyramine binds bile salts in the intestines, which would only help pruritus in extrahepatic bile duct obstructions and not slow the progression of primary biliary cirrhosis.

E. Hepatic or common bile duct stent placement only relieves the symptoms of obstruction caused by malignancies, usually pancreatic carcinoma or cholangiocarcinoma.

332. **D.** Most patients with gestational diabetes do not usually require insulin in the postpartum period. They are, however, given an oral glucose tolerance test (GTT) at 6 weeks to determine possible therapies.

A. This patient requires a GTT to determine if treatment is needed.

B. This is a good possibility, but it is appropriate to perform a GTT to determine if the patient will require diabetic management.

C. Most patients do not need treatment postpartum unless they have a positive GTT.

E. Most patients do not need insulin postpartum.

333. **C.** Nightmares typically occur late in the night during REM sleep. Medications that reduce REM sleep, such as tricyclic antidepressants and benzodiazepines, can be used in treatment.

A. The patient is experiencing nightmares. Patients have no recollection of these events. They frequently awake from sleep after a loud scream.

B. Night terrors occur in slow-wave sleep. Patients have no recollection of these events.

D. Nightmares occur in REM sleep.

E. Tricyclic antidepressants do not reduce the time spent in slow-wave sleep.

334. **A.** Achalasia is characterized by dysphagia and regurgitation of nonacidic material. X-ray appearance of this condition includes a dilated, fluid-filled esophagus and a distal "bird-beaked" stricture. Typical manometric findings include high resting esophageal pressures with abnormal relaxation during swallowing. The esophageal body has continuous low-amplitude contractions after swallowing.

B. Viral esophagitis is common in immunocompromised patients and can present with odynophagia, dysphagia, and fever.

C. Esophageal carcinoma usually occurs in the middle third of the esophagus and is associated with progressive dysphagia and weight loss.

D. Pill-related esophagitis is commonly seen with ingestion of doxycycline, tetracycline, aspirin, ferrous sulfate, and clindamycin. Predisposing factors include recumbency after swallowing pills with small sips of water.

E. Scleroderma is associated with gastroesophageal reflux and dysphagia. X-ray studies often reveal aperistalsis of the esophagus and peptic stricture.

335. **C.** In this patient of greater than 70 years of age, there is a 70% chance that he has benign prostatic hyperplasia. In addition to urinary obstructive symptoms such as nocturia, frequency, urgency, and decreased force of stream, intermittent gross hematuria is also possible.

A. Acute prostatitis can be associated with intermittent gross hematuria but is more frequently associated with fever, low back pain, and a tender prostate upon digital rectal examination.

B. Bladder carcinoma can be associated with either gross or microscopic hematuria as well as irritative or obstructive urinary symptoms. This patient had a normal kidney/bladder sonogram and is a nonsmoker, which places him at low risk for this disease.

D. Renal calculi are usually associated with hydronephrosis or hydroureter as well as the presence of a stone on sonography. Microhematuria is more commonly seen with this condition.

E. Urinary tract infection is unlikely given the urinalysis findings of negative nitrates and leukocytes.

336. **A.** Clomiphene citrate (clomid) is an antiestrogen, so its side effects appropriately remind one of those associated with menopause, or decreased circulating estrogen: hot flashes, emotional lability, changes in vision, and depression. It also has multiple gestational pregnancies as a side effect in 8% of patients.

B. Danocrine is an androgen-derived substance used to treat endometriosis since it decreases follicle-stimulating hormone (FSH) and luteinizing hormone (LH).

C. Human chorionic gonadotropin (hCG) structurally resembles LH and induces ovulation.

D. Lutrepulse is a gonadotropin-releasing hormone agonist and would not have these side effects.

E. Pergonal is purified FSH and LH distilled from postmenopausal women's urine. This drug has multiple gestational pregnancy as a side effect 20% of the time.

337. **E.** The patient has the classic presentation for myasthenia gravis (MG). The mediastinal mass on MRI is most likely a thymoma present in about 10% to 15% of patients with MG. Both the diagnosis and treatment of a thymoma is best done by direct visualization via thoracotomy followed by a thymectomy.

A. Azathioprine is the second-line treatment if prednisone is not effective, but this still does not treat the mediastinal mass.

B. Plasmapheresis is indicated in severe generalized MG refractory to other forms of treatment. It is also very expensive and not suitable for long-term treatment.

C. MG does not lead to respiratory paralysis. This is more associated with Guillain-Barré syndrome.

D. Radiation therapy alone will not be sufficient treatment for the thymoma, although it can be used in conjunction with surgical removal to help prevent 5-year recurrences.

338. **A.** Caput succedaneum is caused by pressure induced from overriding parietal and frontal bones against their sutures, which results in molding and the physical signs described in the question. It is commonly seen in prolonged labor in which the infant is born vaginally in the occiput-anterior position.

B. A cephalohematoma is a traumatic subperiosteal hemorrhage that usually involves the parietal bone and characteristically does not cross suture lines.

C. Hydrocephalus is not consistent with the clinical description of this patient.

D. The clinical history is not suggestive of hydrops fetalis.

E. Renal sonography was not performed thus, one cannot know whether or not this newborn has hydronephrosis.

339. **E.** This patient meets criteria for anorexia nervosa. These patients who are 20% or more below their expected weight should be hospitalized for an inpatient treatment program. If their weight is 30% below expected, they should be hospitalized for 2 to 6 months.

A. Antidepressants are valuable in treating comorbid depression, but have no effect on anorexia alone.

B. Psychotherapy is not valuable during starvation secondary to the cognitive impairment that occurs.

C. Patients should be started on only 500 calories above the amount to maintain their present weight to prevent stomach dilation or circulatory overload; 3000 calories would be nearly twice what this girl would need daily.

D. This patient has lost a significant amount of weight and is at risk for significant medical complications. Following up in the clinic in 1 month would not be aggressive enough treatment.

340. **C.** Patients who are taking diuretics should be aware of several metabolic effects of such agents. Loop diuretics such as furosemide are associated with development of hyperglycemia, hypercholesterolemia, and hypertriglyceridemia. Hypokalemia and hyperuricemia are also possible metabolic derangements.

341. **F.** Terazosin is an alpha-adrenergic blocker and is equivalent to that of the thiazide class of diuretics. This medication has minimal metabolic effects except for a mild reduction of serum triglycerides. This medication has the added benefit of decreasing urinary outflow obstruction in patients with benign prostatic hyperplasia. Thus, in this patient with hypertension and prostatism, terazosin is a reasonable treatment modality.

342. **J.** The most appropriate agent for this individual would be a calcium channel blocker such as verapamil, which will cause bronchodilation as well as decrease blood pressure. Thus, this agent is appropriate in the patient with chronic lung disease who is also hypertensive.

343. **D.** Psychostimulants, such as methylphenidate and pemoline, are often used for attention deficit hyperactivity disorder. The exact mechanism of action is unknown, but it is thought that they work by facilitating the release of endogenous neurotransmitters. Side effects are sympathomimetic in nature, and include tachycardia, hypertension, insomnia, and diaphoresis. The latter of these is much more significant than diaphoresis. It can actually lead to weight loss and inhibition of body growth. Growth curves are often monitored carefully when children are treated with these psychostimulants. One strategy often used is discontinuing the drug on long holidays and summer vacation to allow the child to try to gain some weight.

A–E. Alopecia, bradycardia, decreased appetite, and hypotension are not a typical adverse effect of this agent.

344. **A.** *Pseudomonas aeruginosa* is the most frequent organism to be found growing in hot tubs. It infects the hair follicles, giving it the name hot tub folliculitis. It can potentially infect anybody who enters the hot tub.

B. *Staphylococcus aureus* will not live in the warm water by itself, but it can cause folliculitis. It is not transmitted sexually, but can be transmitted by contact.

C. *Streptococcus pyogenes* is the causative agent of impetigo or rashes seen in scarlet fever (rough areas, areas of desquamation, strawberry tongue, and Pastia lines).

D. Type I neurofibromatosis is transmitted by inheritance, and it presents as papules or plaques not located around hair follicles.

E. Molluscum contagiosum presents as many papules with dense regions either in hairy or bald areas. A tiny central umbilication is also seen. Molluscum contagiosum is transmitted sexually.

345. **C.** Anytime there is possible mixing of fetal and maternal blood, and the mother is Rh negative and the father is Rh positive or unknown, it is necessary to administer RhoGam to prevent isoimmunization.

A. Fetus is stable, checking scalp pH is unnecessary.

B. Serology on this patient denotes resolved infection.

D. Not appropriate management at this time.

E. Starting acyclovir is not indicated at this time.

346. **D.** This case depicts a mechanical small bowel obstruction (SBO) due to adhesions in the abdomen. Adhesions are the number one cause of mechanical SBO followed by incarcerated hernias. A small bowel obstruction is either simple or complicated. This scenario depicts a simple SBO. A complicated SBO means that strangulation of the small bowel has occurred and there will be signs of peritonitis as well as fever and perhaps an elevated WBC count. Treatment for a complicated obstruction is prompt resuscitation of the patient with intravenous fluids and emergency laparotomy. For this patient, who has a simple obstruction, nothing by mouth, intravenous fluids to correct a hypochloremic hypokalemic metabolic alkalosis, and a nasogastric tube to provide bowel rest are sufficient until the patient begins to pass flatus on her own.

A. An adynamic ileus would manifest with multiple distended loops of small and large bowel.

B. A large bowel obstruction presents with a massively dilated colon on abdominal x-ray films.

C. Perforation is impending when the distended colon is about 10 cm in diameter. The small bowel may also be distended if the ileocecal valve is incompetent.

E. Due to the lack of peritoneal signs, fever, or an elevated WBC count, strangulation or perforation is unlikely.

347. **A.** This patient has the symptoms and MRI findings of an acoustic neuroma. A brightly enhancing mass is visible in the internal acoustic meatus. This lesion can be difficult to differentiate from a meningioma of the cerebello-pontine angle. However, this patient likely has an acoustic neuroma because of the unilateral hearing loss.

Figure 347

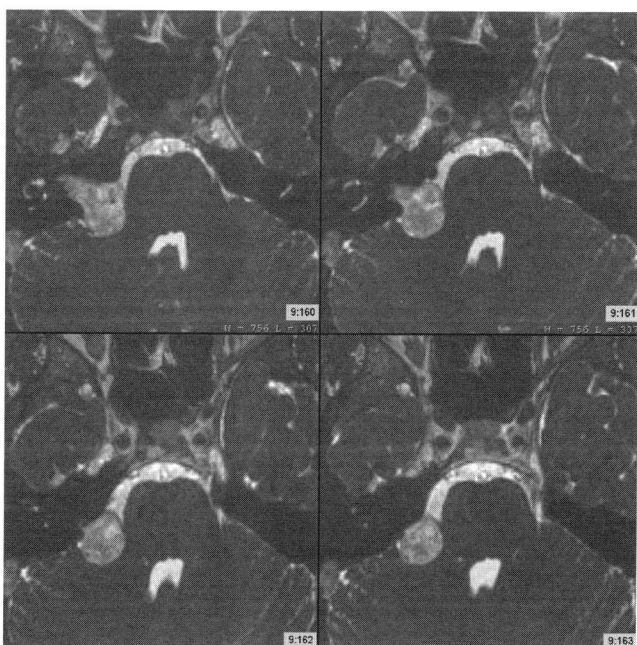

B. There is no diffuse infectious process demonstrated on the MRI.

C. The cerebellar anatomy is normal in the MRI presented.

D. Ménière disease is associated with tinnitus, vertigo, and hearing loss, as is acoustic neuroma. However, in Ménière disease the MRI will be normal.

E. The frontal lobes in this MRI are not visualized.

348. **C.** Infantile spasms usually present between 2 and 7 months in infants with neurodevelopmental disorders or infectious nervous system disease. It is diagnosed by finding the characteristic pattern of hypsarrhythmia on EEG. Corticosteroid therapy has been shown to control the spasms.

A. Cerebral palsy is a nonprogressive disorder of movement and posture, but does not show hypsarrhythmia on EEG.

B. Grand mal (tonic-clonic) seizures are characterized by rhythmic, symmetric contractions of muscles, but EEG does not reveal hypsarrhythmia.

D. Myoclonic seizures are brief jerks that may occur in normal individuals while in light sleep.

E. Petit mal (absence) seizures are brief staring episodes that are diagnosed by a symmetric 3-per-second spike-and-wave pattern on EEG.

349. **B.** This patient has von Willebrand disease, which is diagnosed by clinical manifestations along with laboratory testing (elevated APTT and bleeding time with low levels of vWF:Ag and vWF:Act). Clinical manifestations are similar to those of thrombocytopenia. They include cutaneous bruising, epistaxis, gingival bleeding, menorrhagia, and mucocutaneous bleeding. The mode of inheritance of this condition is autosomal dominant.

A. This disease is not inherited in an autosomal-recessive fashion.

C–E. This disease is inherited in an autosomal-dominant fashion.

350. **B.** Healthy couples experience infertility at a rate of approximately 10%. However, if a woman has endometriosis, the affected couple is likely to experience infertility at a rate of 30% to 40%. Endometriosis is associated with the classic triad of dysmenorrhea, dyspareunia, and dyschezia.

A, C, D, and **E.** Endometriosis is not associated with an increased risk for developing breast cancer, pelvic inflammatory disease, urinary tract infections, or uterine cancer.

351. **B.** Atopic dermatitis in pediatric patients has three clinical phases based on age and distribution. Phase II covers children 2 to 10 years of age, and lesions are visualized over flexor surfaces and sometimes the hands and feet.

A. Phase I, infantile eczema, includes children ages 2 months to 2 years. The rash tends to occur over the extensor surfaces of the extremities, the scalp, face, and neck. Sometimes lesions may appear on the trunk.

C. Phase III of atopic dermatitis is adolescent eczema. This phase mainly involves the hands but may cover the flexor areas as well as the eyelids.

D. This child has evidence of phase II disease. One third of patients with phase I eczema progress to phase II, and one third of patients with phase II move to phase III.

E. This child has evidence of phase II disease.

352. **D.** A second-degree burn is one that effects all of the epidermis and a portion of the dermis, being either deep or superficial. The subcutaneous tissues are not affected in this type of injury. Superficial second-degree burns usually form a blister at the dermal/epidermal junction, below which is sensitive moist pink tissue. This type of burn is sensitive and will blanch will minimal pressure. If infection can be prevented, it will heal spontaneously in 3 weeks. Burn wounds are traditionally treated with débridement and washings with frequent dressing changes. Three antimicrobial agents have been shown to be effective prophylactic agents: silver sulfadiazine, silver nitrate, and mafenide acetate. All are equally effective in controlling burn wound infection if applied before massive colonization. The choice of agent is highly dependent on side effect profile.

A. Amoxicillin is less likely to provide adequate prophylaxis for the burn patient than silver preparations.

B. Ciprofloxacin is less likely to provide adequate prophylaxis for the burn patient than silver preparations.

C. Penicillin is not effective at controlling burn wound infections.

E. Topical steroid preparations may decrease wound healing in the burn patient.

353. **A.** This patient has the avoidant personality disorder. Patients with this disorder exhibit a pervasive pattern of social inhibition, feelings of inadequacy, and hypersensitivity to negative evaluation. They tend to avoid social activities because of fear of rejection or criticism. They generally show restraint with interpersonal relationships, and are often unwilling to become involved with someone unless they are certain of being liked. They may be preoccupied with being rejected or criticized, and view themselves as inept or socially unappealing.

B. Dependent personality disorder, like avoidant personality disorder, is characterized by feelings of inadequacy, hypersensitivity to criticism, and a need for reassurance. However the focus in dependent personality disorder is being taken care of, rather than avoidance of humiliation and rejection.

C. Although social avoidance is also a feature of panic disorder with agoraphobia, it typically starts after the onset of panic attacks.

D. Paranoid personality disorder is usually characterized by a fear of others' malicious intent.

E. Although schizoid personality disorder is also characterized by social isolation, these individuals are usually content with their isolation, whereas people with avoidant personality disorder usually long for meaningful relationships.

354. **C.** Hypoventilation syndrome (or pickwickian syndrome, after a chubby boy in Dickens' *Pickwick Papers*) is a result of morbid obesity and produces the symptoms of constant somnolence, sleep apnea, and increased hematocrit. The presence of so much extra body tissue that needs to be oxygenated makes the individual's body think that it is being oxygen starved, which consequently increases the hematocrit to increase the oxygen-carrying capacity. This is compounded by the sleep apnea, which further decreases the patient's partial pressure of oxygen. The most severe consequence of hypoventilation syndrome (besides the usual sequelae of morbid obesity) is right-sided heart failure.

A. This patient does not meet the criteria of dysthymic disorder because of the limited history given.

B. Hypertension is usually completely asymptomatic. She is more likely to have hypertension due to her morbid obesity, but this cannot be diagnosed until she has three separate readings at least 3 hours apart of blood pressures over 140/90 mm Hg.

D. Although polycythemia will increase the hematocrit, it usually occurs in middle-aged persons and presents as problems related to thrombosis (deep venous thrombosis, stroke, and myocardial infarction), pruritus, venous stasis, and cyanosis.

E. Seasonal allergies would more likely produce symptoms of seasonal rhinitis and postnasal drip.

355. **D.** Hormone replacement therapy is recommended in postmenopausal women who do not have significant contraindications. Women with a history of breast cancer or two first-degree relatives with breast cancer should not receive hormone replacement therapy. Raloxifene has been used in high-risk patients and is not associated with uterine hyperplasia. Vitamin D and calcium should be given to guard against osteoporosis.

A. Raloxifene should also be given to decrease the risk for breast cancer.

B. Premarin should not be given to women with a strong family history of breast cancer.

C. Vitamin D should also be given to this patient to decrease the risk for osteoporosis.

E. Premarin should not be given to women with a strong family history of breast cancer.

356. **B.** This child has juvenile rheumatoid arthritis. More common in girls, this condition is associated with arthritis in more than one joint; the type of onset may be polyarticular, oligoarthritic, or systemic. The most appropriate treatment at this time is inflammatory suppression drugs (nonsteroidal antiinflammatory drugs, immunosuppressive drugs, and steroids) along with physical therapy.

A. Acetaminophen may help with pain, but will not alleviate inflammation.

C. Narcotics are also not indicated. It is not appropriate to start patients on narcotics at such a young age and early stage of disease.

D. Physical therapy alone would not be as effective as physical therapy combined with drug therapy.

E. Surgery may be indicated once the patient has completed growth, but the above patient is still too young to consider this option.

357. **D.** This patient most likely overdosed on her mother's benzodiazepine medicine. Suicidal patients often show an improved mood when they have decided to take their own lives. The most appropriate management is to establish an airway and gain intravenous access. This woman is in a medical emergency, and although flumazenil is the appropriate therapy for benzodiazepine overdose, airway management is a higher priority.

A. This is not an appropriate choice for this patient.

B. Activated charcoal is for tricyclic antidepressant overdose.

C. Serum toxicologies should be sent off in the secondary survey of the patient.

E. Urine drug screen should be sent off in the secondary survey of the patient.

358. **E.** A Meckel diverticulum is a congenital sacculation of the distal ileum. It is usually located within 3 to 6 feet of the ileocecal valve and varies in length from 1 to 6 inches. Normal obliteration of the vitelline duct usually occurs around the seventh week of fetal development. If the ileal portion of this structure is not obliterated, a Meckel diverticulum forms. It is a true congenital diverticulum and therefore contains heterotopic tissue of the digestive tract. Bleeding is often profuse but not life threatening. The most severe complication is intestinal obstruction. Treatment involves surgical resection.

A. A Meckel diverticulum is a congenital sacculation of the distal ileum. The right anterior cardinal vein becomes the superior vena cava.

B. A Meckel diverticulum is a congenital sacculation of the distal ileum. The ductus venosus becomes the ligamentum venosum in adults.

C. A Meckel diverticulum is a congenital sacculation of the distal ileum. Persistence of this duct can lead to infection, obstruction, and bleeding.

D. A Meckel diverticulum is a congenital sacculation of the distal ileum. The Stenson duct carries and releases salivary content just above the upper second molars.

359. **C.** A Smith fracture is also a fracture of the distal radius but with volar angulation of the distal fragment. This fracture also occurs as a result of a fall onto an outstretched hand.

Figure 359

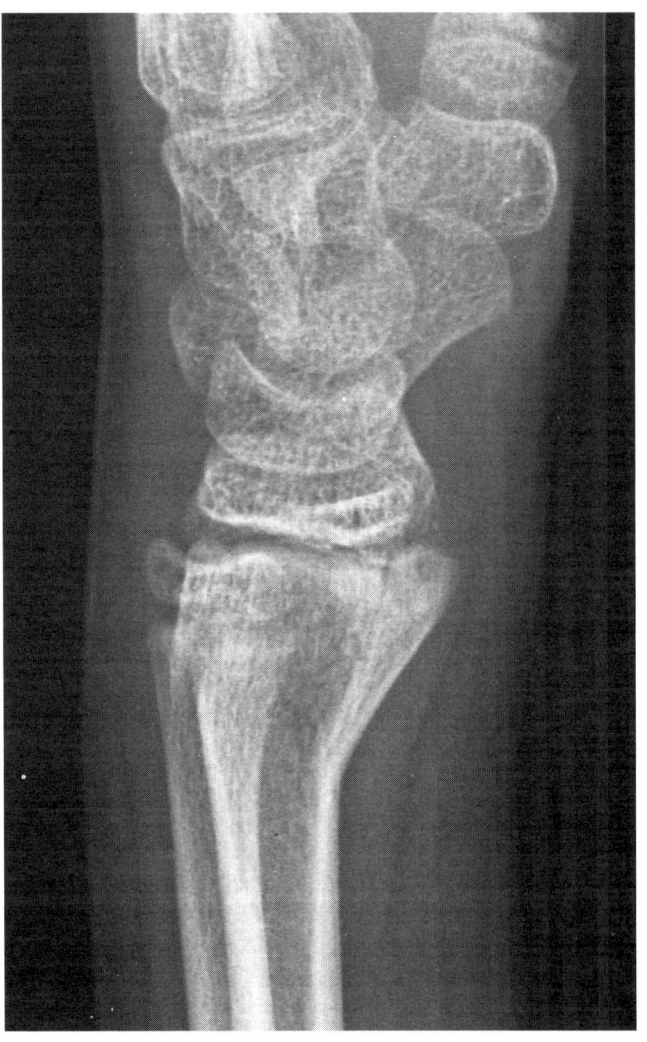

A. The natural response to a fall is to extend a hand in order to decrease the impact to the rest of the body. When the outstretched limb strikes the ground, however, the distal radius is commonly fractured. This is called a Colle fracture. Radiographic assessment of this type of fracture commonly shows fracture of the distal radius with or without a fracture line and dorsal angulation.

B. Like a torus fracture, a greenstick fracture is found in children and is an incomplete break. In this case, the long bone resembles an immature branch that has been broken and is subsequently bowed. One surface will have displacement while the other will have a curved appearance.

D. A torus fracture can be easily differentiated from other fractures of the distal radius. You will find a curve in the straight edge of the distal radius as you trace its edge. Indeed, this curved disruption is the buckle that results from a bending force. This can result from a fall onto an outstretched hand in the upper extremity or in the lower extremity from jumping or falling from greater than 6 feet above the ground. These fractures are frequently found in children.

E. The Salter-Harris Classification defines five types of epiphyseal fractures. Salter-Harris type IV is an epiphyseal break in which the fracture line runs from the joint surface through epiphyseal plate, epiphysis, and metastasis. There is no involvement of the epiphysis in our patient's radiograph.

360. **D.** This patient is at risk for familial adenosis coli, which is an autosomal-dominant disease where colonic polyps are often identified in patients by the age of 25. Polyps usually develop evenly throughout the colon from cecum to anus. Therefore, sigmoidoscopy can appropriately identify individuals with the disease and should be conducted yearly from age 25 to 35. The primary treatment for the disease is total colectomy before the age of 40.

A. Colonoscopy is an effective screening tool for polyps but is unnecessary in screening for polyposis coli since the polyps develop uniformly throughout the colon.

B. Digital rectal examination is a screening regimen commonly used for patients at no increased risk for colon cancer and would not be appropriate in this patient.

C. Occult blood testing of the stool is an ineffective screening tool in patients at risk for familial colon polyps.

E. Total colectomy should be performed before the age of 40 in patients diagnosed with the disease.

361. **C.** The patient is preeclamptic, and because the patient is at term (>37 weeks), it would be appropriate to induce labor to decrease risks to mother and baby. There is no indication to perform a cesarean section.

A. This patient is at term and should be delivered as soon as possible.

B. Induction of labor should proceed and cesarean section performed only for arrest of labor or failure to progress with induction.

D and **E.** Prophylaxis with magnesium sulfate will delay delivery, which should be undertaken sooner rather than later because this patient is at term.

362. **B.** One of the criteria for substance abuse is continued substance use despite having persistent or recurrent social or interpersonal problems caused or exacerbated by the effects of the substance. The rest of the responses are criteria for substance dependence. Other criteria for substance abuse include recurrent use despite physically hazardous situations, legal problems, or failure to fulfill major role obligations at work, school, or home.

A. An increasing alcohol tolerance does not support a diagnosis of alcohol abuse.

C. This criteria does not support a diagnosis of alcohol abuse.

D. Recurrent instances of drinking more than intended does not support a diagnosis of alcohol abuse.

E. These signs and symptoms do not support a diagnosis of alcohol abuse.

363. **E.** Obstructive sleep apnea can be associated with obesity in older children and adults, but is commonly due to anatomic abnormalities in younger children. In this patient, hypertrophied tonsils are the cause. Symptoms include restless sleep, daytime fatigue, snoring or gasping, and morning headache. Symptoms are relieved with tonsillectomy and/or adenoidectomy if enlarged tonsils or adenoids are the cause.

A. Antibiotics may help if the tonsils are infected, but there is no evidence of any underlying infection.

B. The patient's symptoms are not going to improve without some type of therapy.

C. Overnight CPAP is indicated if tonsillectomy does not relieve symptoms.

D. Although sleeping with the head elevated helps for gastroesophageal reflux disease, it has not been effective for obstructive sleep apnea.

364. **E.** This patient has numerous hamartomatous polyps. These polyps are typical of Peutz-Jeghers syndrome. Dense polyps are noted in both the small and large bowel with pigmentation of the buccal mucosa. Gastrointestinal bleeding is common, and there may be an increased risk for development of cancer. However, prophylactic surgery is not recommended. Surveillance colonoscopy is the treatment of choice.

A. Chemotherapy is an inappropriate treatment for this syndrome.

B. Radiotherapy is an inappropriate treatment for this syndrome.

C. Familial polyposis coli should be treated with subtotal colectomy or total colectomy with ileostomy because of its high incidence of leading to colonic malignancy. Hundreds of adenomatous polyps are noted in mainly the large bowel of affected patients; however, small bowel involvement is not uncommon. Familial polyposis is caused by the loss of chromosome q21–q22, the APC gene.

D. Familial polyposis coli should be treated with subtotal colectomy or total colectomy with ileostomy.

365. **A.** Patients with bronchiectasis cannot sufficiently clear airways to prevent recurrent infections. The results of the chest x-ray are consistent with this diagnosis. Classic "tram tracking" of airways is not always seen.

B. Only 4% of cystic fibrosis patients will present in adulthood. Chest x-ray would most likely show upper zone abnormalities.

C. This history does not suggest foreign body obstruction.

D. Chest x-ray findings can be from diffuse infiltrates to lobar consolidation. Effusions may be present.

E. Sarcoidosis is not consistent with this patient's history. In addition, no bilateral hilar lymphadenopathy is noted.

366. **A.** Elevated prostaglandins in the tissues have been associated with primary dysmenorrhea. Primary dysmenorrhea has been the diagnosis established after all organic causes have been ruled out. Often there is a psychological component regarding menstruation that may be acquired from female relatives and friends. Nausea, vomiting, and headaches are also associated.

B. Endometriosis is a cause of secondary dysmenorrhea.

C. An LH:FSH ratio of >2.5 is associated with polycystic ovarian syndrome, not primary dysmenorrhea.

D. In primary dysmenorrhea, pelvic pain is more often associated with day 1 or 2 of menstruation.

E. Pelvic adhesions are a cause of pelvic pain often secondary to surgery.

367. **A.** This is a classic case of acute epiglottitis. The major causative agent is *Haemophilus influenzae,* and patients should be hospitalized and started on intravenous cephalosporins and corticosteroids. Patients often require intubation and continuous pulse oximetry monitoring.

B. Tachypnea, tachycardia, and use of accessory muscles are typical symptoms of asthma.

C. Bronchitis is included in the differential diagnosis but does not explain the rapid onset, difficulty swallowing, or drooling.

D. Difficulty swallowing, cough, and stridor may suggest foreign body aspiration, but the other symptoms do not.

E. Mononucleosis does not have such a rapid onset but may be associated with cervical lymphadenopathy.

F. The rapid onset of symptoms is not consistent with pneumonia. Also, the signs and symptoms described, such as odynophagia, sore throat, drooling, and stridor, signify more upper respiratory tract problems.

368. **B.** A child increases his initiative to explore the world as he develops his control of language and walking. Guilt is refraining from certain activities because you were taught to feel they are wrong. This is normally mastered from 3 to 5 years of age.

A. Our subject already mastered autonomy versus shame. This happens from 18 months to 3 years of age. Autonomy is a sense of mastery over the self's drives and impulses. This leads to exploration of one's surroundings. Shame may be experienced as a consequence of exerting autonomy.

C. Industry versus inferiority is the stage that our subject is working on. This makes sense because it is mastered from 5 to 13 years of age, which is when he experienced his tragedy. The child begins to develop a sense of self based on things he creates. Inferiority involves shunning work, not completing tasks, and not wanting to master any skill.

D. Identity versus role confusion has not been reached by our subject. This normally corresponds to adolescence. One's appearance to others is normally important. Role confusion involves conflicts between the identity and wanting to be accepted.

E. Intimacy versus isolation also has not been reached by our subject, normally achieved from 21 to 40 years of age. This involves the feelings evoked by intimate relationships and the loneliness produced from isolation.

369. **C.** Dysthymic disorder is characterized by a depressed mood most of the day for more days than not for 2 years in adults, but for only 1 year in children and adolescents. At least two of the following symptoms must be present: change in appetite, change in sleep, low energy or fatigue, low self-esteem, poor concentration or difficulty making decisions, or feelings of hopelessness.

A. Cyclothymic disorder is characterized by alternating episodes of hypomania and dysthymia.

B. Major depressive disorder must consist of five out of nine symptoms during the same 2-week period that are different from the normal level of functioning.

D. Minor depressive disorder has a euthymic mood. Between episodes, patients with dysthymic disorder have no euthymic periods.

E. Recurrent brief depressive disorder is characterized by brief periods of less than 2 weeks of depressive episodes. Their symptoms differ from dysthymic disorder because it is an episodic disorder and the severity of symptoms is greater.

370. **A.** This patient has acne because her current birth control pill has significant androgenic activity. Skin cleansers such as benzoyl peroxide may be helpful. However, this patient will benefit from a pill that has less androgenic activity.

B. Change to a pill with less estrogenic activity may not decrease the incidence of acne.

C. Change to a pill with less progestin activity may not alter the incidence of acne.

D. The current dose of this patient's oral contraceptive is causing her acne. This pill should be changed to decrease the incidence of this side effect.

E. This patient can be tried on a different formulation of birth control pill before abandoning this form of contraception.

TEST 2

Board Buster Step 2 was developed to give you the experience of a day of testing. Plan to set aside the time the real examination will take so that you may learn to pace yourself on answering the questions. Each block of questions should be completed in 60 minutes. While working on each block, you may answer the items in any order, review your responses, and change answers. After time expires, you may no longer review test items or change answers.

This section contains a full-length practice test for USMLE Step 2. To simulate the real examination, the test is divided into eight blocks and contains a total of 370 all-new board-format test questions. For your convenience, tear-out answer sheets on which you may record your answers are included in the back of the book.

The Answer Key for Test 2 is listed on p. 226. Complete explanations for each correct and incorrect answer option follow.

371. A 12-year-old boy presents to the pediatrician complaining of bilateral knee pain, which is worse on the right side. He states it has been hurting for the past 2 weeks. No history of trauma is noted, but he started playing basketball regularly about a month ago. Physical examination reveals no limitation in range of motion. However, tenderness is noted with palpation of the tibial tuberosity bilaterally. Radiographs reveal no fracture, but show irregularities of the tibial tubercle contour. What would be the most appropriate next step in the treatment of this patient?

   A. Activity restriction
   B. External fixation
   C. Internal fixation
   D. MRI
   E. Nonsteroidal antiinflammatory drug medication

372. A 5-year-old girl complains of mucous and blood-tinged vaginal discharge for the past 4 days. She also notes perianal pruritus. The mother is the only caretaker of this child and is always with the child. She has no prior medical history. She currently takes no medications. Physical examination findings of the heart, lungs, and abdomen are unremarkable. Pelvic examination reveals perineal erythema. Vaginoscopy reveals a small piece of toilet paper in the lower vaginal vault. Which of the following is the most reliable radiographic study to be obtained in this patient?

   A. CT of the pelvis
   B. MRI of the pelvis
   C. No radiographic study is reliable
   D. Plain film of the abdomen
   E. Transabdominal ultrasonography

373. A 56-year-old alcoholic man comes to the emergency department with complaints of increasing epigastric pain. He says he has had this type of pain before when he suffered from pancreatitis in the past. When asked how often this has occurred, he cannot give a straight answer. Review of systems is positive for weight loss and nonbloody diarrhea that is greasy and floats. Physical examination shows a disheveled male who is uncomfortable. Heart and lungs are normal to auscultation, and abdominal examination reveals tenderness in the epigastric region with no rebound tenderness, as well as a distended abdomen with a fluid shift. Previous abdominal films show pancreatic calcifications. Laboratory values are as follows:

Na, serum	139 mEq/L
K, serum	4.0 mEq/L
Cl, serum	110 mEq/L
CO$_2$	22 mEq/L
Urea nitrogen, serum (BUN)	26 mEq/L

Creatinine, serum	1.1 mg/dL
Glucose (nonfasting)	220 mg/dL
WBC count	7000/mm^3
Hemoglobin	9.8 mg/dL
Hematocrit	29.7%
Platelets	161,000
Aspartate aminotransferase (AST)	275 U/L
Alanine aminotransferase (ALT)	157 U/L
Lactate dehydrogenase	300 U/L
Amylase	3500 U/L
Lipase	2500 U/L

   The man is admitted, given nothing by mouth, and placed on total parenteral nutrition, and is given Demerol to control his pain. What is the next step in the evaluation of this patient?

   A. Wait for pain to go away and for amylase/lipase to normalize, then place on clear fluids
   B. Order a plain film of the abdomen
   C. Send to surgery for dilation of the pancreatic duct
   D. Order endoscopic retrograde cholangiopancreatography (ERCP)
   E. Drain the ascites from his abdomen

374. A young child is brought to the pediatrician for a well-child evaluation. He has a prior medical history of recurrent ear infections. Physical examination of the head, eyes, and ears are within normal limits. The boy is able to pedal a tricycle. He is also able to stand on one foot momentarily. What is his approximate age?

   A. 1 year
   B. 2 years
   C. 3 years
   D. 4 years
   E. 5 years

375. A 30-year-old man complains of a lump on the dorsal side of his wrist that extends into the joint. He has no prior surgical or medical history. Physical examination reveals a cystic lesion on the dorsal side of the wrist that extends into the joint space. Range of motion in flexion, extension, and internal and external rotation appear to be uninhibited. The lesion is 1 cm in diameter and is well circumscribed. There is no evidence of edema or fluctuance. The most appropriate treatment is which of the following?

   A. Bleomycin
   B. Prednisone
   C. Radiotherapy with palladium 103
   D. Splint placement
   E. Surgical removal

376. A 52-year-old black woman presents to her primary care physician with a 4-week history of dry cough, dyspnea, and fatigue. She has no history of tuberculosis or exposure to occupational hazards. Social history is unremarkable. She has a history of hypertension and hyperlipidemia that are controlled with medications. Physical examination reveals that the lungs are clear bilaterally without crackles or rales. She has painless cervical adenopathy and an enlarged parotid gland. Chest x-ray reveals bilateral hilar adenopathy without pulmonary infiltrate. Hilar nodal biopsy reveals noncaseating granuloma with multinucleated giant cells. Results of a purified protein derivative (PPD) skin test are negative for tuberculosis. The above signs and symptoms suggest the diagnosis of idiopathic sarcoidosis. Which of the features are associated with good prognosis for this patient?

- **A.** Elevated angiotensin-converting enzyme
- **B.** Erythema nodosum
- **C.** Hilar adenopathy
- **D.** Ocular involvement
- **E.** Parotid gland enlargement

377. A 9-year-old boy with a history of AIDS presents to the emergency department because of worsening of breathing. Physical examination reveals a room air pulse oximetry of 91%. He is in obvious respiratory distress and is tachypneic. Chest x-ray reveals bilateral infiltrates. Bronchoscopy with biopsy reveals hyaline membranes, cellular infiltrate, and regions of scarring with collagen deposition. What is the most appropriate treatment for this patient?

- **A.** Azithromycin
- **B.** Corticosteroids
- **C.** Erythromycin
- **D.** Racemic epinephrine
- **E.** Surgical resection

378. A 28-year-old G1P0 woman who is pregnant by home pregnancy test presents for evaluation. She denies prior medical or surgical history. Doppler ultrasonography reveals evidence of fetal heart tones. Abdominal examination reveals normoactive bowel sounds with a nonpalpable fundal height. Results of urine beta human chorionic gonadotropin testing in the office are positive. Which of the following pelvic types is most favorable for a vaginal delivery of her newborn?

- **A.** Android
- **B.** Anthropoid
- **C.** Gynecoid
- **D.** Platypelloid
- **E.** Tetroid

379. A 47-year-old man with a history of alcoholic pancreatitis 6 weeks prior to this admission presents with complaints of early satiety, nausea, vomiting, and abdominal pain. Physical examination shows a blood pressure of 100/50 mm Hg and a pulse of 115 beats/min. There is an ill-defined palpable epigastric mass. Results of laboratory studies are shown below:

Blood, plasma, serum

Alanine aminotransferase (ALT)	10 U/L
Amylase, serum	9550 U/L
Aspartate aminotransferase (AST)	10 U/L
Calcium, serum	8.6 mg/dL
Glucose, serum	100 mg/dL
Hematocrit	26%
Urea nitrogen, serum (BUN)	13 mg/dL

Urinalysis

Urine pH	6.5
RBC count	1/HPF
WBC count	1/HPF
Nitrates	Negative
Bacteria	Negative

Rupture of which of the following vessels might explain this patient's symptoms?

- **A.** Common hepatic artery
- **B.** Cystic artery
- **C.** Gastroduodenal artery
- **D.** Left hepatic artery
- **E.** Superior pancreaticoduodenal artery

380. A 56-year-old man is found passed out on the street due to alcohol intoxication. He is brought to the emergency department for evaluation. His health history is unknown. The man is stable but appears malnourished and has multiple bruises throughout his body. He has an open gash on his leg that is stitched up and he is started on cephalexin to avoid infection. Later than evening, the nurse discovers that he is still bleeding from the wound. Laboratory studies reveal a prolonged prothrombin time (PT), normal partial thromboplastin time (PTT), and normal platelets. What is the most likely diagnosis?

- **A.** Hemophilia A
- **B.** Thiamine deficiency
- **C.** von Willebrand's disease
- **D.** Vitamin K deficiency
- **E.** Warfarin therapy

381. A 46-year-old woman presents to her primary care physician with severe abdominal pain, nausea, and vomiting. The pain started 2 days ago and has gradually gotten worse. She cannot locate the pain to a single point, and the pain has kept her from eating or drinking very much for the past 2 days. Her past medical history is significant for an appendectomy at age 26 and a cholecystectomy 3 weeks ago. She began having normal bowel function 2 to 3 days after her latest surgery. She is afebrile. Blood pressure is 90/50 mm Hg, pulse is 90 beats/min, and respirations are 25 breaths/min. Mucous membranes are dry. The abdomen is soft and nontender. There is no rebound or guarding, but the abdomen is somewhat distended. Laboratory studies show a WBC count of 9000/mm³. A CT scan of the abdomen and pelvis was obtained and is shown below (Figure 381) What is the most likely cause of this patient's symptoms?

Figure 381

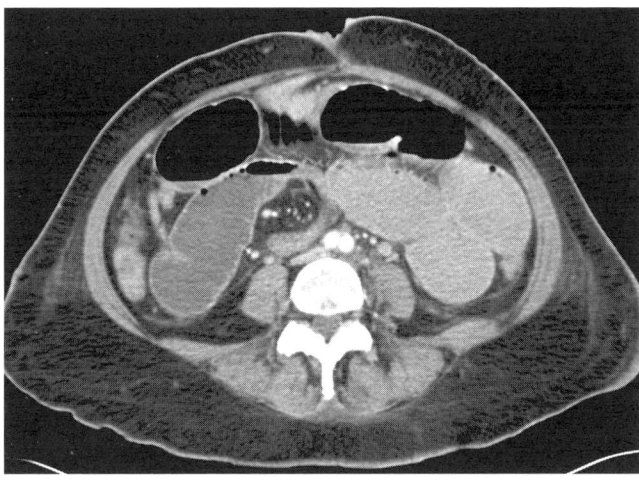

A. Gallstone ileus
B. Intestinal adhesions
C. Intussusception
D. Mesenteric ischemia
E. Paralytic ileus

382. A 17-year-old patient presents to her physician because she is concerned about her cholesterol. Her health class was able to get a laboratory to come to the school and test everyone's cholesterol level. Her total cholesterol was 205, whereas the class average (mean) was 190 with a standard deviation of 9. Even though her cholesterol is high, you try to make her feel a little better by describing normal distribution. If the cholesterols in her class were normally distributed, then 95% of the class should have cholesterols in the range of:

A. 181–199
B. 172–208
C. 163–218
D. 154–227
E. 228–399

383. A 37-year-old woman with a history of chronic pelvic pain secondary to endometriosis underwent hysterectomy. The surgery was performed in an attempt to relieve her chronic use of narcotics for pain. The procedure was uneventful. That same night, the covering resident is called because the patient has a temperature of 104°F. She is sleeping comfortably. Physical examination findings of the heart are normal. Pulmonary auscultation reveals some scattered rales and decreased breath sounds at the bases bilaterally. The wound is clean, dry, and intact. What is the most likely explanation for these findings?

A. Atelectasis
B. Perihepatic abscess
C. Pneumonia
D. Urinary tract infection
E. Wound infection

384. A 2-week-old boy with Down syndrome presents with persistent nonbilious nonprojectile vomiting. Abdominal roentgenograms reveal gastric and duodenal distention with pyloric constriction between the distended segments. Results of laboratory studies are presented below:

Electrolytes, serum

Na, serum	145 mEq/L
Cl, serum	98 mEq/L
K, serum	3.3 mEq/L
Bicarbonate, serum	24 mEq/L
Creatinine, serum	0.5 mg/dL

Leukocyte count and differential

Leukocyte count	8000/mm³
Segmented neutrophils	58%
Bands	5%
Eosinophils	2%
Basophils	1%
Lymphocytes	23%
Monocytes	3%

Blood, plasma, serum

Alanine aminotransferase (ALT)	8 U/L
Amylase, serum	40 U/L
Aspartate aminotransferase (AST)	12 U/L
Hematocrit	33%
Urea nitrogen, serum (BUN)	10 mg/dL

Urinalysis

Urine pH	6.0
RBC count	2/HPF
WBC count	2/HPF
Nitrates	Negative
Bacteria	Negative

What is the most appropriate treatment?

A. Duodenoplasty
B. Enema (gastrograffin)
C. Pyloromyotomy
D. Sigmoid resection
E. Watchful waiting

385. A 25-year-old man presents to the emergency department for evaluation of wrist pain that started approximately 1 week ago. The patient was playing baseball and tried to slide into home plate but tripped and fell onto his hand. Physical examination indicates that the right hand is neurovascularly intact and maintains full range of motion with adequate proximal and distal strength. The patient has tenderness in the anatomic snuffbox. Which of the following is the most appropriate next step in management?

A. Cold ice pack and follow-up
B. CT scan of the injured extremity
C. Immediate immobilization with intrinsic plus cast
D. Mobility exercises and follow-up
E. X-rays of the hand and wrist

386. A 45-year-old man with known HIV infection who has been experiencing insidious fevers, night sweats, and hemoptysis presents to the emergency department. He feels he has also experienced considerable weight loss, but cannot quantify how much. A chest x-ray demonstrates nodular and cavitary abnormalities in the apices bilaterally. Which of the following would be most beneficial in establishing the diagnosis?

A. Physical examination
B. PPD skin test with greater than 5 mm induration
C. PPD skin test with greater than 10 mm induration at 48 hours
D. Purified protein derivative (PPD) skin test with greater than 15 mm induration at 24 hours
E. Sputum culture

387. A 45-year-old woman presents to her primary care physician complaining of nonprogressive, intermittent dysphagia. She admits to a 20-pound weight loss in the absence of dieting. She also has intermittent tongue pain. Her prior medical history is notable for iron deficiency anemia. Her current medications include iron tablets. Upper gastrointestinal endoscopy reveals a distal esophageal ring. Which of the following is the most appropriate treatment for this patient?

A. Esophageal dilation
B. Intralesional corticosteroids
C. Gastroscopic coagulation
D. Surgical resection under general anesthesia
E. No further treatment is necessary

388. A 71-year-old man presents to his primary care physician for evaluation. He was recently diagnosed with a right parietal lobe low-grade tumor. The patient had recently begun experiencing new and frequent headaches. Physical examination reveals left-sided neglect/extinction. What else might you expect to find on physical examination with respect to the visual fields?

A. Bitemporal hemianopsia
B. Left homonymous hemianopsia
C. Left upper quadrant anopsia
D. Left lower quadrant anopsia
E. Macula sparing left homonymous hemianopsia

389. A 30-year-old G3P2 female presents to the emergency department with continued fevers despite broad-spectrum antibiotic therapy for the past 5 days. She delivered her third child 5 days ago by vaginal delivery. Physical examination reveals a temperature of 39.0°C, heart rate of 120 beats/min, blood pressure of 134/80 mm Hg, and respiratory rate of 18 breaths/min. Pelvic examination reveals minimal lochia. Pelvic ultrasonography is negative for pelvic masses. What is the next appropriate step in the treatment of this patient?

A. Antifungal agents
B. Dilation and curettage
C. Exploratory laparotomy
D. Heparin
E. Pelvic examination under anesthesia

390. A 4-year-old boy has recently moved to a new community and is brought by his parents for evaluation with a new pediatrician. The child has a history of mental retardation, tremors, and behavioral problems. Physical examination reveals hypertonicity and skin hypopigmentation. Which of the following is the most likely explanation of these findings?

A. Homocystinuria
B. Hyperuricemia
C. Galactosemia
D. Ornithine transcarbamylase deficiency
E. Phenylketonuria

391. A 45-year-old woman presented to the clinic requesting a surgical age rejuvenation procedure to improve eyelid drooping and wrinkles that have occurred as a result of aging. Her past medical history is significant for hypertension. She does not have previous ophthalmic history. The patient underwent a subciliary blepharoplasty and 4 hours postoperatively had a dilated right pupil and protrusion of the right eyelid with ecchymotic decoloration. Intraocular pressure was 35 mm Hg. She complained of pain and decreased visual acuity as well. What is the next best step in the treatment of this patient?

A. Do a lateral canthotomy and follow with inferior cantholysis
B. Immediately open the incision, drain, and achieve hemostasis
C. Orbital decompression
D. Treat with warm compresses, head elevation, and broad-spectrum antibiotics
E. Wait 7 to 10 days until the blood liquefies and then evacuate it with a large-bore needle.

The response options for items 392–395 are the same. You will be required to select one answer for each item in the set.

A. Analysis of variance
B. Chi-square test
C. Correlation
D. Independent *t* test
E. Paired *t* test

For each clinical study, select the appropriate statistical test.

392. A researcher is interested in comparing body weights of college women in three different age groups.

393. A researcher is interested in evaluating the difference between women who lose weight on a protein-sparing diet versus the percentage of women who fail to lose weight on a regular diet.

394. A researcher is interested in evaluating the differences between initial body weight and final body weight on a protein-sparing diet.

395. A researcher is interested in evaluating the relationship between body weight and systolic blood pressure in a group of 25-year-old women.

396. A 57-year-old black man presents to the ambulatory care clinic for a 6-month follow-up for hypertension. His blood pressure was 175/94 mm Hg at his last visit. No medication was given, but lifestyle modification was initiated for 6 months. Blood pressure today is 172/92 mm Hg. The patient is not diabetic and has no history of cardiac disease. Past medical history is pertinent for appendectomy 12 years ago and depression. The only medication he is currently on is Zoloft for depression. There is a family history of hypertension and myocardial infarction on his mother's side. What is the most appropriate treatment of this patient?

A. Angiotensin converting enzyme (ACE) inhibitor
B. Beta blocker
C. Clonidine
D. Continue lifestyle modifications
E. Thiazide diuretic

397. An 11-day-old boy presents several days early for his 2-week check-up because his mother is worried that he is not feeding well and he seems listless. She reports that he is sleeping well but she is worried that he may be sleeping too much. She also reports that he is quite fussy despite her efforts to console him. On examination, the child is sleeping and has normal vital signs with mildly elevated blood pressure. Cardiac examination reveals a regular rate and rhythm with no murmur, gallop, or rub. Pulmonary examination findings are normal. The abdomen is soft and without peritoneal signs. Examination of the extremities reveals decreased femoral pulses and prolonged capillary refill in

the lower extremities, which are also cool to the touch. Chest x-ray reveals an enlarged aortic knob. Which of the following findings are most likely on ECG?

A. Atrial flutter
B. First-degree atrioventricular block
C. Narrow complex tachycardia
D. Prolonged QT interval
E. Right ventricular hypertrophy

398. A 16-year-old girl presents to her primary care physician for an annual wellness examination. During the history the girl denies having any health concerns, states that she always wears her seatbelt, does not drive with people that have been drinking, does not smoke, and is not sexually active. After discussing all appropriate health care issues pertaining to adolescent girls, including the importance of abstinence and safe sexual practices, she inquires about the rhythm method of contraception. Currently studying human reproductive biology, she asks what day of the menstrual cycle does ovulation begin and what hormones are responsible. Which of the following is the correct response?

A. Ovulation is initiated on approximately day 7 of the menstrual cycle by a luteinizing hormone (LH) spike in response to a preceding estrogen surge from the ovarian follicle
B. Ovulation is initiated on approximately day 7 of the menstrual cycle by a follicle-stimulating hormone (FSH) spike in response to a preceding estrogen surge from the ovarian follicle
C. Ovulation is initiated on approximately day 14 of the menstrual cycle by an LH spike in response to a preceding estrogen surge from the ovarian follicle
D. Ovulation is initiated on approximately day 21 of the menstrual cycle by an LH spike in response to a preceding estrogen surge from the ovarian follicle
E. Ovulation is initiated on approximately day 21 of the menstrual cycle by an FSH spike in response to a preceding estrogen surge from the ovarian follicle

399. A 46-year-old man who presented to the emergency department with right upper quadrant pain, nausea, and vomiting was noted to have an inflamed gallbladder on abdominal ultrasonography. The patient was taken to surgery for laparoscopic cholecystectomy. The patient was given cephalexin and morphine sulfate and started on 110 mL of normal saline with 20 mEq of K intravenously. He was hydrated throughout the procedure and during the first postoperative day. On postoperative day 2, he complained of peripheral muscle weakness. Vital signs are: temperature 97.5°F, blood pressure 135/80 mm Hg, heart rate 83 beats/min, respiratory rate 15 breaths/min, and pulse oximetry 95% on 2 L of nasal cannula. His chest x-ray was normal. ECG showed normal sinus rhythm with peaked T waves in leads V1–V6. Which of the following would be the next appropriate course of action?

A. Obtain two-dimensional echo sonogram and consult cardiology

B. Stop antibiotics and administer benadryl and epinephrine

C. Stop intravenous fluids and administer sodium gluconate, sodium bicarbonate, and insulin with glucose

D. Obtain cardiac enzymes, repeat electocardiogram every 8 hours, and administer aspirin, nitroglycerin, and beta blocker

E. Give K intravenously

400. A 32-year-old woman who recently returned from her honeymoon in Mexico presents to her primary care physician complaining of right upper quadrant pain accompanied by a spiking fever and malaise. She also complains of bloody diarrhea while in Mexico. Physical examination of the heart, and lungs are within normal limits. The liver span is 16 cm in the midclavicular line. There is no guarding or rebound tenderness. Bowel sounds are present in all four quadrants. Results of laboratory studies are shown below:

WBC count	20,000/mm^3
Differential	
Neutrophils	78%
Lymphocytes	15%
Monocytes	7%
Hemoglobin	11 mg/dL
Hematocrit	35%
Platelets	300,000
Chest x-ray	Right hemidiaphragm elevation
CT of the abdomen	Cavitating lesion in right lobe of liver

What is the most appropriate treatment for this patient?

A. Amphotericin B

B. Metronidazole

C. Penicillin G

D. Surgical removal of the lesion

E. Trimethoprim-sulfamethoxazole

401. A 60-year-old woman presents to her primary care physician with several episodes of rectal bleeding over the past 2 weeks, which are not associated with pain. She reports no other recent complaints. Her past medical history is significant for hypertension, hypercholesterolemia, and easy bleeding. She reports that she has always eaten well, with a diet mostly consisting of fruits, vegetables, cereals, and very little fat. Her family history is significant for hypertension, paternal myocardial infarction at age 54, and diabetes in her mother. She also says that her mother and sister bleed easily. Physical examination findings are normal except for a positive Hemoccult. What is the most likely diagnosis?

A. Antithrombin III deficiency

B. Arteriovenous malformation

C. Colon cancer

D. Diverticulosis

E. Diverticulitis

402. A 45-year-old man is brought in to the emergency department by the police after being found unconscious on the sidewalk. His clothes are dirty, and it appears he has not bathed in several days. You are able to smell alcohol on his breath. During the interview, he tells you he drove here to the hospital himself. He is unable to recall distant memories such as the street where he grew up, or the name of his first pet. He tells you that both of his feet are quite painful. Which nutrient is this patient most likely to be lacking?

A. Vitamin B$_1$

B. Vitamin B$_2$

C. Vitamin B$_6$

D. Vitamin B$_9$

E. Vitamin B$_{12}$

403. A 39-year-old woman comes to the clinic complaining of mastodynia in her right breast. The patient thinks that she has a rapidly growing breast mass on her right breast. Physical examination of the right breast reveals a large, mobile 7-cm mass. The skin is erythematous, shiny, and warm. What is the most likely diagnosis?

A. Cystosarcoma phyllodes

B. Duct ectasia

C. Fibroadenoma

D. Intraductal papilloma

E. Sqamous cell carcinoma

404. A 31-year-old G2P1 woman is pregnant with her second child. She is currently in labor on the labor and delivery floor. Physical examination reveals full cervical dilatation. For the past 2 hours she has been in the second stage of labor and is exhausted. The head is at station 3+ and is visible at the introitus. The occiput is straight anterior. She is contracting every 2 minutes with strong amplitude. What is the most appropriate next step in the management of this patient?

A. Administer an epidural anesthetic

B. Explain to the patient to push harder

C. Oxytocin drip

D. Outlet forceps delivery

E. Transabdominal sonogram

405. A 27-year-old man presents to the emergency department complaining of a red external ear for the past 12 hours. The pain has become more intense, as has the redness. He denies any prior medical or surgical history. He takes no medications. Physical examination reveals erythema, induration, and thickening of the right pinna. Pulling and pinching the affected ear reveals exquisite tenderness. The left ear is without erythema, edema, or induration. Otoscopy is undertaken for both ears and reveals tympanic membranes that are without effusion and move well to pneumatomassage. Results of laboratory studies are shown below:

Leukocyte count and differential

Leukocyte count	17,000/mm^3
Segmented neutrophils	75%
Bands	6%
Eosinophils	2%
Basophils	1%
Lymphocytes	24%
Monocytes	4%

Which of the following is the most appropriate treatment?

A. Intravenous ampicillin and gentamicin

B. Oral ampicillin

C. Oral fluconazole

D. Oral prednisone

E. Surgical exploration with débridement

406. A 65-year-old male smoker with a lung mass on CT scan is found to have a serum Na of 128 mEq/L. Serum osmolality is 265 mOsm/kg. Volume status gives no indication of either hypovolemia or hypervolemia. A urine osmolality is 950 mOsm/kg. Urine Na is 35 mEq/L. What is the most likely diagnosis?

A. Adenocarcinoma

B. Large cell cancer

C. Mesothelioma

D. Small cell cancer

E. Squamous cell cancer

407. A 10-year-old boy presents to his pediatrician with complaints of abdominal pain. The patient states he has had abdominal pain for the past week. He has also noticed some blood in his stool, and he had an episode of emesis last night. The patient also complains of fatigue for the past 2 weeks. His oral temperature is 38.8°C. Physical examination reveals bowel sounds are present in all quadrants, the abdomen is diffusely tender to palpation, and no masses are appreciated. A complete blood count (CBC) reveals leukocytosis, thrombocytopenia, and anemia. An abdominal CT scan reveals enlarged lymph nodes in the retroperitoneum. Which of the following is the most likely diagnosis?

A. Acute lymphocytic leukemia (ALL)

B. Acute myelogenous leukemia (AML)

C. Hodgkin lymphoma

D. Non-Hodgkin lymphoma (NHL)

E. Neuroblastoma

408. A 29-year-old G1P0 woman presents to the primary care clinic. She states that she is pregnant. She has not had any prenatal care and states that she "is past her due date." She is a smoker and an occasional drinker during her pregnancy. The date of her last menstrual period was 42 weeks ago. Pelvic examination reveals a fetal head that is fixed in the pelvis. Her cervix is soft, 2 cm dilated, and 40% effaced. What is the most appropriate intervention for this patient?

A. Epidural anesthetic

B. Induction of labor

C. Non-stress testing

D. Oxytocin challenge test

E. Watchful waiting

409. A 68-year-old woman presents to her primary care physician with a 1-month history of morning stiffness, mainly in her hands, wrists, ankles, and feet. The stiffness lasts for about an hour and a half each morning and is always worse in the morning than in the evening. On examination, she is afebrile and in no acute distress. Her ankles and feet are nonedematous and display a full range of motion. Her wrists are edematous and warm to touch, as are her proximal interphalangeal joints and metacarpophalangeal joints bilaterally. Figure 409 shows a radiograph of the hand. What is the most appropriate treatment for this condition?

Figure 409

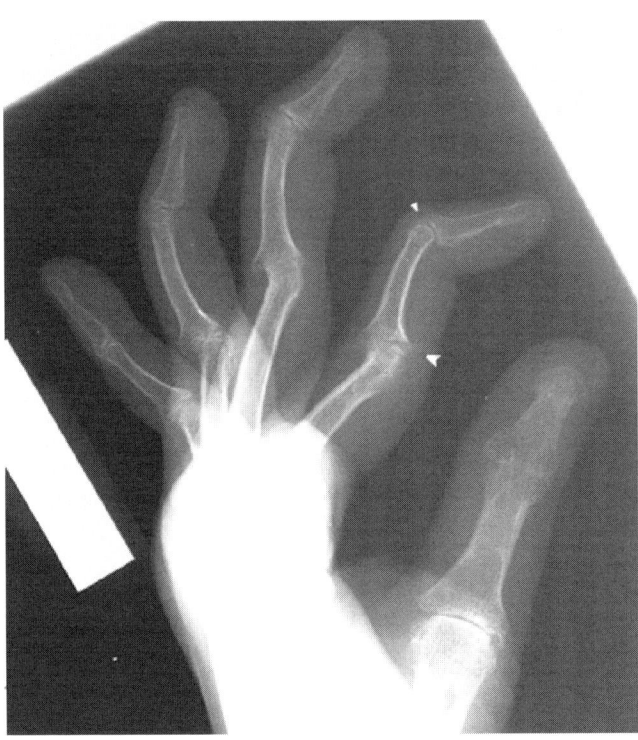

A. Aspirin
B. D-penicillamine
C. Gold salts
D. Methotrexate
E. Prednisone

410. A 63-year-old man with anorexia and a 30-pound weight loss over the past 4 months presents for evaluation. He has a 40 pack/year smoking history and drinks three beers per day. Physical examination reveals a regular rate and rhythm. Pulmonary auscultation reveals good breath sounds bilaterally. Gastrointestinal examination reveals normoactive bowel sounds with a palpable mass in the midepigastrium. Peritoneal signs are absent. Rectal examination reveals stool in the vault, and results of guaiac testing are positive. Upper gastrointestinal x-ray studies reveal thickening of the gastric antrum with a filling defect. Which of the following is the most likely diagnosis?

A. Adenocarcinoma
B. Leiomyoma
C. Leiomyosarcoma
D. Lymphoma
E. Melanoma

411. A 51-year-old man presents to the emergency department complaining of a 6-hour history of left-sided chest pain. Which of the following statements will elicit the most information from this patient?

A. "Is there a family history of heart disease in your family?"
B. "Point to the area in your chest that hurts."
C. "Tell me about the pain."
D. "Tell me about the pain in your chest."
E. "When did the pain begin?"

412. A 46-year-old woman presents to her gynecologist for a second opinion regarding heavy vaginal bleeding. She has been passing large blood clots along with heavy menstrual periods for the past 6 months. She has a history of stress urinary incontinence and has been treated with pseudoephedrine. She wears two pads per day. Physical examination reveals blood in the vaginal vault. Diagnostic laparoscopy, hysteroscopy, and biopsy are normal. Results of urinalysis and urine cytology are negative. What is the most likely cause for this patient's bleeding?

A. Anovulation
B. Coagulation defect
C. Multiple ovulations
D. Transitional cell carcinoma of the bladder
E. Uterine polyps

413. A 55-year-old man with no prior medical history begins a diet rich in fruits, vegetables, wine, and tea in hopes of preventing cancer. Physical examination findings of his heart, lungs, and abdomen are within normal limits. Both testicles are descended bilaterally and the prostate is 30 g and without masses. Results of laboratory studies are shown below:

Electrolytes, serum

Na, serum	145 mEq/L
Cl, serum	102 mEq/L
K, serum	3.6 mEq/L
Bicarbonate, serum	25 mEq/L
Magnesium, serum	2.0 mEq/L
Creatinine, serum	1.0 mg/dL

Leukocyte count and differential

Leukocyte count	5000/mm³
Segmented neutrophils	45%
Bands	5%
Eosinophils	3%
Basophils	1%
Lymphocytes	24%

This patient's dietary habits might have a possible action in cancer reduction by

A. Bacteriostasis

B. Blockade of nitrosamine formation

C. Detoxification of enzymes against bacteria

D. Pump-mediated efflux of carcinogens from cells

E. Suppression of carcinogenic action of estrogen

414. A change occurs in the oncogenes that lead to colon cancer. The change results in a much more rapid progression of the disease, leading to a higher rate of death for people who develop colon cancer. What will this do to the incidence and the prevalence of the disease?

A. Incidence no change, prevalence no change

B. Incidence increases, prevalence decreases

C. Incidence no change, prevalence decreases

D. Incidence decreases, prevalence decreases

E. Incidence increases, prevalence increases

415. A 46-year-old obese woman presents to her primary care physician with right upper quadrant pain that has been worsening over the past month. Her pain is sharp in nature and occurs after meals. The pain goes away approximately 2 to 3 hours after meals. She typically eats fried, fatty foods. She has occasional diarrhea. The patient denies having fevers, chills, or discoloration of her skin. She has never had this pain in the past. What would be the best test to help confirm the diagnosis?

A. Abdominal x-ray

B. Bladder and renal ultrasonography

C. CT scan of her abdomen/pelvis

D. Hepatic ultrasonography

E. Upper gastrointestinal endoscopy

416. A 16-year-old high school volleyball player presents for evaluation of right knee pain which is worse after practice or games. He has no prior medical or surgical history. Physical examination reveals point tenderness over the right infrapatellar pole. There is also tenderness of the right quadriceps tendon at the superior attachment to the patella. What is the most appropriate statement to make to this patient regarding this condition?

A. Antibiotics and analgesics are important modes of therapy

B. Complete rest for 6 months is required

C. Continuation of activities will lead to recovery

D. Pain becomes resistant to treatment with scarring of the tendon

E. Surgical resection is curative

417. Allison is a freshman in college and a pledge of the Phi Gamma Phi sorority. She lives in a dormitory room with two other girls, Michele and Kristy. She participates in sports and worked as a lifeguard at the local pool, but she has no close friends. All of her roommates are pledging the same sorority as she is. Allison often sabotages her roommates by making up false stories and telling them to the sorority members to ruin their reputation and hurt their chances of becoming a member. However, when she talks to her mother on the phone, she tells her that her roommates are the ones making up stories about her. Allison also told one roommate, Michele, that she caught Kristy having sex with Rob, a star football player, and that she was only doing it to help her popularity with the sorority. However, Allison was the person who had sex with Rob. Which defense mechanism best describes Allison's actions?

A. Displacement
B. Projection
C. Reaction formation
D. Splitting
E. Undoing

418. A 39-year-old woman with a history of sarcoidosis is applying for a job as a teacher in the community that she and her husband have just moved to. She does have some dyspnea on exertion. She is an avid treadmill runner but can only walk 2 miles per hour (pace of 30 min/mile) without difficulty. This new job requires that she have a complete history and physical examination prior to beginning work. Physical examination findings of the heart, lungs, and abdomen are unremarkable. Chest x-ray reveals hilar adenopathy. What is the most appropriate intervention at this time?

A. Antibiotics for 10 days with follow-up at 6 weeks
B. High-dose corticosteroids for 6 weeks
C. Low-dose corticosteroids until adenopathy resolves
D. Lung transplantation should be anticipated and patient should be immediately placed on transplant list
E. No treatment is required at this time

419. A 26-year-old woman presents with a 2-day history of excruciating pain in her right groin region. Blood pressure is 120/76 mm Hg and pulse is 68 beats/min. Physical examination reveals painful swelling inferior to the inguinal ligament. Results of laboratory studies are shown below:

Urinalysis

Urine pH	6.0
Color	Yellow
Odor	Slight
RBC count	2/HPF
WBC count	2/HPF
Nitrates	Negative
Bacteria	Negative

What is the most likely diagnosis?

A. Femoral hernia
B. Inguinal hernia
C. Obturator hernia
D. Umbilical hernia
E. Vertebral disc herniation

420. A 49-year-old migrant farmer who recently arrived from Mexico presents to the emergency department accompanied by his son. His son said that he witnessed his father have a seizure this morning. It began with a twitching in his right arm that then turned into a loss of consciousness with diffuse twitching and grunting. The seizure lasted about 2 minutes. His father regained consciousness after the seizure but was groggy for about a half an hour. His father has no prior history of seizures. He complains of a recent weight loss of 10 pounds over the past 2 months. The remainder of the review of systems is negative. He has a 35 pack/year history of smoking, no history of alcohol or drug abuse, and formerly farmed pigs in Mexico. Physical examination findings, including those of a detailed neurologic examination, are normal. A CT of his head is ordered and at least 10 calcified cysticerci are found. A fecal examination reveals proglottids and eggs. What is the most appropriate treatment for this patient?

A. Albendazole
B. Diethylcarbamazine
C. Ivermectin
D. Metronidazole
E. Mebendazole
F. Praziquantel
G. Pyrantel pamoate
H. Thiabendazole

421. An obese 37-year-old G4P4004 woman presents to her primary care physician complaining of recurring, steady right upper quadrant pain that occurs mostly after meals. These episodes have been going on for approximately a week and are sometimes associated with vomiting. Physical examination reveals an obese white female who is in acute distress, afebrile, and has a normal skin tone. Bilateral sclera are not jaundiced, and pupils are equally round and reactive to light. Oropharynx is nonerythematous. There are no neck masses, cervical lymphadenopathy, or supraclavicular lymphadenopathy. The heart has a regular rate and rhythm without murmur. Lungs are clear to auscultation bilaterally. Bowel sounds are present. Abdominal examination reveals guarding with pain to palpation in the right upper quadrant without rebound tenderness. The Murphy sign is positive.

There is no swelling of her bilateral lower extremities. Results of laboratory studies are shown below:

WBC count	19,000/mm^3
Hemoglobin	13.1 mg/dL
Hematocrit	40.5%
Platelet count	360,000/mm^3
Aspartate aminotransferase (AST)	38 U/L
Alanine aminotransferase (ALT)	15 U/L
Alkaline phosphatase	218 U/L
Serum bilirubin	6.9 mg/dL

Ultrasonography of the gallbladder reveals gallstones. What is the most likely diagnosis?

A. Cholelithiasis
B. Cholecystitis
C. Cholangitis
D. Choledocholithiasis
E. Gallbladder adenocarcinoma

422. A 28-year-old G1P0 woman is 35 weeks pregnant. She tells you that she does not desire to become pregnant again upon completion of the present delivery. Her prenatal care has been up to date. She has a history of hypertension in pregnancy but takes no medications. She is currently in labor and was contracting regularly at 10-minute intervals during the past 3 hours. She complains of sudden onset of suprapubic pain and vaginal discharge. Electronic fetal monitoring reveals the absence of uterine contractions. Her blood pressure is 70/40 mm Hg and pulse is 140 beats/min. Cardiac examination reveals faint heart tones. Pulmonary examination reveals good breath sounds bilaterally. Abdominal examination reveals tenderness to palpation in the right and left lower quadrants. Bloody vaginal discharge is noted. Ultrasonography reveals extension of fetal extremities and an abnormal fetal position. Which of the following is the most appropriate treatment for this individual?

A. Embolization of the hypogastric artery
B. Embolization of the uterine artery
C. Hysterectomy
D. Vaginal packing
E. No further treatment is necessary

423. A mother brings her 2-week-old girl to her pediatrician for evaluation. The birth history reveals an uncomplicated spontaneous vaginal delivery at 39 weeks' gestation. The patient had Apgar scores of 9 at 9 minutes and weighed 6 pounds 6 ounces at birth. The mother states the child has been breast-feeding without any difficulties. Physical examination reveals normal vital signs. Primitive reflexes are present. There is an absent red reflex in the left eye. What is the most appropriate next step in the treatment of this patient?

A. CT scan of the head
B. MRI of the head
C. Observation

D. Ophthalmologic consultation
E. Topical therapy with erythromycin

424. You are a neurologist practicing in an area with very few pediatric subspecialists. Therefore, you are asked to see most pediatric patients with neurologic concerns in addition to your adult patients. One child is referred to you with a chief complaint of a poor attention span. From the history given by the patient's mother, you suspect that this may be secondary to a seizure disorder. You therefore order electroencephalography (EEG), which shows the characteristic 3-Hz spike-and-wave pattern. What is the most appropriate treatment for this patient?

A. Carbamazepine
B. Ethosuximide
C. Phenobarbital
D. Phenytoin
E. Valproic acid

425. A 41-year-old woman with multiple myeloma treated with chemotherapy complains of a 3-month history of progressive low back pain. She denies history of recent trauma. Her pain is unrelieved by rest and minimally relieved with oral antiinflammatory agents. She has a prior surgical history of hysterectomy for endometriosis. Physical examination of the heart, lungs, and abdomen are unremarkable. Examination of the spine reveals no evidence of scoliosis. Her skin is intact without obvious abnormalities. MRI is remarkable for sparing of the disk space. Which of the following is the most likely diagnosis?

A. Low back strain
B. Lumbar arachnoiditis
C. Metastasis to the spine
D. Spondylolisthesis
E. Vertebral osteomyelitis

426. A 58-year-old man with an 80 pack/year history of smoking presents to his primary care physician complaining of night sweats and a 35-pound weight loss in the past 5 months. He also complains of generalized weakness. Physical examination reveals an emaciated man who fatigues easily. He has bilateral rales and rhonchi on auscultation of the chest. Chest x-ray demonstrates central hilar nodules. Urine osmolality is 400 mOsm/L; serum osmolality is 200 mOsm/L. Serum Na is 130 mEq/L. Which of the following can potentially be associated with this condition?

A. Lambert-Eaton syndrome
B. Lymphangioleiomyomatosis
C. Metastatic renal carcinoma
D. Myasthenia gravis
E. Superior vena cava syndrome

427. A newborn male infant was delivered approximately 20 minutes ago by the obstetrician/gynecologist. He is now being examined by the pediatric resident. Apgar score was 9 at 5 minutes. Examination reveals cleft palate, small abnormally shaped ears, and hypoplasia of the mandible. What is the most likely exposure that would explain these findings?

    A. Alcohol

    B. Amphetamines

    C. Diethylstilbestrol

    D. Isotretinoin

    E. Norethisterone

The response options for items 428–432 are the same. You will be required to select one answer for each item in the set.

    A. Acute cholecystitis

    B. Acute pancreatitis

    C. Cholelithiasis

    D. Choledocholithiasis

    E. Chronic cholecystitis

    F. Chronic pancreatitis

    G. Pancreatic carcinoma

    H. Primary sclerosing cholangitis

For each patient with abdominal pain, select the most appropriate diagnosis.

428. A 75-year-old man with a 35-pound weight loss complains of a 6-month history of abdominal pain that radiates to the back. He also notes clay-colored stools and a darkening of the color of his urine. His sclera are icteric. The gallbladder is palpable. Laboratory studies are shown below:

Blood, plasma, serum

Alanine aminotransferase (ALT)	110 U/L
Amylase, serum	90 U/L
Aspartate aminotransferase (AST)	110 U/L
Calcium, serum	8.8 mg/dL
Glucose, serum	120 mg/dL
Hematocrit	31%
Urea nitrogen, serum (BUN)	17 mg/dL

429. A 39-year-old man with ulcerative colitis complains of pruritus, right upper quadrant pain, fever, and weight loss. Laboratory studies reveal elevation of serum alkaline phosphatase and bilirubin. Endoscopic retrograde cholangiography reveals stenosis and dilatation of the intrahepatic and extrahepatic bile ducts.

430. A 44-year-old woman has a long history of dyspepsia and fatty food intolerance associated with right upper quadrant pain. Ultrasonography reveals gallstones within a contracted gallbladder. Serum transaminases are normal.

431. A 33-year-old woman complains of a 3-hour history of right upper quadrant pain, nausea, vomiting, and a fever of 101.5°F. Examination reveals right upper quadrant pain upon deep inspiration and coughing. A right upper quadrant mass is palpable. The WBC count is elevated, as are serum bilirubin and alkaline phosphatase levels.

432. A 38-year-old woman complains of right upper quadrant pain occurring 60 minutes after meals and lasting for several hours, occasionally radiating to the right scapula. She also notes occasional nausea and vomiting. Physical examination of the abdomen reveals mild midepigastric tenderness to deep palpation without peritoneal signs. Bowel sounds are normoactive. Laboratory studies obtained are shown below:

Blood, plasma, serum

Alanine aminotransferase (ALT)	19 U/L
Amylase, serum	75 U/L
Aspartate aminotransferase (AST)	18 U/L
Calcium, serum	9.2 mg/dL
Glucose, serum	115 mg/dL
Hematocrit	37.5%
Urea nitrogen, serum (BUN)	12 mg/dL

433. A 27-year-old woman, who notes her desire to conceive, has had spontaneous abortions during the second trimester of her last three pregnancies. The patient's mother took diethylstilbestrol (DES) while pregnant with her. Physical examination reveals the cervix is 0.6 cm long. What is the best treatment that will increase her chance of maintaining her next pregnancy?

    A. Cervical cerclage

    B. Clomiphene citrate

    C. Human chorionic gonadotropin (hCG) injections

    D. Leuprolide acetate

    E. Progesterone supplement

434. A first-year medical student's mother dies of pancreatic cancer. He attends the funeral and goes right back to school. Instead of mourning, he studies pancreatic cancer extensively and eventually publishes a paper on the subject during his third year. The defense mechanism he is portraying is:

    A. Altruism

    B. Dissociation

    C. Intellectualization

    D. Rationalization

    E. Sublimation

435. A 35-year-old man presents to his primary care physician complaining of a painless testicular mass that he reports having for the past 8 months. The patient now is experiencing back pain in the lower lumbar spine. Physical examination reveals bilateral gynecomastia and a 3-cm solid right testicular mass. Scrotal ultrasonography confirms a solid testicular mass. What is the next best step to be taken in this patient?

A. Alpha-fetoprotein

B. Begin chemotherapy

C. CA 27.29

D. Percutaneous biopsy

E. Radical orchiectomy

436. A 3-year-old boy presents to the emergency room with a sudden onset of respiratory distress. Temperature is 39°C. The patient appears to be most comfortable when sitting up and leaning forward. He is drooling and has difficulty speaking and swallowing. Results of laboratory studies are presented below:

Electrolytes, serum

Na, serum	141 mEq/L
Cl, serum	98 mEq/L
K, serum	3.9 mEq/L
Bicarbonate, serum	24 mEq/L
Creatinine, serum	0.6 mg/dL

Leukocyte count and differential

Leukocyte count	19,000/mm³
Segmented neutrophils	75%
Bands	5%
Eosinophils	3%
Basophils	1%
Lymphocytes	24%
Monocytes	4%

Blood, plasma, serum

Hematocrit	33%

Urinalysis

Urine pH	6.5
RBC count	1/HPF
WBC count	1/HPF
Nitrates	Negative
Bacteria	Negative

Which of the following is the most appropriate treatment?

A. Epinephrine (racemic)

B. Laryngoscopy (flexible)

C. Oxygen administered by nasal cannula

D. Intravenous corticosteroids

E. Intubation and intravenous antibiotics

437. A newborn is transferred from a rural hospital to a tertiary care center for evaluation. He is found to have cutis aplasia, a sloping forehead, holoprosencephaly, polydactyly, and clindactyly. Which of the following is the most likely explanation of these findings?

A. Cri-du-chat syndrome

B. Prader-Willi syndrome

C. Trisomy 13

D. Trisomy 18

E. Trisomy 21

438. A 17-year-old girl presents to the emergency department complaining of abdominal pain in the lower abdomen for 4 weeks. Physical examination reveals no evidence of guarding or rebound tenderness. A soft tissue mass is felt in the left lower quadrant. Abdominal x-rays shows a mass lesion in the left lower quadrant that reveals toothlike structures and areas of calcifications. What is the most likely diagnosis?

A. Choriocarcinoma

B. Cystic teratoma

C. Endodermal sinus tumor

D. Follicular cyst

E. Mucinous cystadenoma

439. A 68-year-old man presents with a 3-month history of cough, weight loss, and increasing fatigue. He has a 30 pack/year history of smoking. Physical examination reveals that he is febrile and you note a dry cough. Breath sounds are clear, but you notice he becomes dyspneic after 6 deep breaths. A CT of the chest is ordered and is shown below (Figure 439). What is the most likely diagnosis?

Figure 439

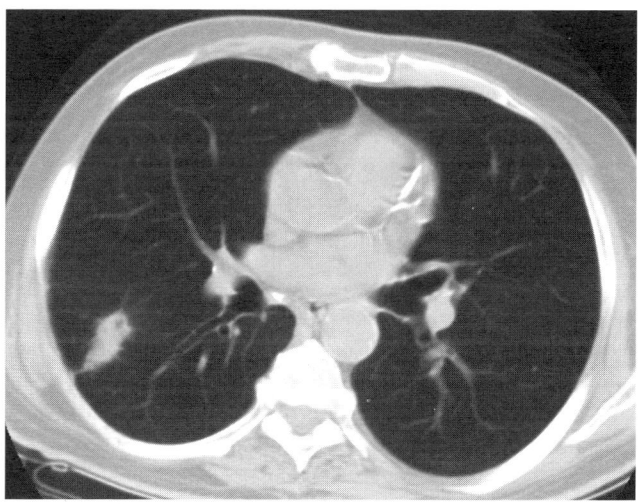

A. Adenocarcinoma

B. Carcinomatosis (metastases)

C. Chronic obstructive pulmonary disorder

D. Small cell carcinoma

E. Squamous cell carcinoma

440. A 53-year-old man presents to his primary care physician with symptoms of right upper quadrant abdominal pain that is worsened 30 minutes after eating. He has no symptoms of fever, heartburn, melena, or hematochezia. He does report a history of weight loss and early satiety. Physical examination reveals a nonjaundiced man in considerable pain with a positive Murphy sign. Ultrasonography is performed on his abdomen, and several stones are seen in his gallbladder. He signs a consent for the performance of a laparoscopic cholecystectomy in addition to any other procedures should a complication occur. After removal of the gallbladder, the surgeon visually examines the abdominal cavity and sees that the patient's stomach appears abnormal and leathery. Knowing that the patient did not consent for any other procedures to occur, the surgeon closes up the patient and then feels for supraclavicular lymphadenopathy. Virchow node is palpated. What is the most likely explanation of these findings?

A. Linitis plastica

B. Metastatic breast cancer

C. Normal anatomic variant

D. Superficial spreading gastric carcinoma

E. Systemic sclerosis

441. A 55-year-old woman comes to the emergency department complaining of a 10-hour history of progressive gastric distress. She seems agitated and says that she is afraid that she has cirrhosis of the liver and then stops speaking. Which of the following will best encourage her to continue speaking?

A. "Do you drink?"

B. "How much beer do you drink?"

C. "I can see that you are very upset."

D. "Please go on."

E. "Why did you take so long to come in for evaluation?"

442. A 25-year-old man who is a law student presents to the clinic with a 3-week complaint of lower left quadrant abdominal pain and alternating constipation and diarrhea. The pain is relieved with bowel movements. The patient notes that lately he has been under increased stress because his girlfriend has broken up with him. The patient's past medical history is remarkable for a left inguinal hernia repair 5 years ago. He takes no medications except for a daily multivitamin. Physical examination reveals a regular heart rate and rhythm, clear lungs bilaterally, hypoactive bowel sounds and some mild tenderness to deep palpation of the left lower quadrant without guarding or rebound. Rectal examination reveals some small internal hemorrhoids. Results of laboratory studies are presented below:

Electrolytes, serum

Na, serum	139 mEq/L
Cl, serum	102 mEq/L
K, serum	3.9 mEq/L

Bicarbonate, serum	24 mEq/L
Creatinine, serum	1.1 mg/dL

Leukocyte count and differential

Leukocyte count	5000/mm³
Segmented neutrophils	55%
Bands	5%
Eosinophils	2%
Basophils	2%
Lymphocytes	23%
Monocytes	2%

What kind of disorder does this patient suffer from?

A. Hematologic

B. Infectious

C. Peristaltic

D. Psychological

E. Psychosomatic

443. A previously healthy 14-year-old girl presents to the pediatric clinic with a 1-week history of low-grade fever, malaise, and dry cough. Physical examination reveals diffuse crackles, wheezing, and rales. Chest x-ray reveals a bronchopneumonia with a small pleural effusion. The patient is subsequently sent home with a prescription for erythromycin. What is the organism most likely responsible for this patient's pneumonia?

A. *Chlamydia pneumoniae*

B. *Haemophilus influenzae*

C. *Legionella pneumophila*

D. *Mycoplasma pneumoniae*

E. *Pseudomonas aeruginosa*

444. A 38-year-old G4P4004 married woman presents to her gynecologist for her annual wellness examination. Her history is significant for anxiety disorder, fibrocystic changes of the breast, and oligomenorrhea with menstrual cycles lasting 41 to 42 days. She declares that her mother went through menopause when she was 35 years old and now she worries that she, too, has begun having symptoms of menopause. "I have been having every symptom found on the Internet for the last 2 months." She complains of hot flashes, nausea, mood changes, and breast tenderness. Additionally, she complains that her long menstrual cycles are worsening, with her last menstruation being 10 weeks ago. Physical examination reveals fibrocystic changes and breast tenderness. Pelvic examination reveals bluish discoloration of the vagina and cervix without signs of atrophy. What is the most appropriate next step in the treatment of this patient?

A. Begin exogenous estrogen replacement therapy to prevent coronary artery disease, stroke, and loss of bone mineral content

B. Council patient on importance of finding reputable sources of health information on the Internet

C. Obtain serum follicle-stimulating hormone levels

D. Obtain serum beta human chorionic gonadotropin levels

E. Perform chromosomal studies to investigate genetic basis for family history

445. Cindy, a mother of three children, is extremely afraid of the dark. One day while driving her kids home from school, her 5-year-old son, Mark, opens his window so that he can pretend his toy airplane is really flying in the wind. As they pull into the driveway, Cindy can hear the phone ringing in the house. She quickly turns off the car without rolling the window up and runs inside to get the phone. That night, it starts to rain. She remembers that the window is still down in the car but cannot bring herself to go out into the dark and role up her window. She proceeds to scream at Mark that he forgot to role up the window, and it is his job to go outside, turn on the car, and close the window. Which defense mechanism best describes Cindy's actions?

A. Denial

B. Displacement

C. Rationalization

D. Reaction formation

E. Regression

446. A 48-year-old woman presents to her primary care physician because of intermittent right lower quadrant pain. She has a history of type II diabetes mellitus, hypertension, and hypothyroidism. She takes several medicines but does not know their names, doses, or frequencies of administration. Upon further questioning, she mentions that her right knee began to hurt at the same time. Vital signs are stable. Physical examination reveals a mildly distended abdomen with no obvious tenderness. No masses are felt in the abdomen or groin. What is the likely diagnosis?

A. Femoral hernia

B. Inguinal hernia

C. Obturator hernia

D. Spigelian hernia

E. Umbilical hernia

447. A 37-year-old woman with long-standing multiple sclerosis complains of worsening spasticity. Physical examination of the heart, lungs, and abdomen are within normal limits. Results of urinalysis are normal. Which of the following is the most appropriate medication to include in her treatment regimen?

A. Azathioprine

B. Baclofen

C. Methotrexate

D. Immunoglobulin

E. Interferon B

448. A 6-month-old infant is brought to the emergency department because of a 2 day history of wheezing, a mild fever (38.5°C) and rhinorrhea. The child has no known history of allergies but there is a history of allergies in the family. Physical examination reveals a respiratory rate of 60/minute. Pulmonary auscultation reveals rhonchi and moist rales bilaterally. Chest x-ray reveals evidence of hyperaeration. What is the most appropriate treatment for this patient?

A. Ampicillin

B. Cold, humidified oxygen

C. Erythromycin

D. Inhaled albuterol

E. Inhaled corticosteroids

449. A 42-year-old man presents to his primary care physician because of severe diarrhea that started suddenly this morning. He describes the diarrhea as profuse and watery. He also complains of vomiting and abdominal pain. He states that he just returned from visiting family in India. Physical examination shows decreased capillary refill and dry mucous membranes. Mild abdominal tenderness is present. Results of laboratory studies are shown below:

WBC count	12,100/mm^3
Hemoglobin	15.2 mg/dL
Hematocrit	45.5%
Platelet count	320,000/mm^3
Na, serum	152 mEq/L
Cl, serum	92 mEq/L
K, serum	4.2 mEq/L
Bicarbonate	14 mEq/L
Urea nitrogen, serum (BUN)	24 mg/dL
Creatinine	1.4 mg/dL
Stool examination	Rice-water appearance
O1 antigen	Positive
Stool culture	Positive for *Vibrio cholerae*

What is the best treatment for this patient?

A. Hydration and metronidazole

B. Hydration and tetracycline

C. Hydration and trimethoprim

D. Hydration and amphotericin B

E. Hydration and penicillin G

450. A 23-year-old G1P0 woman presents to her primary care physician for her first prenatal visit at 10 weeks' gestation. She complains of nausea lasting most of the day and vomits two to three times per day. These symptoms have been present for the past 10 days. What is the most likely explanation for these findings?

A. Estrogen

B. Human chorionic gonadotropin

C. Progesterone

D. Testosterone

E. Thyroxine

451. A 39-year-old woman has a 2-week history of catatonic behavior, delusions, and auditory hallucinations after being fired from her job as an executive of a corporation. She appears to be in emotional turmoil and is confused. Conversations with her are notable for rapid shifts from one intense affect to another. She is emotionally labile with confused and incoherent speech. She appears to be transiently disoriented and cannot remember events from her recent past. Which of the following is the most likely diagnosis?

A. Brief reactive psychosis
B. Posttraumatic stress disorder
C. Psychotic disorder not otherwise specified
D. Schizoaffective disorder
E. Schizophrenia

452. A 22-year-old woman presents to her primary care physician with a 3-month history of diarrhea, abdominal pain, and anorexia. She has lost 12 pounds in the past 3 months. Occasionally her diarrhea is blood-tinged. She mentions that her mother has lived with chronic diarrhea and crampy abdominal pain on and off for years. Physical examination reveals mild abdominal tenderness and hemepositive stool. Spot film from a fluoroscopic small bowel examination is shown below (Figure 452). What is the most likely diagnosis?

Figure 452

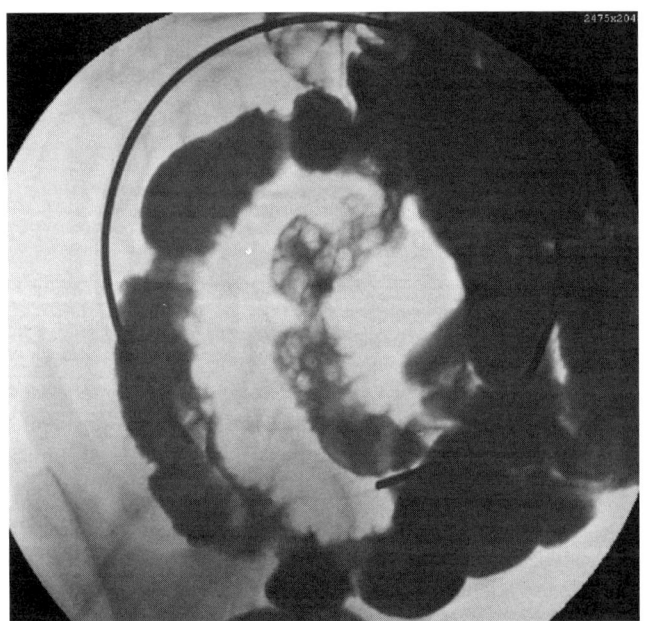

A. Crohn disease
B. Irritable bowel syndrome
C. Mesenteric adenitis with appendicitis
D. Small bowel obstruction
E. Ulcerative colitis

453. A 62-year-old woman complains of painless gross hematuria. She presents to her primary care physician for further evaluation. She has no prior history of stone disease or urologic abnormalities. She has a 40 pack/year history of smoking and still smokes occasionally. Results of her purified protein derivative (PPD) test are positive. Her prior surgical history is notable for a splenectomy for trauma and an elective cholecystectomy. Physical examination findings of the heart, lungs, and abdomen are unremarkable. Laboratory values reveal a blood urea nitrogen of 19 mg/dL and creatinine level of 0.9 mg/dL. What is the most likely diagnosis?

A. Bladder cancer
B. Bladder stone with obstruction
C. Chronic urinary retention
D. Interstitial cystitis
E. Ureteral calculus

454. A 51-year-old morbidly obese man with a history of sleep apnea presents to a new physician for a second opinion regarding management. His most significant problem is that he struggles to draw air through his nose and mouth. Review of prior records indicates that sleep studies were obtained and showed increased sleep-induced resistance. Examination of the oropharynx reveals no evidence of obstruction. What is the most effective long-term treatment for this patient?

A. Exercise program
B. Hypnosis
C. Positive airway pressure
D. Tonsilectomy and adenoidectomy
E. Tracheostomy

455. A 70-year-old man with a history of a abdominal aortic aneursym presents to the emergency department complaining of sharp back pain. While interviewing the patient, he becomes unresponsive and his blood pressure decreases to 60/20 mm Hg. What is the most appropriate intervention to take?

A. Emergent surgical intervention
B. Bolus of normal saline
C. Blood transfusion
D. Call for help, assess the airway, and initiate cardiopulmonary resuscitation
E. Perform an exploratory laparotomy in the emergency department

456. A somnolent 13-year-old female type 1 diabetic presents to the clinic with a 4-day history of a sinus infection. She reports frequent urination over the past 24 to 36 hours. The patient complains of abdominal pain, nausea, and vomiting. On physical examination, temperature is 98.1°F, abdominal examination is unremarkable, the patient appears to be breathing in a slow, deep pattern, and an acetone scent is detected on the patient's breath. Plasma glucose is 548 mg/dL with a pH of 7.28. The K level is 4.7 mEq/L and the Na level 131 mEq/L. What is the most appropriate treatment for this patient?

A. Bicarbonate administration
B. Glucose administration
C. Oral hypoglycemics
D. Potassium (K) administration
E. Rehydration/insulin administration

457. A 26-year-old woman presents to the emergency room with sudden onset of generalized, moderate severity abdominal pain. She reports that she has no medical conditions and takes no medications except for birth control pills. The patient denies the possibility of being pregnant because she is meticulous about taking her birth control pills daily and has done so for 10 years. The patient is afebrile, blood pressure is 90/50 mm Hg, and pulse is 120 beats/min. Abdominal examination reveals right upper quadrant tenderness to palpation. The skin of the right upper and lower quadrants are ecchymotic. What is the most likely diagnosis?

A. Acute appendicitis
B. Ruptured hepatic adenoma
C. Ruptured spleen
D. Tuboovarian abscess
E. Uremia

458. A 25-year-old man has been suffering from a long-standing irritation of his face. The condition is confined to the beard area, is occasionally pruritic, and appears to be aggravated by shaving. The patient has tried a number of over-the-counter remedies, including witch hazel and antiseptic soap. Examination of the skin reveals numerous firm papules and occasional pustules on the cheeks, chin, and neck. Results of laboratory studies are shown below:

Electrolytes, serum

Na, serum	144 mEq/L
Cl, serum	102 mEq/L
K, serum	4.4 mEq/L
Bicarbonate, serum	26 mEq/L
Magnesium, serum	1.9 mEq/L
Creatinine, serum	1.2 mg/dL

Leukocyte count and differential

Leukocyte count	5000/mm^3
Segmented neutrophils	55%
Bands	6%
Eosinophils	3%
Basophils	1%
Lymphocytes	24%
Monocytes	4%

Blood, plasma, serum

Alanine aminotransferase (ALT)	12 U/L
Amylase, serum	540 U/L
Aspartate aminotransferase (AST)	13 U/L
Calcium, serum	9.2 mg/dL
Glucose, serum	110 mg/dL
Hematocrit	39%
Urea nitrogen, serum (BUN)	11 mg/dL

Urinalysis

Urine pH	6.0
RBC count	2/HPF
WBC count	2/HPF
Nitrates	Negative
Bacteria	Negative

Which of the following is the most appropriate treatment for this patient?

A. Amphotericin B
B. Laser ablation
C. Retinoic acid
D. Surgical ablation
E. Watchful waiting

459. A 7-year-old boy is brought to the pediatrician in the summer for evaluation of a rash. He has no prior medical or surgical history. Physical examination reveals painful ulcers on the roof of the mouth. Vesicles are present on the palms and soles of the feet that have a linear appearance. What is the most appropriate treatment for this patient?

A. Antibiotics
B. Corticosteroids
C. Surgical excision
D. Topical mupirocin cream
E. Watchful waiting

460. A 16-year-old female high school track runner presents to her primary care physician because of a 6-month history of lower midabdominal pain that is colicky in nature. The pain radiates to her back and thighs. Pain begins within a few hours of the onset of her menstrual period and lasts for several hours to up to 2 days. She began her periods at age 13 and is not currently sexually active. Physical examination of the heart, lungs, and abdomen are unremarkable. Pelvic examination reveals an intact hymen. What is the most likely diagnosis?

A. Dysmenorrhea (primary)
B. Dysmenorrhea (secondary)
C. Endometriosis
D. Pelvic inflammatory disease
E. Psychogenic pain syndrome

461. A 9-year-old boy has a 1-year history of recurrent eye blinking, head jerking, and facial grimacing. Recently he has progressed to multiple coughing attacks as well as grunting and sniffling. During the past week he has begun to repeat his own words and the words of his family members. Teachers in school have noted that the child has difficulty concentrating and occasionally hits himself and jumps up and down. Which of the following is the most appropriate treatment for this individual?

A. Clonidine
B. Haloperidol
C. Pimozide
D. Propranalol
E. Thorazine

462. A 26-year-old female graduate student presents to the university health service for her annual physical examination. She has no medical or surgical history. She is sexually active with several partners and occasionally uses birth control. Pelvic examination is normal and the cervix appears to be healthy. Papanicolaou (Pap) smear reveals cervical intraepithelial neoplasia grade I. What is the most appropriate intervention at this point?

A. Follow-up Pap smear in 3 months
B. Follow-up Pap smear in 6 months
C. Follow-up Pap smear in 1 year
D. Referral for colposcopy
E. Referral for cone biopsy

463. A 45-year-old woman presents to the clinic with nausea, vomiting, and severe upper abdominal pain for 1 day. The pain radiates to the middle of her back. She has a history of hypertriglyceridemia, hypertension, and coronary artery disease. She has a body mass index of 31. She has mild tenderness of the epigastrium, diaphoresis, and appears pale. Her laboratory studies reveal a serum triglyceride level of 2356 mg/dL. CT scan of the abdomen is shown in Figure 463. What is the next best step in the evaluation/treatment of this problem?

Figure 463

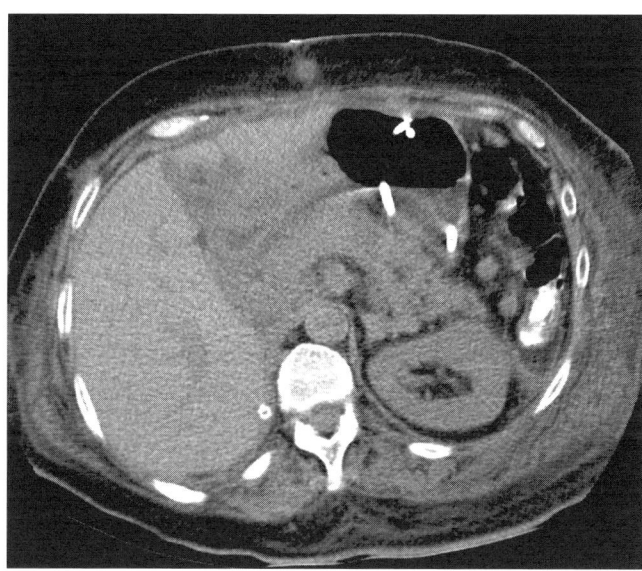

- **A.** Blood levels of serum amylase
- **B.** Maintain nothing by mouth status
- **C.** Normal saline via intravenous line
- **D.** Restriction of fluids
- **E.** Watchful waiting and pain medications

464. A 14-year-old boy presents to the emergency department with complaints of right knee pain. He states he has had the pain for 2 days, and notes no history of trauma. His mother says he had a tactile fever last night, but has not recently had any infection. Physical examination reveals normal range of motion of the joints of the lower extremities. However, tenderness is noted to light palpation of the soft tissue overlying the distal femur. Erythema and edema are also noted within this same area. Radiographs are normal. Joint aspiration reveals osteomyelitis. What is the most likely organism found on aspiration?

- **A.** *Escherichia coli*
- **B.** Group A *Streptococcus*
- **C.** Group B *Streptococcus*
- **D.** *Salmonella*
- **E.** *Staphylococcus aureus*

465. A 21-year-old woman presents for evaluation of painful breasts. She complains of bilateral, multiple breast masses that fluctuate in size and discomfort in relation to the menstrual cycle. Her pain is most intense just prior to menses. Physical examination of both breasts reveals no evidence of mass, dimpling, skin retraction, or nipple inversion. Both axillae are without palpable adenopathy. Cardiovascular examination reveals a regular rate and rhythm with no evidence of rubs, murmurs, or gallops. Pulmonary auscultation reveals good breath sounds bilaterally, and abdominal examination reveals no evidence of peritoneal signs. Which of the following is the most likely diagnosis?

- **A.** Fat necrosis
- **B.** Fibrocystic change
- **C.** Galactocele
- **D.** Infiltrating ductal cell carcinoma
- **E.** Macromastia

466. A 9-year-old girl is brought to the pediatric clinic for a routine examination. Her mother is concerned that her daughter lags behind in development as compared with other girls in school. Her daughter has not begun menses yet. Developmental history reveals that her speech and language are age appropriate. She is in the twenty-fifth percentile for height and weight. Physical examination reveals a well-developed child with no evidence of sexual hair or breast development. She has limited presence of axillary hair. Cardiovascular examination reveals a regular rate and rhythm. Which of the following is the most appropriate statement to make to the child's mother?

- **A.** "Her sexual maturation is age appropriate"
- **B.** "Her axillary hair growth is dampened"
- **C.** "Her breast development is delayed"
- **D.** "Her pubic hair development is delayed"
- **E.** "Her growth spurt should have occurred"

467. A 23-year-old man is involved in a motorcycle accident. He was not wearing a helmet. The patient arrives at the emergency department conscious in a cervical collar. Blood pressure is 130/78 mm Hg, pulse 90 beats/min, and respirations 16 breaths/min. The patient is conversant. Physical examination reveals ecchymoses around both eyes and a thin chalky white discharge dripping from his nose. What is the most appropriate next step in the management of this patient?

A. CT scan
B. Evaluation of the cervical spine
C. Immediate intubation to begin hyperventilation
D. Prophylactic antibiotics
E. Watchful waiting

468. Allison is a 21-year-old woman who was raped in high school by a football player. Her parents are getting a divorce in the near future and she often has to hear about her awful father whenever she calls her mother. Her father left town when her mother recently gave birth to a child who is mentally retarded. These events worry Allison throughout most of the day. These stresses would be listed on which DSM-IV axis?

A. Axis I
B. Axis II
C. Axis III
D. Axis IV
E. Axis V

469. A 28-year-old woman is found dead on the scene after a hit-and-run accident. She is brought to the local coroner for autopsy. No information regarding prior history is available. At autopsy it is discovered that she was pregnant with a male fetus and had a placenta weighing approximately 1000 g. Which of the following is a likely explanation for these findings.

A. Anemia
B. Hypoglycemia
C. Immune deficiency state
D. Leukemoid reaction
E. Percocet abuse

470. A 58-year-old white woman presents to her primary care physician complaining of pain, stiffness, and weakness. Her shoulders and pelvic girdle are involved, and she has difficulty arising from a chair. Symptoms have been present for 6 weeks. She also states that she has been feeling under the weather and fatigued. Social history is unremarkable. She denies chest pain or shortness of breath. Blood pressure has been controlled with propranolol and hydrochlorothiazide for 5 years. She denies experiencing nausea, vomiting, diarrhea, constipation, or abdominal discomfort. She denies having dysuria, hematuria, or vaginal discharge. She has no bowel or bladder incontinence. She has received appropriate health-care maintenance with a negative Papanicolaou

smear and mammogram within the past year and has no complaints of depression or anxiety. She also takes fexofenadine for seasonal allergies and a daily multivitamin. Physical examination reveals a temperature of 38.3°C, blood pressure of 132/86 mm Hg, pulse of 86 beats/min, and weight of 57 kg (61 kg on previous examination). Cardiac examination reveals a regular rate and rhythm without murmur. Lungs were clear to auscultation bilaterally. Abdomen was soft and nontender, with good bowel sounds. No rashes are appreciated. There is no adenopathy or thyromegaly. There is no edema or orthostatic hypotension. Musculoskeletal examination does not reveal effusion or erythema of any joints. Gait is normal. There is pain with elevation of arms above the head but no impairment in range of motion. Results of a Yerginson test are negative. No weakness is appreciated in the upper or lower extremities bilaterally. Laboratory studies are significant for normochromic, normocytic anemia and a sedimentation rate of 45 mm/h. Plain x-rays of the shoulder and pelvic girdles are without lesion or joint space narrowing. The patient is treated with prednisone 10 mg daily and shows significant improvement in all symptoms at follow-up visit. What is the most likely diagnosis?

A. Fibromyalgia
B. Osteoarthritis
C. Osteosarcoma
D. Polymyalgia rheumatica
E. Rheumatoid arthritis

471. A 60-year-old previously healthy man accompanied by his wife and one of his children comes to his primary care physician because of a recent onset of blood-streaked, thin stools. He worked as an engineer and ate a mostly high-fat, low-fiber diet throughout his life, but he was always active and maintained a reasonable body weight. He has a normal digital rectal examination, but Hemoccult testing is positive. Carcinoembryonic antigen is elevated, and barium enema reveals an apple-core filing defect in the mid-descending colon. What is the best statement to make to the patient and family?

A. "Your tests have come back suspicious"
B. "Your family should leave us alone"
C. "I'm terribly sorry, but you have colon cancer"
D. "I think you have cancer, so I want you to get a colonoscopy right away"
E. "Would your family please excuse us for a moment?"

472. A 24-year-old man is involved in a high-speed motor vehicle accident. He arrives at the emergency department with fixed, dilated pupils. He has a small scalp laceration and bilateral fractures of the lower extremity. His blood pressure is 80/60 mm Hg, with a barely perceptible pulse rate of 150 beats/min. Results of laboratory studies are shown below:

Electrolytes, serum

Na, serum	141 mEq/L
Cl, serum	99 mEq/L
K, serum	5.2 mEq/L
Bicarbonate, serum	26 mEq/L
Creatinine, serum	1.3 mg/dL

Leukocyte count and differential

Leukocyte count	8000/mm^3
Segmented neutrophils	55%

Blood, plasma, serum

Alanine aminotransferase (ALT)	15 U/L
Amylase, serum	60 U/L
Aspartate aminotransferase (AST)	12 U/L
Calcium, serum	9.2 mg/dL
Glucose, serum	100 mg/dL
Hematocrit	37%
Urea nitrogen, serum (BUN)	10 mg/dL

Urinalysis

Urine pH	5.0
RBC count	3/HPF
WBC count	1/HPF
Nitrates	Negative
Bacteria	Negative

What is the most likely explanation of these findings?

A. Diffuse axonal injury

B. Epidural hematoma

C. Lower extremity fracture

D. Subarachnoid hemorrhage

E. Subdural hematoma

473. A 24-year-old man presents to the emergency department complaining of new-onset severe headaches. He just had an episode and decided that it was time to seek medical attention even though it spontaneously resolved. He states that these headaches are located around his left eye and have been occurring for about 1 week. He states that they normally happen when he lies down to go to bed in the evening. He rates them as a 9 on a scale from 1 to 10, with 10 being the worst. He also complains of "uncontrollable crying" and a stuffy nose when the headaches occur. Physical examination reveals no focal neurologic deficits. What approach to treatment would you use at this time?

A. Initiate abortive therapy

B. Initiate prophylactic therapy

C. Initiate both abortive and prophylactic therapy

D. Only follow-up is needed at this time

E. Only reassurance is needed; no further treatment or follow-up is required

474. A 12-year-old boy is brought to the pediatric specialty clinic after referral from his primary care pediatrician. He complains of weakness and left-sided abdominal fullness. Physical examination shows a boy who appears to be his stated age. Cardiac and pulmonary evaluations are normal. Abdominal examination reveals a palpable, nontender, spleen. The remainder of the abdominal examination is without evidence of peritoneal signs. Results of laboratory studies are shown below:

Electrolytes, serum

Na, serum	137 mEq/L
Cl, serum	104 mEq/L
K, serum	3.9 mEq/L
Bicarbonate, serum	24 mEq/L
Magnesium, serum	1.7 mEq/L
Creatinine, serum	0.7 mg/dL

Leukocyte count and differential

Leukocyte count	170,000/mm^3

Blood, plasma, serum

Alanine aminotransferase (ALT)	20 U/L
Amylase, serum	40 U/L
Aspartate aminotransferase (AST)	20 U/L
Glucose, serum	100 mg/dL
Hematocrit	33%
Urea nitrogen, serum (BUN)	10 mg/dL

Urinalysis

Urine pH	6.0
RBC count	2/HPF

Blood smear analysis and staining reveals an increased number of myeloid cells with all maturational forms present. A 9–22 chromosomal translocation is suggested. Which of the following is the most appropriate treatment for this patient?

A. Busulfan and hydroxyurea

B. Doxorubicin

C. Interferon-alpha

D. Methotrexate

E. Radiation therapy to the lumbar spine

475. A 63-year-old woman presents to her primary care physician with syncope, mild angina, and occasional dyspnea on exertion. She has otherwise been in good health. She takes calcium supplements, glucosamine, and chondroitin sulfate. Physical examination reveals a woman who appears to be her stated age and is afebrile, and her vital signs are stable. There is a murmur present on cardiac auscultation. No edema or jugular venous distention is present; no carotid bruits are noted. Echocardiography reveals a hypertrophied ventricular septum inferior to the aortic valve and mild left ventricular hypertrophy. What is the most likely diagnosis?

A. Aortic regurgitation

B. Aortic stenosis

C. Mitral stenosis

D. Mitral valve prolapse

E. Mitral valve regurgitation

476. A 15-year-old girl presents to her primary care physician for a health history and physical examination required by her school to participate in softball. She has an unremarkable past medical history except for a left femur fracture 3 years ago resulting from an 8-foot fall from a tree. During the interview, the patient confides in her physician that she is sexually active and is worried after hearing about something referred to as "PID" during health class. What statement below is true concerning adolescents and pelvic inflammatory disease?

A. Adolescent females who are sexually active are more likely to acquire PID when compared with the general female population

B. Adolescent females who are sexually active tend to have a greater tendency to seek out early diagnostic screening for sexually transmitted infections when compared with the general female population

C. Adolescent females who are sexually active tend to have a greater tendency to seek out treatment services for sexually transmitted infections when compared with the general female population

D. Adolescent females who are sexually active have greater mucosal immunity to sexually transmitted infections when compared with the general female population

E. Adolescent females who are sexually active tend to have sexual relationships with partners with a lower prevalence of chlamydial and gonococcal infection when compared with the general female population

477. A 3-year-old boy with a history of multiple upper respiratory tract infections, three episodes of pneumonia, and failure to thrive is admitted to the hospital with dyspnea, tachypnea, and productive cough. The patient's pulse oximetry is 90% on room air, and chest x-ray suggests pneumonia. Results of a sweat Cl test are positive. What is the most likely organism responsible for this patient's pneumonia?

A. *Mycobacterium avium-intracellulare*

B. *Mycobacterium tuberculosis*

C. *Mycoplasma pneumoniae*

D. *Pneumocystis carinii*

E. *Pseudomonas aeruginosa*

478. An 8-year-old child is hit by a hockey puck while watching a hockey game. The puck strikes him on the left side of his head anterior to his ear. The child slowly regains consciousness and is able to speak clearly and walk unaided. While being transported to the emergency department, the patient loses consciousness again. This time he cannot be aroused. The pupils are asymmetric, the left being significantly larger than the right. Which of the following is the most likely explanation for the symptoms the patient is displaying?

A. Diffuse axonal injury

B. Epidural hematoma

C. Rupture of an arteriovenous malformation

D. Subarachnoid hemorrhage

E. Subdural hematoma

479. A 35-year-old woman presents to her primary care physician with symptoms of lethargy, headache, and confusion that seem to wax and wane over minutes. She appears pale with multiple spots of purpura on asymmetric patches throughout her body. Results of laboratory studies are shown below:

Electrolytes, serum

Na, serum	144 mEq/L
Cl, serum	99 mEq/L
K, serum	3.9 mEq/L
Bicarbonate, serum	27 mEq/L
Magnesium, serum	1.6 mEq/L
Creatinine, serum	1.1 mg/dL

Leukocyte count and differential

Leukocyte count	14,000/mm^3
Segmented neutrophils	75%
Bands	7%
Eosinophils	3%
Basophils	1%
Lymphocytes	27%
Monocytes	4%
Platelet count	100,000/mm^3
Reticulocytes	4%

Blood, plasma, serum

Alanine aminotransferase (ALT)	10 U/L
Amylase, serum	50 U/L
Aspartate aminotransferase (AST)	10 U/L
Calcium, serum	9 mg/dL
Glucose, serum	100 mg/dL
Hematocrit	27%

Urea nitrogen, serum (BUN) 10 mg/dL

Blood smear Schistocytes, helmet cells, and triangle forms

What is the most likely diagnosis?

A. Evans syndrome

B. Disseminated intravascular coagulation

C. Hemolytic uremic syndrome

D. Idiopathic thrombocytopenic purpura

E. Thrombotic thrombocytopenic purpura

480. You are a third year medical student starting your first day at the state psychiatric hospital. The resident gives you a new patient workup form and asks you to see someone in the triage room. All he tells you is that the person is psychotic. You ask the patient, "What brings you in today?" Your ability to redirect patients is not yet defined, and the patient proceeds to tell you a 20-minute story about how he got there. It starts by telling you at length about what his mother had talked to him about that morning and some background about her. He then includes his entire day at work and the thoughts he had at work. However, he does manage to include the important detail that he forgot to take his medicine and he started to have "other thoughts" and he didn't feel safe anymore. This type of speech is best described by:

A. Circumstantial

B. Echolalia

C. Echopraxia

D. Tangential

E. Thought insertion

481. A 28-year-old woman is 4 days post partum. She presents to her primary care physician complaining of insomnia, restlessness and thoughts of wanting to harm her newborn. Her brother is a paranoid schizophrenic. Which of the following is the most important statement to make to this patient's husband regarding this condition?

A. Electroconvulsive therapy is the mainstay of treatment

B. Hormonal changes are likely to contribute to this condition

C. In-patient psychiatric hospitalization with restraints is required

D. Psychodynamic conflicts regarding fatherhood are likely

E. Underlying systemic infection predisposes to this condition

482. A 48-year-old woman presents to her primary care physician with a breast that she states seems to be growing over the past few months. There is no distinctly palpable mass and no nipple discharge but the skin over approximately half of the breast is erythematous, edematous, and warm. The patient states that she was given antibiotics for a breast infection but it never healed. What is the most likely diagnosis?

A. Cystosarcoma phyllodes

B. Ductal carcinoma in situ

C. Inflammatory carcinoma

D. Lobular carcinoma in situ

E. Paget disease

483. A 35-year-old G1P1002 presents to her gynecologist for her yearly wellness examination with hopes of becoming pregnant within the year. A thorough history reveals that her menstrual cycle has increased from every 28 days to every 31 days for the past 6 months. She denies any pelvic discomfort, weight loss, or abdominal distention. Her past medical history is remarkable for identical twins delivered by cesarean section. Her family history is significant for an aunt who died of breast cancer at age 73. Physical examination is unremarkable except for bimanual examination revealing a left sided 8-cm mobile adnexal mass. What is the most appropriate next step in this patient's treatment?

A. Long-term management through use of oral contraceptives

B. Obtain CA-125 level

C. Pelvic ultrasonography

D. Surgical exploration (laparoscopy)

E. Watchful waiting and reevaluate after next menstrual cycle

484. A 47-year-old alcoholic man presents to his primary care physician because of memory impairment. He is able to remember very remote events better than more recent events. He also has impairment in short-term memory. When asked to remember the names of three items and repeat them 5 minutes later, he is only able to remember one of the items. He also has impaired memory of past presidents and well-known dates. Physical examination findings of the heart, lungs, and abdomen are within normal limits. What is the most appropriate treatment for this patient?

A. Amoxicillin

B. Electroconvulsive therapy

C. Labetalol

D. Thiamine

E. Watchful waiting

485. A 73-year-old woman presents to her primary care physician complaining of a 5-year history of waking up at nights gasping for air. She also complains of dyspnea on exertion and general fatigue. Physical examination reveals an S_3 gallop. Chest x-ray is obtained and is shown in Figure 485. What laboratory value is most likely to be elevated in this patient?

Figure 485

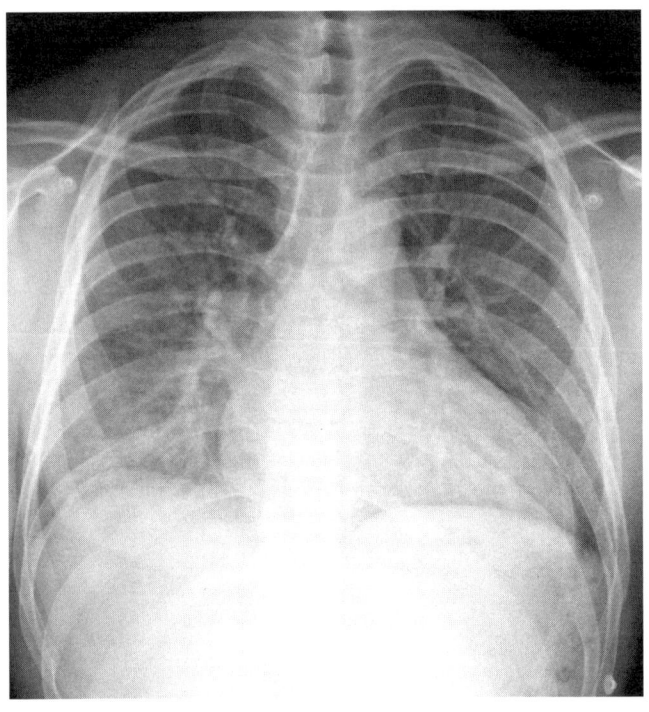

A. Brain natriuretic peptide
B. Creatinine kinase (CK)
C. Isoenzyme of creatinine kinase with muscle and brain subunits (CK-MB)
D. Myoglobin
E. Troponin I

486. A local community is preparing a suicide prevention program for area teens. Which of the following individuals would be most likely to benefit from such services?

A. 13-year-old girl, white, with no medical problems
B. 13-year-old girl, Asian-American, with sickle cell anemia
C. 14-year-old boy, white, with asthma
D. 15-year-old boy, white, with asthma
E. 15-year-old boy, black, with no medical problems

487. A 23-year-old woman presents to her family physician complaining of a painless, single lump in the medial portion of her right breast around her nipple. The patient says that the size of the lump varies throughout the month but she is unaware of its relationship to her menstrual cycle. Physical examination reveals that the lump is 3 cm in diameter, oval, and freely movable. Ultrasonography shows a circumscribed, oval, homogeneous, hypoechoic mass with a smooth, thin echogenic capsule. What is the most likely diagnosis?

A. Cystosarcoma phyllodes
B. Fibroadenoma
C. Hamartoma
D. Intraductal papilloma
E. Simple cyst

488. A 6-year-old boy is brought to the emergency department because of a 10-day history of vomiting and diarrhea. The child has vomited three to five times per day and has had diarrhea bouts four times per day. The parents have expressed a concern that their child is dehydrated. Which of the following is the earliest manifestation of dehydration?

A. Dry mucous membranes
B. Hyperpnea
C. Hypotension
D. Tachycardia
E. Urine output cessation

489. A 16-year-old girl comes to the emergency department desiring birth control. While obtaining the history you find that she is not dating anyone and that her mother will not allow her to socialize outside of her house. She says that her mother keeps her from running away to have sex with boys at her school. She says that she has had five or six partners in the past year and that she needs contraception "in case her mother can't prevent her." When the girl's mother arrives, she pulls you aside to tell you that boys are pursuing her daughter and that despite all of her attempts to prevent it, her daughter is sleeping with them several times a week. The girl cannot name any of her partners. Results of her physical examination is normal, and her pelvic examination reveals an intact hymen. Laboratory studies are negative for beta human chorionic gonadotropin, *Chlamydia*, and gonorrhea. What is the best course of action?

A. Admit mother for psychiatric evaluation and alert child protective services for the daughter
B. Deny daughter oral contraceptives since she is not sexually active
C. Obtain a rape kit to look for signs of abuse
D. Obtain separate psychiatric consults of mother and daughter
E. Provide the girl with oral contraceptives and discharge from the emergency department

490. A 20-year-old girl who delivered via cesarean section 5 days ago develops abdominal pain and a persistent temperature of 39.2°C. Broad-spectrum antibiotic coverage is initiated, but her fever persists over the next 3 days. The patient is then placed on intravenous heparin, with resolution of fever and pain within 48 hours. What is the most likely diagnosis?

A. Acute endometritis
B. Chorioamnionitis
C. Pelvic abscess
D. Pelvic inflammatory disease
E. Septic pelvic thrombophlebitis

491. A 19-year-old male immigrant from South America presents to the ambulatory care clinic with sudden onset of severe headache, tachycardia, high fever, generalized aches and pains, nausea, and vomiting. After a short remission of 1 to 2 days he develops bradycardia, hypotension, and jaundice. He also has profuse coffee-ground emesis. Physical examination reveals a temperature of 39.2°C, blood pressure of 90/60 mm Hg, icteric sclera, and hepatomegaly. Results of laboratory studies are shown below:

WBC count	4700/mm³
Hematocrit	45.1%
Platelet count	310,000/mm³
Na	140 mEq/L
Cl	102 mEq/L
K	4.0 mEq/L
Bicarbonate	25 mEq/L
Urinalysis	Increased albumin, positive for blood

What is the most likely diagnosis?

A. Chagas disease
B. Cryptosporidiosis
C. Echinococcosis
D. Lymphatic filariasis
E. Yellow fever

492. A 60-year-old obese postmenopausal woman with a history of hypertension and diabetes mellitus presents to her primary care physician with the complaint of vaginal bleeding. Results of pelvic examination are normal. After endometrial biopsy, she is diagnosed with stage I endometrial cancer. She undergoes a total abdominal hysterectomy and bilateral salpingo-oophorectomy and has postoperative radiation treatment. What is the most appropriate follow-up regimen?

A. Follow-up every 3 months for a year, then every 6 months for 2 years, then every year
B. Follow-up every 3 months for 2 years, then every 6 months for 3 years, then every year
C. Follow-up every 6 months indefinitely and treat with high-dose progestins
D. Follow-up every 6 months indefinitely and treat with estrogen replacement therapy
E. Follow-up is not necessary after definitive therapy

493. A 7-year-old boy is brought to the emergency department for evaluation of a dog bite that occurred 24 hours ago. He has no prior medical or surgical history. He has no known drug allergies. Vital signs are stable. The child is comfortable. Physical examination of the bite site on the left leg reveals pain, swelling, and a watery-gray odorous discharge. Gram stain of the discharge reveals small, motile gram-negative rods. What is the most appropriate treatment for this patient?

A. Incision, drainage, and débridement
B. Penicillin (intravenous), hospital admission
C. Penicillin (oral), outpatient follow-up
D. Tetracycline (oral), outpatient follow-up
E. Watchful waiting

494. A 66-year-old woman presents to her primary care physician with a 1-month history of poor sleep. She states that she has been waking up much earlier than usual, and has been feeling more tired than usual. She has lost 10 pounds in the past month. She states that she has been feeling down since her husband died of a stroke 6 weeks ago. She has not been participating in bingo or church activities since his death. What is the most likely diagnosis?

A. Bipolar disorder
B. Dysthymic disorder
C. Major depressive disorder
D. Normal bereavement
E. Schizoaffective disorder

495. A 22-year-old female college student presents to the university health service for her annual physical examination and to obtain a prescription for birth control pills. She has a history of seasonal allergic rhinitis. She is sexually active with several partners and occasionally uses birth control. Pelvic examination is normal and the cervix appears to be healthy. Papanicolaou (Pap) smear reveals class II *Trichomonas* present. What is the most appropriate intervention for this patient?

A. Metronidazole, repeat Pap smear in 2 weeks
B. Metronidazole, repeat Pap smear in 6 months
C. Metronidazole, repeat Pap smear in 1 year
D. Referral for colposcopy
E. Referral for cone biopsy

The response options for items 496–499 are the same. You will be required to select one answer for each item in the set.

A. Aortic regurgitation
B. Aortic stenosis
C. Mitral regurgitation
D. Mitral stenosis
E. Tricuspid regurgitation

For each patient with cardiac arrhythmia, select the most appropriate diagnosis.

496. A 65-year-old man presents to his primary care physician with exertional dyspnea and fatigue, palpitations, and 2+ ankle edema. Jugular venous pressure is elevated and there is evidence of hepatomegaly. There is a palpable right-sided thrill and a pansystolic murmur at the left substernal border. ECG findings demonstrate right atrial enlargement with possible right ventricular enlargement.

497. A 65-year-old man presents to his primary care physician with significant dyspnea on exertion. He complains of chronic cough and occasional hemoptysis. He has a history of atrial fibrillation. Crackles are auscultated diffusely over both lungs. There is a loud first heart sound and a diastolic rumble. Chest x-ray shows enlargement of the cardiac silhouette, pulmonary congestion, double density of the right heart border, and loss of retrosternal space.

498. A 65-year-old man presents to his primary care physician with chest pain and lightheadedness with exertion. Physical examination reveals a crescendo-decrescendo systolic murmur and pulsus tardus et parvus. An S_4 is audible, S_2 is muffled. ECG demonstrates evidence of left ventricular hypertrophy. Chest x-ray shows enlargement of the cardiac silhouette.

499. A 65-year-old man presents to his primary care physician with chest pain, orthopnea, and occasional lightheadedness. Physical examination reveals a high-pitched, diastolic decrescendo murmur and widened pulse pressure. An apical diastolic rumble is appreciated, as is a pistol shot at the femoral artery. There is a sharp rapid carotid upstroke. ECG findings are nonspecific. Chest x-ray shows enlargement of the cardiac silhouette with mildly widened mediastinum.

500. A 60-year-old man with a history of hemorrhoidectomy at age 50 presents to the primary care clinic complaining of blood in the stool for 4 to 5 days. Family history is negative for cancers. He is currently taking baby aspirin once a day. Temperature is 98.1°F, blood pressure 138/86 mm Hg, respirations 14 breaths/min, and heart rate 80 beats/min. Abdominal examination reveals no evidence of peritoneal signs. Rectal examination reveals bright red blood on the glove with normal sphincter tone. What is the next most appropriate step in the management of this patient?

A. Abdominal CT scan
B. Colonoscopy (right sided)
C. Flexible sigmoidoscopy
D. Radiographic evaluation of the sigmoid colon and rectum (barium enema)
E. Watchful waiting—send the patient home with fecal occult blood test cards and follow up in 1 week

501. A 33-year-old woman presents to her gynecologist for a prenatal examination. She is 12 weeks pregnant with her first child. She complains of a 2-week history of constipation. She has had only one bowel movement during the past week. Physical examination findings of the heart, lungs, and abdomen are unremarkable. What is the most appropriate treatment for this patient?

A. Begin oral iron therapy
B. Begin oral iron therapy and intramuscular iron injections
C. Limit fluid intake
D. Psyllium supplementation
E. Watchful waiting

502. A 5-year-old boy has an 8-month history of passing feces in inappropriate places such as in his clothing and onto the floor. This behavior occurs approximately twice a month and appears to be unintentional. The child was continent of stools for approximately 1 year prior to these events. He is in the thirty-fifth percentile for height, weight, and head circumference. Physical examination reveals a well-developed child. Cardiovascular examination reveals a regular rate and rhythm. Pulmonary auscultation reveals no evidence of rales, rhonchi, or wheezes. Gastrointestinal examination reveals normoactive bowel sounds. Anorectal examination reveals good sphincter tone with soft stool in the vault. Which of the following is the most likely associated condition to be seen in this individual?

A. Anal fissure
B. Anal fistulas
C. Functional enuresis
D. Hemorrhoids
E. Hirschsprung disease

503. A 42-year-old male physician presents to his primary care physician because of a 3-month history of depressed mood. He states that he feels stressed at work. He has recently taken a new position in a practice where he is on call every other night and every third weekend. His office schedule is busy, and he sees as many as 50 patients per day. He is also having difficulty with one of his partners, who appears to be having an affair with one of the office staff members. He has no prior medical, surgical, or psychiatric history. He takes no medications. Physical examination findings of the neck, heart, lungs, and abdomen are within normal limits. What is the most likely diagnosis?

A. Adjustment disorder
B. Depression

C. Dysthymia

D. Organic affective disorder

E. Thyroid dysfunction

504. A 21-year-old man has a 10-hour history of right and left lower quadrant pain, nausea, anorexia, and fever to 100.5°F. Physical examination reveals a young man who is lying in a fetal position on the examination table. He has a regular rate and rhythm. Pulmonary auscultation reveals good breath sounds bilaterally. Gastrointestinal examination reveals normoactive bowel sounds with right lower quadrant tenderness to deep palpation and localized guarding and rebound tenderness. Rectal examination reveals tenderness to deep pressure on the right side. Laboratory findings are presented below:

Electrolytes, serum

Na, serum	143 mEq/L
Cl, serum	100 mEq/L
K, serum	3.3 mEq/L
Bicarbonate, serum	24 mEq/L
Creatinine, serum	1.0 mg/dL

Leukocyte count and differential

Leukocyte count	12,000/mm³
Segmented neutrophils	72%
Bands	6%
Eosinophils	4%
Basophils	2%
Lymphocytes	28%
Monocytes	4%

Blood, plasma, serum

Alanine aminotransferase (ALT)	15 U/L
Amylase, serum	45 U/L
Aspartate aminotransferase (AST)	10 U/L
Calcium, serum	9 mg/dL
Glucose, serum	100 mg/dL

Urinalysis

Urine pH	6.0
RBC count	2/HPF
WBC count	2/HPF
Nitrates	Negative
Bacteria	Negative

Which of the following conditions should receive the lowest priority in terms of workup of this patient?

A. Appendicitis

B. Gastroenteritis

C. Mesenteric adenitis

D. Regional enteritis (Crohn disease)

E. Testicular torsion

505. A 19-year-old man without prior medical or surgical history suffers a C2 fracture while diving into a swimming pool that was only partially filled with water. His acute care hospitalization has been completed and he is now transferred for rehabilitation therapy. Which of the following is an expected functional outcome for this patient?

A. Independent bladder function

B. Independent bowel function

C. Independent dressing

D. Independent feeding

E. Mechanical ventilation with assisted cough

506. A 59-year-old woman with a history of recurrent, superficial, multifocal bladder cancer presents to her physician for further evaluation. At last transurethral resection, she had four small superficial tumors. She currently works as a physician's assistant and wants to continue working during treatment. Physical examination findings of the heart, lungs, and abdomen are unremarkable. What is the most appropriate treatment for this patient?

A. Bacillus Calmette-Guérin (BCG; full dose)

B. Bacillus Calmette-Guérin (reduced dose)

C. Mitomycin C

D. Radical cystectomy

E. Watchful waiting

507. A 60-year-old man who presents to his primary care physician with a fear of dying after the recent loss of his wife 6 months ago reports new onset of weight loss, dry mouth, and hip pain. Review of systems is positive for nausea and vomiting for a few months, with no blood seen. He takes no medications. He reports that he has been taking four to six megavitamins each day because he feels that they will help him live longer the more he takes. Physical examination reveals cracked, dry oral mucosa and hepatomegaly. What is the most likely explanation for these findings?

A. Vitamin A toxicity

B. Vitamin B_1 toxicity

C. Vitamin B_2 toxicity

D. Vitamin B_3 toxicity

E. Vitamin C toxicity

F. Vitamin K toxicity

508. A 48-year-old woman presents to the emergency department with sudden onset of pain in her left groin. She works for a postal service and has to constantly load heavier packages into the delivery truck. Physical examination reveals the patient has a temperature of 101.7°F and has a heart rate of 120 beats/min. Lungs are clear to auscultation, and no murmurs, rubs, or gallops are appreciated. The abdomen is distended, tympanic to percussion, and diffusely tender to palpation. A nonreducible painful mass is felt in her left groin, accompanied by some skin discoloration in the area. What is the next most appropriate management course for this patient?

A. Administer oral antibiotics

B. Administer intravenous antibiotics

C. Emergent surgical repair

D. Fine-needle aspiration of the mass

E. Inguinal lymph node biopsy

509. A 42-year-old man with a history of insulin-dependent diabetes mellitus presents to the emergency department after arising in the morning. He complains that he is unable to perceive light in his left eye. There is no history of trauma or foreign body. He is otherwise healthy. Funduscopic examination of the left eye reveals disc neovascularization. Results of laboratory studies are shown below:

Blood, plasma, serum

Alanine aminotransferase (ALT)	10 U/L
Amylase, serum	45 U/L
Aspartate aminotransferase (AST)	10 U/L
Calcium, serum	9.1 mg/dL
Glucose, serum	300 mg/dL
Hematocrit	37%
Urea nitrogen, serum (BUN)	12 mg/dL

Urinalysis

Urine pH	6.5
RBC count	0–2/HPF
WBC count	0–2/HPF
Nitrates	Negative
Bacteria	Negative

Which of the following is the most likely explanation?

A. Acute narrow angle glaucoma

B. Acute retinal detachment

C. Dense intraocular hemorrhage from unrecognized neovascularization

D. Infarction of the optic nerve

E. Macular degeneration

510. A 13-year-old boy presents to his primary care physician for evaluation of knee pain. The patient states that he has been experiencing pain for 3 months that is not relieved by oral analgesics. Physical examination reveals exquisite tenderness and swelling of the left knee joint with pain localized to the distal femur. Some limitation of motion is detected. An x-ray reveals a preemptive lesion in the metaphysis that does not cross the epiphysis. New periosteal bone formation is also appreciated at the diaphyseal end of the lesion. Results of laboratory studies are shown below:

Electrolytes, serum

Na, serum	139 mEq/L
Cl, serum	101 mEq/L
K, serum	4.1 mEq/L
Bicarbonate, serum	24 mEq/L
Creatinine, serum	0.8 mg/dL

Leukocyte count and differential

Leukocyte count	5000/mm^3
Segmented neutrophils	55%
Bands	6%
Eosinophils	2%
Basophils	2%
Lymphocytes	24%
Monocytes	4%

Blood, plasma, serum

Alanine aminotransferase (ALT)	14 U/L
Aspartate aminotransferase (AST)	10 U/L
Calcium, serum	9 mg/dL
Glucose, serum	110 mg/dL
Hematocrit	38%
Urea nitrogen, serum (BUN)	10 mg/dL

Urinalysis

Urine pH	7.0
RBC count	1/HPF
WBC count	1/HPF
Nitrates	Negative
Bacteria	Negative

What is the most likely diagnosis?

A. Juvenile rheumatoid arthritis
B. Meniscal tear
C. Osgood-Schlatter disease
D. Osteogenic sarcoma
E. Stress fracture of tibial plateau

511. A prospective study is comparing two chemotherapeutic agents for the treatment of colon cancer. Cases were selected from one group of patients who had yearly Hemoccult card readings for at least 5 years before their diagnosis of cancer, and another group of patients who never had Hemoccult testing. Selection of cases from these groups may result in what type of bias?

A. Confounding
B. Interviewer bias
C. Lead time bias
D. Recall bias
E. Unknown bias

512. An obese 26-year-old white female pediatric nurse who is well known to your primary care practice presents with increasing generalized body aches and fatigue that worsens when stressed and is somewhat relieved by exercise. Symptoms are not relieved with acetaminophen or ibuprofen. She complains of weakness but denies having joint swelling. There is no morning stiffness. She denies having upper respiratory infection symptoms or recent trauma. She denies having vision changes, seizure history, or syncopal episodes. She denies having chest pain, shortness of breath, orthopnea, or paroxysmal nocturnal dyspnea. She denies having dysuria, hematuria, or vaginal discharge. She denies having nausea, vomiting, hematochezia, or hemoptysis. You are currently treating her for depression and irritable bowel syndrome. She states that she feels depressed but that her depression has improved significantly with sertraline. She states that she usually feels tired upon waking, although she sleeps 8 to 10 hours at night. Physical examination reveals that she is afebrile, with blood pressure of 120/82 mm Hg, pulse of 82 beats/min, height of 64 inches and weight of 98 kg. Cranial nerves II through XII are grossly intact. Skin is without rash or lesion. Physical examination findings of heart and lungs are normal, and there are no carotid bruits or jugular venous distention. Musculoskeletal examination is negative for impaired range of motion, joint swelling, or erythema. Strength is within normal limits in all four extremities. Deep tendon reflex is 2+ in triceps, biceps, and patellar tendons. Toes are downward pointing on examination. Gait is normal. Pain is reproducible with palpation of 12 standard trigger points. Laboratory studies reveal a normal erythrocyte sedimentation rate and a normal hemoglobin. Electrolytes are also within normal limits. ECG reveals normal sinus rhythm. What is the most appropriate initial therapy for this patient?

A. Acetaminophen
B. Alprazolam
C. Prednisone
D. Rofecoxib
E. Supportive therapy including rest and physical therapy

513. A 20-year-old woman with a history of substance abuse has delivered a child whose weight is less than the tenth percentile. Other findings include microcephaly, short palpebral fissures, flat midface, and hypoplastic philtrum. On auscultation of the heart, a systolic ejection murmur near the upper left sternal border with a fixed, split S_2 is appreciated. These findings are most associated with which of the following substances?

A. Alcohol

B. Cocaine

C. Marijuana

D. Opioids

E. Tobacco

514. A 39-year-old morbidly obese woman presents to her primary care physician with complaints of fever and chills. She has no pain, no cough, no nausea/vomiting/diarrhea, no dysuria, and no vaginal discharge. Physical examination reveals a morbidly obese, nondiaphoretic woman with a temperature of 38.8°C. She has an area of erythema over her left proximal anterior thigh measuring $3 \times 8\,cm$. The area is warm to the touch, nontender, numb, and flat, and crepitus is appreciated while palpating the region. The patient does not know how long the redness and numbness have been present. What is the most likely diagnosis?

A. Cellulitis

B. Factitious disorder

C. Nectrotizing fasciitis

D. Shingles

E. Superficial candidiasis

515. A 2-day-old infant has yet to pass meconium. She begins to vomit a bilious mixture, and a distended abdomen is suggestive of dilated loops of bowel. Abdominal x-rays reveal multiple dilated loops of bowel. Which of the following is the next most appropriate step in management?

A. Administer hypertonic solution orally

B. Administer simethicone suppositories

C. Nasogastric tube to suction and intravenous fluids before and during a gastrograffin enema

D. Receive nothing by mouth until meconium passes

E. Watchful waiting

516. A 16-year-old boy presents to his pediatrician for his annual evaluation. The patient complains of decreased energy for the past few months. He also has noted an 11-pound weight loss during the past 2 months. He denies any recent infections, but states he has felt feverish lately. Physical examination reveals a nontender, palpable 2-cm cervical lymph node. CBC reveals a WBC count of 24,000/mm³ with 7% eosinophils. Tissue biopsy reveals numerous Reed-Sternberg cells. What is the most appropriate next step in the treatment of this patient?

A. Bone marrow biopsy

B. Chest radiograph and CT scan of retroperitoneum

C. Multiagent chemotherapy

D. Radiotherapy

E. Radiation and chemotherapy

517. A 25-year-old woman complains of vulvar itching and vaginal discharge for 2 weeks. The discharge has a cottage cheese appearance and is without odor. Anorectal examination reveals small internal hemorrhoids that prolapse with Valsalva maneuver. Vaginal speculum examination reveals vulvar edema and erythema with white, curdlike connections of exudate on saline mount. Which of the following is the most appropriate treatment?

A. Acyclovir

B. Erythromycin

C. Metronidazole

D. Miconazole

E. Tetracycline

518. A patient presents with a clinical picture characteristic for an ischemic stroke. Hemorrhage was ruled out with the appropriate brain imaging studies. The neurologist decides that this patient is an appropriate candidate for tissue plasminogen activator therapy (TPA). What is the time window for intravenous TPA therapy from the onset of clinical signs of ischemic stroke?

A. 30 minutes

B. 60 minutes

C. 90 minutes

D. 180 minutes

E. 360 minutes

519. A 30-year-old woman is seen on the floor 2 days after undergoing a thyroidectomy to remove a cancerous lesion. Pathology report is pending. On morning rounds, you notice that her voice continues to sound hoarse. Which of the following structures was most likely injured during the operation?

A. Accessory laryngeal nerve

B. Internal laryngeal nerve

C. Recurrent laryngeal nerve

D. Superficial branch of the laryngeal nerve

E. Superior thyroid nerve

520. A 31-year-old man who is trying out for an adult semi-professional basketball team presents to his primary care physician for a physical examination. He has no prior medical or surgical history. Cardiac auscultation reveals an S_4 heart sound, and a harsh systolic murmur heard best at the left sternal border. Echocardiography reveals left ventricular hypertrophy with asymmetric septal hypertrophy. Which of the following is the most appropriate treatment?

A. Digitalis

B. Furosemide

C. Valvoplasty

D. Verapamil

E. Watchful waiting

521. A 2-month-old boy is brought to his pediatrician for evaluation. He has a history of poor feeding and constipation for the past 6 weeks. Physical examination of the heart reveals a systolic ejection murmur. Pulmonary and gastrointestinal examinations are unremarkable. Testicles are descended bilaterally. The penis is uncircumcised. Results of laboratory studies are shown below:

Blood, plasma, serum

Calcium, serum	12.1 mg/dL
Glucose, serum	111 mg/dL
Hematocrit	31%
Urea nitrogen, serum (BUN)	7 mg/dL

What is the most appropriate treatment for this condition?

A. Calcitonin
B. Furosemide
C. Hydrocortisone
D. Low calcium diet
E. Rehydration with 0.9% saline

522. A 21-year-old man presents to the emergency department with right lower quadrant pain for 2 hours. While on first base in his collegiate baseball game he experienced periumbilical discomfort. After attempting to steal home, he had the sudden onset of severe right lower quadrant pain. He is febrile but in obvious discomfort. There is no rebound tenderness, and the psoas sign is negative. Results of laboratory studies include a WBC count of 21,000/mm³, hemoglobin of 14 mg/dL, hematocrit of 48%, and platelet count 300,000/mm³. A CT scan of the abdomen is ordered and is show below (Figure 522). What is the treatment of choice in this patient?

Figure 522

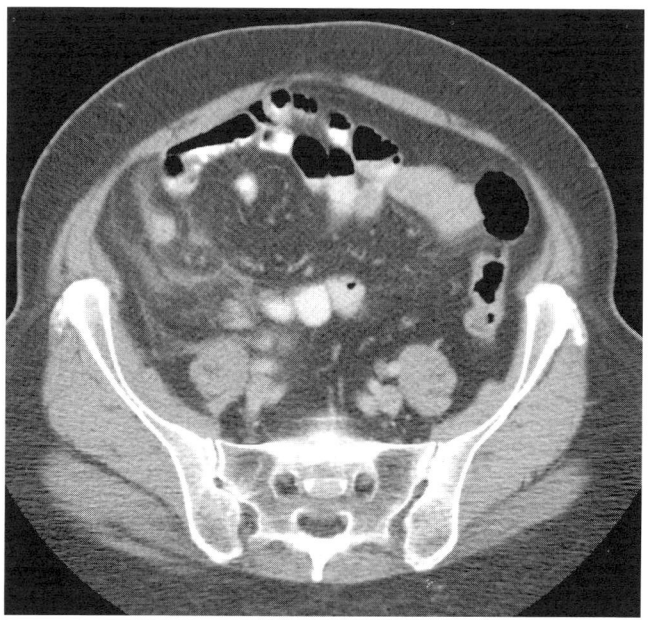

A. Appendectomy
B. Intravenous fluids
C. Morphine
D. Nothing by mouth
E. Vancomycin

523. A 53-year-old man complains of recurrent headaches. He describes the pain as stabbing and lasting approximately 30 seconds. The distribution of pain is over his right cheek and lower jaw. He often notes a focal point of pain in his gums that limits his ability to eat. Auscultation reveals no bruits bilaterally. The remainder of the physical examination findings are within normal limits. Laboratory studies obtained are shown below:

Electrolytes, serum

Na, serum	141 mEq/L
Cl, serum	101 mEq/L
K, serum	3.9 mEq/L
Bicarbonate, serum	27 mEq/L
Magnesium, serum	1.9 mEq/L
Creatinine, serum	1.1 mg/dL

Leukocyte count and differential

Leukocyte count	8000/mm³
Segmented neutrophils	65%

Which of the following is the most likely diagnosis?

A. Classic headache (migraine type)
B. Common migraine
C. Cluster headache
D. Hypertension
E. Trigeminal neuralgia

524. A 17-year-old unmarried student gives birth to a newborn at term by vaginal delivery. She did not present for prenatal care because of fear of her parents finding out about her pregnancy. At birth, the newborn has Apgar scores of 4 and 7 at 1 and 5 minutes, respectively. Further examination of the umbilical cord reveals the presence of a single umbilical artery. Which of the following conditions could manifest in this newborn?

A. Rectal fistula
B. Tracheoesophageal fistula
C. Ureteral fistula
D. Urethral fistula
E. Vaginal fistula

525. A 1-month-old infant has dyspnea, tachypnea, poor feeding, and diaphoresis. Maternal prenatal history reveals a reactive rapid plasma reagin test. Auscultation reveals a pansystolic murmur with a thrill. Pulmonary auscultation reveals no evidence of rhonchi or rales, but scattered bilateral wheezes were audible. Gastrointestinal evaluation reveals normoactive bowel sounds with absence of peritoneal signs. ECG reveals left atrial enlargement and left ventricular hypertrophy. Which of the following is the most likely diagnosis?

- **A.** Dextrocardia
- **B.** Ectopia cordis
- **C.** Situs inversus
- **D.** Transposition of the great arteries
- **E.** Ventricular septal defect

526. A third year medical student on the obstetrics and gynecology rotation is preparing to vaginally deliver her first life birth. Which of the following anatomic landmarks determines the necessary diameter for the fetal head during delivery?

- **A.** Ischial tuberosity and inferior surface of the pubis
- **B.** Ischial tuberosity and superior surface of the pubis
- **C.** Sacral promontory and closest part of the pubis
- **D.** Sacral promontory and inferior surface of the pubis
- **E.** Sacral promontory and superior surface of the pubis

527. A 39-year-old woman has recently discovered a solitary thyroid nodule. She denies having any tenderness or pain on palpation. She also denies having hoarseness, dysphagia, or any recent fevers. Family history is negative for thyroid disease or cancer. Physical examination reveals a small nodule on the right inferior side of the gland. No other neck masses were palpated. The remaining examination findings were normal. Fine-needle aspiration results were indeterminate, but suspicious. Serum thyroid-stimulating hormone was low. What is the next step in the treatment of this patient?

- **A.** Obtain a thyroid scan
- **B.** Obtain a thyroid ultrasound
- **C.** Recommend follow-up in 6 months for repeat evaluation on the nodule
- **D.** Repeat the fine-needle aspiration
- **E.** Surgical resection

528. A new patient enters the office of her primary care physician because she is interested in antidepressant medications. She feels that she has been depressed for quite some time. You manage to work in most of the mental status examination during the first 15 minutes of the conversation. After she gives you an answer to "What would you do if you smelled smoke in a movie theater?" she asks you what that tells you about her. You tell her that the question gives you information about the patient's:

- **A.** Accuracy
- **B.** Insight
- **C.** Judgment
- **D.** Reliability
- **E.** Thought process

529. A 40-year-old woman presents to her primary care physician for follow-up after undergoing a total thyroidectomy for papillary carcinoma. The patient reports irritability and muscle cramps. Physical examination reveals that the patient exhibits spasms of her hands when her blood pressure is taken and facial muscle contraction when tapping over the facial nerve. What is the most appropriate therapy for this patient?

- **A.** Furosemide
- **B.** Hydrochlorothiazide
- **C.** Phenytoin
- **D.** Phosphate supplementation
- **E.** Rapid infusion of normal saline

530. A 32-year-old man presents to his primary care physician with a 1-day history of inflammation and pain in his right knee. He underwent cholecystectomy 2 weeks ago. There is no family history of rheumatoid arthritis or systemic lupus erythematosus. He has a temperature of 99.7°F, blood pressure of 132/84 mm Hg, and pulse of 78 beats/min. The patient's right knee is warm, red, and inflamed. The rest of the musculoskeletal examination findings are normal. The heart is regular in rate and rhythm, and the results of lung examination are unremarkable. Abdominal examination findings are also unremarkable, except for some tenderness around his surgical scar. Laboratory values are as follows:

WBC count	14,000/mm^3
Erythrocyte sedimentation rate	41 mm/h
Uric acid, serum	9.1 mg/dL
Na, serum	142 mEq/L
K, serum	4.1 mg/dL
Cl, serum	102 mmol/L
Synovial fluid aspirate	Calcium pyrophosphate dihydrate crystals

What is the most likely diagnosis?

- **A.** Gout
- **B.** Osteoarthritis
- **C.** Pseudogout
- **D.** Rheumatoid arthritis
- **E.** Trauma

531. A 79-year-old man with malignant lymphoma and metastatic adenocarcinoma of the prostate is receiving end of life care in a hospice. He has refused to eat food for the past 3 days. The patient's spouse believes that her husband is "giving up" and urges the physician to intervene. Which of the following is the most appropriate course of action for the physician to take?

A. Administer an appetite stimulant
B. Forced feeding
C. Parenteral nutrition
D. Tube feeding
E. No intervention

The response options for items 532–534 are the same. You will be required to select one answer for each item in the set.

A. Behçet syndrome
B. Bowenoid papulosis
C. Bullous pemphigoid
D. Contact dermatitis
E. Crohn disease
F. Herpes simplex
G. Lichen sclerosus
H. Perineal pseudoverrucous papules
I. Pinworms
J. Psoriasis

For each child with an anogenital skin lesion, select the most likely diagnosis.

532. A 5-year-old boy is brought to his pediatrician for evaluation of an anogenital rash and intermittent genital pain. He has no prior medical or surgical history. Physical examination findings of the heart, lungs, and abdomen are within normal limits. The anogenital area has bilateral edema and erythema. Groups of vesicles and blisters are noted. He has similar lesions on his face, neck, palms, and soles. Skin biopsy reveals dermal inflammation.

533. A 9-year-old boy with a long history of intermittent right lower quadrant pain and diarrhea presents to his pediatrician complaining of rectal pain with defecation. Cardiac examination reveals a regular rate and rhythm. Pulmonary auscultation reveals good breath sounds bilaterally. Anogenital examination reveals marked anal dilation. A small perirectal fistula is noted in the left lateral quadrant. A small skin tag is noted in the right inferior quadrant. There is no evidence of internal or external hemorrhoids.

534. A 12-year-old girl with a history of uveitis and recurrent oral ulcers presents to her pediatrician for evaluation of vulvar pain and skin rash. Physical examination reveals multiple small oral aphthous ulcers. Examination findings of the heart, lung, and abdomen are within normal limits. The vulva has several discrete areas of ulceration, with the largest measuring 0.5 × 0.5 cm. The ulcers appear to be deep but are painless to palpation.

535. A 51-year-old man comes into the ambulatory care clinic complaining of epigastric pain that has been present for the past 4 months. He describes the pain as dull, achy, constant, and worsened by eating. He denies smoking or aspirin use but has a history of alcoholism. He currently denies alcohol use. Physical examination reveals that he is a thin, frail man with a blood pressure of 140/90 mm Hg, pulse of 70 beats/min, and respirations of 16 breaths/min. Abdominal examination is significant for midepigastric tenderness on deep palpation. No masses or organomegaly are noted. Stool is guaiac positive. What is the next most appropriate step in the diagnosis/evaluation of this patient?

A. Cimetidine prescription and follow-up in 3 months
B. Esophagogastric duodenoscopy
C. Colonoscopy
D. Surgical exploration
E. Testing for *Helicobacter pylori*

536. A 45-year-old woman with a history significant for poorly controlled diabetes mellitus presents to her primary care physicians with a 4-month history of vaginal pruritus, dyspareunia, and thick, white discharge. She states that symptoms are worse several days after menstruation ends. She had been seen previously 2 months ago with similar complaints, a complete and thorough workup was performed, and she was placed on an appropriate course of miconazole. Physical examination demonstrates vulvar erythema and edema as well as a small amount of white curdy vaginal discharge. Wet-mount preparation with KOH of the discharge is performed, and microscopic examination reveals branching hyphae and spores and a vaginal pH of 4.5. What is the most likely cause of failure of this patient's previous medical management?

A. Development of drug-resistant *Candida albicans*
B. Elevated blood glucose levels secondary to poorly controlled diabetes
C. Incorrect diagnosis of infecting organism
D. Incorrect choice of pharmacologic agent
E. Patient's noncompliance with use of miconazole

537. A 9-year-old girl is walking her dog when the dog breaks loose and is hit by a bicycle. Following the accident, the dog can only walk with a bad limp. Her father brings her to the pediatric clinic for evaluation. For several days, the little girl walks with a limp, too, and says her entire lower leg is numb. What is the most likely diagnosis?

A. Conversion disorder
B. Factitious disorder
C. Hypochondriasis
D. Normal guilt reaction
E. Somatization disorder

538. A 24-year-old woman presents to her primary care physician complaining of dysuria, urinary frequency, pelvic pain, and vaginal discharge. Temperature is 37.2°C, blood pressure 114/78 mm Hg, pulse 80 beats/min, and respiratory rate 14 breaths/min. Pelvic examination reveals vulvar edema and erythema. The vaginal walls are inflamed and vaginal discharge is present. Punctate hemorrhages are present on the cervix. What is the most likely diagnosis?

A. Bacterial vaginosis
B. Candidiasis
C. *Chlamydia*
D. Gonorrhea
E. Herpes simplex virus
F. Human immunodeficiency virus
G. Human papilloma virus
H. Syphilis
I. *Trichomonas*

539. A 71-year-old man with a history of hypertension has been doing well after aortic aneurysm resection and tube graft 2 years ago. He has been followed by his primary care physician for routine examinations and blood tests. His most recent examination, 1 month ago, yielded the following results:

History	No significant interval change
Interval physical examination	
Blood pressure	180/90 mm Hg
Pulse	92 beats/min
Respirations	16 breaths/min
Coronary	Regular rate and rhythm
Chest	Clear bilaterally
Abdomen	Soft, nontender, nondistended
Extremities	No cyanosis or clubbing
Rectal examination	No hemorrhoids
Prostate	Normal size, guaiac negative

During the past month the man has been in good health with no new symptoms. One day, after defecation, he noted a streak of bright red blood on the toilet paper. He then phoned his primary care physician to tell him of this finding. Which of the following interventions is most appropriate?

A. Aortogram
B. Barium enema
C. Colonoscopy
D. Observation
E. Oral psyllium and docusate

540. During a total colectomy, a 48-year-old man with a history of diabetes mellitus and hypertension requires a blood transfusion due to moderate blood loss. He is administered 3 units of packed RBCs over 4 hours, after which the patient's vital signs were found to be stable. An hour postsurgery, the patient becomes tachycardic and develops an arrhythmia. What is the most likely explanation for these findings?

A. ABO blood type mismatch
B. Excessive citrate in the blood
C. Hypovolemia
D. RBC damage during storage
E. Rh antigen mismatch

541. A 25-year-old G1P1 female is in the delivery suite in active labor for the past 8 hours. Fetal weight is 4000 grams. Her cervix is dilated 9 cm, and she has been at this point for the last 2 hours despite strong, regular contractions 2 to 3 minutes apart. Fetal rhythm shows a reactive fetal heart with no decelerations. Membranes have been ruptured for 4 hours. Fetal position is left occiput anterior. Significant caput formation is evident. Ischial spines are prominent. What is the most appropriate treatment for this patient?

A. Continue to observe the progression of labor
B. Epidural anesthesia and follow-up
C. Oxytocin infusion
D. Surgical intervention (cesarean section)
E. Watchful waiting for 24 hours

542. A 75-year-old woman underwent cardiac catheterization yesterday. She has a history of congestive heart failure for which she takes atenolol and propranolol. This morning she complains of difficulty breathing and a heaviness in her chest. She becomes agitated with your questioning and refuses to answer any more questions. Physical examination reveals that she is afebrile and has a blood pressure of 160/95 mm Hg. Rales are heard throughout the left lower lung field. She is coughing copious amounts of clear sputum. A chest x-ray is ordered and is shown in Figure 542. What is the best next step in the management of this patient?

A. Change beta blocker to be administered intravenously with fluids
B. Diagnostic thoracentesis
C. Flexible bronchoscopy
D. Intravenous normal saline
E. Observation

Figure 542

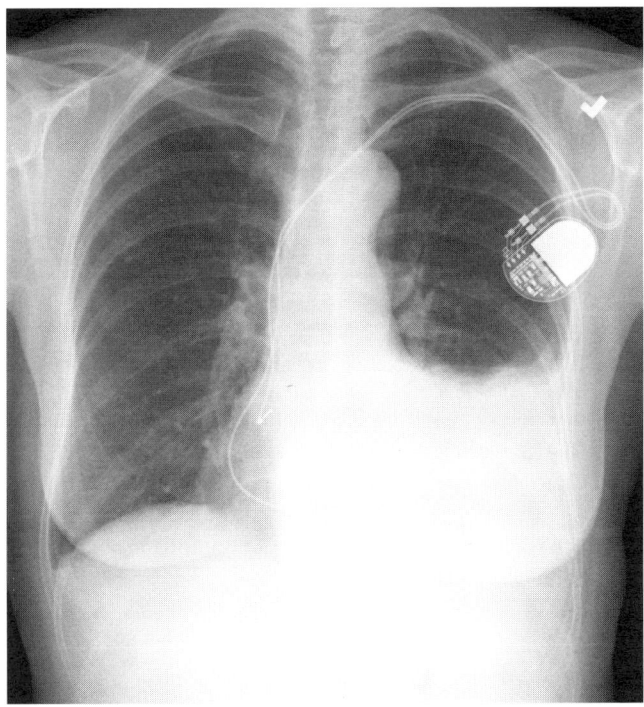

543. A 22-year-old woman presents with a rapidly growing adnexal mass and abdominal pain. She has a prior medical history of dyspareunia and dysmenorrhea. She has a past surgical history of tonsillectomy. Physical examination findings of the heart, lungs, and abdomen are unremarkable. The CA-125 level is negative and the beta human chorionic gonadotropin level is positive. What is the most likely diagnosis?

A. Epithelial cell tumor

B. Granulosa-theca cell tumor

C. Immature teratoma

D. Nongestational choriocarcinoma

E. Squamous cell carcinoma

544. A 34-year-old woman with schizophrenia is brought in to the emergency department by her mother with a 2-hour history of sustained muscle spasms of her neck and jaw. She is extremely uncomfortable, and finds it difficult to speak with the spasm. After obtaining a history from her mother, you learn that her medication had been changed from chlorpromazine to haloperidol 2 days ago. You instruct her not to take any more haloperidol. What is the next best step in this patient's management?

A. Benztropine (intravenous)

B. Benztropine (oral)

C. Dantrolene

D. Diphenhydramine (intravenous)

E. Diphenhydramine (oral)

545. An 18-year-old female freshman college student is brought to the university clinic by her roommate after an apparent suicide attempt. Physical examination of the heart, lung, and abdomen are unremarkable. She is alert, awake, and oriented, but smells of alcohol on her breath. Further questioning reveals that the patient has a prior history of a major depressive episode after the death of a best friend at age 13. Which of the following conditions is associated with the highest risk for successful suicide attempts?

A. Bipolar disorder

B. Borderline personality disorder

C. Major depression

D. Panic disorder

E. Schizophrenia

546. A 25-kg child is hospitalized overnight after undergoing an appendectomy. He has no pertinent prior medical or surgical history. Gross pathology at surgery suggested an enlarged, inflamed appendix with suppuration. The child is able to drink fluids postoperatively. How much maintenance intravenous fluid is required per day for this child?

A. 1400 mL

B. 1500 mL

C. 1600 mL

D. 1700 mL

E. 1800 mL

547. A 31-year-old woman presents to her primary care physician for evaluation of sexual and voiding dysfunction. She voids 18 times per day and 4 times per night with a weak force of stream. She also has chronic pelvic pain. She has been evaluated by numerous physicians and all are baffled by her complaints. She complains of numerous urinary tract infections but review of her records indicates that all urine cultures are negative. Physical examination findings of the heart, lungs, and abdomen are unremarkable. Pelvic examination reveals no evidence of pelvic prolapse. She does have anterior vaginal wall tenderness. Which of the following sexual dysfunctions is this patient most likely to exhibit?

A. Arousal

B. Desire

C. Lubrication

D. Orgasm

E. Pain

548. A 33-year-old man with a history of ulcerative colitis was admitted to the hospital for exacerbation of bloody diarrhea and abdominal pain. Endoscopy revealed friable colonic mucosa and multiple colonic pseudopolyps. He is being treated with intravenous steroids. On hospital day 4, he noticed tender, red pustules that progressed to an ulcer with a purulent base on his forearm and neck. Biopsy of the lesion reveals acute inflammatory exudate with fragments of inflamed granulation tissue. Laboratory studies obtained are shown below:

Leukocyte count and differential

Leukocyte count	19,000/mm^3
Segmented neutrophils	84%
Bands	9%
Eosinophils	3%
Basophils	1%
Lymphocytes	27%
Monocytes	4%

Which of the following is the most likely diagnosis?

A. Erythema
B. Erythema nodosum
C. Herpetiform dermatitis
D. Pyoderma gangrenosum
E. Steroid-induced dermatitis

549. A 4-year-old boy presents to the pediatric clinic with a rash. The patient's mother notes that the rash initially started on the patient's head and progressed caudally. The patient's mother also notes that her son has had a cough associated with the rash. Physical examination reveals a confluent erythematous maculopapular rash, conjunctivitis, and Koplik spots. What is the most likely diagnosis?

A. Fifth disease
B. Measles
C. Roseola
D. Rubella
E. Varicella

550. A 36-year-old man was sent to a specialist by his primary care doctor complaining of episodic headaches, flushing, and anxiety. He has recently been diagnosed with high blood pressure and thinks this is the cause of his anxiety. Otherwise he is without any other complaints. What is the first test to order to help confirm your diagnosis?

A. MRI of the abdomen/pelvis
B. Methyl-iodo-benzyl-guanidine scan
C. Metanephrine, normetanephrine, and vanilmandelic acid studies of the urine
D. Sestamibi scan
E. Watchful waiting, then order an MRI of the head in 1 week

551. A 59-year-old man with a 50-pound weight loss during the past 6 months presents to his physician complaining of fatigue and malaise. CT scan of the abdomen reveals a 3-cm pancreatic mass with liver and lung metastases. The patient is unaware of the CT findings and his prognosis. Which of the following is the physician's best strategy in delivering these findings to the patient?

A. Accomplish a complete discussion in a single interview
B. Answer questions concisely and compassionately
C. Delegate the task to the hospital social worker
D. Formal description using technical jargon
E. Liberal use of euphemism with some optimism

552. A 41-year-old obese woman presents to the emergency department with abdominal pain in her right upper quadrant that often radiates to her right scapula. She states that pain is worse after eating meals. Temperature is 38.2°C, blood pressure 135/88 mm Hg, pulse 102 beats/min, and respirations 15 breaths/min. Physical examination reveals that the lungs are clear to auscultation, and the abdomen is tender to palpation in the right upper quadrant. While palpating in the right subcostal area, you ask the patient to take a deep breath and notice that she immediately stops her deep inspiration. No rebound tenderness is appreciated. Upon pelvic examination no cervical motion tenderness, mass, or discharge is appreciated. What is the next best step that should be taken in the management of this patient?

A. Administer antibiotics and obtain nuclear scan in 1 week
B. Angiography
C. CT of the abdomen
D. MRI of abdomen
E. Ultrasonography of the abdomen

553. A 44-year-old woman presents to her primary care physician because of heavy menstrual periods with blood clots for the past month. She has a prior medical history of hypertension. Her current medications include a calcium channel blocker. Physical examination reveals blood and clots in the vaginal vault. Diagnostic laparoscopy, hysteroscopy, and biopsy are normal. What is the most likely diagnosis?

A. Adenomatous hyperplasia
B. Adenomyosis
C. Dysfunctional uterine bleeding
D. Submucosal fibroma
E. Uterine polyp

554. A 64-year-old man with a 10-year history of chronic obstructive pulmonary disease (COPD) presents to the clinic with warm, erythematous, painful distal extremities. He also complains of a 15-pound weight gain over the past 2 months. Physical examination reveals decreased breath sounds at the left lower lung base. Bilateral clubbing of his digits is also noted. X-ray of his ankles shows periosteal thickening. Chest x-ray reveals a lesion suspicious for malignancy. What is the most likely diagnosis?

A. Behçet syndrome

B. Hypertrophic osteoarthropathy

C. Osteomyelitis

D. Reiter syndrome

E. Rheumatoid arthritis

555. A 63-year-old man with prostate cancer undergoing external beam radiation complains of diarrhea, rectal bleeding, and the sensation of incomplete evacuation of stools. Physical examination reveals a regular rate and rhythm. Pulmonary auscultation reveals good breath sounds bilaterally. Abdominal examination reveals normoactive bowel sounds without peritoneal signs. Anorectal examination reveals hemorrhagic and inflamed mucosa of the distal rectum. Laboratory values are shown below:

Blood, plasma, serum

Alanine aminotransferase (ALT)	16 U/L
Amylase, serum	42 U/L
Aspartate aminotransferase (AST)	14 U/L
Calcium, serum	9 mg/dL
Glucose, serum	110 mg/dL
Hematocrit	39%
Prostate-specific antigen	4.0 ng/mL
Urea nitrogen, serum (BUN)	10 mg/dL

Urinalysis

Urine pH	6.0
RBC count	25/HPF
WBC count	2–5/HPF
Nitrates	Negative
Bacteria	Negative

What is the most likely diagnosis?

A. External hemorrhoids (thrombosed type)

B. Fissure (chronic type)

C. Fistula (transsphincteric)

D. Internal hemorrhoids (prolapsing type)

E. Radiation proctitis

556. A 43-year-old man is found to have multiple renal cysts and a mass that is thought to be renal cell carcinoma on CT scan. Because of persistent dizziness, CT scan of the head was ordered and revealed a cerebellar hemangioblastoma. The patient had been complaining of trouble with his vision and was later diagnosed with an angioma in his right retina. What is the most likely diagnosis?

- **A.** Autosomal-dominant polycystic kidney disease
- **B.** Bartter syndrome
- **C.** Neurofibromatosus 1 (von Recklinghausen disease)
- **D.** Tuberous sclerosis
- **E.** von Hippel-Lindau disease

557. A 34-year-old G1P0 woman who is determined to be pregnant by home pregnancy test presents for evaluation. She has a history of systemic lupus erythematosus and takes prednisone daily. Doppler ultrasonography reveals evidence of fetal heart tones. Abdominal examination reveals normoactive bowel sounds with a fundal height at 5 cm below the umbilicus. Her serum electrolytes are normal. Which of the following is a possible fetal cardiac defect in pregnancy?

- **A.** Coarctation of the aorta
- **B.** Complete heart block
- **C.** Transposition of the great vessels
- **D.** Tricuspid atresia
- **E.** Ventricular septal defect

558. A 7-year-old mentally retarded boy is brought to his pediatrician for evaluation of a seizure episode. The patient's mother states that the child had a significant seizure 3 days ago. No recent history of any fever was noted. Physical examination reveals no focal neurologic deficits. However, multiple hypopigmented macules with areas of thickened skin are noted on the trunk. What is the most likely diagnosis?

- **A.** Down syndrome
- **B.** Neurofibromatosis
- **C.** Sturge-Weber disease
- **D.** Tuberous sclerosis
- **E.** von Hippel-Lindau disease

559. A 14-year-old boy presents to the pediatric clinic for evaluation following a motor vehicle accident. His parents tell you that since the accident 2 months ago, he has had trouble concentrating in school, and his grades have dropped significantly. He also has had a harder time verbalizing his thoughts, and his mother tells you that he "just doesn't seem himself." What is the most appropriate next step in this patient's management?

- **A.** Admit patient to the hospital for further evaluation
- **B.** Administer a Wechsler Intelligence Scales for Children test
- **C.** Reassure the parents
- **D.** Tell parents to carefully monitor patient's behavior, and schedule another appointment in 4 weeks
- **E.** Watchful waiting

560. A 25-year-old man presents to the emergency department with nausea, vomiting, and severe abdominal pain. The patient appears to try to stay as motionless as possible. Blood pressure is 128/88 mm Hg, pulse 112 beats/min, and temperature 101.5°F. On physical examination the patient has diminished bowel sounds with right lower quadrant abdominal pain and rebound tenderness. The patient expresses pain on passive extension of the hip while lying on his left side with the knee extended. No pain is appreciated on passive internal rotation of the hip. Laboratory data shows the following:

WBC count	15,000/mm^3
Neutrophils	81%
Lymphocytes	10%
Monocytes	7%
Eosinophils	2%

What is the most likely diagnosis?

- **A.** Appendicitis (appendix in the anterior pelvis)
- **B.** Appendicitis (retrocecal)
- **C.** Diverticulum of the cecum
- **D.** Pancreatitis
- **E.** Testicular torsion

561. A 49-year-old man is found unresponsive by family members one morning. They reported him acting slightly confused before he went to bed the previous night. Family members state that he undertook his normal routine the day before of working on the family farm. He is brought by the rescue squad to the hospital. He had some convulsions in the ambulance on the way to the hospital. The patient is tachypneic and pale looking. His past medical history is significant for depression, alcoholism, and previous knee surgery. Arterial blood gas assessment reveals metabolic acidosis with increased anion gap. There is a high osmolar gap. Electrolytes are normal but the blood urea nitrogen level is 50 mg/dL, serum creatinine 6.5 mg/dL, and serum calcium 6.5 mg/dL. Urinalysis reveals crystal-like structures. Serum aspartate aminotransferase and alanine aminotransferase are normal. What is the most likely diagnosis?

- **A.** Chlorinated insecticide poisoning
- **B.** Ethanol intoxication
- **C.** Ethylene glycol ingestion

D. Methanol ingestion

E. Mushroom ingestion

562. A 14-year-old boy presents to the emergency department after falling on an outstretched hand while attempting to catch a pass thrown during a football game. He complains of right wrist pain. Physical examination reveals exquisite tenderness in the right anatomic snuffbox and decrease in right wrist range of motion, especially with flexion and extension. Examination of the left wrist reveals good range of motion in flexion, extension, and internal and external rotation. Radiographs reveal no evidence of a fracture. What is the most likely diagnosis?

A. Endochondroma

B. Nonossifying fibroma

C. Perilunate dislocation

D. Scaphoid fracture

E. Smith fracture

563. A 35-year-old woman desires to undergo elective sterilization. A laparoscopic tubal ligation is planned. She has no prior medical or surgical history. Preoperative laboratory studies including hepatic function tests and coagulation profiles are normal. Which of the following is the most appropriate method of preventing development of deep vein thrombosis during the procedure?

A. Giving a dose of intravenous heparin prior to pneumoperitoneum

B. Giving a dose of warfarin to the patient the night prior to surgery

C. Maintaining less than 15 mm Hg pneumoperitoneum

D. Use of pneumatic compression devices on the lower extremities

E. Use of spinal anesthesia

564. A 35-kg child with a history of intractable nausea and vomiting is brought to the emergency department for evaluation. The child attends a day-care center at which several other children are suffering from the same symptoms. Physical examination suggests that this child is 10% dehydrated. What is the total fluid replacement he should receive in mL/h during the first 8 hours?

A. 75 mL/h

B. 95 mL/h

C. 195 mL/h

D. 295 mL/h

E. 395 mL/h

565. You are called to evaluate a preterm infant with a heart murmur. Physical examination reveals a continuous machinelike murmur in the left second intercostal space. Two-dimensional echocardiography confirms that the child has a patent ductus arteriosus. The patient is treated with indomethacin. After 1 week of therapy the infant is still feeding poorly and is in respiratory distress. Workup reveals a patent ductus arteriosus. What is the most appropriate definitive treatment?

A. Attempt a trial of another antiprostaglandin inhibitor

B. Continue indomethacin treatment

C. Discontinue indomethacin and observe patient

D. Embolization

E. Surgical repair

566. An obese 50-year-old white man presents to his primary care physician for evaluation of bilateral lower extremity pain and cramping with exertion. He claims it occurs after walking approximately 50 yards; symptoms subside with rest. He takes no medications. He has attempted to quit smoking on three occasions and currently has a 30 pack/year history. Physical examination reveals a man who appears to be his stated age. He is afebrile. His heart rate is 80 beats/min, and blood pressure is 160/100 mm Hg in both arms. He has decreased peripheral pulses bilaterally and an absent dorsalis pedis on the right. There are no ulcerations or discolorations present. His nonfasting glucose level is 126 mg/dL. What is the most likely diagnosis?

A. Buerger disease

B. Lumbar spinal stenosis

C. Peripheral vascular disease

D. Popliteal artery entrapment

E. Thromboangiitis obliterans

The response options for items 567–570 are the same. You will be required to select one answer for each item in the set.

A. Adjustment disorder with depressed mood

B. Bipolar disorder

C. Cyclothymia

D. Dysthymia

E. Intoxication with pharmacologic-induced psychosis

F. Major depression

G. Schizophrenia

H. Uncomplicated bereavement

For each patient vignette below, select the best answer.

567. A 21-year-old woman with a family history of major depression in her father has a 1-year history of job instability, occasional suicide attempts, and multiple short hospitalizations over the past 2 years. She experiences mild depression and hypomania. She is an intermittent drug and alcohol abuser.

568. A 68-year-old man is anhedonic, sad, and tearful after the death of his wife due to a chronic illness. After intense mourning and resolution, his symptoms improve within 2 weeks.

569. A 59-year-old woman is anhedonic, sad, and tearful after the death of her husband due to a chronic illness. She is now unable to work, forgets to eat three meals per day, and has lost 10 pounds over the past month. She rarely goes outside to be with friends or relatives.

570. A 29-year-old woman has a 2-year history of tearfulness and difficulty falling asleep but is less symptomatic in the morning. She is usually despondent in the afternoon and evening. She suffered the loss of her mother when she was 5 years old and was recently beaten by her boyfriend.

571. A 12 year-old boy presents to the emergency department 2 days after returning from a camping trip with new onset of frequent, foul-smelling, watery diarrhea. He also complains of abdominal pain, nausea, and flatulence. Physical examination reveals some mild tenderness in all quadrants without evidence of guarding or rebound tenderness. What is the most likely cause of this patient's diarrhea?

  A. *Clostridium difficile*
  B. *Giardia lamblia*
  C. *Salmonella*
  D. *Shigella*
  E. *Vibrio cholerae*

572. A 15-year-old girl presents to her primary care physician because of fear of pregnancy. She has had unprotected sexual intercourse with several partners during the past 6 months. Her menses are regular. Her last menstrual period was 3 months ago. Physical examination findings of the heart, lungs, and abdomen are within normal limits. Which of the following is the most compelling evidence of pregnancy?

  A. Blue violet hue to the cervix
  B. Cervical softening
  C. Cessation of menses
  D. Fetal heart rate detection by transvaginal ultrasonography
  E. Nausea

573. A 27-year-old man is being treated in the trauma center after a motor vehicle accident in which he was not seriously injured. During secondary evaluation the medical student inquires as to why the patient's left arm appears shorter than his right. The patient states that when he was a child he fell and suffered a serious injury that crushed his growth plate. Which of the following is the most likely type of growth plate injury that occurred?

  A. Salter I fracture
  B. Salter II fracture
  C. Salter III fracture
  D. Salter IV fracture
  E. Salter V fracture

574. A 28-year-old man with AIDS presents to his primary care physician complaining of fever, chills, hemoptysis, and pleu-

ritic chest pain. He complains of worsening shortness of breath and productive cough over the past few days. On physical examination, bilateral rales are noted. Laboratory values are as follows:

WBC count	3200/mm^3
Absolute neutrophil count	472/mm^3
Blood cultures	No growth after 3 days
Sputum cultures	No growth after 3 days
Chest x-ray	Necrotizing bronchopneumonia
Lung biopsy	Septate, acutely branching hyphae

What is the most likely diagnosis?

  A. Anthrax
  B. Aspergillosis
  C. Coccidioidomycosis
  D. Cytomegalovirus
  E. *Pneumocystis carinii* pneumonia

575. A 47-year-old woman is preparing to have elective reconstructive surgery of her breasts. She has a history of idiopathic thrombocytopenia. Physical examination of the heart, lungs and abdomen are within normal limits. There is no evidence of ecchymosis. Preoperative laboratory studies are shown below:

WBC count	14,000/mm^3
Hemoglobin	12.3 mg/dL
Hematocrit	38.1%
Platelet count	55,000/mm^3

Which of the following is the most appropriate next step?

  A. Administer fresh frozen plasma on call to surgery
  B. Cancel the surgery until the platelet count increases
  C. Continue as planned with the operation, repeat laboratory studies postoperatively
  D. Delay surgery and repeat laboratory studies in 1 hour
  E. Transfuse the patient 1 hour before with whole blood

576. A 31-year-old mother and her newborn boy are prepared to be discharged from the hospital after a normal delivery course. The newborn was born at term via spontaneous vaginal delivery. Prenatal care was completed without event. Physical examination of the newborn was within normal limits. The mother plans to bottle feed the newborn. What are the appropriate recommendations regarding number of feedings and volume/feedings/day?

Number of feedings/day	*Volume (mL)*
A. 6–10	30–90
B. 7–8	60–120
C. 5–7	120–180
D. 4–5	180–210
E. 3–4	210–240

577. A 20-year-old woman in college presents to the university health service for her yearly wellness examination and is requesting information on available types of oral contraceptives. She reports having had sexual intercourse for the first time 4 weeks ago with a fellow dormitory resident whom she just met. She reports occasional use of condoms during sexual intercourse but wishes to try an alternative means of pregnancy prevention. Physical examination reveals bilateral inguinal lymphadenopathy and a well-demarcated 5-mm circumferential erythematous lesion on her vulva of which she was not aware. What is the most appropriate next step in the treatment of this patient?

- **A.** Establish diagnosis by identifying motile spirochetes under dark-field microscopy
- **B.** Establish diagnosis through use of rapid plasmin reagin (RPR)
- **C.** Establish diagnosis through use of Venereal Disease Research Laboratory (VDRL) test
- **D.** Have patient closely monitor lesion and return for follow-up
- **E.** Treat empirically with a 15-day course of tetracycline

578. A 58-year-old alcoholic man complains of epigastric pain radiating toward his back. He presents to the emergency department for evaluation. The pain began while watching television yesterday. Eating makes the pain worse, and nothing seems to make it better. He has never had this pain in the past. He has no associated fevers, chills, nausea, or vomiting. He had some mild constipation within the past 2 weeks. Physical examination is remarkable for epigastric tenderness. Laboratory studies reveal a WBC count of 13,000/mm^3 with elevated amylase and lipase levels. What is the most appropriate treatment for this patient?

- **A.** Exploratory laparotomy
- **B.** Broad-spectrum antibiotics

- **C.** Hospital admission, nothing by mouth, and follow the patient conservatively
- **D.** Low-fat/low-cholesterol diet
- **E.** Ultrasonography to rule out a leaking abdominal aortic aneurysm

579. A 90-year-old woman presents to her family physician for a 6-month check-up. Her past medical history is significant only for cholecystectomy at age 45, and she currently lives at home by herself. She has started walking every day and denies having any dyspnea or chest pain. Physical examination is insignificant, except for a heart rate of 95 beats/min. Figure 579 shows the results of a routine ECG. What is the next best step in the treatment of this patient?

- **A.** Cardioversion
- **B.** Atropine
- **C.** Follow-up
- **D.** Pacemaker insertion
- **E.** Studies of cardiac electrophysiology

580. A 38-year-old man with a past medical history of gout comes into the emergency department complaining of a sharp left flank pain radiating to his groin. There are no alleviating or exacerbating factors to his pain. He has been without fevers, chills, nausea, or vomiting. He has had increased urinary frequency and diarrhea for the past week. What is the first radiologic test to order to confirm the diagnosis?

- **A.** Abdominal x-ray
- **B.** Bladder and renal ultrasonography
- **C.** Intravenous pyelography
- **D.** Pelvis and abdominal CT scan with intravenous contrast
- **E.** Pelvis and abdominal CT scan without intravenous contrast

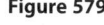

Figure 579

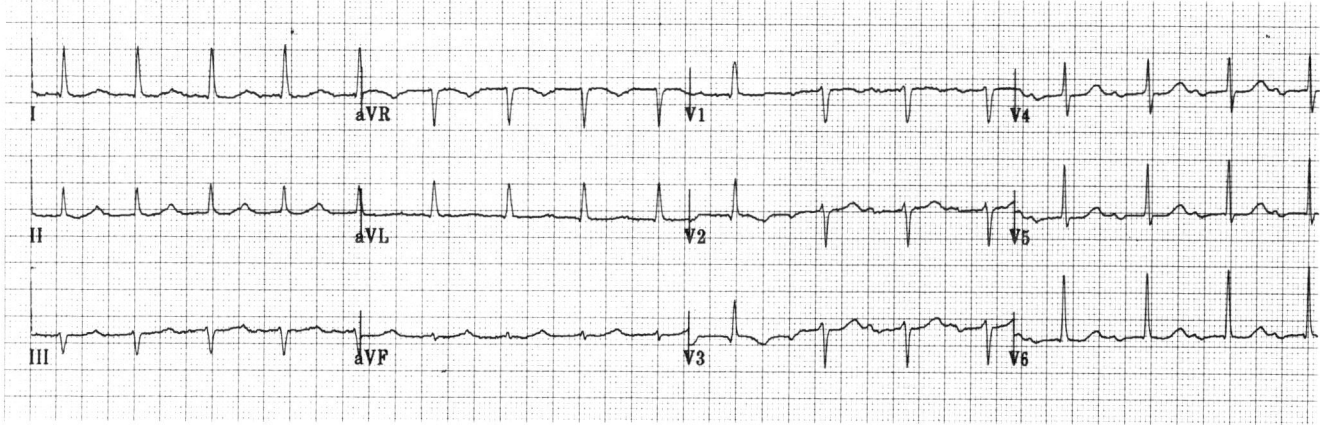

581. A 40-year-old woman presents to the emergency room with a chief complaint of dizziness. On further questioning, you are able to clarify her complaint as vertigo as opposed to presyncope. She denies any recent injury to her head. She states that the dizziness is so severe that it has led to vomiting on a number of occasions. She states that she has had multiple recurrences of the same episodes that each last approximately a couple of days. Review of systems reveals that the vertigo is accompanied by unilateral tinnitus and decreased auditory acuity. In the differential diagnosis, what medications must you consider as a possible cause of this clinical picture?

A. Aminoglycosides and carbonic anhydrase inhibitors
B. Carbonic anhydrase inhibitors and beta blockers
C. Loop diuretics and aminoglycosides
D. Loop diuretics and beta blockers
E. Loop diuretics and carbonic anhydrase inhibitors

582. A 34-year-old woman comes to the primary care physician with no past medical history. She has noticed epigastric pain for the past 5 months that she describes as intermittent burning discomfort. She notices it particularly after eating a heavy meal. She denies having any nausea or vomiting. She currently is not taking any medications, but has occasionally taken calcium carbonate tablets with some relief of symptoms. Physical examination findings of the heart, lungs, and abdomen are unremarkable. Which of the following is the most appropriate next step in the evaluation/treatment of this patient?

A. Cholecystectomy
B. Diagnostic laparoscopy
C. Endoscopic retrograde cholangiopancreatography (ERCP)
D. Prescription of an H2 blocker and follow-up in 4 weeks
E. Upper gastrointestinal endoscopy

583. A 2-year-old boy is brought to the emergency department by paramedics after being struck by a motor vehicle while crossing the street with his mother. Upon arrival in the emergency department, the child is breathing and has a palpable femoral pulse. The fastest location to obtain intravenous access is via which route?

A. Antecubital left arm vein
B. Dorsal right hand vein
C. Femoral vein cannulation
D. Internal jugular venous cannulation
E. Intraosseous cannulation

584. A 22-year-old G1P0 woman who is 16 weeks pregnant and her 23-year-old sister who is not pregnant present to their primary care physician for routine care. Of the following laboratory parameters, which would be unchanged in both the pregnant and nonpregnant woman?

A. Alkaline phosphatase
B. Creatinine

C. Hemoglobin
D. Lactate dehydrogenase
E. Total cholesterol

585. A 41-year-old woman notes a 4-year history of episodes of feeling short of breath and dizzy with trembling and shaking when she is in crowded places such as a shopping mall or a train station. During such episodes she notes nausea and abdominal pain, chills, and tingling sensations in her hands. Physical examination findings of the heart, lungs, and abdomen are within normal limits. Results of laboratory studies are shown below:

Electrolytes, serum

Na, serum	141 mEq/L
Cl, serum	99 mEq/L
K, serum	4.2 mEq/L
Bicarbonate, serum	24 mEq/L
Creatinine, serum	1.0 mg/dL

Leukocyte count and differential

Leukocyte count	6000/mm³
Segmented neutrophils	65%

Blood, plasma, serum

Alanine aminotransferase (ALT)	10 U/L
Amylase, serum	50 U/L
Aspartate aminotransferase (AST)	10 U/L
Calcium, serum	9 mg/dL
Glucose, serum	100 mg/dL
Hematocrit	33%
Urea nitrogen, serum (BUN)	10 mg/dL

Urinalysis

Urine pH	6.0
RBC count	2/HPF
WBC count	2/HPF
Nitrates	Negative
Bacteria	Negative

Which of the following physiologic findings might be noted in this patient?

A. Decreased levels of neurepinephrine
B. Hyperactive center in the temporal cerebral cortex
C. Increased levels of gamma-aminobutyric acid
D. Increased REM sleep latency
E. Increased urinary flow rate

586. A 33-year-old woman who is 3 weeks postpartum presents to her primary care physician complaining of body aches, fatigue, and pain during breast-feeding. Physical examination reveals an erythematous, warm left breast. No masses were palpated. No discharge from the breast was appreciated. Temperature is 38.3°C, heart rate 77 beats/min, blood pressure 135/72 mm Hg, and respiratory rate 15 breaths/min. What would the most appropriate next step in the treatment of this patient?

A. Continue to breast-feed and start antibiotics

B. Perform breast biopsy

C. Perform fine-needle aspiration

D. Stop breast-feeding and start antibiotics

E. Stop breast-feeding and give Tylenol

587. A 29-year-old primigravid woman with a history of hypothyroidism is expecting her first child; she is 12 weeks pregnant by dates. The woman has a history of alcohol and drug abuse and currently lives at a women's shelter. Her blood pressure is mildly elevated at this visit and she complains of feeling "more jittery and shaky than usual." Physical examination reveals vaginal bleeding, and the uterus is palpable at 18 cm above the symphysis pubis. What is the most likely diagnosis?

A. Endometrial adenocarcinoma

B. Hydatidiform mole

C. Normal pregnancy with acute alcohol withdrawal symptoms

D. Placental abruption

E. Botryoid sarcoma

588. A 25-year-old woman is diagnosed with a dysgerminoma germ cell tumor. She presents to your clinic for a second opinion. Her previous physician recommended an experimental protocol and appeared to anger this patient. What is the most appropriate treatment?

A. Chemotherapy and radiation

B. Removal of the involved ovary with radiation treatment

C. Removal of the involved ovary without radiation treatment

D. Total abdominal hysterectomy and bilateral oophorectomy (TAHBSO)

E. Watchful waiting

589. A 23-year-old woman presents to the ambulatory care clinic with a 2-week history of sore throat with neck tenderness that is getting worse over time. She has also felt hot lately, with episodes of sweating but has not checked her temperature. She reports feeling tired the past few weeks. Her pain started on the left side but has now settled on the right. She reports having a cough with runny nose and congestion about a month ago. On physical examination an asymmetric, firm, tender goiter is appreciated. Oropharynx is clear without redness or exudates. Tympanic membranes are unremarkable. Lungs are clear to auscultation without wheezes. Heart is regular in rate and rhythm. Laboratory values are as follows:

WBC count	12,000/mm^3
Erythrocyte sedimentation rate	42 mm/h
Thyroid-stimulating hormone level	0.3 μIU/mL
Total thyroxine level	18 μg/dL
Radioactive iodine uptake	0

What is the most likely diagnosis?

A. de Quervain thyroiditis

B. Graves disease

C. Hashimoto thyroiditis

D. Lymphocytic thyroiditis

E. Medullary carcinoma

590. In the year 2000, Anytown, USA, had 1000 live births. Thirty of these were twins. Four mothers died, and there were 45 stillbirths, which were delivered at greater than or equal to 20 weeks' gestation. Thirteen deaths occurred in the first year of life. Six of those died in the first 28 days of life. What was the infant mortality rate in Anytown, USA, in the year 2000?

A. 13/1051

B. 13/1000

C. 63/1045

D. 6/1000

E. 6/1045

591. A 42-year-old man presents to the ambulatory care clinic with abdominal pain, diarrhea, a 10-pound weight loss, polyarthralgia, and pleuritic pain. Lung examination reveals crackles. Changes in skin pigmentation are also noted. Overall, the patient appears malnourished. Chest x-ray reveals hilar lymphadenopathy. Lymph node biopsy shows foamy macrophages that stain with periodic acid-Schiff. The most likely diagnosis is:

A. Celiac disease

B. Crohn disease

C. Intestinal lymphangiectasia

D. Tropical sprue

E. Whipple disease

592. A 36-year-old woman presents to her gynecologist at 16 weeks' gestation. She has no prior medical history. She has a surgical history of tonsillectomy. Physical examination reveals blood pressure of 160/100 mm Hg after 5 minutes of rest. A repeat measurement 1 week later is 154/98 mm Hg. What is the most likely diagnosis?

A. Chronic hypertension

B. Chronic hypertension with preeclampsia

C. Labile hypertension

D. Preeclampsia

E. Transient hypertension

593. A 66-year-old woman presents to her primary care physician with intermittent bright red blood per rectum for 1 month. Yesterday she experienced left lower quadrant pain, nausea, and vomiting. She says she felt feverish. Physical examination reveals that she is afebrile, and vital signs are stable. The abdomen is soft, nontender, and nondistended. A CT scan of the abdomen is ordered (Figure 593). What is the most plausible explanation of these findings on CT scan?

Figure 593

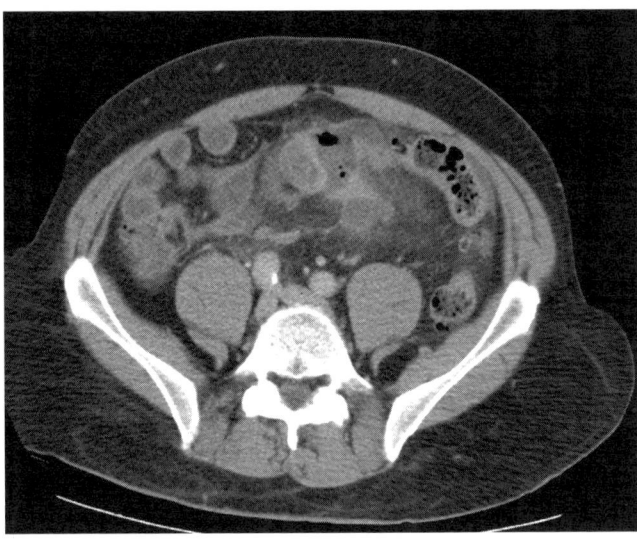

A. Bowel wall thickening
B. Colonic diverticula
C. Increased soft tissue density within pericolic fat
D. Pericolic fluid collections
E. Soft tissue mass

594. A 4-year-old boy is brought to his pediatrician for evaluation of simple coryza of 3 days duration. He has no prior medical or surgical history. He was born at term by spontaneous vaginal delivery. He is afebrile and comfortable. Physical examination of the ears, nose, and throat are normal. Cardiac, pulmonary, and abdominal examinations are within normal limits. What is the most appropriate treatment for this patient?

A. Amoxicillin
B. Doxycycline
C. Erythromycin
D. Interferon
E. Supportive therapy

595. A 42-year-old woman complains of nausea after receiving a dose of morphine sulfate for a 4-mm renal stone identified on CT scan. Her current medications are haloperidol and acetaminophen with codeine. Physical examination reveals

left flank tenderness. Physical examination findings of the heart, lungs, and abdomen are unremarkable. Which of the following medications could cause irreversible side effects in this patient when used as an antiemetic?

A. Cimetidine
B. Metoclopramide
C. Ondansetron
D. Prochlorperazine
E. Trimethobenzamide

596. A 63-year-old man with bronchogenic carcinoma that is scheduled for resection presents to his primary care physician for preoperative clearance. He has a chronic cough and sometimes coughs up bloody sputum. He reports no nausea, vomiting, seizures, headache, or pain. He has no other medical problems. He has no history of bleeding disorders. Social history is positive for a 60 pack/year history of smoking cigarettes. What is the next most appropriate test for this patient?

A. Bone scan
B. Chest x-ray
C. Liver ultrasonography
D. MRI of the brain
E. Pulmonary function tests

597. An 80-year-old woman presents to her primary care physician with a 3-week history of fatigue and shortness of breath, especially when she is walking. She often gets up at night to get a breath of air. She denies experiencing weight gain, edema, or other symptoms. Physical examination reveals bilateral rales. What is the most likely diagnosis?

A. Asthma
B. Cor pulmonale
C. Left ventricular heart failure
D. Right ventricular heart failure
E. Both ventricles have failed

598. A 38-year-old G2P2002 woman presents to her gynecologist for her yearly wellness examination. This patient does not want to have more children. She has a past medical history significant for hypertension and a family history significant for hypothyroidism. She is without any complaints and reports compliance with routine monthly breast self-examinations. Bimanual vaginal examination reveals a firm, nontender 8-week gestational sized irregularly enlarged uterus with bosselated midline protrusions from the uterine wall. The remainder of the physical examination findings are unremarkable. Results of laboratory studies are shown below:

Electrolytes, serum

Na, serum	145 mEq/L
Cl, serum	101 mEq/L
K, serum	3.9 mEq/L
Bicarbonate, serum	24 mEq/L

Magnesium, serum	2.0 mEq/L
Creatinine, serum	1.0 mg/dL

Leukocyte count and differential

Leukocyte count	5000/mm^3
Segmented neutrophils	50%
Bands	4%
Eosinophils	3%
Basophils	1%
Lymphocytes	24%
Monocytes	4%

What is the most appropriate management recommendation?

A. Expectant management

B. Exogenous estrogen to inhibit further growth of the lesion

C. Patient should be placed on gonadotropin-releasing hormone (GnRH) agonists

D. Surgical removal (hysterectomy)

E. Uterine myomectomy

599. A 15-year-old boy is brought for evaluation of recurrent focal generalized seizures and ataxia of gait. He is currently unable to walk. His prior medical history is notable for measles at the age of 12. Electroencephalographic studies in this individual are most likely to reveal

A. Diffuse flat waves

B. High-voltage sharp waves

C. High-voltage slow waves

D. Periodic bursts of high-voltage waves and a flat pattern

E. Transient low-voltage sharp waves

600. A 14-year old boy is brought to the pediatrician for evaluation. He appears to have a wasted appearance and complains of fatigue and irritability. He has diarrhea two to three times per week. His diet consists primarily of junk food. Physical examination findings of the heart, lungs, and abdomen are within normal limits. No neurologic abnormalities are found. Laboratory studies reveal serum folate levels of 2 ng/mL and elevated lactate dehydrogenase. Microscopic examination of the peripheral smear reveals macrocytic RBCs. What is the most appropriate treatment for this patient?

A. Diet change to include fruits and vegetables

B. Erythropoietin

C. Plasmapheresis

D. Platelet transfusion

E. Vitamin D supplementation

601. A 41-year-old male executive from a local bank presents to his primary care physician because of multiple complaints over the past 4 months. He is present with his wife for this evaluation. He complains of a 10-pound weight loss, fatigue, insomnia, inability to concentrate, and a lack of interest in his wife. He thinks that his symptoms are due to financial difficulties that the bank is having. He has no prior medical history. His surgical history is notable for endoscopic sinus surgery. Physical examination findings of the heart, lungs, and abdomen are unremarkable. What is the most likely diagnosis?

A. Adjustment disorder

B. Dysthymia

C. Generalized anxiety disorder

D. Major depression

E. Organic affective disorder

602. A middle-aged, premenopausal female presents to her gynecologist with complaints of dyspareunia and localized vaginal pain. She also states having discomfort with walking, but denies any abnormal vaginal bleeding. She reports having a similar, but smaller, mass about 1 year ago that resolved on its own, and reports having a recent Papanicolaou smear approximately 6 months ago, which was normal. Temperature is 99.5°F, heart rate 78 beats/min, blood pressure 128/88 mm Hg, and respirations 16 breaths/min. There is a 3 × 4 cm mass protruding from the labia majora, just external to the hymenal ring. What is the next appropriate step in management of this patient?

A. Antibiotic therapy

B. Biopsy mass

C. Excision of mass and labia, and laboratory analysis

D. Incision and drainage

E. Warm compresses and sitz baths

603. A 39-year-old G3P2103 has just given birth to a healthy 3800-g boy by cesarean section. On postpartum day 2 she begins complaining of chills and pelvic discomfort. Her temperature is 38.2°C, blood oxygen saturation 97%, and respiratory rate 14 breaths/min. She has no marked breast tenderness or costovertebral angle tenderness. Her abdominal incision is without signs of infection. Bimanual examination result is positive for uterine tenderness. Results of laboratory studies are shown below:

Leukocyte count and differential

Leukocyte count	19,000/mm³
Segmented neutrophils	75%
Bands	7%
Eosinophils	3%
Basophils	1%
Lymphocytes	27%
Monocytes	4%

What is the most appropriate next step in this patient's evaluation and treatment?

A. Begin empiric antibiotic treatment with ampicillin and gentimicin

B. Begin triple antibiotic therapy with ampicillin, gentimicin, and clindamycin

C. Obtain aerobic and anaerobic cultures of blood, endocervix, and uterine cavity, as well as a catheterized urine specimen

D. Perform helical CT scan of chest

E. Surgical exploration of the uterine cavity

604. A 35-year-old woman with mental retardation and angiofibromas of the face is brought to the emergency department for evaluation of unexplained seizures. Physical examination reveals an ash-leaf hypopigmented macule on her back as well as yellowish thickenings of the skin over the lumbosacral region. MRI scan reveals hydrocephalus from obstruction of the foramen of Monroe from a benign giant cell astrocytoma. What is the most likely diagnosis?

A. Central nervous system lymphoma

B. Craniopharyngioma

C. Neurofibromatosis type 2

D. Tuberous sclerosis

E. von Hippel-Lindau syndrome

605. A 20-month-old girl is brought to the pediatric clinic by her parents because she has been increasingly socially withdrawn and has become clumsy. In the past several months she has been less interested in talking to her parents and friends. Her parents have also noticed that she has begun to "walk funny," and she is wringing her hands frequently. Looking at her chart, you find that her birth and developmental history are completely normal up until a few months ago. Her head circumference at birth was in the fifty-fourth percentile, but currently her head circumference is in the third percentile for her age. Physical examination reveals poorly coordinated gait. She does not speak during the course of the visit. What is the most likely diagnosis?

A. Asperger disorder

B. Autistic disorder

C. Childhood disintegrative disorder

D. Mental retardation

E. Rett disorder

606. A boy is brought to his pediatrician for a well-baby evaluation. His birth history is unremarkable. Physical examination findings of the heart, lungs, and abdomen are within normal limits. Genital examination reveals descended testicles and a small reactive hydrocele on the right side. The boy can now walk up and down steps without assistance from his nanny. He is also able to climb on furniture. What is his approximate age?

A. 18 months

B. 24 months

C. 36 months

D. 48 months

E. 60 months

The response options for items 607 and 608 are the same. You will be required to select one answer for each item in the set.

A. Bacteremia

B. Refractory shock

C. Sepsis

D. Sepsis syndrome

E. Septicemia

F. Septic shock

G. Tuberculosis

H. Viral syndrome

I. Uremia

For each patient with fever, select the most likely diagnosis.

607. A 29-year-old man with a history of inflammatory bowel disease underwent small bowel resection 2 days ago. His prior surgical history is notable for anal fistulectomy and fulgeration of urethral valves as a child. He now has a temperature of 102°F, pulse of 88 beats/min, respirations of 14 breaths/min, and blood pressure of 140/70 mm Hg. Blood cultures are drawn and reveal gram-negative rods in both aerobic and anaerobic bottles.

608. A 77-year-old man with a history of myocardial infarction and cerebrovascular accident has been intubated for 3 weeks in the intensive care unit. His vital signs are as follows: temperature 102°F, blood pressure 96/60 mm Hg, pulse 128 beats/min, and respirations 12 breaths/min on a ventilator. Urine output has been 0.2 mL/kg/h over the past 6 hours and serum lactate 5.0 mg/dL. Blood cultures have been drawn, but the results are not available yet.

609. A 53-year-old man is diagnosed with hepatocellular carcinoma following development of alcoholic cirrhosis. He is treated with cryotherapy to ablate a 3.5-cm tumor. The procedure is uneventful and he has no complications in the postoperative period. What is the most appropriate regimen to monitor this patient for possible recurrence?

A. Monitor alpha-fetoprotein (AFP)

B. Monitor human chorionic gonadotropin (hCG)

C. Monitor 5-hydroxyindole acetic acid (5-HIAA)

D. Monitor CA-125

E. Monitor carcinoembryonic antigen (CEA)

610. A 38-year-old obese woman undergoes a radical hysterectomy for intractable uterine bleeding because of fibroids. On postoperative day 3 she complains of an inability to adduct her right thigh. Physical examination of the heart, lungs, and abdomen are unremarkable. The abdominal wound is clean, dry, and intact. Physical examination of the legs reveals no obvious abnormality other than loss of power in internal and external rotation of the right thigh. What is the most likely explanation for these findings?

A. Injury to the genitofemoral nerve

B. Injury to the hypogastric plexus

C. Injury to the obturator nerve

D. Injury to the sacral plexus

E. Injury to the sciatic nerve

611. An elderly Asian patient presents to the emergency room because of severe pain in her left eye. She also complains of blurred vision. Physical examination reveals that her left pupil is larger than the right and does not react to light. The eye is inflamed and on palpation feels firm. Ophthalmology consultation is ordered. What aspect of the physical examination should be avoided in this patient?

A. Assessing visual acuity

B. Dilating the pupils

C. Everting the eyelids

D. Performing a funduscopic examination

E. Testing for a near reaction

612. A 32-year-old woman with mitral valve prolapse without regurgitation is about to undergo wisdom tooth extraction. She has no other prior medical or surgical history. She has no known allergies. Physical examination of the heart reveals no evidence of murmur. What is the appropriate prophylactic treatment for this patient?

A. Amoxicillin

B. Clindamycin

C. Cefazolin

D. Vancomycin

E. No treatment is needed

613. A 55-year-old man who works as a shipbuilder complains of a 6-month history of progressive dyspnea and dry cough. He also complains of fatigue, anorexia, and a 5-pound weight loss over the past 3 months. Physical examination of the heart is within normal limits. Pulmonary auscultation reveals late inspiratory crackles at the posterior lung bases. Abdominal examination is within normal limits. Chest x-ray reveals diffuse reticulonodular markings prominent in the lower lung zones. Laboratory studies are shown below:

Blood, plasma, serum

Alanine aminotransferase (ALT)	13 U/L
Amylase, serum	55 U/L
Aspartate aminotransferase (AST)	18 U/L
Calcium, serum	9.2 mg/dL
Glucose, serum	110 mg/dL
Hematocrit	39%
Urea nitrogen, serum (BUN)	12 mg/dL

Urinalysis

Urine pH	6.5
RBC count	1/HPF
WBC count	0/HPF
Nitrates	Negative
Bacteria	Negative

The physician elects to perform pulmonary function tests in this patient. Which of the following findings would be most likely?

A. Decreased total lung capacity

B. Increased forced expiratory volume

C. Increased residual volume

D. Increased vital capacity

E. Unchanged vital capacity

614. A 67-year-old diabetic man has recently been placed on the kidney transplant list. A kidney is found that is an ABO group match and has satisfactory HLA histocompatability. A serum cross-match is completed and no reaction was detected. Which of the following tests performed should receive highest priority, be done first, and is an absolute contraindication to transplantation if abnormal?

A. ABO group matching

B. HLA histocompatability

C. Serum cross-match test

D. Serum cross-match test and HLA compatibility are equally weighted in terms of transplant eligibility

E. Serum cross-match test, HLA compatibility, and ABO group matching—any abnormal result in any of the tests is a contraindication to transplantation

615. A 22-year-old obese woman presents for evaluation of amenorrhea. Her last full menstrual period was 9 months ago, but she has been having intermittent vaginal spotting for the past 6 months. She is sexually active with multiple partners. She uses birth control on some occasions. Physical examination of the heart and lungs are within normal limits. Abdominal examination reveals a fundal height palpable at the ensiform cartilage. Urine beta human chorionic gonadotropin (beta-hCG) is positive. Serum beta-hCG is sent off to the laboratory. Which of the following is the best estimate of gestational age?

A. 8 weeks

B. 12 weeks

C. 16 weeks

D. 20 weeks

E. 36 weeks

616. A 10-year-old boy is hospitalized in the pediatric ward because of diabetic ketoacidosis. He is clinically stable and looks to be improving. Most recent laboratory studies show a serum sodium of 132 mEq/L and serum glucose of 550 mg/dL. Review of laboratory studies obtained yesterday shows that the serum glucose was 150 mg/dL. What is the most appropriate next step in the treatment of this patient?

A. Observation

B. Salt administration

C. Salt restriction

D. Water administration

E. Water restriction

617. A 32-year-old male Peace Corps worker presents to his primary care physician with severe headache, fever, shaking chills, cough, and fatigue. He has just returned from a 2-week mission in Africa. He has felt weak for the past few days. Physical examination reveals profuse sweating, tachycardia, splenomegaly, and lymphadenopathy. Laboratory studies reveal anemia, thrombocytopenia, hyperbilirubinemia, and hypoglycemia. What is the most appropriate next step in the evaluation?

A. Chest x-ray

B. CT of the brain

C. Enzyme-linked immunosorbent assay (ELISA)

D. Giemsa-stained thick and thin peripheral blood smears

E. No further evaluation is necessary. Treat with chloroquine

618. A 75-year-old female presents to the clinic with her daughter. Her daughter complains that her mother began seeing "pink dogs coming out of the walls" a few days ago. The daughter brings her mother's medications in a bag. She takes medications for blood pressure, heart, arthritis, stomach, depression and insomnia. Her current medications include: hydrochlorothiazide, propranolol, digoxin, ibuprofen, cimetidine, Maalox, amitryptiline and triazolam. Physical examination reveals that the patient is agitated and confused. She is pointing to the ceiling and yelling "get the pink dogs." Cardiac examination reveals a grade III/VI systolic ejection murmur at the left sternal border. What is the most likely explanation for these findings?

A. Cimetidine

B. Digoxin

C. Hydrochlorothiazide

D. Ibuprofen

E. Propranolol

619. A 60-year-old woman presents to her primary care physician with a 1-month history of anorexia, weight loss, lethargy, and abdominal distention. She also complains of abdominal pain but cannot localize it to any particular area. She is postmenopausal. Physical examination reveals that the patient is cachectic and has less than normal muscle bulk and tone. She has diffuse abdominal tenderness to palpation with more on the right than the left. An adnexal mass is palpated on the right side. Laboratory evaluation shows an elevated CA-125 level and a decreased albumin level. Pelvic ultrasonography is performed (Figure 619). What is the next best step?

Figure 619

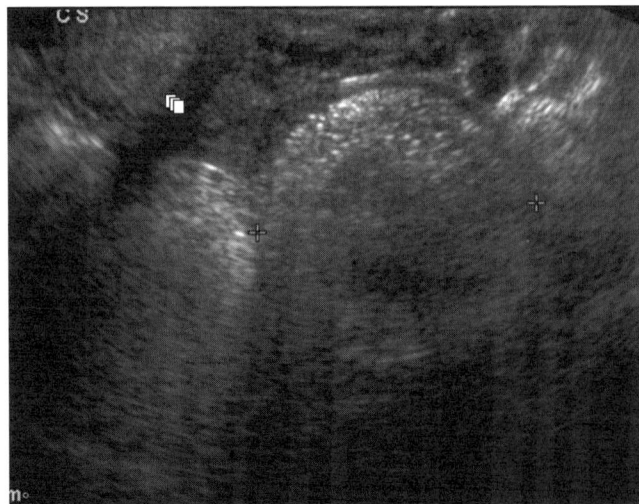

A. Abdominal hysterectomy and bilateral salpingo-oophorectomy

B. Serial CA-125 levels at 3, 6, 9, and 12 months

C. Serial pelvic examinations at 3, 6, 9, and 12 months

D. Surgical laparotomy

E. Ultrasonography at 3, 6, 9, and 12 months

620. A 50-year-old female secretary presents to her primary care physician with a chief complaint of cough. She has recently had a purified protein derivative (PPD) test for her job as a health professional. Findings were negative. Physical examination reveals that she is afebrile with stable vital signs. Pulmonary auscultation reveals crackles in upper zones of the lungs during auscultation. Chest x-ray reveals a diffuse interstitial pattern in the upper lung zones bilaterally as well as hilar and paratracheal adenopathy. There is no evidence of decreased lung volumes and cardiomegaly on the chest x-ray. What is the most likely diagnosis?

A. Asbestosis

B. Blastomycosis

C. Sarcoidosis

D. Silicosis

E. Tuberculosis

621. A 25-year-old black man presents to the emergency department with a 2-day history of neck pain, fever, and difficulty swallowing. Temperature is 101.7°F, pulse 118 beats/min, respirations 24 breaths/min, and blood pressure 122/65 mm Hg. Physical examination reveals decreased range of motion of the neck, cervical lymphadenopathy, and pharyngeal edema. Lateral neck x-rays show an increased retropharyngeal space. CT scan of the neck demonstrates a hypodense lesion in the retropharyngeal space with peripheral ring enhancement. What is the best treatment for this patient?

A. Cricothyrotomy

B. Endotracheal intubation

C. Incision and drainage

D. Nasopharyngolaryngoscopy

E. Tracheostomy

622. A 79-year-old man with an unknown prior medical history is brought to the emergency department by paramedics. He is comatose. Blood pressure is 96/60 mm Hg and pulse is 90 beats/min. Physical examination findings of the heart and lungs are unremarkable. Paralysis of all extremities is noted. Paralysis of conjugate lateral and vertical gaze is noted along with vertical nystagmus bilaterally. Which of the following is the most likely diagnosis?

A. Basilar artery syndrome

B. Medullary syndrome (unilateral)

C. Infarction of the cerebellar peduncle

D. Infarction of the medial lemniscus

E. Pontine syndrome (unilateral)

623. A 6-year-old boy is undergoing treatment for acute lymphocytic leukemia (ALL). He has just completed a 4-week course of induction chemotherapy consisting of prednisone, vincristine, and L-asparaginase. What is the next step in the treatment of this patient?

A. Bone marrow transplantation

B. Chemotherapy over the next 2 years

C. Intrathecal methotrexate

D. Intravenous antibiotics

E. Observation only

624. A 25-year-old woman who is 14 weeks pregnant with her second child presents for a pulmonary evaluation at the request of her primary care physician. She suffers from acute asthma attacks and has required intubation once secondary to a severe attack precipitated by a food intolerance. Physical examination findings of the heart and abdomen are within normal limits. Which of the following physiologic processes might be expected to increase during pregnancy?

A. Blood pressure

B. Creatinine

C. Free thyroxine

D. Minute ventilation

E. pco_2

625. A 5-year-old boy with gait abnormality presents for evaluation. He complains of fever, pain, and tenderness over the left femur. Massive soft tissue edema and induration are noted. Physical examination reveals tenderness and soft tissue swelling over the lateral aspect of the left femur. The right femur is without erythema, edema, or mass lesion. Biopsy reveals small blue, round cells with little cytoplasm and abundant glycogen. Which of the following is the most appropriate treatment for this patient?

A. Antibiotics (intravenous)

B. Antibiotics (oral)

C. Multiagent chemotherapy and radiation

D. Surgical excision

E. Surgical excision and pelvic reconstruction

626. A 27-year-old man presents to the ambulatory care clinic with a 1-week history of penile discharge. After further questioning and laboratory tests, he is diagnosed with gonorrhea. Due to the history of a sexually transmitted disease he is tested for other diseases. Laboratory values are as follows:

Rapid plasma reagin	Negative
Gram stain for *Chlamydia*	Positive
Hepatitis B surface antigen (HBsAg)	Negative
Hepatitis B surface antibody (HBsAb)	Positive
Hepatitis B core antigen (HBcAg)	Negative
Hepatitis B core antibody (HBcAb)	Negative
Hepatitis B e antigen (HBeAg)	Negative
Hepatitis B e antibody (HBeAb)	Negative
Hepatitis D antigen (HDAg)	Negative

What is the most likely diagnosis?

A. Acute hepatitis B
B. Chronic hepatitis B
C. Hepatitis D infection
D. Patient has hepatitis B vaccine
E. Prior hepatitis B infection now resolved

627. A 14-year-old boy is seen in the pediatric clinic for a follow-up visit. His parents are concerned because Joseph is unable to form friendships at school. While in your office, he only reluctantly answers your questions. He says he wants to go home and watch television. His mother says he has never had any friends, and that he has frequent outbursts of anger at home. "He just doesn't seem to be happy with his family," she says. Joseph is enthralled with a drawer in the examination room and pulls it out repeatedly. What is the most likely diagnosis?

A. Asperger disorder
B. Autistic disorder
C. Pervasive development disorder
D. Schizoid personality disorder
E. Tourette disorder

628. A 16-year-old high school boy is brought to the emergency department 3 hours after suffering an injury during football practice. The patient was tackled from behind and his helmet became dislodged. He then complained of right ear pain and swelling. No pressure dressing was applied by either school officials or ambulance attendants. Physical examination reveals erythema and edema of the right helix, tragus, and antitragus. Otoscopy of the right ear reveals fresh blood within the external auditory canal. The tympanic membrane is intact and moves well to pneumatic otoscopy. The left ear is without deformity. Otoscopy of the left ear reveals a small area of tympanosclerosis without effusion. Which of the following is the most appropriate treatment for this individual?

A. Amoxicillin
B. Corticosteroids

C. Needle aspiration and application of a pressure dressing
D. Pressure dressing, admission to the hospital for observation
E. Surgical exploration with Robinson catheter drainage

629. A 3-week-old boy is brought to the emergency department by his parents, who complain that he is not keeping any of his feeds down. He continually vomits his formula across the room within minutes of his feeds. His parents state that he has lost weight since birth. He has been playful at home and has not had any recorded fevers. What is the most appropriate next step in the evaluation of this patient?

A. Abdominal flat and upright plain films
B. Colonoscopy
C. CT scan of the abdomen/pelvis
D. Ultrasonography of the pylorus
E. Upper gastrointestinal endoscopy

The response options for items 630 and 631 are the same. You will be required to select one answer for each item in the set.

A. Atrial septal defect
B. Coarctation of the aorta
C. Congenital mitral stenosis
D. Ebstein anomaly
E. Eisenmenger syndrome
F. Hypoplastic left heart syndrome
G. Pulmonary atresia
H. Tetrology of Fallot
I. Transposition of the great vessels
J. Ventricular septal defect

For each child with cardiac symptomatology, select the appropriate associated condition.

630. A 3-year-boy is brought to the pediatrician for evaluation. He has difficulty at day care because he gets tired easily and cannot participate in all activities. Physical examination reveals a pulmonic ejection murmur audible at the left sternal border. The wide splitting of the second heart sound is noted, as is a soft, middiastolic rumble. Pulmonary evaluation reveals soft wheezes scattered in both lung bases. Results of laboratory studies are shown below:

Urinalysis

Urine pH	6.0
RBC count	0/HPF
WBC count	1/HPF
Nitrates	Negative
Bacteria	Negative
Color	Yellow

631. A 9-month-old boy with failure to thrive and poor feeding is brought to his pediatrician for evaluation. Physical examination reveals decreased blood pressure in both legs as compared with both arms. Cardiac evaluation reveals a systolic murmur heard best at the left sternal border that radiates to the back. Femoral pulse pressures feel weak bilaterally.

632. A 44-year-old woman with a history of breast carcinoma underwent a left segmental mastectomy 3 years ago. In the past 3 months she has noted induration of tissue in her right axilla. She is scheduled to undergo a right axillary lymph node dissection. Which lymph nodes provide the majority of lymphatic drainage of the breast?

    A. Axillary

    B. Interpectoral

    C. Internal mammary

    D. Supraclavicular

    E. Thoracic

633. A 19-year-old man is brought in to the emergency department by his parents after he began shouting at the family dog. He is insisting that the dog is actually an alien, planted here to spy on him. He sometimes hears the aliens' conversations in his head. You learn from talking with his parents that the boy has previously performed very well academically, but for the past few months his grades have been declining, and about 7 months ago he started to become suspicious of the dog. He has also become more and more reclusive recently, spending lots of time in his room, and has not been going out with friends as much. Physical examination reveals that the boy appears confused, and his speech is disorganized and at times incoherent. He is lying comfortably on the bed. Results of a urine toxicology screen are negative. What is the most appropriate next step in this patient's treatment?

    A. Clozapine

    B. Diazepam

    C. Haloperidol

    D. Psychotherapy

    E. Reassurance and follow-up with psychiatry

634. A 53-year-old man has been having intermittent chest pain for the past 3 months. He describes it as a deep substernal pain that lasts 35 minutes and then resolves. This episode occurs a couple of times a week. He presents to his primary care physician for further evaluation. He has a family history of coronary artery disease. He is generally healthy for his age and eats healthy and exercises daily without exertional chest pain. Physical examination findings of the heart, lungs, and abdomen are noncontributory. A stress test and upper gastrointestinal endoscopy were performed and results were normal. What is the next best step in the evaluation of this patient?

    A. CT of the chest

    B. Esophageal motility test

    C. MRI of the chest

    D. pH probe

    E. Upper gastrointestinal series

635. A 48-year-old man has had a lump on his left groin for the past 2 years and presents to his primary care physician because he can usually "push the lump back" but now he can't move the lump. He has increased pain around the mass. There is increasing erythema of the mass. He was lifting 50 pound crates when he noticed the mass today. Examination reveals an afebrile male in obvious pain with a nonreducible mass in his left groin. What is the next step in the management of this patient?

    A. Immediate surgical exploration for hernia reduction

    B. Hospital admission, observation, and serial abdominal examinations

    C. Narcotics to control his pain and follow-up in 1 week

    D. Narcotics, local anesthetics to try to reduce his hernia; if unsuccessful, then take the patient for surgical exploration

    E. Watchful waiting; send the patient home with an abdominal binder

636. A 14-month-old boy is brought to a pediatrician for a new patient evaluation. His parents are new to this community and are seeking care for their child. The boy has had a long history of difficulty walking. Physical examination reveals the left forefoot is rotated 90 degrees in all planes. A deep crease is present on the medial border of the foot, and range of motion is limited in all planes. Leg muscles are underdeveloped. X-ray studies reveal abnormal parallelism of the left talus and calcaneus. What is the most appropriate first-line treatment for this patient?

    A. Casting

    B. Exercises to increase stretch

    C. Orthotic shoes

    D. Surgical lysis and amputation

    E. Watchful waiting

637. A 33-year-old woman presents to her gynecologist at 10 weeks' gestation. She has no prior surgical history. She has a history of hypertension and is treated with amiloramide. Blood pressure is 125/85 mm Hg. What is the most appropriate treatment for this patient?

    A. Begin atenolol, stop amiloramide

    B. Begin methyldopa, stop amiloramide

    C. Continue amiloramide

    D. Stop amiloramide

    E. Watchful waiting

638. A 63-year-old woman presents to her primary care physician because of a chronic, erythematous, scaly and oozing rash of her right breast involving the nipple. She has no prior medical or surgical history. There is no palpable mass, and mammography showed no suspicious lesions. What is the most appropriate next step in the management of this patient?

    A. Advise her to change her detergent since this is likely an allergic reaction

    B. Biopsy the lesion

    C. Oral therapy with vitamin E and topical aloe vera cream

    D. Referral to a dermatologist

    E. Topical therapy with 5-fluorouracil

639. A 12-year-old boy with a history of diabetes mellitus is brought to his pediatrician for a follow-up examination. He is currently taking glucophage. He has no prior surgical history. Physical examination findings of the heart, lungs, and abdomen are within normal limits. Glycosylated hemoglobin (A1C) levels are drawn and likely reflect the blood concentration of glucose during the preceding

    A. 4 hours

    B. 36 hours

    C. 7 days

    D. 30 days

    E. 60 days

640. An 18-year-old female junior university student is brought to the student health clinic by her roommate after an apparent suicide attempt. Physical examination findings of the heart, lungs, and abdomen are unremarkable. She is alert, awake, and oriented but smells of alcohol on her breath. You attempt to assess the patient's risk for violence. Which of the following indicators is most suggestive of a patient that is at risk to undertake violent behavior?

    A. Age over 25 years

    B. Good impulse control

    C. Few social supports

    D. Past history of anorexia nervosa

    E. Upper socioeconomic status

641. A 41-year-old man presents with the sudden onset of dyspnea. He recently returned home on a 10-hour bus ride. While walking to his door he had the sudden onset of dyspnea, began sweating, and then collapsed. Inside, his wife immediately called 911. In the emergency department, his vital signs are as follows: temperature 38.5°C, pulse 106 beats/min, blood pressure 128/88 mm Hg, and respiration rate 30 breaths/min. On examination, breath sounds are vesicular with no added sounds. Heart is tachycardic with no murmur, rubs, or gallops. The ECG is shown below (Figure 641). What is the best next step in the management of this patient?

    A. Aspirin

    B. Celecoxib

    C. Heparin

    D. Placement of inferior vena cava filter

    E. Warfarin

642. A 25-year-old G1P0 woman presents to the primary care clinic. She is new to this community and states that she is pregnant. She has not had any prenatal care and states that she "is past her due date." She wants to be admitted to the hospital for labor induction. Postterm pregnancy is defined as how many days of gestation?

    A. 240

    B. 250

    C. 270

    D. 290

    E. This information is not possible to determine

643. A 28-year-old man presents to the emergency department after a motor vehicle accident in which he was not wearing his seatbelt and was thrown from the car. Past history is significant for asthma. Family history is positive for coronary artery disease, and his father died from a heart attack at the age of 45. Physical examination in the emergency depart-

Figure 641

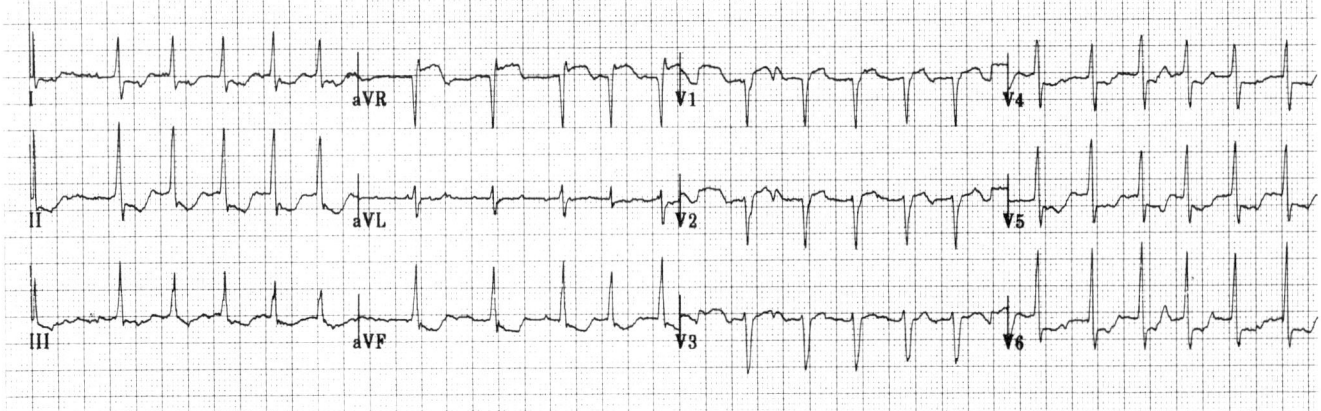

ment reveals vital signs as follows: blood pressure 82/46 mm Hg, heart rate 155 beats/min, and temperature of 98.0°F. The patient is unconscious with a fixed, dilated left pupil, and no external signs of bleeding. Neck veins are nondistended. What is most appropriate next step in the management of this patient?

A. Brain MRI
B. Brain CT
C. Fluid resuscitation
D. Peritoneal lavage
E. Watchful waiting and follow-up neurologic examination

644. A 59-year-old man is brought to his primary care physician for evaluation of progressive mental status changes. His wife states that although he has had gait abnormalities for several months, during the past 3 weeks his cognition has become impaired and his short-term memory has become clouded. He has a history of hypertension and coronary artery disease. Physical examination findings of the heart, lungs, and abdomen are within normal limits. What is the most appropriate treatment for this patient?

A. Further identification of the cause
B. Imipramine
C. Prednisone
D. Thiamine
E. Tolterodine

645. A 3-year-old boy is brought to the pediatrician for evaluation of pruritus and perineal irritation. He has a prior medical history of recurrent otitis media infections. Past surgical history is unremarkable. Physical examination of the anorectum reveals a whitish yellow thread. Microscopic evaluation of adhesive tape applied to the anorectum reveals the presence of eggs. What is the most appropriate treatment for this patient?

A. Amoxicillin
B. Erythromycin
C. Mebendazole
D. Metronidazole
E. Trimethoprim

646. A 47-year-old Asian man complains of a 1-year history of erectile dysfunction. His past medical history is significant for hypertension and bipolar disorder. He also admits to a 30 pack/year history of smoking. He states that his wife has recently cheated on him with a 26-year-old man. He complains of having difficulty obtaining an erection and achieving an orgasm, climax, and ejaculation. Physical examination findings of the heart, lungs, and abdomen are unremarkable. The testes are descended bilaterally and are without masses. The prostate is 30 g in size and is smooth and without nodules. Results of laboratory studies are shown below:

Testosterone, serum	375 mg/dL
Glucose, serum	111 mg/dL
Cholesterol, serum	218 mg/dL
Triiodothyronine, serum	0.4 ng/dL
Thyroxine, serum	8 µg/dL
Triglycerides, serum	100 mg/dL
Prostate-specific antigen	2 ng/mL
Penile duplex ultrasonography	No arterial narrowing
Nocturnal Penile Tumescence (NPT) test	Positive

What is the most appropriate treatment?

A. External vacuum device to produce an erection
B. Hormone replacement therapy
C. Injection therapy with papaverine
D. Sexual counseling
E. Slidenafil citrate

647. A 25-year-old woman presents to her primary care physician for evaluation of chronic pelvic pain and urinary frequency. She voids 25 times per day and 4 times per night with a weak force of stream. She also has chronic pelvic pain. She has been evaluated by numerous physicians and all are baffled by her complaints. Her current medications include trimethoprim, Xanax, ibuprofen, and Celebrex. She complains of numerous urinary tract infections, but review of her records indicates that all urine cultures are negative. Physical examination findings of the heart, lungs, and abdomen are unremarkable. Pelvic examination reveals no evidence of pelvic prolapse. She does have anterior vaginal wall tenderness. Urinalysis reveals trace microhematuria. Urine pregnancy test result is negative. What is the next most appropriate step in the evaluation of this patient?

A. Cystoscopy
B. Diagnostic laparoscopy
C. Hysteroscopy
D. MRI
E. Transvaginal ultrasonography

648. A 45-year-old man presents to his primary care physician as a new patient. He weighs 260 pounds, has a 40 pack/year history of smoking, and drinks one beer per day. He works in a local supermarket 12 hours a day, 6 days a week. He has no prior medical or surgical history. Physical examination reveals a blood pressure of 180/100 mm Hg, pulse of 86 beats/min, and respirations of 14 breaths/min. He is obese and appears to be his stated age. Physical examination findings of the heart, lungs, and abdomen are within normal limits. His blood pressure is rechecked three times and is still 180/100 mm Hg. What would be a realistic goal in terms of blood pressure reduction for this patient?

A. 160/100
B. 150/90
C. 140/90
D. 130/80
E. 120/80

649. A 51-year-old man is brought to the emergency department after being struck by a car while crossing the street. The patient is breathing on his own. Oxygen saturation is 95% on room air. Physical examination findings of the heart, lungs, and abdomen are within normal limits. He does have some pelvic instability and pain. An x-ray and CT scan reveal an open book fracture of the pelvis and a formed hematoma. Blood pressure has decreased to 90/55 mm Hg and heart rate has increased to 130 beats/min. The patient is started on intravenous fluids and transfused with 2 units of packed RBCs. Which of the following is the most appropriate next step in management?

   A. Admission to the hospital and repeat examination in a few hours
   B. Continue expectant management
   C. Drainage of the pelvic hematoma
   D. Surgical placement of an external fixator
   E. Upper and lower gastrointestinal endoscopy to determine bleeding source

650. A 6-year-old girl with mild mental retardation presents to the emergency department with a 3-day history of vomiting and abdominal pain. She is given intravenous fluids and admitted, but continues to vomit whenever she tries to drink anything. On endoscopy, a bezoar consisting of hair is found. The patient states that she has been eating strands of her own hair for the past 2 months. What is the patient's most likely DSM-IV diagnosis?

   A. Bulimia nervosa
   B. Enuresis
   C. Feeding disorder of early childhood
   D. Pica
   E. Rumination disorder

651. A 3-month-old boy who attends day care is noted by caretakers to be restless and feeding poorly during the past 24 hours. The infant is brought to the emergency department for evaluation. The child appears tired and vomits during the physical examination. Temperature (rectal) is 104.1°F. A bulging fontanel is palpable. Cardiovascular and pulmonary examination findings are within normal limits. Bowel sounds are normoactive and there is no evidence of rebound tenderness. Latex agglutination testing is positive. Good prognostic indicators for successful therapy of this child include

   A. Bacteria present in the cerebrospinal fluid
   B. Human immunodeficiency state
   C. Late-onset seizures
   D. Older age
   E. Presence of gram-negative enteric bacteremia

652. A 24-year-old female graduate student presents to her primary care physician for a routine examination. She has no prior medical or surgical history. She has a 10 pack/year history of cigarette smoking. Physical examination reveals moderately thick, vaginal discharge. The vulva is normal. There is no discharge present at the introitus. However, there is some vaginal discharge that is white and curd-like. Secretion analysis reveals a pH of 4.0 and has no odor. Microscopic evaluation reveals epithelial cells. What is the most appropriate treatment for this patient?

   A. Ampicillin
   B. Cotrimazole
   C. Miconazole
   D. Tetracycline
   E. Watchful waiting

653. A 30-year-old woman presents to her primary care physician for a check-up. She has no major complaints. However, family history indicates that the patient's father had colon cancer at age 55. Results of recent laboratory studies are shown below:

Electrolytes, serum

Na, serum	138 mEq/L
Cl, serum	97 mEq/L
K, serum	3.8 mEq/L
Bicarbonate, serum	27 mEq/L
Magnesium, serum	1.8 mEq/L
Creatinine, serum	0.7 mg/dL

Leukocyte count and differential

Leukocyte count	6000/mm^3
Segmented neutrophils	55%
Bands	4%
Eosinophils	1%
Basophils	1%
Lymphocytes	24%
Monocytes	4%

Blood, plasma, serum

Alanine aminotransferase (ALT)	16 U/L
Amylase, serum	60 U/L
Aspartate aminotransferase (AST)	14 U/L
Calcium, serum	9.1 mg/dL
Glucose, serum	110 mg/dL
Hematocrit	39%
Urea nitrogen, serum (BUN)	10 mg/dL

Urinalysis

Urine pH	6.0
RBC count	2/HPF

WBC count	2/HPF
Nitrates	Negative
Bacteria	Negative

When should this patient be evaluated for colon cancer?

A. Immediately

B. Age 40

C. Age 45

D. Age 50

E. Age 55

654. A 65-year-old man presents to his primary care physician with a 2-month history of flushing, diarrhea, abdominal pain, 8-pound weight loss, and rectal bleeding. Barium swallow reveals a mass causing partial obstruction of the midgut. Physical examination of the heart reveals a blowing holosystolic ejection murmur. Examination of the lungs and abdomen are unremarkable. What is the next most appropriate diagnostic evaluation for this patient?

A. Erythrocyte sedimentation rate

B. HLA-B27 testing

C. Serum protein electrophoresis/urine protein electrophoresis (SPEP/UPEP)

D. Urinary 5-hydroxyindole acetic acid (5-HIAA)

E. 24-hour urine for vanilmandelic acid (VMA), and metanephrines or catecholamines

655. You are called for a consultation of a 16-year-old girl who has been admitted to the hospital following an automobile accident. Before you see the patient, you review her laboratory studies and note that her toxicology screen was positive for cannabinoids. As you walk into the room, you see both of her parents standing by her bed. The most appropriate next step in dealing with this patient is to:

A. Admit her to the substance abuse unit of the psychiatry ward

B. Ask her parents to leave the room

C. Ask her how long she has been using drugs

D. Explain to her that her urine test was positive for drugs

E. Perform a thorough physical examination

656. A 31-year-old G1P0 woman who tested positive by home pregnancy test presents for evaluation. She has a history of deep venous thrombosis and takes coumadin daily. Doppler ultrasonography reveals evidence of fetal heart tones. Abdominal examination reveals normoactive bowel sounds with a nonpalpable fundal height. Results of urine beta human chorionic gonadotropin testing in the office are positive. Which of the following is a possible fetal defect in this pregnancy?

A. Clear cell carcinoma of the vagina

B. Congenital heart disease

C. Nasal hypoplasia

D. Neonatal jaundice

E. Stained teeth

657. A 10-week-old female neonate was brought to her pediatrician for a routine clinical evaluation. The mother states that her baby is doing well. Vitals signs are as follows: temperature 36.4°C, pulse 135 beats/min, respirations 50 breaths/min, and blood pressure 85/55 mm Hg. Physical examination reveals that when the femur is flexed and adducted with posterior pressure applied, the neonate's left hip is displaced from the acetabulum. When the two flexed thighs are held together, asymmetric skin folds are detected. Plain radiographs of the pelvis reveal displacement of the femoral head out of the joint space and disruption of the Shenton line. What is the most appropriate next step in the treatment of this patient?

A. Brace that maintains hip flexion and abduction

B. Closed reduction under general anesthesia

C. No further treatment is required; this condition will resolve

D. Open reduction of the hip

E. Open reduction with pelvic osteotomy

658. A 51-year-old man with type 2 diabetes mellitus, depression, and chronic diarrhea presents to his primary care physician with postprandial epigastric pain that radiates to the back. He also notes decreased appetite and occasional unexplained pains in his legs that come and go over about 2 weeks on average. Physical examination reveals slight jaundice and a palpable gallbladder. What is the most likely diagnosis?

A. Acute cholecystitis

B. Choledocholithiasis

C. Hepatocellular carcinoma

D. Pancreatic carcinoma

E. Peptic ulcer

659. A 3-week-old boy is brought to the emergency department because of projectile vomiting of solids and liquids. Birth history is notable for a term delivery by cesarean section. Maternal history is positive for crack cocaine use. Physical examination of the heart and lungs are within normal limits. Examination of the abdomen reveals a palpable bulge in the midepigastrium. Abdominal sonography reveals a dilated gastric bulb and hypertrophy of the antrum. Which of the following is the most likely diagnosis?

A. Abscess formation

B. Chalasia

C. Esophagitis (viral)

D. Obstruction by foreign body

E. Pyloric stenosis

660. A 29-year-old woman with dysfunctional uterine bleeding for consecutive months undergoes diagnostic hysteroscopy with endometrial biopsy. She has no prior medical history. Preoperative physical examination reveals minimal anterior wall vaginal tenderness. Pelvic ultrasonography reveals a 3-cm right ovarian cyst. Pathology report from the endometrial biopsy reveals hypertrophy of endometrial glands and an increase in stromal ground substance. What is the most likely explanation for these findings?

A. Early proliferative endometrium

B. Late proliferative endometrium

C. Leiomyosarcoma

D. Botryoid sarcoma

E. Squamous cell carcinoma

661. Your 68-year-old history teacher from high school commits suicide. You think about the risk factors that you were taught in medical school for suicide, and you realize that he actually had a fairly high risk for trying to commit suicide. Some factors are listed in the table below. Please choose what will happen to the person's risk for committing suicide for each of the factors listed in Table 661.

A. Row A

B. Row B

C. Row C

D. Row D

E. Row E

662. A 28-year-old female lawyer who has been studying furiously for the bar examination presents to her primary care physician with the complaints of a sore throat, fatigue, swollen glands, and fever over the past three weeks. She states that she has not taken good care of herself recently because of her upcoming examinations. She notes a weight loss of 20 pounds. She has been self-medicating herself with caffeinated beverages to stay awake during her studies. She has no prior medical or surgical history. Temperature is 101.5°F, blood pressure 110/70 mm Hg, pulse 68 beats/min, and respirations 14 breaths/min. She has several cervical lymph nodes that are soft, rubbery, and tender. These nodes are located along the course of the sternocleidomastoid muscle bilaterally. The remainder of the physical examination is normal except for a liver span of 18 cm in the midax-

illary line. What is the next most appropriate step in the evaluation of this patient?

A. CT of the abdomen

B. CBC

C. Lymph node biopsy

D. MRI of the abdomen

E. Ultrasonography of the abdomen

663. A 55-year-old woman comes to her primary care physician for her annual examination. She reports no new problems. Past history is significant for asthma and hypertension. Physical examination reveals moderate fibrocystic changes in both breasts and a 2-cm localized thickening in the upper outer quadrant of the left breast. Mammography reveals fibrocystic changes in both breasts, but no masses or suspicious changes were seen. What is the next most appropriate step in the management of this patient?

A. Check CA-125 level

B. Consult surgery for a fine-needle aspiration

C. Follow-up in clinic if mass becomes larger or symptomatic

D. Mammography in 6 months

E. Tamoxifen therapy

664. A 60-year-old white man is asked to return to the clinic for a follow-up appointment after laboratory results are completed following a routine visit. The patient is being started on some new medications, so a CBC and liver enzyme panel are ordered along with cholesterol studies. After further questioning, the patient admits to a 10-pound weight loss and some fatigue over the past few months. Physical examination shows mild hepatosplenomegaly and generalized lymphadenopathy. Laboratory values are as follows:

WBC count	16×10^3/mL
	(32% lymphocytes)
Lymphocytes	32%
Neutrophils	60%
Basophils	0%
Eosinophils	1%
Monocytes	5%
Bands	2%
Hemoglobin	9 g/dL
Hematocrit	34%

Table 661

	INCREASING AGE	BEING CATHOLIC	HIGHER EDUCATION	HAVING A MENTAL ILLNESS	HAVING A TERMINAL ILLNESS
A.	Increased risk	Increased risk	Increased risk	Increased risk	Increased risk
B.	Increased risk	Decreased risk	Increased risk	Increased risk	Increased risk
C.	Increased risk	Decreased risk	Decreased risk	Increased risk	Increased risk
D.	Decreased risk	Decreased risk	Increased risk	Increased risk	Increased risk
E.	Increased risk	Decreased risk	Increased risk	Increased risk	Decreased risk

Cholesterol

Total	232
Low-density lipoprotein	150
High-density lipoprotein	42
Amylase	75 U/dL
Alkaline phosphatase	50 U/dL
Albumin	5.2 gm/dL

What is the most likely diagnosis?

A. Acute lymphoblastic leukemia

B. Acute myelogenous leukemia

C. Chronic lymphocytic leukemia

D. Chronic myelocytic leukemia

E. Myelodysplastic syndrome

665. Of 200 patients in a local community hospital, 50 have lung cancer. Of these 50 patients, 45 are smokers. Of the remaining 150 hospitalized patients who do not have lung cancer, 60 are smokers. What is the odds ratio for smoking and the risk for lung cancer?

A. 5

B. 13.5

C. 18.5

D. 45

E. 60

666. A 32-year-old woman presents for a health maintenance examination. She has no significant past medical history. She is a nonsmoker and she exercises once a week. Physical examination shows an oral temperature of 37.2°C, blood pressure of 178/100 mm Hg, heart rate of 80 beats/min, and respirations of 20 breaths/min. Renal angiography indicates renal artery stenosis on the right in a string of pearls pattern. Which of the following is the most likely treatment for this condition?

A. Angiotensin-converting enzyme inhibitors

B. Calcium channel blockers

C. Simvastatin

D. Trial of diet and exercise

E. No treatment is indicated

667. A 67-year-old woman with a history of congestive heart failure presents with increasing dyspnea and left lower extremity edema. Physical examination reveals that she is afebrile but breathing laboriously. There are crackles throughout the posterior chest. Her heart demonstrates a regular rate and rhythm with no murmur, rubs, or gallops. ECG is obtained (Figure 667). Which diuretic does she take for her congestive heart failure?

A. Acetazolamide

B. Ethacrynic acid

C. Furosemide

D. Hydrochlorothiazide

E. Spironolactone

668. A 25-year-old female G3PO presents to the emergency department with vaginal bleeding. She is approximately 3 months pregnant. She complains of mild cramps. Her previous two pregnancies ended in miscarriages. Physical examination of the heart, lungs and abdomen are within normal limits. Pelvic examination reveals evidence of aborted fetal tissue. Most of the placental tissue is present. What is the most appropriate course of action to take?

A. Antibiotic therapy

B. Corticosteroid infusion

C. Ergonovine infusion

D. Surgical intervention (dilation and curettage)

E. Watchful waiting with follow-up in 1 week

Figure 667

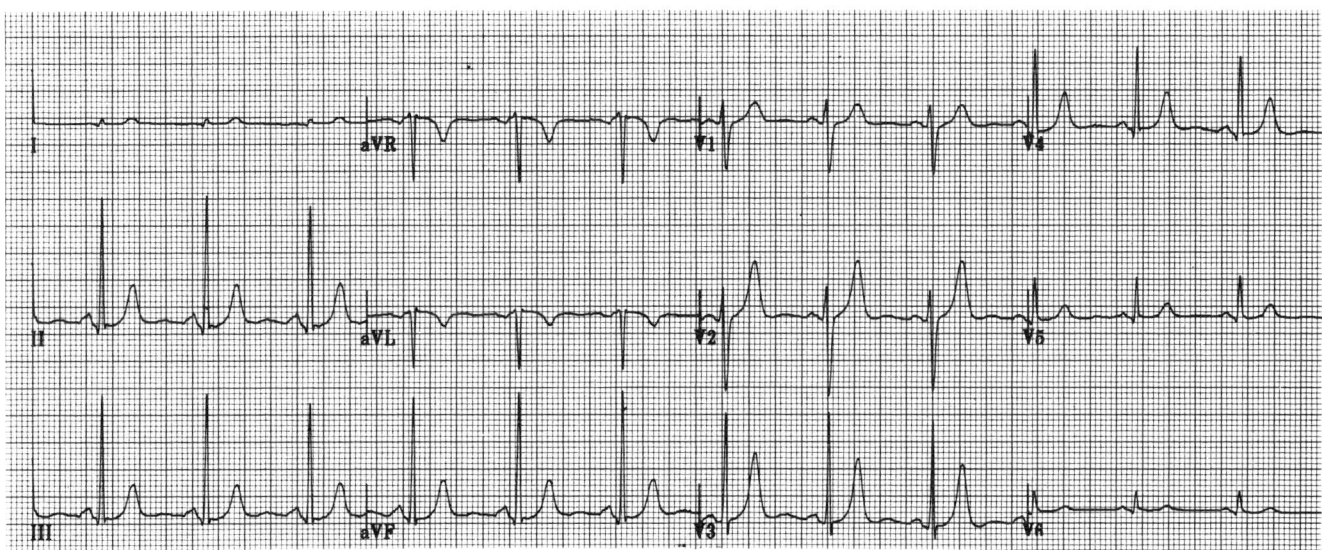

669. A 23-year-old man presents to the emergency department after being hit by a vehicle as he was walking across the street. He has a history of alcoholism and was coming home from a bar when he was hit. On arrival in the emergency department, blood pressure was 83/45 mm Hg, heart rate 130 beats/min, and respiratory rate 32 breaths/min. Intravenous fluids were started. The patient was agitated and showed no signs of external blood loss and was able to move all four extremities. Lungs were clear with normal breath sounds bilaterally, and abdomen was soft and nontender. X-ray findings of the cervical spine, chest, and pelvis were all normal. Hematocrit was 35% and his blood alcohol level was 430 mg/dL. After 30 minutes, blood pressure was 90/60 mm Hg, heart rate 125 beats/min, and respiratory rate 30 breaths/min. What is the most appropriate next step in the management of this patient?

A. Exploratory laparotomy
B. Diagnostic arteriography of the abdominal aorta
C. Diagnostic peritoneal lavage
D. Radiologic study (CT scan of chest)
E. Watchful waiting with decrease in intravenous fluids

670. A child with lower abdominal pain and bloody stools is brought to the emergency department for evaluation. The consulting surgeon orders a radiologic imaging study. A technetium 99 pertechnetate scan is performed, which may elucidate which of the following diagnoses?

A. Appendicitis
B. Hirschsprung disease
C. Malrotation
D. Meckel diverticulum
E. Pyloric stenosis

671. A 49-year-old man presents for evaluation of progressive right radial palsy. He also complains of intermittent flank pain. He denies history of trauma. His past medical history is unremarkable. Social history is remarkable for beer drinking of home-produced products. The home brew is stored in vessels and pipes. Physical examination reveals a decrease in sensation and motor function of the right wrist. There is no evidence of edema, erythema, or trauma. Examination of the abdomen is unremarkable. Which of the following is the most likely diagnosis?

A. Lead intoxication
B. Mercury intoxication
C. Methotrexate intoxication
D. Thallium intoxication
E. Vincristine neurotoxicity

672. A 72-year-old man with diabetes, hypertension, coronary artery disease, and a 110 pack/year smoking history presents to his primary care physician complaining of sharp epigastric pain every time he eats. The pain is so bad that he only eats one time per day. There is no radiation of the pain. Eating makes the pain worse, and the pain only presents when he eats. He has lost 30 pounds in the past

2 months. He gets nauseous when he eats but does not vomit. He does not have any diarrhea or constipation. What test would you order to confirm your diagnosis?

A. Barium swallow
B. CT scan of the abdomen/pelvis
C. Flat and upright plain films of the abdomen
D. Mesenteric angiography
E. Upper gastrointestinal endoscopy

673. A 40-year-old man is referred to his primary care physician for elevated liver function tests on routine laboratory studies obtained 3 months earlier. He denies having a family history of liver cancer, but has a history of intravenous drug use 20 years ago. Physical examination reveals splenomegaly and spider angioma. He has slight right upper quadrant pain on deep palpation. Results of laboratory studies are shown below:

Blood, plasma, serum

Alanine aminotransferase (ALT)	90 U/L
Amylase, serum	70 U/L
Aspartate aminotransferase (AST)	70 U/L
Calcium, serum	9 mg/dL
Glucose, serum	100 mg/dL
Albumin, serum	3.3 g/dL
Anti–hepatitis C virus	Positive

Which of the following statements is most correct?

A. A bone marrow biopsy should be performed secondary to thrombocytopenia
B. He is at considerable risk for hepatocellular cancer, and screening is advised
C. Hepatitis D is usually positive with hepatitis C
D. Liver biopsy is the next step in management
E. Splenectomy should be performed secondary to thrombocytopenia

674. A 17-year-old adolescent girl presents to her primary care physician for a health history and physical examination required by her school to participate in basketball. During the physician interview the patient confides that she has been sexually active for the past year. She complains of abdominal pain described as "crampy" mostly on the right side for the past 6 weeks during intercourse, and she reports having a vaginal discharge. Physical examination shows a temperature of 37.4°C and diffuse lower abdominal pain without rebound tenderness. Pelvic examination reveals a mucopurulent cervical discharge, cervical motion tenderness, and right-sided adnexal tenderness. Blood tests demonstrate leukocytosis, elevated C-reactive protein, and no evidence of pregnancy. What is the most appropriate course of management for this patient?

A. Patient should be admitted to hospital for direct observation and treated with cefoxitin until she is asymptomatic for 48 hours with a concomitant course of doxycycline for 14 days

B. Patient should undergo laparoscopy to obtain a definitive diagnosis of pathology and then management should subsequently begin based on findings

C. Patient should be screened for sexually transmitted diseases and placed on antiinflammatory treatments including low-dose corticosteroids to reduce the likelihood of fallopian tube adhesions until results of the screening are obtained

D. Patient should be treated with ceftriaxone and probenecid followed by a 14-day course of doxycycline and instruction to contact the office if no improvement is noted within 24 to 48 hours

E. Patient should be given approval to participate in softball but instructed to contact the clinic immediately if fever persists

675. A 42-year-old woman presents with fever, malaise, weight loss, and chronic sinusitis. She complains of a bloody nasal discharge. She reports dyspnea on exertion, and an occasional cough productive of blood-tinged sputum. The patient reports intermittent hematuria. These symptoms have been progressing over the past year or so. Physical examination reveals pain over the sinuses, nasal and oral ulcerations, tachypnea, and granulomatous skin lesions. Laboratory tests show an elevated erythrocyte sedimentation rate, leukocytosis, and anemia. Urinalysis reveals hematuria, proteinuria, and RBC casts. C-ANCA is positive. What is the most likely diagnosis?

A. Churg-Strauss syndrome

B. Giant cell arteritis

C. Polyarteritis nodosa

D. Takayasu arteritis

E. Wegener granulomatosis

676. A 39-year-old woman with cholelithiasis has multiple episodes of right upper quadrant pain associated with ingestion of a fatty meal. Physical examination findings of the heart, lungs, and abdomen are within normal limits. She desires to undergo a cholecystectomy in hopes of eliminating her symptoms of colic. She can choose either a laparoscopic or an open cholecystectomy. Should she choose to undergo a laparoscopic cholecystectomy, which of the following is the most likely postoperative complication she might encounter?

A. Adynamic ileus

B. Diarrhea

C. Foreign body–impacted stool bolus

D. Phlebitis

E. Residual lithiasis

677. A 52-year-old man is brought to the emergency department because of chest pain. He was shopping in the local mall for a gift for his wife. He collapsed but did not lose consciousness. He appears in the emergency department within 1 hour of the onset of his pain. He still has a heaviness in the midportion of his chest. He weighs 190 pounds, has a 40 pack/year history of smoking, and drinks excessively. Physical examination reveals a man who appears to be his stated age. His blood pressure is 160/100 mm Hg, pulse 110 beats/min, and respirations 16 breaths/min. ECG reveals a Q wave in leads II, III, and AVF as well as ST elevation in the same leads. What is the most appropriate treatment for this patient?

A. Admission and observation

B. Heparin infusion

C. Lidocaine infusion

D. Morphine infusion

E. Streptokinase infusion

678. A 37-year-old woman presents with right-sided nipple discharge. She has a prior medical history of interstitial cystitis and hypertension. Medications include pentosan polysulfate and atenolol. The discharge began spontaneously. It is green and sticky and is not related to her menstrual cycle. What is the most likely diagnosis?

A. Breast abscess

B. Duct ectasia

C. Intraductal papilloma

D. Pituitary adenoma

E. Tuberculosis

679. You have a patient in your psychiatric clinic who is always late to his appointments. You have repeatedly requested that he make efforts to be on time, but he has thus far responded by saying that it cannot be that bad—only 15 minutes late. When he says this, he reminds you of your ex-husband, who was always late for your dates. You begin to consider canceling this patient's appointments if he cannot be on time next week. What explains this thought process you have?

A. Countertransference

B. Projection

C. Reaction formation

D. Transference

E. Triangulation

The response options for items 680–683 are the same. You will be required to select one answer for each item in the set.

A. *Bacillus cereus*

B. Cholera

C. *Cryptosporidium*

D. *Giardia lamblia*

E. Norwalk viruses

F. *Rotavirus*

G. Shigellosis

H. *Vibrio cholerae* (mutant type)

I. *Vibrio parahemolyticus*

J. *Yersinia* species

For each entity listed above, select the appropriate patient who presents with diarrhea.

680. A 26-month-old boy has a 24-hour history of fever and vomiting. He is brought to the pediatric clinic on a cold January morning. He has had diarrhea five times per day for the past 4 days. Physical examination reveals dry mucous membranes. The child is crying during the examination but is unable to express tears. The abdominal examination is unremarkable. Stool is not palpable in the rectal vault.

681. A 13-year-old boy is brought to his pediatrician for evaluation of a chronic, intermittent history of diarrhea one to two times per day for the past 6 months. He states that several other classmates have similar symptoms and have consulted their doctors regarding care. Physical examination findings of the heart, lungs, and abdomen are unremarkable. Rectal examination reveals a small formed stool in the rectal vault.

682. A 5-year-old boy is brought to the emergency room with a 1-week history of fever and a 9-day history of diarrhea. The child attends day care, and several other children have had similar symptoms. He has dry skin and lips. Cardiac and pulmonary examination findings are within normal limits. Stool culture reveals fecal leukocytes and the presence of a nonmotile gram-negative rod. Results of other laboratory studies are shown below:

Leukocyte count and differential

Leukocyte count	13,000/mm^3
Segmented neutrophils	71%
Bands	5%
Eosinophils	3%
Basophils	2%
Lymphocytes	23%
Monocytes	4%

683. A 16-year-old boy goes with a group of friends to a sushi restaurant for a celebratory meal. Six hours later he and several others who attended the dinner complain of abdominal cramps, nausea, and vomiting. They also complain of bouts of watery diarrhea during the past 2 hours.

684. A 35-year-old woman presents with eczematous changes of the nipple of her right breast. She has a prior medical history of fibroadenoma of her right breast approximately 3 years ago. Physical examination reveals that the right nipple appears crusty and there is a bloody discharge coming from it. What is the most likely diagnosis?

A. Ductal carcinoma in situ
B. Inflammatory breast carcinoma
C. Infiltrating ductal carcinoma
D. Paget disease of the nipple
E. Tuberculosis

685. A 40-year-old woman arrives in the emergency department complaining of worsening shortness of breath. She admits to a 25 pack/year history of smoking. Physical examination

reveals distant S$_1$ and S$_2$ heart sounds without rubs or gallops. Breath sounds are decreased bilaterally. ECG reveals low voltage in all leads. Chest x-ray reveals an enlarged cardiac silhouette with unremarkable pulmonary vasculature. There is a linear hyperlucency along the left cardiac border. What is the most likely diagnosis?

A. Anxiety
B. Pneumothorax
C. Pneumomediastinum
D. Pneumopericardium
E. Tension pneumothorax

686. A 17-year-old girl presents to her primary care physician with a 6-month history of weight loss. Her body weight is 72% of what would be expected for her age and height. She appears emaciated and cachexic. You learn from speaking to her that she feels that she is "fat" and is afraid of gaining weight because she will "look like a hog." Her last menstrual period was 4 months ago. You learn from her parents that she has been caught on many occasions using laxatives inappropriately to purge herself after a meal. What is the most likely diagnosis?

A. Anorexia nervosa
B. Body dysmorphic disorder
C. Bulimia
D. Superior mesenteric artery syndrome
E. The patient does not fit criteria for any of the above diagnoses

687. A 37-year-old obese man with hypertension presents for an annual examination. He has no new complaints. His current medications include hydrochlorothiazide and propranolol. Family history is negative for coronary artery disease, hypertension, and diabetes mellitus. Physical examination reveals a blood pressure of 140/80 mm Hg, pulse of 80 beats/min, and respirations of 12 breaths/min. Cardiac, pulmonary, and abdominal examination findings are within normal limits. Random cholesterol is 244 mg. What is the most appropriate treatment for this patient?

A. Cholestipol
B. Dietary modification
C. Gemfibrozil
D. Lovastatin
E. Nicotinic acid

688. A 2-week-old newborn is brought to the pediatric clinic because of fever to 103°F. Maternal and birth history are remarkable for a term birth at 37 weeks by spontaneous vaginal delivery. Prenatal care was uneventful. Otologic examination reveals erythema and effusion of the right tympanic membrane. Pneumatic otoscopy of the right ear reveals decreased mobility and on the left reveals a tympanic membrane that moves well. The left tympanic membrane is without erythema or effusion. Results of laboratory studies are as follows:

Electrolytes, serum

Na, serum	143 mEq/L
Cl, serum	100 mEq/L
K, serum	3.7 mEq/L
Bicarbonate, serum	24 mEq/L
Creatinine, serum	0.3 mg/dL

Leukocyte count and differential

Leukocyte count	18,000/mm^3
Segmented neutrophils	75%
Bands	7%
Eosinophils	2%
Basophils	1%
Lymphocytes	27%
Monocytes	4%

Urinalysis

Urine pH	6.0
RBC count	2/HPF
WBC count	2/HPF

Which of the following is the most appropriate disposition and treatment plan for this child?

A. Hospital admission

B. Oral outpatient antibiotic therapy

C. Outpatient observation

D. Percutaneous antibiotics administered at home

E. Watchful waiting

689. A 19-year-old G1P0 woman is being followed by her gynecologist for a small-for-gestational-age baby. She is at 34 weeks' gestation and has noticed decreased fetal movements for the past 2 days. Her score is 4/10 on a biophysical profile. Blood pressure is 160/100 mm Hg. An oxytocin challenge is administered and reveals deep decelerations. What is the most appropriate intervention for this patient and her baby?

A. Bed rest, antihypertensive agents, and periodic reevaluation

B. Cesarean section

C. Furosemide infusion

D. Oxcytocin infusion

E. Prostaglandin gel

690. A 40-year-old man is brought to the emergency department by his wife because has been acting strange lately. Over the past month, he has become increasingly irritable, angry, and suspicious. He has not slept in the past 4 nights and was found in the garage working on his laptop computer. He states that God has made him the new leader of computer development at his company. He thinks that his work might be stolen by leaders of other countries and has tried to hide his work in books written in Japanese. He has also changed his appearance in the past 2 weeks. He now wears a long overcoat, sunglasses, and a top hat. He states that his attire will help elude others from stealing his ideas. During the interview with the physician, he paces the floor and makes an advance at a nurse assistant who walks into the room. The patient has never had a drug or alcohol dependency problem. What is the most likely diagnosis?

A. Adult-onset brain attention deficit disorder

B. Mania

C. Organic brain syndrome

D. Schizoaffective disorder

E. Schizophrenia, paranoid type

691. A 7-year-old girl presents to her primary care physician with a right abdominal mass. The child's mother noticed the mass while dressing her this morning. She has no other complaints. Her past medical history is significant only for rheumatic fever at age 3. Physical examination reveals that she is thin and appears her stated age. She is afebrile and vital signs are stable. Abdomen is nontender with normoactive bowel sounds throughout. A mass is palpated in the right lower adnexa but exhibits no tenderness. Transabdominal ultrasonography of the pelvis is ordered (Figure 692). What is the next best step in the treatment of this patient?

Figure 691

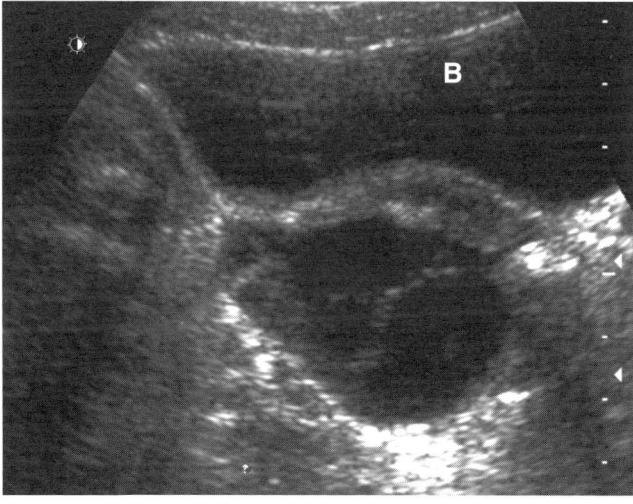

A. Follow-up physical examination in 4 weeks

B. Oophoropexy of involved ovary

C. Follow-up ultrasonography in 4 weeks

D. Oophoropexy of involved ovary and contralateral ovary

E. Reassurance

692. A 31-year-old woman complains of a 3-day history of left otalgia. She has no prior medical or surgical history. Physical examination of the left ear reveals grouped vesicles in various stages of development on the pinnae. Motor function of the facial nerve is intact. Which of the following is the most appropriate treatment for this individual?

A. Acyclovir

B. Metronidazole

C. Methylprednisolone

D. Methylprednisolone and acyclovir

E. Tetracycline, methylprednisolone, and acyclovir

693. A 41-year-old woman presents to her primary care physician because of urinary dribbling, dysuria, and dyspareunia. She has had these problems for several years but her symptoms have gotten progressively worse in the past 6 months. She is now unable to have sexual intercourse because of the vaginal pain. Her current medications include trimethoprim. Pelvic examination reveals a bulge in the anterior vaginal wall along the course of the urethra. The bulge has a cystic feel, and palpation causes expression of urine from the urethra. What is the most likely diagnosis?

A. Bartholin cyst

B. Cystocele

C. Rectocele

D. Spasm of the levator muscles

E. Urethral diverticulum

694. A 25-year-old woman with hypothyroidism who is 18 weeks pregnant with her second child presents to the emergency department with a 3-hour history of vaginal bleeding. She states that she had some crampy abdominal pain and then noticed blood in her panties. Her first pregnancy was uncomplicated. Pelvic examination reveals blood in the vaginal vault with a nondilated cervix. Ultrasonography reveals a viable fetus. What is the most likely diagnosis?

A. Incomplete abortion

B. Inevitable abortion

C. Missed abortion

D. Threatened abortion

E. Spontaneous abortion

695. A new screening test for diabetes involves using tears to measure the person's serum glucose. This screening test has been put through many trials. Your colleague tells you that the null hypothesis for the most recent trial has been rejected. Which of the following statements below regarding the rejection of a null hypothesis is true?

A. The *p* value must be greater than 0.05

B. There is a risk for a type I error

C. There is a risk for a type II error

D. There is not a risk for a type I or type II error

E. There is a risk for a type III error

696. A 29-year-old man presents to his primary care physician with generalized malaise. He says this has been progressing for years and he cannot remember the last time he felt like he had a lot of energy. Review of systems is positive for weight loss, several months of nausea and vomiting, as well as years of watery/nonbloody diarrhea. He has tried many things to control the diarrhea, including over-the-counter antidiarrheals, fiber, and avoiding milk products. Physical examination shows a man with hyperactive bowel sounds, nontender abdomen, and Hemoccult-negative test results. All other findings are normal. Laboratory values are as follows:

Na	136 mEq/L
K	2.2 mEq/L
Cl	84 mEq/L
Urea nitrogen, serum (BUN)	24 mEq/L
Creatinine	0.9 mg/dL
Glucose	76 mg/dL

The patient is admitted and given normal saline with K. His condition does not improve and the serum K continues to drop. What is the next step in the workup?

A. Check serum gastrin/vasoactive intestinal peptide

B. Check serum insulin/glucagon

C. Colonoscopy

D. Esophogastroduodenoscopy

E. Laparotomy

697. A 50-year-old woman presents for evaluation of new-onset bloody vaginal discharge as well as urinary frequency and dysuria. She notes that sexual intercourse has become painful. Vaginal speculum examination reveals a mass lesion in the upper portion of the vaginal vault. Laboratory values include a hematocrit of 29%. Which of the following is the primary treatment option for this patient?

A. Intravenous chemotherapy

B. Intravesicular chemotherapy

C. Radiotherapy

D. Surgical excision

E. Watchful waiting

698. A 54-year-old man presents to the emergency department with a sudden onset of a severe frontal headache, nausea, and vomiting earlier in the day. His past medical history is significant for hypertension and diabetes mellitus. Vitals signs are temperature 36.1°C, blood pressure 190/72 mm Hg, pulse 118 beats/min, respirations 42 breaths/min. He is awake but has a decreased level of consciousness and complains of vertigo. Physical examination reveals loss of sensation and paralysis in his right extremities. He also has right gaze preference. What is the next most appropriate step in the management of this patient?

A. Assess airway

B. Establish intravenous access

C. Nitroprusside

D. Obtain serum glucose levels

E. Obtain ECG and institute cardiac monitoring

699. A young girl is brought to her pediatrician for a well-child evaluation. Her immunizations are up to date. Physical examination findings of the heart, lungs, and abdomen are within normal limits. Examination of the genitalia reveals minimal labial fusion. She is able to jump over several blocks and "skip" while walking. What is her approximate age?

A. 1 year

B. 2 years

C. 3 years

D. 4 years

E. 5 years

700. A 55-year-old man presents for a new patient visit with a primary care physician. He has a history of hypertension and congestive heart failure. His hypertension has been refractory to most medical interventions. He has stable angina that occurs with exertion but no history of myocardial infarct. Surgical history is notable for carotid endarterectomy and femoral-popliteal bypass. His creatinine level is 2.1 mg/dL. He takes an aspirin, a beta blocker, an angiotensin-converting enzyme (ACE) inhibitor, a thiazide diuretic, and a calcium channel blocker. Which medicine will the patient likely need to stop taking?

A. ACE inhibitor

B. Aspirin

C. Beta blocker

D. Calcium channel blocker

E. Thiazide diuretic

701. A 34-year-old man comes to the emergency department with a 1-hour history of severe muscle rigidity, diaphoresis, dysphagia, and tremor. Vital signs are respirations 20 breaths/min, pulse 116 beats/min, temperature 38.4°C, and blood pressure 150/96 mm Hg. He has a 4-year history of schizophrenia. What is most likely to have precipitated this patient's condition?

A. Alcohol ingestion
B. Benzodiazepine ingestion
C. Cocaine ingestion
D. Ethylene glycol ingestion
E. Phenothiazine ingestion

The response options for items 702–704 are the same. You will be required to select one answer for each item in the set.

A. Balanced electrolyte solution (Ringer lactate)
B. Dextrose 5% solution
C. Isotonic saline (0.9% solution)
D. Hydroxyethyl starch (Hetastarch)
E. Human serum albumin
F. Normal saline (Normosol)

For each resuscitation solution, select the appropriate statement.

702. A 49-year-old man with end-stage renal disease on hemodialysis is admitted to the hospital with chest pain. ECGs are unchanged from prior studies. He is started on intravenous fluids and is later found unresponsive by nurses. CT of the head suggests infarct in the distribution of the right middle cerebral artery. His serum lactate level is now 9 mg/dL and serum osmolarity is 600 mOsm/L.

703. A 44-year-old man with chronic renal insufficiency presents to the emergency room with chest pain. ECG reveals T-wave inversion in the precordial leads. He is placed on intravenous fluids. Twelve hours later his serum K is 5.4 mEq/L and serum calcium is 12.5 mg/dL.

704. A 56-year-old man with dehydration and diverticulitis has a blood pressure of 90/50 mm Hg, pulse of 110 beats/min, and urine output of 0.8 mL/kg/h despite intravenous fluids running at a rate of 120 mL/h. An additional intravenous solution is added. Three days later his serum amylase is 300 U/L and his creatinine level increases to 1.6 mg/dL.

705. A 33-year-old man with AIDS is hospitalized on the medicine service with *Pneumocystis carinii* pneumonia. He is currently being treated with zidovudine, ganciclovir, trimethoprim-sulfamethoxazole, and delavirdine. Pulmonary auscultation reveals rhonchi bilaterally with decreased breath sounds at the bases. Which of the following adverse reactions is most concerning to the physician who is treating this patient?

A. Anemia
B. Headache
C. Malaise
D. Nausea
E. Neutropenia

706. A 25-year-old G1P0 woman who is pregnant by home pregnancy test presents for evaluation. She denies prior medical or surgical history. Doppler ultrasonography reveals evidence of fetal heart tones. Abdominal examination reveals normoactive bowel sounds with a nonpalpable fundal height. Urine beta human chorionic gonadotropin testing in the office is positive. Which of the following nutrients requires the highest percentage increase in supplementation during pregnancy?

A. Calcium
B. Niacin
C. Vitamin A
D. Vitamin D
E. Vitamin E

707. A 3-year-old boy presents to his pediatrician for evaluation of an abdominal mass found by his parents during his nighttime bath. Parents note that the child has recently had some bouts of vomiting and intermittent right-sided abdominal pain. The patient appears well. Physical examination findings of the heart, lungs, and abdomen are within normal limits. However, palpation of the right upper quadrant reveals a hard mass. Laboratory studies obtained are shown below:

Electrolytes, serum

Na, serum	143 mEq/L
Cl, serum	100 mEq/L
K, serum	3.7 mEq/L
Bicarbonate, serum	24 mEq/L
Creatinine, serum	1.1 mg/dL

Leukocyte count and differential

Leukocyte count	7000/mm³
Segmented neutrophils	55%
Bands	4%
Eosinophils	3%

Blood, plasma, serum

Calcium, serum	9 mg/dL
Glucose, serum	100 mg/dL
Urea nitrogen, serum (BUN)	10 mg/dL

Urinalysis

Urine pH	6.0
RBC count	4/HPF
WBC count	2/HPF
Nitrates	Negative
Bacteria	Negative

Which of the following is the most appropriate next step in the evaluation of this patient?

A. Barium upper gastrointestinal series
B. Cystoscopy
C. Retrograde urethrography
D. Sonography
E. Ureteroscopy and biopsy

708. A 22-year-old female college student is brought to the emergency department by university police because of a suspected suicide attempt. The patient was observed to take a handful of aspirin by mouth. She complains of vertigo, nausea, and vomiting. The patient is given activated charcoal in the emergency department and is admitted to the medicine ward for observation. Six hours later, laboratory studies are obtained that reveal an anion gap of 14. What is the most appropriate treatment?

A. Dialysis
B. Ethanol infusion
C. Insulin
D. N-acetylcysteine
E. Sodium bicarbonate

709. The systolic blood pressure in a community is normally distributed with a mean of 120 mm Hg and a standard deviation of 10. What percentage of people have a systolic blood pressure at or above 140 mm Hg?

A. 1.9%
B. 2.5%
C. 13.5%
D. 34%
E. 64.2%

710. An 18-year-old man presents to his primary care physician with 1½ weeks of runny nose, sore throat, and diarrhea. He says the runny nose and sore throat are improving, but the diarrhea is not resolving. In fact, when he drinks milk or eats cheese, the symptoms are worse and he experiences cramps, gas, and increased diarrhea. He says he has not lost any weight during this period and has no significant stress in his life. He has not left home and has not drunk any stream or well water recently. Physical examination reveals rhinorrhea, nonboggy nasal turbinates, nonerythematous pharynx, no cervical adenopathy, nontender abdomen, and increased bowel sounds. What is the most likely diagnosis?

A. *Bacillus cereus* infection
B. *Giardia lamblia* infection
C. Irritable bowel syndrome
D. Lactose intolerance
E. Viral gastroenteritis

711. A 2-week-old infant presents with recurrent regurgitation of feeds without vomiting. Physical examination reveals tachycardia and a holosystolic murmur heard best at the base. Pulmonary auscultation reveals bilateral scattered wheezes without rales or rhonchi. Gastrointestinal examination reveals normoactive bowel sounds and encrustations over the umbilicus. Barium swallow and endoscopy reveal dilatation of the lower esophageal sphincter without inflammation. Which of the following is the most appropriate strategy in the management of this patient?

A. Cimetidine
B. Metoclopramide
C. Supine positioning after feeding
D. Surgical fundoplication, Nissen type
E. Thinning of feeds

712. A previously healthy 30-year-old G1P1 female athlete comes to the emergency department with sudden onset of abdominal pain. She is a bodybuilder. She admits to using anabolic steroids and oral contraceptives that were prescribed by her gynecologist. She has a blood pressure of 90/55 mm Hg and generalized abdominal tenderness. CT of the abdomen shows large amounts of free fluid in the abdomen and a solitary 4-cm mass in the liver. The CT scan also reveals a 1.5-cm right ovarian cyst and a small amount of fluid in the cul-de-sac. What is the most likely diagnosis?

A. Hemangioma
B. Hepatic abscess
C. Hepatocellular adenoma
D. Metastatic adenocarcinoma
E. Ruptured hepatic cyst

713. A 55-year-old man presents to his primary care physician with complaints of chest pain that has been increasing in frequency and duration for the past several months. The pain worsens with activity and is relieved by rest. Physical examination reveals a high-volume water-hammer (collapsing pulse) and a widened pulse pressure. Other findings include a murmur over the femoral artery, a pronounced S_2, and III/VI early diastolic murmur indicating aortic involvement. Additionally, there is a middiastolic murmur best heard over the cardiac apex. ECG findings include cardiomegaly with left ventricular hypertrophy. A chest x-ray demonstrates a widened mediastinum and a large cardiac silhouette. There are calcifications in the aorta in a tree bark pattern. Which of the following is the most likely diagnosis?

A. Idiopathic chest pain
B. Myocardial infarction
C. Rheumatic heart disease
D. Tertiary stage syphilis
E. Unstable angina

714. A 46-year-old man is brought to the emergency department unconscious. The patient smells of alcohol, and no further history is available. Vital signs are pulse 60 beats/min, blood pressure 100/50 mmHg, and respirations 14 breaths/min. Physical examination shows an unkempt man looking much older than his stated age. Pupils are dilated and reactive to light. Chest examination reveals bilateral crackles. Cardiac examination findings are normal. The abdomen is mildly distended, soft, with bowel sounds present. Extremity, genitalia, and rectal examination findings are normal. Laboratory values are:

Na, serum	145 mEq/L
K, serum	3.5 mEq/L
Cl, serum	109 mEq/L
Carbon dioxide, serum	15 mEq/L
Glucose, serum	119 mg/dL
Urinalysis	
pH	5.5
WBC count	2–5/HPF
RBC count	1–2/HPF with calcium oxalate crystals seen

Which of the following is the most likely etiology of this patient's condition?

A. Acetaminophen overdose
B. Cocaine overdose
C. Diabetic ketoacidosis
D. Ethanol ingestion
E. Ethylene glycol ingestion

715. A 26-year-old woman delivers a newborn male at term. Apgar scores are 8 and 9 at 1 and 5 minutes, respectively. The woman has a persistent headache after receiving her epidural anesthetic with a 16-gauge needle approximately 12 hours ago. Physical examination findings of the head, ears, eyes, nose, and throat are within normal limits. Which of the following is the most appropriate treatment?

A. Acetaminophen
B. Amoxicillin
C. Encourage ambulation
D. Intravenous fluids at 35 mL/h
E. Patch (blood)

716. A 28-year-old man presents to the emergency department complaining of severe abdominal pain, nausea, and vomiting for 8 hours. Temperature is 101.7°F, pulse 90 beats/min, and blood pressure 130/80 mmHg. Abdominal examination reveals periumbilical to left lower quadrant pain with rebound tenderness. He was started on intravenous fluids and taken to the operating room for exploration. Surgical findings at laparoscopy include colonic erythema and inflammation with fat accumulating on the antimesenteric order of the bowel wall. Biopsy was taken of the affected area and revealed epithelioid histocytes surrounded by lymphocytes and giant cells. What is the most likely diagnosis?

A. Carcinoma of the colon
B. Crohn disease
C. Ischemic bowel disease
D. Tuberculosis
E. Ulcerative colitis

717. An 11-year-old girl presents to the emergency department complaining of right lower quadrant pain. She also had three bouts of emesis and fever up to 102°F. On further questioning, she states that the pain began about 10 hours ago around her umbilicus and has since traveled to the right lower quadrant. A few hours after the pain began, she developed nausea and vomiting. The patient has not eaten anything since the pain began because it hurt too much. Examination findings of her heart and lungs are benign. Her abdomen is tender to palpation, especially in the right lower quadrant. She is most tender when you remove your hands from her abdomen. What would be the next step in managing this patient?

A. CT scan to confirm diagnosis
B. Emergency appendectomy
C. Hospital admission, broad-spectrum antibiotics, and perform serial abdominal examinations
D. Hospital discharge; have her follow-up with you in 1 week
E. Radiographic evaluation with barium enema

718. A 38-year-old woman with a family history of breast cancer presents to the ambulatory care clinic because she found a lump in her breast on self-examination 4 months ago. The lump has not changed in size since she first noticed it. There is no variation of the lump with her menstrual cycle. She denies having any breast tenderness, skin color changes, or nipple discharge. What is the next step in managing this mass?

A. Fine-needle aspiration
B. Mammography
C. Monitor the mass with serial examinations
D. Surgical excisional biopsy
E. Surgical incisional biopsy

719. The mother of an 11-year-old boy has become aggravated because her son continues to miss school because of constipation. Recent physical examination by her pediatrician reveals a normal cardiac, pulmonary, and abdominal examination. Rectal examination reveals impacted stool in the rectal vault. The patient's mother wants to treat constipation by moving the stool along (peristalsis). Which of the following agents will satisfy this goal?

A. Docusate sodium
B. Mineral oil
C. Senekot
D. Simple carbohydrates
E. Vincristine

720. A 54-year-old G3P3003 woman presents to her gynecologist for her annual wellness examination. All children were delivered vaginally, with her last child being born 20 years ago and requiring forceps extraction. Her medical history is significant hypertension diagnosed at age 47 and type II diabetes diagnosed at age 52. Her hypertension is managed with hydrochlorothiazide and her diabetes is currently managed through diet modification. She has a 20 pack/year history of smoking. She also complains of worsening symptoms of involuntary urinary leakage that occurs when she coughs or strains to lift a heavy object. She denies having dysuria, urgency, nocturia, or constant dribbling. She reports this problem has occurred for 10 years but states it has gotten significantly more troublesome the past 3 years. What is the likely etiology of her urinary incontinence?

   A. Adverse reaction to the use of hydrochlorothiazide for the management of hypertension
   B. Chronic urinary tract infections with cystitis resulting in lower urinary tract irritability
   C. Detrusor insufficiency or detrusor areflexia resulting from autonomic neuropathy secondary to her diabetes mellitus
   D. Urethral resistance to urinary flow is overcome by an increase in intraabdominal pressure
   E. Urinary fistula between the bladder and the vagina secondary to obstetric trauma resulting from operative delivery (forceps)

721. A 77-year-old woman presents with right hip pain after a fall 3 hours ago. While coming from her garden she tripped over the garden hose in her driveway. When she fell she struck her right hip. Physical examination reveals that she is afebrile but breathing deeply and heavily at a rate of 35 breaths/min. There is point tenderness over the right trochanter, and any movement of the right hip causes pain. A radiograph of the right hip is shown in Figure 721. What is the most likely diagnosis?

   A. Femoral diaphysis fracture
   B. Femoral neck fracture
   C. Femoral head fracture
   D. Intertrochanteric fracture
   E. Subtrochanteric fracture

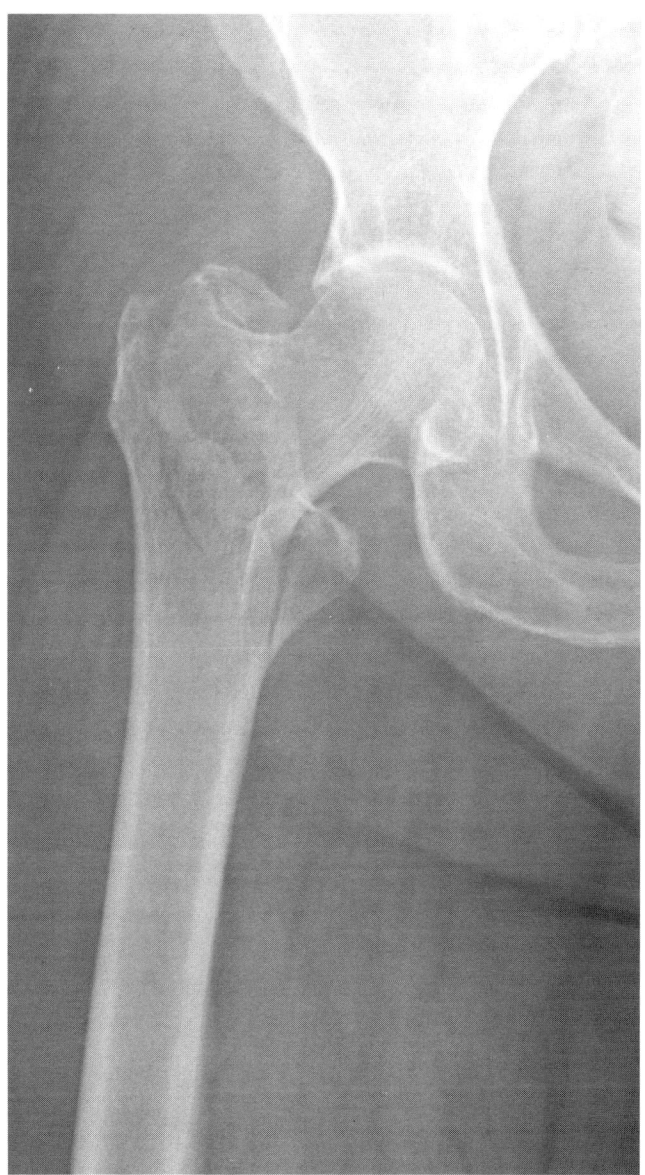

Figure 721

722. A 26-year-old woman presents to the ambulatory care clinic with a 10-day history of worsening fatigue, sore throat, and cough productive of blood-tinged sputum. Physical examination is unremarkable except for some faint crackles on lung examination. Chest x-ray reveals a lower lobe bronchopneumonia. Gram stain of sputum shows neutrophils. The patient is diagnosed with atypical community acquired pneumonia. What is the most appropriate treatment for this patient?

A. Acyclovir
B. Erythromycin
C. Penicillin
D. Supportive care only
E. Trimethoprim

723. In the year 2000, Anytown, USA, had 1000 live births. Thirty of these were twins. Four mothers died, and there were 45 stillbirths delivered after greater than or equal to 20 weeks' gestation. Thirteen deaths occurred in the first year of life. Six of those died in the first 28 days of life. What would be the perinatal mortality rate in Anytown, USA, in the year 2000?

A. 51/1000
B. 6/1000
C. 51/1045
D. 45/1045
E. 45/1000

724. A 40-year-old woman has a palpable cystic lesion in her left breast. She has a prior history of fibrocystic disease of the breasts. Her mother also had a history of fibroadenoma. The mass was drained via needle aspiration, but the fluid reaccumulated after 1 week. What is the most appropriate next step?

A. Drain the fluid again and reevaluate again for recurrence
B. Excise the mass with a 5-mm edge of normal tissue around the perimeter
C. Excise the mass with a 1-cm edge of normal tissue around the perimeter
D. Obtain a mammogram of the breast
E. Watchful waiting

725. A 4-day-old boy presents to the emergency department for evaluation of red eyes. His mother states that she noticed both eyes turned red yesterday evening. Birth history was uncomplicated, and the patient and mother were discharged 24 hours postpartum. Temperature is 39.1°C. Physical examination reveals purulent discharge in both eyes. Conjunctival eye culture demonstrates *Neisseria gonorrhoeae*. What is the most appropriate treatment for this patient?

A. Observation only
B. Oral erythromycin
C. Saline eye drops

D. Tetracycline ointment and oral erythromycin
E. Topical and intravenous penicillin

726. A 52-year-old woman has been complaining of abdominal pain for the past 6 months. She presents to her primary care physician for further evaluation. She has a history of hypertension for the past 6 years and has been well controlled with antihypertensives. Her current medications include a calcium channel blocker and a thiazide diuretic. She is an obese woman with predominantly upper abdominal obesity. Her vitals signs are temperature 37.2°C, blood pressure 165/97 mm Hg, pulse 83 beats/min, and respirations 15 breaths/min. Physical examination shows proximal muscle weakness. Abdominal examination findings were within normal limits. A CT scan of the abdomen revealed a small left adrenal mass. Results of laboratory studies are shown below:

Electrolytes, serum

Na, serum	141 mEq/L
Cl, serum	99 mEq/L
K, serum	4.7 mEq/L
Bicarbonate, serum	24 mEq/L
Magnesium, serum	2.2 mEq/L
Creatinine, serum	1.1 mg/dL

Leukocyte count and differential

Leukocyte count	9000/mm^3
Segmented neutrophils	61%
Bands	7%
Eosinophils	3%
Basophils	1%
Lymphocytes	24%
Monocytes	4%

Blood, plasma, serum

Glucose, serum	100 mg/dL
Hematocrit	37%
Urea nitrogen, serum (BUN)	10 mg/dL

Urinalysis

Urine pH	6.0
RBC count	2/HPF

What is the most appropriate next step in the management of this patient?

A. Insulin-hypoglycemic test
B. MRI of the abdomen
C. Percutaneous adrenal biopsy
D. Plasma aldosterone and renin activity
E. Urinary free cortisol

727. A 20-year-old woman presents to the emergency room with a complaint of recent-onset unilateral facial paralysis. She also complains of numbness in the same distribution as the facial paralysis. Physical examination is noncontributory aside from the unilateral facial paresis and decreased sensory acuity. What can you tell the patient about her prognosis?

A. Most patients never recover full function

B. Less than half will recover full function

C. Greater than two thirds will recover full function

D. Ninety percent of patients will recover completely

E. Ninety-nine percent of patients will recover completely

728. A 60-year-old man is brought to the emergency department because of chest pain. His wife states that the chest pain developed 3 hours ago while shoveling snow. The patient characterized the pain as a heaviness in the mid-portion of his chest, but it has now gone away. He weighs 230 pounds, has a 50 pack/year history of smoking, and drinks 3 beers per week. Physical examination shows an obese male who appears to be his stated age. He has vomited once since arrival and is diaphoretic. His blood pressure is 150/110 mm Hg, pulse 125 beats/min, and respirations 16 breaths/min. ECG reveals a Q wave in leads V1–V4 as well as ST elevation in the same leads. What is the most likely diagnosis?

A. Anterior wall myocardial infarction

B. Chest wall pain

C. Inferior wall myocardial infarction

D. Myocardial ischemia

E. Pericarditis

729. A 15-year-old boy who is a runner on the school cross country team presents to his pediatrician for evaluation of vague left lower extremity pain. He has been running approximately 100 miles per week in order to train for an upcoming track meet. Physical examination reveals nonlocalizing vague thigh pain. Oblique x-rays reveal a periosteal reaction. What is the most appropriate treatment for this patient?

A. Arthroscopy

B. Corticosteroids

C. Crutches

D. Dimethylsulfoxide

E. Watchful waiting with continuation of running regimen

730. A 28-year-old G1P0 woman at 36 weeks' gestation presents to the emergency department with contractions occurring every 5 minutes. She has a prior medical history of type II diabetes mellitus. She takes no medications. Physical examination reveals that her cervix is dilated 3 cm. She is admitted to the obstetrics floor for observation. She is reevaluated 6 hours later and her cervix is found to be dilated 4 cm and 75% effaced and is at station 0. Amnionic membranes are bulging. She has walked around the floor several times but has not had more frequent contractions. Fetal heart rate tracing is reactive. What is the most appropriate course of action for this patient?

A. Amniotomy

B. Begin oxytocin via intravenous drip

C. Epidural anesthetic

D. Jogging regimen around the hospital floor

E. Walking regimen around the hospital floor

731. A 71-year-old man presents to the emergency department because of an acute onset of left-sided paralysis. The paralysis seemed to evolve over several hours and now he is unable to walk. He has a past medical history of hypertension that is treated with hydrochlorothiazide. Blood pressure is 150/95 mm Hg, pulse 90 beats/min, and respirations 12 breaths/min. Neurologic examination reveals left-sided hemiplegia with decreased sensation to pain and light touch on the left side. Ocular examination reveals left homonymous hemianopsia. His head and eyes are deviated to the right side. What is the most appropriate next step in the evaluation of this patient?

A. Angiography

B. CT scan of the head

C. Digital subtraction angiography

D. Lumbar puncture

E. MRI scan

732. You are asked in the clinic to see a 45-year-old woman who underwent an abdominoplasty 12 days ago by your partner to control morbid obesity. She was discharged home on postoperative day 4. The patient is complaining of pain that is not adequately controlled. Physical examination of the wound reveals some purulent and serous discharge leaking from the incision. The wound edges are erythematous. The incision feels warm to the touch. Which of the following is an appropriate medication to start at this time?

A. Ampicillin

B. Clindamycin

C. Cephalexin

D. Ketoconazole

E. Metronidazole

733. A 5-year-old boy is brought to the emergency department because of a 1-week history of unilateral purulent nasal discharge. He has no pertinent past medical or surgical history. Physical examination reveals a foreign body in the left nostril (pencil eraser) obscured by dried secretions. What is the most appropriate treatment for this patient?

   A. Direct laryngoscopy
   B. Flexible laryngoscopy
   C. Removal with grasping forceps
   D. Trial of inhaled corticosteroids
   E. Watchful waiting

734. A 17-year-old G1P0 female high school student is brought to the emergency department by her boyfriend because she cannot feel her baby moving. She was out "partying" with friends and admits to doing some things that she should not have done. She has a small-for-gestational-age baby. She is a smoker. She is at 33 weeks' gestation and has noticed decreased fetal movements for the past 2 days. Her score is 4/10 on a biophysical profile. Physical examination reveals a blood pressure of 130/90 mm Hg. Pitocin challenge is administered and reveals deep decelerations. What is the most likely explanation of these findings?

   A. Alcohol abuse
   B. Cigarette smoking
   C. Hypertension
   D. Illicit drug use
   E. Malnutrition

735. A 63-year-old man presents to the medical clinic for annual follow-up. Specifically, he is being evaluated for adjustment of his current congestive heart failure medications. ECG is ordered (Figure 735). It is noted that he has had no worsening of symptoms since the level was changed 1 year ago. Which statement is true about this medication?

   A. It is causing the arrhythmia shown
   B. The level is inadequate
   C. The level is therapeutic
   D. The level is toxic
   E. Hyperkalemia is the most serious electrolyte disorder to have while on this medication

736. A 38-year-old woman notes a 4-year history of episodes of feeling short of breath and shaking when she is in crowded places such as a concert hall. She states that these symptoms are also accompanied by nausea, abdominal pain, chills, and tingling sensations in her hands. During these episodes she feels as if she is going crazy. Physical examination shows a well-developed, well-nourished woman in no apparent distress. Her thyroid gland is palpable without masses. Cardiovascular examination reveals a regular rate and rhythm. Pulmonary auscultation reveals no evidence of rales, rhonchi, or wheezing. Which of the following is the most appropriate treatment for this individual?

   A. Alprazolam
   B. Clonidine
   C. Imipramine
   D. Propranolol
   E. Trazodone

Figure 735

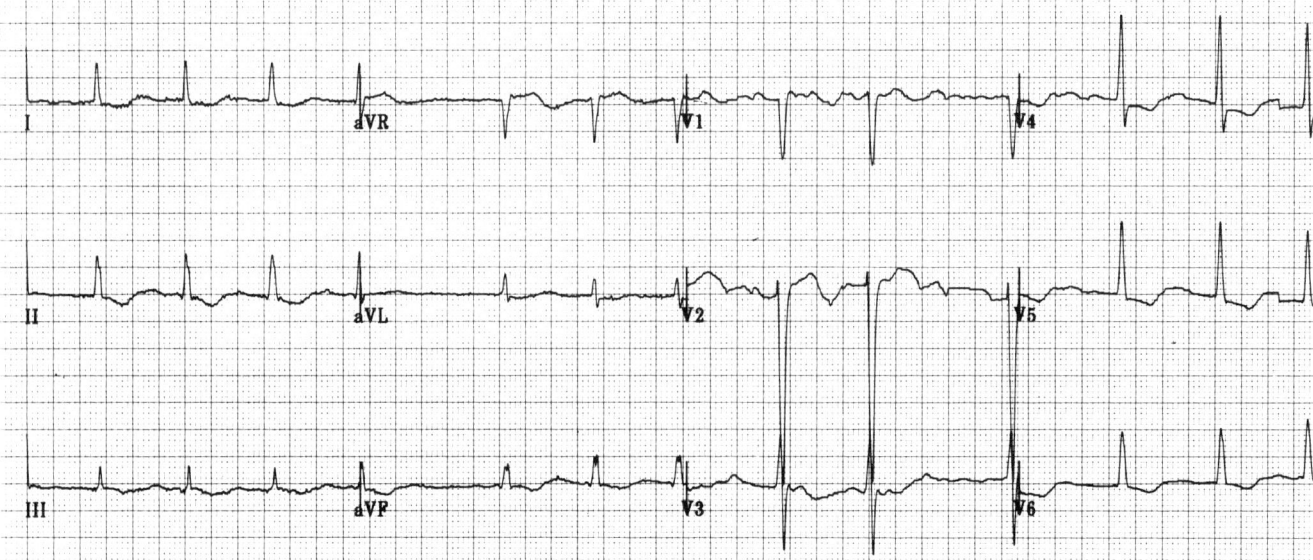

737. A 39-year-old man with a history of diabetes mellitus, hypertension, smoking, and polysubstance abuse presents to the emergency department complaining of nausea, vomiting, and epigastric pain for 5 days. His current medications include a beta blocker and cimetidine. Physical examination reveals pale yellow eruptive papules on the skin, predominantly over the trunk and buttocks. Physical examination findings of the heart, lungs, and abdomen are unremarkable. Results of laboratory studies are shown below:

Amylase, serum	59 U/L
Lipase, serum	699 U/L
Triglycerides, serum	5793 mg/dL
Bilirubin, direct	0.5 mg/dL
Na, serum	135 mEq/L
K, serum	4.1 mEq/L

What is the most appropriate treatment for this patient?

A. Dietary fats

B. Heparin

C. Lipid emulsion

D. Plasmapheresis

E. Stop cimetidine and beta blocker administration

738. A 32-year-old man is brought to the emergency department after being stabbed in the neck. The knife blade was 6 cm long and half the blade entered the neck. The patient is alert and oriented with a normal voice and normal breath sounds bilaterally. His vital signs are stable. Physical examination reveals that the stab wound of the neck was 2 cm inferior to the left mandible. The wound entry site is measured to be 3 cm in diameter. Before the patient goes for surgical exploration, which diagnostic test should be ordered?

A. Bronchoscopy

B. Esophagography

C. Laryngoscopy

D. Pulmonary angiography

E. No further testing is required

739. A 40-year-old obese man presents to his primary care physician because of daytime sleep attacks. He states that these sleep attacks occur several times per week and lately have been associated with a sudden loss of muscle tone resulting in a fall to the ground. At other times, he feels weak. These attacks are often brought on by feelings of anger or laughter. Physical examination findings of the heart, lungs, and abdomen are within normal limits. What is the most appropriate treatment for this patient?

A. Corticosteroids

B. Imipramine

C. Methylphenidate

D. Tonsilectomy

E. Watchful waiting

740. A 7-year-old boy presents to his pediatrician for evaluation of visual difficulties. He is having difficulty seeing the blackboard in school, and his grades have declined over the past few months. His mother has a history of bilateral cateracts. Ophthalmologic examination reveals bilateral clouding of the lens. What is the most appropriate next step in the evaluation of this patient?

A. CT scan of the head

B. MRI scan of the head

C. Ocular ultrasonography

D. Vertebral artery angiography

E. Visual acuity testing

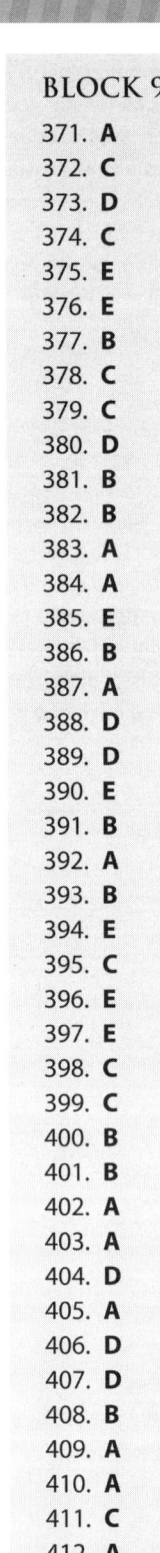

✳ TEST 2 ANSWER KEY

BLOCK 9	BLOCK 10	BLOCK 11	BLOCK 12
371. **A**	417. **B**	463. **C**	510. **D**
372. **C**	418. **B**	464. **E**	511. **C**
373. **D**	419. **A**	465. **B**	512. **E**
374. **C**	420. **F**	466. **A**	513. **A**
375. **E**	421. **B**	467. **B**	514. **C**
376. **E**	422. **C**	468. **D**	515. **C**
377. **B**	423. **D**	469. **A**	516. **B**
378. **C**	424. **B**	470. **D**	517. **D**
379. **C**	425. **C**	471. **E**	518. **D**
380. **D**	426. **A**	472. **E**	519. **C**
381. **B**	427. **D**	473. **C**	520. **D**
382. **B**	428. **G**	474. **A**	521. **D**
383. **A**	429. **H**	475. **B**	522. **A**
384. **A**	430. **E**	476. **A**	523. **E**
385. **E**	431. **A**	477. **E**	524. **B**
386. **B**	432. **C**	478. **B**	525. **E**
387. **A**	433. **A**	479. **E**	526. **D**
388. **D**	434. **E**	480. **C**	527. **A**
389. **D**	435. **A**	481. **B**	528. **C**
390. **E**	436. **E**	482. **C**	529. **B**
391. **B**	437. **C**	483. **C**	530. **C**
392. **A**	438. **B**	484. **D**	531. **E**
393. **B**	439. **A**	485. **A**	532. **C**
394. **E**	440. **A**	486. **B**	533. **E**
395. **C**	441. **D**	487. **B**	534. **A**
396. **E**	442. **C**	488. **D**	535. **B**
397. **E**	443. **D**	489. **D**	536. **E**
398. **C**	444. **D**	490. **E**	537. **A**
399. **C**	445. **B**	491. **E**	538. **I**
400. **B**	446. **C**	492. **B**	539. **A**
401. **B**	447. **B**	493. **C**	540. **D**
402. **A**	448. **B**	494. **D**	541. **D**
403. **A**	449. **B**	495. **A**	542. **B**
404. **D**	450. **B**	496. **E**	543. **D**
405. **A**	451. **A**	497. **D**	544. **D**
406. **D**	452. **A**	498. **B**	545. **C**
407. **D**	453. **A**	499. **A**	546. **C**
408. **B**	454. **E**	500. **C**	547. **D**
409. **A**	455. **D**	501. **D**	548. **E**
410. **A**	456. **E**	502. **C**	549. **B**
411. **C**	457. **B**	503. **A**	550. **C**
412. **A**	458. **C**	504. **C**	551. **B**
413. **D**	459. **E**	505. **E**	552. **E**
414. **C**	460. **A**	506. **C**	553. **C**
415. **D**	461. **B**	507. **A**	554. **B**
416. **D**	462. **D**	508. **C**	555. **E**
		509. **C**	

BLOCK 13	BLOCK 14	BLOCK 15	BLOCK 16
556. **E**	602. **D**	649. **D**	695. **B**
557. **B**	603. **C**	650. **D**	696. **E**
558. **D**	604. **D**	651. **D**	697. **C**
559. **B**	605. **E**	652. **E**	698. **A**
560. **B**	606. **B**	653. **C**	699. **E**
561. **C**	607. **A**	654. **D**	700. **A**
562. **D**	608. **D**	655. **B**	701. **E**
563. **C**	609. **A**	656. **C**	702. **B**
564. **D**	610. **C**	657. **A**	703. **A**
565. **E**	611. **B**	658. **D**	704. **D**
566. **C**	612. **E**	659. **E**	705. **E**
567. **C**	613. **A**	660. **B**	706. **A**
568. **H**	614. **C**	661. **B**	707. **D**
569. **A**	615. **E**	662. **B**	708. **E**
570. **D**	616. **A**	663. **B**	709. **B**
571. **B**	617. **D**	664. **C**	710. **E**
572. **D**	618. **E**	665. **B**	711. **B**
573. **E**	619. **D**	666. **A**	712. **C**
574. **B**	620. **C**	667. **E**	713. **D**
575. **C**	621. **C**	668. **D**	714. **E**
576. **A**	622. **A**	669. **C**	715. **E**
577. **A**	623. **C**	670. **D**	716. **B**
578. **C**	624. **D**	671. **A**	717. **B**
579. **C**	625. **C**	672. **D**	718. **B**
580. **E**	626. **D**	673. **B**	719. **C**
581. **C**	627. **A**	674. **A**	720. **D**
582. **D**	628. **C**	675. **E**	721. **D**
583. **E**	629. **D**	676. **D**	722. **B**
584. **D**	630. **A**	677. **E**	723. **C**
585. **B**	631. **B**	678. **B**	724. **C**
586. **A**	632. **A**	679. **A**	725. **E**
587. **B**	633. **C**	680. **F**	726. **E**
588. **B**	634. **B**	681. **E**	727. **C**
589. **A**	635. **D**	682. **G**	728. **A**
590. **B**	636. **A**	683. **I**	729. **C**
591. **E**	637. **D**	684. **D**	730. **A**
592. **A**	638. **B**	685. **D**	731. **B**
593. **C**	639. **E**	686. **A**	732. **C**
594. **E**	640. **C**	687. **B**	733. **C**
595. **D**	641. **C**	688. **A**	734. **B**
596. **E**	642. **D**	689. **B**	735. **C**
597. **C**	643. **C**	690. **B**	736. **C**
598. **A**	644. **A**	691. **C**	737. **E**
599. **D**	645. **C**	692. **D**	738. **E**
600. **A**	646. **D**	693. **E**	739. **B**
601. **D**	647. **A**	694. **D**	740. **E**
	648. **C**		

371. **A.** Osgood-Schlatter disease is inflammation of the tibial tuberosity. It occurs most commonly in children 10 to 17 years of age, and is associated with repetitive stress or trauma. Tenderness and swelling may be present over the tibial tuberosity. Most cases are treated with activity restriction.

B. External fixation (casting) may be useful in more severe cases in which activity restriction is ineffective.

C. Internal fixation has no role in the management of Osgood-Schlatter disease.

D. An MRI would not be beneficial for the management of this patient.

E. The use of nonsteroidal antiinflammatory drugs are not indicated in the management of Osgood-Schlatter disease.

372. **C.** Although the most common foreign body found in the vagina in vulvovaginitis is toilet paper, other objects such as beads and toys can be found. Radiographs are not reliable for diagnosis because most objects are not radiopaque. Therefore, no radiographic study should be performed on this child.

A. CT of the pelvis will not provide reliable information in children with vulvovaginitis.

B. MRI of the pelvis will not provide reliable information in children with vulvovaginitis.

D. Plain films of the abdomen will not provide reliable information in children with vulvovaginitis.

E. Transabdominal ultrasonography of the pelvis will not provide reliable information in children with vulvovaginitis.

373. **D.** ERCP is indicated at this point in time because it can be used to establish the diagnosis of chronic pancreatitis, which this man does not yet have. Such a diagnosis is likely because these patients will have a history of weight loss and steatorrhea due to malabsorption as well as symptoms of diabetes mellitus and pancreatic insufficiency. ERCP will show a stenosed pancreatic duct due to the multiple prior episodes of pancreatic inflammation. ERCP is useful in this case because according to the Ranson criteria, he is at increased risk for mortality, and establishing a diagnosis of chronic pancreatitis would prompt a more aggressive treatment.

A. Although this would be the standard treatment for acute pancreatitis, more should be done in this man's case given the recurrent nature of his pain.

B. Previous films have already established the presence of calcifications on his pancreas, and seeing an increase in calcifications would not alter the treatment.

C. Pancreatic duct dilation is an aggressive approach and would not be warranted for a patient who does not have an established diagnosis of chronic pancreatitis. If his ERCP does show signs of chronic pancreatitis, then surgery could be indicated. Pancreatic duct dilation can be palliative.

E. This patient's ascites is likely to have been present for an extended period of time, and drainage is not of the utmost priority at the moment.

374. **C.** Gross motor skills of the 3-year-old child include the ability to easily pedal a tricycle. Children at this age are often able to alternate their feet when going up stairs. The ability to stand on one foot momentarily is also noted at this age. Visual motor skills that are apparent at this age include the ability to dress and undress partially. This child should also be able to copy simple figures such as a circle or an "x."

A. A child of this age can walk alone or with assistance.

B. A child of this age can walk up or down stairs with help.

D. A child of this age can walk and run well.

E. A child of this age can walk, run, and jump over small obstacles.

375. **E.** This patient has a ganglion tumor. These tumors occur in four locations on the hand. One typical location is on the dorsal side of the wrist extending into the joint. The treatment of choice is surgical excision to include the entire cyst and its origin.

A. Chemotherapy is an ineffective treatment for ganglion tumor.

B. Corticosteroids are an ineffective treatment for ganglion tumor.

C. Radiotherapy is an ineffective treatment for ganglion tumor.

D. Splinting might relieve the pain associated with ganglion tumor because of immobilization. Surgical excision is the treatment of choice.

376. **E.** Sarcoidosis is a chronic, systemic, idiopathic, granulomatous disease, primarily affecting the lungs. Most patients have a benign course, and many have spontaneous remissions. Sarcoidosis is also associated with lacrimal and parotid gland enlargement, uveitis, and cranial nerve palsy. Parotid involvement is a good prognostic indicator for this patient.

A. The angiotensin-converting enzyme level is elevated in 60%, but has no prognostic indication.

B. Erythema nodosum is the typical cutaneous manifestation in sarcoidosis, and skin involvement in these patients is associated with excellent prognosis.

C. Cervical and hilar adenopathy are common in sarcoidosis.

D. Ocular involvement is a poor prognostic indicator.

377. **B.** This child has interstitial lung disease. Diffuse interstitial pneumonia is noted on biopsy with inflammation and collagen deposition. This condition can occur in immunocompromised patients. Treatment involves high-dose corticosteroids. The mortality rate can be as high as 50%.

A. Interstitial lung disease is treated with corticosteroids.

C. Erythromycin is unlikely to be of benefit in interstitial lung disease.

D. Racemic epinephrine may be an adjunctive treatment but is not considered to be a first-line treatment of interstitial lung disease.

E. There is no indication for surgery in this patient.

378. **C.** The gynecoid pelvis is the most favorable pelvis for vaginal delivery. This pelvis type is seen in 50% of women and is characterized by an oval inlet, straight sidewalls, nonprominent ischial spines, a wide subpubic arch and a concave sacrum.

A. The android pelvis is wedge shaped with convergent pelvic sidewalls and prominent ischial spines.

B. The anthropoid pelvis is common in African-American women and is marked by an oval inlet with divergent pelvic sidewalls.

D. The platypelloid pelvis is rare and characterized by a wide transverse diameter of the inlet.

E. Tetroid is not a description of the female pelvis.

379. **C.** This patient is suffering from a pancreatic pseudocyst, which is a complication of pancreatitis. A pseudocyst draws it name from the absence of a true capsule surrounding the cyst. Ultrasonography and CT can be used to image pseudocysts. Treatment usually involves a period of observation to allow the pseudocyst capsule to mature so that a surgical treatment can be performed. Percutaneous drainage can be performed, but more definitive procedures include anastomosing the cyst wall to the stomach to allow its contents to drain into the stomach. Usually the symptoms of a pseudocyst are due to the compression of adjacent structures. In this clinical scenario, the cyst has eroded into the gastroduodenal artery, which, along with the splenic arteries, have been found to occur with pancreatic pseudocysts.

A, B, D, and **E.** Erosion occurred into the gastroduodenal artery.

380. **D.** Vitamin K is required for synthesis of factors II, VII, IX, and X. The PTT assesses all coagulation proteins except factors VII and XII. The PT is elevated when there is a deficiency in factors I, II, V, VII, or X. Factor VII has the shortest half-life; a deficiency in factor VII is the usual cause in generalized problems such as liver disease. This patient may have liver disease, but it should be recognized that the most frequent setting for vitamin K deficiency is a malnourished patient receiving antibiotics. Thus, the malnourished patient had a lack of vitamin K leading to decreased production of the above factors creating a prolonged PT and excessive bleeding.

A. Hemophilia A is an X-linked recessive disorder. Patients often present with hemarthoses, and excessive bleeding with surgery/trauma. Laboratory findings would show prolonged PTT, not PT. Bleeding time is normal.

B. Although thiamine deficiency is common in alcoholics and this patient could likely be an alcoholic, it does not cause this abnormality. Thiamine deficiency is responsible for Wernicke-Korsakoff syndrome, not a coagulopathy.

C. von Willebrand disease is an autosomal-dominant condition resulting in defective von Willebrand factor, which is produced by megakaryocytes and endothelial cells. It is the only clotting factor not produced by the liver. Examination would show easy bruising, mucosal bleeding, and postincisional bleeding. Laboratory studies would show no disorders of PT, PTT, or platelets.

E. It is possible that coumadin therapy can prolong the patient's PT. However, we have no reason to suspect that the patient has been taking coumadin. Given the malnourished state of the patient and the fact that he was found unconscious on the street and drunk makes liver disease or vitamin K deficiency a more likely diagnosis.

381. **B.** The patient's presentation is consistent with small bowel obstruction (SBO), and the two most common causes of this condition are postoperative adhesions and hernias. With our patient's history of significant intra-abdominal surgery, presence of adhesions is the best diagnosis. A history of nonspecific symptoms such as abdominal pain, nausea, and vomiting may not seem very helpful in making the diagnosis until put face to face with the physical examination findings. Nonlocalized pain out of proportion to physical examination findings is in fact a hallmark sign of SBO. The upright radiograph finding of an air-fluid level and dilated intestinal loops confirm the diagnosis. This is an important diagnosis to make in our patient because of the dehydration sequelae that accompany this problem. In our patient, low blood pressure and dry mucous membranes are signs of dehydration that will need to be addressed with intravenous fluids.

Figure 381

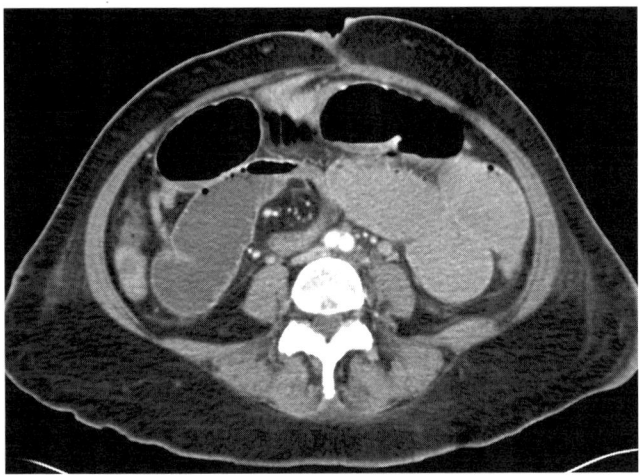

A. Approximately 1% to 2% of SBOs are caused by gallstones. With the gallbladder removed, however, the source for a stone becomes difficult to imagine. Also, radiographic evidence of a stone is not present, which along with signs of obstruction and pneumobilia (air in the biliary tree) is present in 50% of radiographs of patients with gallstone ileus.

C. Intussusception can occur in adult patients but most commonly occurs in the pediatric population, peaking at 5 to 9 months of age; therefore, this is an unlikely diagnosis in our patient who has a history of prior intra-abdominal surgery. However, this is the most common cause of SBO in children.

D. Although mesenteric ischemia can cause SBO, this patient does not have any risk factors for this problem, such as coronary artery disease, thromboembolism, or hypercoagulable state.

E. Postoperative paralytic ileus can be distinguished from postoperative adhesions by the history. With ileus the patient will never regain bowel function after the surgery. With adhesions the patient will have a period of postoperative ileus, the regaining of normal bowel function, and then bowel function decline as the obstruction occurs.

382. **B.** In the normal, or gaussian, distribution the values fall into a bell-shaped curve. Sixty-eight percent fall within 1 standard deviation. Ninety-five percent fall within 2 standard deviations of the mean. Ninety-nine percent fall within 3 standard deviations of the mean.

383. **A.** The most common source of same-day fever following an operation is atelectasis, which is caused by the inadequate breathing effort postsurgery. It is more commonly seen with surgeries in the abdomen and pelvis.

B. Perihepatic abscess does not develop in under 24 hours. They usually form 5 to 7 days postsurgery.

C. Pneumonia usually takes 2 to 3 days to develop and is most often secondary to the atelectasis if the atelectasis is not treated.

D. Urinary tract infections are usually catheter related and take more than 24 hours to develop. They can occur 3 to 5 days postsurgery.

E. Wound infections do not occur in under 24 hours. They usually take 5 to 8 days postsurgery to occur.

384. **A.** This child has symptoms suggestive of duodenal atresia. This condition is frequently associated with Down syndrome. Symptoms include nonbilious vomiting and a "double-bubble" sign on abdominal x-rays, which is a result of gastric and duodenal distention with a thickened pylorus between them. Treatment includes surgical duodenoplasty.

B. Gastrograffin enema is appropriate in the treatment of meconium ileus syndrome.

C. Pyloromyotomy is appropriate to treat pyloric stenosis.

D. Sigmoid resection is not necessary because this condition does not occur in the sigmoid colon.

E. Watchful waiting is inappropriate in this condition.

385. **E.** This patient appears to have suffered a scaphoid fracture. Hand and wrist injuries are common in the population but nonetheless deserve a great deal of attention due to the importance of the hands in everyday life. This patient has fallen on an outstretched hand and now has pain in the anatomic snuffbox, a classic description of a scaphoid fracture. This patient should be sent for x-rays, which will be taken in three views (oblique, lateral, anteroposterior). The scaphoid fracture is a very worrisome injury due to the increased likelihood of avascular necrosis. With suspicious mechanisms of injury and point tenderness, one should always request films.

A. Ultimately this patient can be treated with cold packs and follow up after x-rays are taken.

B. CT scan is costly and unlikely to be of benefit in this patient.

C. Casting is not necessary for this type of injury.

D. X-rays should be taken of this patient to be sure of the diagnosis.

386. **B.** This patient presents with secondary tuberculosis, as evidenced by his classic symptoms and radiographic findings in the lung apices. The criteria for diagnosis in patients with known HIV is a purified protein derivative (PPD) of greater than 5 mm induration. Nonimmunocompromised patients will need larger areas of induration to be present before establishing a diagnosis because their bodies can mount a relatively larger response to the PPD skin test, so using a criteria of greater than 5 mm would decrease specificity too much.

A. Although certainly the physical examination can lead to suspicion of tuberculosis, it is not diagnostic in a patient with known HIV infection, who may have several possibilities for lung infection.

C. Ten millimeters induration is the criteria used in higher risk patients, such as those who are homeless, imprisoned, or malnourished.

D. This is the criteria used for low-risk patients. Having HIV excludes the patient from this criteria.

E. A sputum culture takes weeks to grow tuberculosis.

387. **A.** This patient has evidence of an esophageal web. This is a mucosal stricture located anywhere along the esophagus. Intermittent dysphagia is a typical presentation. Plummer-Vinson syndrome is associated with iron deficiency anemia, achlorhydria, glossitis, and stomatitis. Treatment involves endoscopic dilation.

B. Intravenous corticosteroids may be useful in the treatment of caustic ingestions.

C. Monopolar coagulation can be useful in the management of bleeding esophageal varices.

D. Surgical resection is not indicated in this patient.

E. Watchful waiting is inappropriate in this individual with symptoms and a significant weight loss.

388. **D.** A tumor in the right parietal lobe interfering with the optic radiations would produce a left lower quadrant anopsia.

A. A lesion compromising the optic chiasm would produce a bitemporal hemianopsia.

B. A lesion interrupting the right optic tract would lead to a left homonymous hemianopsia.

C. A left upper quadrant anopsia would result from a lesion in the inferior portion of the right optic radiation within the temporal lobe.

E. Such a clinical picture would occur with a lesion further posterior within the optic radiation.

389. **D.** The most likely diagnosis if pelvic abscess is ruled out is septic pelvic thrombophlebitis. Intravenous heparin is the most appropriate treatment for this condition. The pregnant woman's predispositions to thrombophlebitis include stasis, vascular damage, and hypercoagulability. Venous thrombi usually develop in relatively small veins and then extend centrally as far as the inferior vena cava.

A. Antifungal agents are unlikely to be of benefit in patients with septic pelvic thrombophlebitis.

B. Dilation and curettage is unlikely to be of benefit in the patient with septic thrombophlebitis.

C. Exploratory laparotomy would not contribute to management.

E. Results of pelvic examination were normal. Repeating this step is unnecessary.

390. **E.** This child has phenylketonuria. Symptoms often begin in childhood and include hypertonicity, tremors, mental retardation and behavioral problems. These occur as a result of increased levels of toxic metabolites. The hypopigmentation occurs secondary to decreased tyrosine, which is needed for melanin production.

A. Symptoms of homocystinuria are also observed in childhood. They include a Marfan body habitus, mental retardation, dislocated lenses, and vascular thromboses.

B. There is no evidence to suggest hyperuricemia in this patient. There is no evidence of destructive behavior or renal stones.

C. Galactosemia, or deficiency of galactose-1-phosphate uridyl transferase, becomes evident a few days to weeks after initiation of feedings. Symptoms include emesis, anorexia, poor growth, hepatomegaly, liver failure, acidosis, and declining renal function. Later in life those affected may have learning disabilities and premature ovarian failure or ovarian hypofunction.

D. Ornithine transcarbamylase deficiency appears 24 to 48 hours after initiation of protein-containing feeds. Infants appear lethargic and may have seizures at high ammonia levels. Female carriers, who exhibit lionization, may also be symptomatic. They may suffer from emesis, headaches, and even learning disabilities.

391. **B.** Treatment should take place as soon as the retrobulbar hematoma is diagnosed. Sutures should be opened immediately to relieve the pressure. Head elevation and compresses should be continued. Give 20% mannitol intravenously as well as corticosteroids.

A. Lateral canthotomy is performed only if there is no improvement after incision and drainage.

C. This is performed only if there is no improvement after incision, drainage, and canthotomy.

D. Warm compresses, head elevation, and antibiotics are treatments for eye infection. This is not recommended treatment for hemorrhage.

E. Evacuation of hematoma with a large bore needle is only done if the hematoma is of moderate size and non-expanding, which would be determined clinically by the patient's symptoms.

392. **A.** Analysis of variance allows for the researcher to determine the differences between the means of more than two samples. Two-way analysis of variance tests differences between the mean body weights of men and woman and among mean body weights of different groups.

393. **B.** The chi-square test allows the researcher to assess the differences between frequencies in a sample. This will test the difference between the percentage of people with body weight at or under 140 pounds and the percentage of people with body weight over 140 pounds in a second group at a second time.

394. **E.** The *t* test allows for the determination of differences between the means of two samples. The dependent *t* test (paired) tests the differences between mean body weights at time 1 and time 2 of the people in group 1 (i.e., the same people sampled on two occasions).

395. **C.** Correlation tests the mutual relationship between two continuous variables. For example, this can test the relationship between blood pressure and body weight at time 2.

396. **E.** African Americans respond best to thiazide diuretics and calcium channel blockers for treatment of hypertension. Thiazide diuretics may cause hypokalemia, hyperuricemia, hyperglycemia, and elevated low-density lipoprotein.

A. Whites respond best to ACE inhibitors and beta blockers. African Americans do not respond as well to ACE inhibitors.

B. Beta blockers are effective in reducing long-term mortality in patients after myocardial infarction. They are also effective in patients with diabetes.

C. Clonidine is not as effective as most of the other antihypertensive medications and would not be a good first-line choice in this patient.

D. It was appropriate to try lifestyle modifications for 3 to 6 months, but because no improvement has been seen, pharmacologic therapy should be initiated.

397. **E.** Coarctation of the aorta results in upper extremity hypertension and lower extremity hypotension. This hypertension leads to aortic dilatation, pulmonary hypertension, and right ventricular hypertrophy. The left ventricle may become inadequate, and an echocardiogram for left ventricular function is indicated.

A. Atrial flutter is not associated with coarctation of the aorta.

B. First-degree atrioventricular block is not associated with coarctation of the aorta.

C. Narrow complex tachycardia is not associated with coarctation of the aorta.

D. Prolonged QT interval is not associated with coarctation of the aorta.

398. **C.** The menstrual cycle begins as the follicular phase at day 0 with the end of menstruation. During the follicular phase, the pituitary releases FSH and results in the development of a primary ovarian follicle. This follicle produces estrogen, which is responsible for the proliferation of the uterine lining. Midway through the cycle, at approximately day 14, the estrogen levels reach a critical point that leads to a pituitary-driven LH spike, which stimulates the release of the ovum from the follicle, or ovulation. Ovulation marks the end of the follicular phase and the beginning of the luteal phase.

399. **C.** This patient has hyperkalemia. Examination findings and ECG results show the classic peaked T waves. Treatment involves stopping potassium intake and administering sodium gluconate, sodium bicarbonate, and insulin with glucose.

A. Two-dimensional echocardiography is not necessary in the evaluation of hyperkalemia.

B. There is no reason to give epinephrine because this patient is not having an anaphylactic reaction.

D. Cardiac enzymes and repeat ECG would be indicated if this patient were having chest pain with unstable angina.

E. Potassium should not be given because this patient already has hyperkalemia.

400. **B.** Metronidazole is the correct treatment for amebic liver abscess. Travel to an endemic area is a risk factor for this disease. The patients usually present with the triad of fever, hepatomegaly, and right upper quadrant pain. Multiple ulcers are present on the enlarged liver with a large abscess that may contain chocolate-colored pus. *Entamoeba histolytica* may spread to the lungs or brain. Leukocytosis with neutrophilia is seen on CBC. A complement-fixation test will have a positive reaction to *E. histolytica*. Metronidazole is first-line treatment followed by surgery if the abscess ruptures or treatment fails.

A. Amphotericin B is not effective against amebic liver abscess.

C. Penicillin G is not effective against amebic liver abscess.

D. Surgery is reserved for treatment failure or abscess rupture.

E. Trimethoprim-sulfamethoxazole is not effective against amebic liver abscess.

401. **B.** Arteriovenous malformation (AVM) along with diverticulosis are the most common causes for asymptomatic rectal bleeding in adults. AVM is more likely in her case because her risk for diverticulosis is lessened due to her diet high in fiber and low in fat. AVM is also associated with von Willebrand factor deficiency (hence the easy bleeding) and aortic stenosis.

A. Antithrombin III deficiency would be associated with a history of hypercoagulability, not easy bleeding.

C. Although colon cancer should certainly be in the differential diagnosis of this patient's painless rectal bleeding, it is not as likely as an AVM or diverticulosis.

D. Diverticulosis is the second most likely cause of painless rectal bleeding in her case.

E. Diverticulitis would present with acute abdominal pain associated with left lower quadrant tenderness. She would also likely present with a history of a high-fat, low-fiber diet because the presence of diverticulosis is necessary before diverticulitis can occur.

402. **A.** The patient is suffering from Korsakoff psychosis, which is caused by vitamin B_1 (thiamine) deficiency. Patients with this psychosis present with signs of anterograde and/or retrograde amnesia with confabulation. It is often also associated with alcoholic neuropathy. The treatment is administration of vitamin B_1 intravenously.

B–E. This patient is lacking vitamin B_1.

403. **A.** Cystosarcoma phyllodes is a variant of fibroadenoma. The lesions are typically 4 to 5 cm in diameter and grow rapidly. The mass is usually mobile, with a smooth, well-circumscribed border. The skin above the lesion is engorged, warm, shiny, and erythematous. They are uncommon and most are benign; however, some have a sarcomatous potential.

B. Duct ectasia is associated with multicolored, sticky nipple discharge. Patients may present with breast pain, subareolar masses, or a retracted nipple. This occurs most often after menopause and is caused by ductal inflammation. Patients need a mammogram and an excisional biopsy to rule out cancer. Local excision is the definitive treatment.

C. Fibroadenomas are the most common breast lesions in patients under 30 years of age. The lesions are firm, rubbery, and nontender. They are mobile and well circumscribed and typically 1 to 5 cm in diameter. Any lesion larger than 5 cm is a giant fibroadenoma and must be evaluated to rule out cystosarcoma phyllodes. They usually change with a woman's menstrual cycle or with oral birth control pills and pregnancy. If the patient is stable and has no family history of breast cancer, these lesions may be followed clinically. In other patients, the lesion needs to be differentiated from phyllodes and cancer by fine-needle aspiration or excised if the lesion is suspicious.

D. Intraductal papilloma is associated with bloody nipple discharge. This is a benign lesion, but the discharge should be sent for analysis to rule out invasive papillary carcinoma, which can present with similar symptoms. The lesions are usually solitary and do not usually turn malignant. The treatment is ductal excision.

E. Squamous cell carcinoma is unlikely to occur in the breast. In the female, this tumor can occur in the cervix, urethra, and bladder.

404. **D.** This woman is in labor and is exhausted. Her contractions are strong and 2 minutes apart. Because the baby's head is at station +3 and is visible at the introitus, delivery by outlet forceps is an acceptable choice. This baby could also be delivered by vacuum extractor.

A. Epidural anesthetic may arrest labor and is not indicated at this point.

B. If a mother has been pushing for 2 hours and is exhausted, it is not advisable to tell her to push harder.

C. Oxytocin drip is inappropriate for this patient because she has strong contractions at frequent intervals.

E. Transabdominal ultrasonography is unlikely to benefit the management of this patient.

405. **A.** This patient has a red pinna characteristic of chondritis. The affected ear is usually red, thickened, and indurated, sometimes with areas of purulent discharge. The best clinical test to distinguish cellulitis or external otitis from chondritis is that pulling the ear and pinching the ear will be quite painful in the latter condition. Treatment involves intravenous antibiotics, and some patients may require surgical débridement.

B. Oral antibiotics are inappropriate for patients with chondritis.

C. This condition is not caused by a fungus; therefore, treatment with antifungal agents is inappropriate.

D. Oral corticosteroids as a sole means of therapy for this condition are inappropriate because antibiotics are needed to treat the underlying infection.

E. Following a course of intravenous antibiotics, surgical débridement of infected cartilage may be necessary.

406. **D.** Fifteen percent of patients with small cell carcinoma of the lung will develop syndrome of inappropriate antidiuretic hormone secretion (SIADH). There is high urine osmolality (normal 500–850 mOsm/kg), urine sodium greater than 20 mEq/L, hyponatremia, and decreased serum osmolality. Small cell cancer is the type most associated with paraneoplastic conditions in lung cancer and most commonly produces SIADH and adrenocorticotropic hormone.

A. Adenocarcinoma is not as likely to be found in smokers and is the most common lung cancer of nonsmokers. It would not be as likely as small cell cancer in this situation.

B. Large cell cancer is associated with smoking and may produce a paraneoplastic syndrome, but small cell is more likely in this case.

C. The risk for mesothelioma is increased with smoking but usually is associated with exposure to asbestos.

E. Squamous cell cancer is associated with smoking but is more noted for producing hypercalcemia from pro-thrombin hormone–related peptide production.

407. **D.** NHL in children is diffuse and highly malignant. It normally occurs between 7 and 11 years of age, and is three times more likely in males. The abdomen is the most common site of initial manifestation, which produces symptoms of abdominal pain, ascites, or obstruction by serving as the lead point for an intussusception. Treatment consists of aggressive multidrug chemotherapy.

A. ALL normally presents with fatigue, fever, and pallor, and a CBC reveals neutropenia.

B. AML presents with the same symptoms as ALL.

C. Hodgkin lymphoma often presents with painless lymphadenopathy, normally of the supraclavicular and cervical nodes.

E. Neuroblastoma often presents as an abdominal mass with pain, and hypertension may be present.

408. **B.** This patient is at 42 weeks' gestation by dates. She should have induction of labor with oxytocin. By inducing labor in this patient, there should be a decrease in this infant's risk for perinatal mortality.

A. Epidural anesthetic will slow labor progression in this patient.

C. Non-stress testing should be checked periodically if the dates are not firm.

D. Oxytocin challenge should be performed periodically if the dates are not firm.

E. This patient has a postterm pregnancy and should deliver as soon as possible.

409. **A.** The history and radiograph describe rheumatoid arthritis (RA). A key features that differentiates it from osteoarthritis is morning stiffness lasting for more than 1 hour that is worse in the morning. The radiographic appearance of RA includes narrowing of the joint space, which results from a decrease in the articular cartilage, and a decrease in the radiodensity of the periarticular bone, which results from a decrease in bone mineral density. First-line therapy for RA is aspirin or nonsteroidal antiinflammatory drugs.

Figure 409

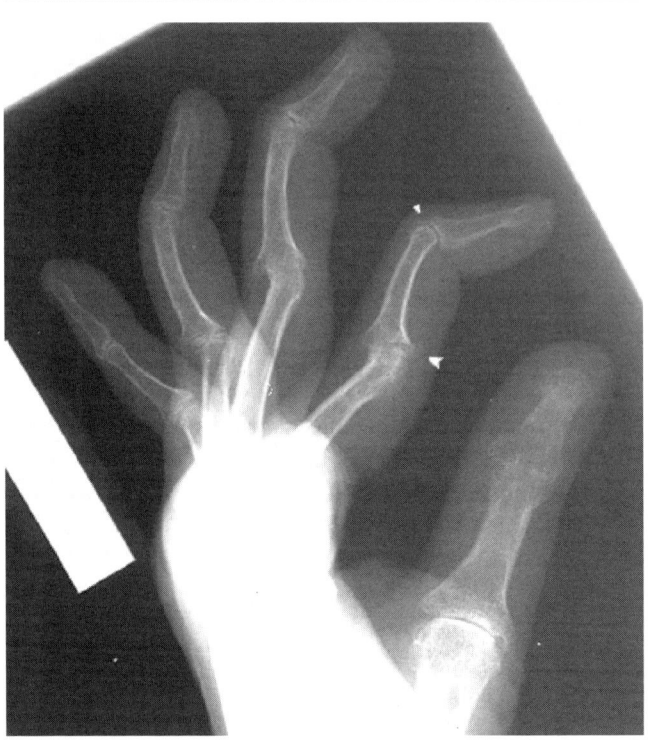

B–E. This agent is second-line therapy for RA. Other second-line agents include sulfasalazine, antimalarials, and azathioprine. Together with the salicylates these second-line agents are effectively called disease-modifying antirheumatic drugs.

410. **A.** This patient has symptoms of gastric carcinoma. Signs and symptoms include anorexia and weight loss. Nausea, vomiting, and dysphagia are also common. Examination may reveal an abdominal mass in 50% of patients. Adenocarcinoma is the most common variety, seen in 95%. This tumor demonstrates infiltration of the gastric mucosa on the accompanying upper gastrointestinal series.

B. Leiomyoma is a smooth muscle tumor that can ulcerate when large. This tumor is benign.

C. Leiomyosarcoma is an uncommon tumor with muscular elements that can occur in the stomach.

D. Gastric lymphoma may be isolated or from widespread disease. Thickened rugal folds are noted on endoscopy.

E. Melanoma rarely occurs in the stomach, even when the disease is metastatic.

411. **C.** Although direct questioning can elicit information, the open-ended type of question and interview is most likely to produce a good clinical relationship, aid in obtaining information about the patient, and not close off potential areas of pertinent information.

A, B, D, and **E.** These are examples of direct questions.

412. **A.** The most common cause of dysfunctional uterine bleeding is anovulation. Anovulation can be associated with heavy menstrual bleeding or scant menstrual bleeding. This condition is common in puberty and before menopause.

B. Coagulation defect is unlikely in this patient.

C. Ovulation dysfunction is more common in the reproductive years.

D. Transitional cell carcinoma is unlikely in this patient with a negative urinalysis result.

E. Uterine polyps are uncommon in this age group.

413. **D.** This patient is consuming a diet rich in flavonoids, which are phytochemicals. These agents are antioxidants and reduce cell proliferation. They also increase the pump-mediated efflux of certain carcinogens from cells. Isoflavones of soy may also lower low-density lipoprotein cholesterol.

A. Flavonoids are not bacteriostatic.

B. Chlorogenic acid blocks nitrosamine formation.

C. Allylic sulfides detoxify enzymes against bacteria.

E. Triterenoids suppress carcinogenic activity of estrogen.

414. **C.** The incidence rate is the number of new events that occur in a specific period of time divided by the population at risk. The prevalence is all of the cases of the disease at a specific point in time divided by the number of people at risk. The incidence will not change because the same number of people will be getting cancer. However, fewer people will have cancer at a specific period in time (the prevalence) because there will be fewer survivors.

A. The prevalence will decrease.

B. The incidence will not change.

D. The incidence will not change.

E. The incidence will not change and the prevalence will decrease.

415. **D.** This patient has symptomatic cholelithiasis. Upper abdominal (hepatic) ultrasonography may reveal the presence of gallstones, thickened gallbladder wall, and pericholecystic fluid.

A. Abdominal x-ray is inappropriate because only about 15% of gallstones are visualized on plain film.

B. Renal and bladder ultrasonography is inappropriate because the kidneys are not the culprit in this case.

C. CT scan of the abdomen would also confirm the diagnosis but it is more expensive and does not offer a significant advantage over ultrasonography.

E. Upper gastrointestinal endoscopy will not give any information about the gallbladder.

416. **D.** This patient has patellar tendonitis. This condition is usually seen in basketball or volleyball players and is characterized by chronic anterior knee pain from microscopic fatigue tears at the insertion of the patella tendon into the inferior pole of the patella. Treatment includes rest, ice, antiinflammatory medication, and frequent stretching of the quadriceps muscle. Pain becomes resistant to treatment with scarring of the tendon.

A. Antibiotics are not likely to be helpful in patellar tendonitis.

B. Complete rest for 6 to 8 weeks is required to maximize treatment response.

C. Continuation of activities will lead to recurrence of symptoms.

E. There is no role for surgical resection for the treatment of patella tendonitis.

417. **B.** Projection is when feelings that are distressing to an individual are attributed to others.

A. Displacement is when feelings or ideas that are distressing to someone are redirected to a substitute that evokes a less intense emotional response.

C. Reaction formation is transforming an unacceptable impulse to the opposite.

D. Splitting is when one says something is all good or all bad to avoid thinking about living in contradictory states.

E. Undoing is trying to prevent or undo consequences from an irrationally anticipated event.

418. **B.** Corticosteroids should be considered in patients with severe or progressive lung disease, hypercalcemia, cardiac involvement, uveitis, or neurosarcoidosis. Such a patient would be started on prednisone 40 mg daily for a few months then tapered to avoid side effects.

A. There is no indication for antibiotics in this patient.

C. This patient needs therapy with high-dose steroids and a taper.

D. Lung transplantation is not eminent for this patient.

E. In a patient with asymptomatic hilar adenopathy no therapy is required.

419. **A.** Femoral hernias are about five times more common in women than in men. The borders of a femoral hernia are inferior to the inguinal ligament, lateral to the lacunar ligament, and medial to the femoral vein. These hernias are more prone to incarceration and strangulation of viscera.

B. Inguinal hernias are more common in males.

C. Obturator hernias occur when the hernia sac protrudes through the obturator canal.

D. There are no findings to suggest an umbilical hernia, which often protrudes through the umbilicus.

E. There is no evidence to suggest a vertebral hernia, which could cause nerve root compression and cause signs of neurologic deficiency.

420. **F.** Praziquantel (or niclosamide) is the primary treatment for either cestodes (tapeworms) or trematodes (flukes). When the eggs of the pork tapeworm (*Taenia solium*) are consumed (rather than the cysts from infected meat), the cysts mature in the human gastrointestinal tract and then migrate into either the muscle or brain. Brain infection of the cysticercus can cause either seizures, focal neurologic deficits, or obstructive hydrocephalus. Diagnosis is made by fecal sample or biopsy of the infected tissue.

A. Although albendazole does treat *Taenia solium* in addition to the worms treated by mebendazole, it is not the treatment of choice for *Taenia solium*.

B. Diethylcarbamazine is used for filariasis, which causes elephantiasis, or swelling of the extremities due to lymphatic blockage by the filarial worm.

C. Ivermectin is used against intestinal nematodes and *Onchocerca volvulus*.

D. Metronidazole is used for infections of *Giardia, Entamoeba, Trichomonas,* or *Clostridium difficile*.

E. Mebendazole is used for worms such as nematodes, *Ascaris,* hookworms (*Necator*), pinworms, whipworms, or *Trichinella spiralis*.

G. Pyrantel pamoate is an alternative to mebendazole, thiabendazole, and albendazole in case the side effects of those drugs are not tolerated, which may include abdominal pain.

H. Thiabendazole is used to treat the same worms that mebendazole treats.

421. **B.** Cholecystitis is inflammation of the gallbladder most commonly due to the presence of gallstones. Biliary colic often occurs (episodic right upper quadrant pain associated with nausea and vomiting) after a fatty meal. Pain can be quite severe and radiate posteriorly to the right scapula. A low-grade fever can be present as well. Laboratory studies often show leukocytosis and elevated serum bilirubin and elevated alkaline phosphatase. Ultrasonography is accurate, but hepato-iminodiacetic acid (HIDA) scans are the gold standard.

A. Cholelithiasis implies the presence of gallstones, but does not necessarily cause symptoms. More than half of the stones are made of cholesterol, and thus cannot be seen on x-ray, as with bile pigment stones. Calcium stones are visible on plain films of the abdomen.

C. Cholangitis is a bacterial infection of the bile ducts usually due to stone obstruction. It classically presents with the Charcot triad: biliary colic, jaundice, and fever. Laboratory values will be similar to those of cholecystitis. Ultrasonography will often show stones obstructing the bile ducts. Endoscopic retrograde cholangiopancreatography is more sensitive.

D. Choledocholithiasis is the presence of stones in the common bile duct, which is not present in this patient.

E. Although prolonged cholecystitis is a risk factor for gallbladder adenocarcinoma, cancer is not the most likely diagnosis in this patient. Her symptoms are of short duration. She denies experiencing jaundice, weight loss, anorexia, or fever.

422. **C.** This patient has signs and symptoms of uterine rupture. Rupture may be spontaneous or traumatic. Symptoms include bleeding during labor, suprapubic pain, and cessation of uterine contractions. Hemoperitoneum and hypovolemic shock can result. Treatment involves abdominal exploration and may require hysterectomy.

A. Embolization of the hypogastric artery is an inappropriate treatment for rupture of the uterus.

B. Embolization of the uterine artery is an inappropriate treatment for rupture of the uterus.

D. Vaginal packing is inappropriate for a patient with hypovolemic shock and uterine rupture.

E. Observation is inappropriate for a patient with hypovolemic shock and uterine rupture.

423. **D.** Leukocoria (white pupil) in a child may be caused by a number of entities. Cataracts are the most common cause of leukocoria, but retinoblastoma is the most lifethreatening cause. Leukocoria may be detected by routine screening of the red reflex and, if found, requires immediate referral to an ophthalmologist.

A. CT scan of the head would not be indicated for this patient.

B. MRI of the head would not be indicated for this patient.

C. Leukocoria requires prompt evaluation due to the possibility of a life-threatening cause.

E. Erythromycin eye drops are the treatment of choice for bacterial conjunctivitis, but are not indicated for leukocoria.

424. **B.** The scenario describes a patient with absence seizures. The 3-Hz spike-and-wave pattern on EEG is a classic finding. Ethosuximide is the treatment of choice.

A. Carbamazepine is not used to treat absence seizures.

C. Phenobarbital is the preferred treatment of tonicclonic seizures in the pediatric population.

D. Phenytoin is not used to treat absence seizures.

E. Although valproic acid is a potential treatment for absence seizures, ethosuximide is now the preferred treatment.

425. **C.** Back pain is the most common neurologic symptom in patients with systemic cancer. Metastatic carcinoma, multiple myeloma, and lymphoma can involve the spine. Pain is often unrelieved with rest. MRI reveals metastasis with sparing of the disc space.

A. Without a history of trauma, low back strain is not a likely diagnosis.

B. Lumbar arachnoiditis may follow inflammatory response to local tissue injury in the subarachnoid space.

D. Spondylolisthesis is slippage of the anterior spine while leaving the posterior elements behind. Lumbar radiculopathy can result.

E. Vertebral osteomyelitis is associated with low back pain that is unrelieved by rest, focal spine tenderness, and an elevated erythrocyte sedimentation rate.

426. **A.** This patient has small cell (oat cell) carcinoma of the lung. It is a primary tumor that is often metastatic at presentation. The disease is linked to endocrine syndromes such as Cushing disease and syndrome of inappropriate antidiuretic hormone secretion (SIADH). In addition, Lambert-Eaton syndrome is a myasthenia gravis–like syndrome that may occur in patients with small cell lung carcinoma. The mechanism is induction of autoantibodies that cross-react with the presynaptic calcium channel.

B. Lymphangiolyomyomatosis is a progressive disease nearly always found in menstruating women. It can be associated with pneumothorax, not small cell carcinoma of the lung.

C. Metastatic renal carcinoma may secondarily metastasize to the lung. It would be expected to present with secondary polycythemia due to ectopic erythropoietin production.

D. Although it has symptoms similar to those of Lambert-Eaton syndrome, myasthenia gravis is not known to be associated with small cell carcinoma of the lung. However, it does have an association with anterior mediastinal tumors of the thymus.

E. Although superior vena cava syndrome can be present with bronchogenic carcinoma or lymphoma, it would present as a swelling of the head and upper extremities due to physical blockage of the superior vena cava.

427. **D.** Isotretinoin (vitamin A) is associated with several congenital malformations. Physical examination of exposed individuals may reveal small, abnormally shaped ears, hypoplasia of the mandible, cleft palate, and cardiac defects.

A. Fetal alcohol syndrome results from maternal ingestion of alcohol during pregnancy. Features of this condition include short palpebral fissures, maxillary hypoplasia, and cardiac defects.

B. Amphetamines are associated with several congenital malformations, including cleft lip and palate, as well as cardiac defects. This teratogen is not associated with mandibular hypoplasia or otologic abnormalities.

C. Diethylstilbestrol exposure is associated with limb abnormalities.

E. Norethisterone is associated with gynecomastia.

428. **G.** Pancreatic carcinoma has an insidious onset with abdominal pain that radiates to the back in 75% of patients. Peak incidence is in the seventh decade of life, with a male to female ratio of 5:1. Anorexia, weight loss, dark urine, clay-colored stools, and pruritus can also occur. Examination may reveal jaundice and a palpable gallbladder. Ultrasonography will show a mass in 75% of patients.

429. **H.** This patient has primary sclerosing cholangitis. This condition is more common in men between the ages of 25 and 45. Sixty percent of cases occur in patients with ulcerative colitis. Signs include pruritus, right upper quadrant pain, jaundice, fever, weight loss, and malaise. Elevations of bilirubin and alkaline phosphatase are common. Endoscopic retrograde cholangiopancreatography studies will reveal stenosis and dilatation of the intra- and extrahepatic bile ducts.

430. **E.** Chronic cholecystitis is usually caused by gallstones. Patients complain of nonspecific right upper quadrant pain and dyspepsia associated with intake of fatty foods. Serum transaminases are normal. Ultrasonography reveals gallstones within a contracted gallbladder. Treatment is generally supportive, but surgery should be considered if the patient is symptomatic.

431. **A.** Acute cholecystitis is an inflammation of the gallbladder usually secondary to cystic duct obstruction by an impacted stone. Ninety percent of cases are associated with gallstones. Signs and symptoms include right upper quadrant pain, nausea, vomiting, and fever. Examination may reveal a palpable mass in 20% of patients as well as a positive Murphy sign. This sign is present when deep inspiration during palpation of the right upper quadrant produces inspiratory arrest. Laboratory findings in this condition include elevations of WBC count, alkaline phosphatase, and serum transaminases.

432. **C.** This patient has symptoms of cholelithiasis. Typical symptoms include biliary colic, which is constant, and right upper quadrant pain that occurs approximately 60 minutes after meals, lasts for several hours, and occasionally radiates to the back or right scapula. Nausea and vomiting are typical. Physical examination may reveal epigastric pain to deep palpation or be completely normal. Mild elevation of transaminases is frequently seen.

433. **A.** History of DES exposure has been linked to incompetent cervix. Management includes elective, prophylactic cerclage at 12 to 14 weeks' gestational age. DES exposure is also linked to clear cell carcinoma of the cervix or vagina. Other vaginal abnormalities include vaginal adenosis, incomplete septa, fibrous bands, and segmental vaginal narrowing.

B and **C.** DES exposure is associated with incompetent cervix. The problem is not hormonal or endocrine in nature.

D. This problem is not endocrine in nature. Thus, leuprolide acetate is unlikely to be of benefit.

E. Progesterone supplement is not appropriate management for DES exposure.

434. **E.** Sublimation is a mature defense and involves taking feelings that are distressing to the ego and converting them to something more acceptable.

A. Altruism is a benign, constructive reaction formation to an emotion that usually benefits others.

B. Dissociation is another neurotic defense involving a modification of a person's character to avoid personal distress.

C. Intellectualization is actually a neurotic defense; it involves excessive stress placed on irrelevant details.

D. Rationalization is offering rational explanations to justify attitudes that may be unacceptable.

435. **A.** Alpha-fetoprotein (AFP), beta human chorionic gonadotropin, and imaging studies such as CT scan of the abdomen and pelvis are useful to obtain first before any invasive intervention. This allows for proper diagnosis and staging of the tumor. AFP helps exclude a seminoma as an etiology. Therefore it may be useful diagnostically.

B. Diagnostic and staging steps should be taken before treatment with chemotherapy. Chemotherapy is usually implemented in cases of recurrence, retroperitoneal spread, or distant metastasis.

C. CA 27.29 is a tumor marker useful in breast cancer.

D. Percutaneous biopsy should never be performed due to risk of spreading cancer cells.

E. Radical orchiectomy confirms the diagnosis of testicular cancer. Metastasis should first be ruled out with imaging studies.

436. **E.** Epiglottitis is an acute swelling of the epiglottis typically seen in children 2 to 7 years of age. Clinical presentation includes respiratory distress and high fever. Individuals may complain of aphonia, dysphagia, and drooling. Treatment includes emergency placement of an endotracheal tube and intravenous antibiotics active against *Haemophilus influenzae*.

A. Alpha-adrenergic drugs have no place in the treatment of acute epiglottitis.

B. Direct laryngoscopy in this patient may precipitate spasm and closure of the airway and therefore is contraindicated.

C. Oxygen mist has no place in the treatment of acute epiglottitis.

D. Intravenous corticosteroids have no place in the treatment of acute epiglottitis.

437. **C.** This newborn has trisomy 13. This condition is associated with features like microcephaly, holoprosencephaly, a sloping forehead, cleft lip or palate, cutis aplasia, microophthalmia, hypoplastic nails, clinodactyly, polydactyly, congenital heart disease, and renal anomalies.

A. Cri-du-chat syndrome (catlike cry) is associated with cataracts, optic atrophy, and profound mental retardation. Unlike trisomy 13 and 18, most of those affected survive into adulthood.

B. Children with Prader-Willi syndrome have a narrow bifrontal diameter, a downturned mouth, almond-shaped palpebral fissures, central obesity, short stature, small hands and feet, small genitalia, obstructive sleep apnea, mild mental retardation, and impulse control problems

D. Characteristics of trisomy 18 include prominent occiput, a narrow bifrontal diameter, a narrow nose, micrognathia, cleft lip or palate, hypoplastic nails, clinodactyly, rocker-bottom feet, congenital heart disease, and developmental delays.

E. Children with trisomy 21 have a much higher life expectancy than children with trisomy 13 or 18. Down syndrome includes features like excess skin on the posterior neck, a flat occiput, epicanthic folds, upslanted palpebral fissures, low-set ears, a flat nasal bridge, a small mouth, protruding tongue, sandal gap toe, small genitalia, endocardial cushion defects, duodenal atresia, Hirschsprung disease, and hypothyroidism.

438. **B.** Cystic teratomas are characterized by tissues from multiple germ layers, such as cartilage, bone, thyroid tissue, and other organoid formations. These are the most common ovarian tumors during the early reproductive years (age 18–30 years). Overall, they comprise approximately 25% of primary ovarian tumors, and about 15% are bilateral. Cysts can be filled with heavy, greasy sebaceous material.

A. Choriocarcinomas have areas of hemorrhage and necrosis.

C. Endodermal sinus tumors are rare. They occur in young women and can even affect small children.

D. This lesion does not characterize a follicular cyst.

E. Mucinous tumors comprise 15% to 25% of ovarian neoplasms and account for 6% to 10% of ovarian cancers. They can be bilateral in 8% to 10%.

439. **A.** The history of smoking along with the symptoms commonly associated with a cancerous process (weight loss and increasing fatigue) should raise suspicions of lung cancer as the diagnosis. Of the types of lung cancer that have been histologically classified by the World Health Organization, adenocarcinoma, squamous cell carcinoma, large cell carcinoma, and small cell carcinoma account for approximately 95% of all cases of lung cancer. Thirty percent to 40% of the cases are adenocarcinoma, making it the most common type diagnosed. The radiograph shown supports this diagnosis because of the peripherally located nodule in the costophrenic angle of the right lower lobe.

Figure 439

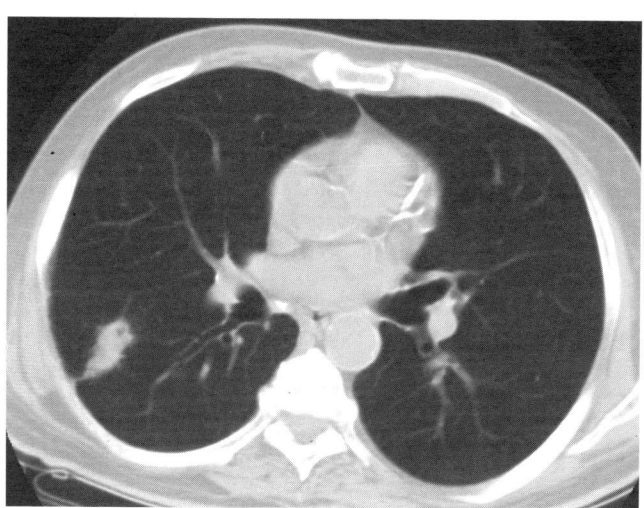

B. No elements of the history point to another location as the primary tumor site. Also, the radiograph provided does not show diffuse, round, well-demarcated nodules of a metastatic lung cancer.

C. Although many patients with lung cancer do have some component of obstructive pulmonary disease, the presence of a nodule on the radiograph should steer you toward lung cancer as the best diagnosis.

D and **E.** Both squamous cell and small cell carcinoma are important causes of lung cancer, representing 20% to 30% and 20% of all cases, respectively; however, the radiographic picture of these cancers would most likely show centrally positioned nodules.

440.   **A.** Linitis plastica is the presence of gastric carcinoma throughout the entire wall of the stomach. The symptoms of early satiety and weight loss correlate with gastric carcinoma, as does the presence of a Virchow node. Gastric carcinoma is more prevalent in Japan, China, and Russia. Carcinoma accounts for approximately 90% of gastric carcinomas. Risk factors include consumption of nitrates or salted/pickled foods, presence of *Helicobacter pylori*, history of partial gastrectomy, Barrett esophagus, gastric adenomas, family history of gastric cancer, and hereditary nonpolyposis colon cancer.

B. Although metastasized breast cancer to the stomach can give it the appearance of a leather bottle and cause the presence of a Virchow node, it is not likely in a man without a history of breast mass.

C. A leathery looking stomach is not likely to be a normal anatomic variant.

D. Superficial spreading gastric carcinoma occurs on the interior mucosa and submucosa of the stomach and does not penetrate the rest of the wall. It has the best prognosis of all gastric carcinomas.

E. Systemic sclerosis would more likely present as dysphagia due to its affinity for the esophagus rather that the stomach. The patient would also lack a Virchow node if this were the case.

441.   **D.** This question illustrates the concept of facilitation. This is a basic interviewing technique used by the physician to encourage the patient to elaborate on an answer. For example, "please go on."

A and **B.** These responses do not encourage facilitation.

C. This response illustrates the concept of empathy.

E. This response illustrates the concept of confrontation.

442.   **C.** This patient presents with typical signs of irritable bowel syndrome. It classically affects young people who are under a great deal of stress from jobs or family situations who complain of alternating constipation and diarrhea and vague tenderness in the right or left lower quadrant. It is suggested that the clinician take stool specimens for ova and parasites to rule out infectious causes. Irritable bowel syndrome is felt to be a peristaltic disorder because of alteration of the normal cholinergic mediated contractions of the small and large bowel musculature. For this reason, some patients with this syndrome respond well to antispasmodic agents. Although this disorder is stress related, it is not psychosomatic or psychological.

A. Irritable bowel syndrome is not a hematologic disorder.

B. Irritable bowel syndrome is not an infectious disorder although infectious causes for these symptoms should be considered initially.

D. Irritable bowel syndrome is not a psychological disorder.

E. Irritable bowel syndrome is not a psychosomatic disorder.

443.   **D.** This patient has a community-acquired atypical pneumonia. *Mycoplasma pneumoniae* is the most common cause of atypical community acquired pneumonia in adolescent population.

A. *Chlamydia pneumoniae* is more common in the neonatal population.

B. *Haemophilus influenzae* would be treated with amoxicillin and is more common in smokers and older patients with community acquired pneumonia.

C. *Legionella pneumophila* is also more common in older patients who have been exposed to poor ventilation systems.

E. *Pseudomonas aeruginosa* is not a common pathogen in patients with community-acquired pneumonia. When this type of pneumonia is seen in a young patient, consider cystic fibrosis or immunocompromised patients.

444.   **D.** The most appropriate next step in this patient's treatment is to test for pregnancy. This patient feels that she is experiencing menopause because of her family history and "hot flashes," and although it is always important to listen to the patient, there are other signs and symptoms that necessitate ruling out or ruling in pregnancy. Although her menstrual cycles are longer than average, they are regular at 41 to 42 days, and her last menstrual period was 70 days ago. She also has symptoms of nausea and breast tenderness. Signs of pregnancy include the Chadwick sign and breast tenderness.

A. The most appropriate next step in this patient's treatment should be to first rule out pregnancy. Although it is true that exogenous estrogen replacement has been found to prevent the loss of bone mineral content, the Women's Health Initiative and other recent randomized controlled trials have failed to confirm beliefs of other potential benefits in reducing the risk of coronary artery disease and stroke.

B. Although it is important to council patients on the importance of discerning correct information found on the Internet from incorrect and finding reputable sources, this should not be the first issue addressed with this patient.

C. The diagnosis of menopause can be made largely by way of a thorough history and physical examination. Confirmation of this diagnosis can be made through the finding of elevated serum follicle-stimulating hormone levels. However, in the scenario above, it is more important to first establish whether or not the patient is pregnant.

E. Women who reach menopause before the age of 40 years are considered to have premature menopause. This is often the result of idiopathic premature ovarian failure (POF). However, if menopause occurs before age 35, chromosomal studies can be obtained to rule out a genetic basis such as Turner syndrome. Turner syndrome typically results in the most severe and irreversible POF, often clinically evident prior to menarche. In Turner syndrome, menopause typically precedes menarche, and there is no evidence of ovarian function. However, cases with multiple tissues diagnosed as 45,X have been reported to result in ovarian function and even pregnancy.

445. **B.** Displacement is the shifting of emotions from an undesirable situation to one that is personally tolerable. To Cindy, it is more tolerable to have Mark go outside and get angry at him, even though she is unhappy with herself.

A. Denial is not accepting reality because it is too painful.

C. Rationalization is creating explanations of an event to justify a behavior.

D. Reaction formation is doing the opposite of an unacceptable impulse. An example is falling in love with your wife's sister and then making fun of her.

E. Regression is using behaviors from an earlier stage of development to avoid tension. Although her actions are immature, they do not fit this definition.

446. **C.** In some cases, bowel loop can manage to herniate through the obturator foramen. This can cause small bowel obstruction and pressure on the obturator nerve, which causes ipsilateral knee pain. The hernia cannot be palpated because the obturator canal is located deep within the pelvis.

A. Femoral hernias come through the femoral canal and should be palpable if symptomatic. Knee pain is not associated with this.

B. Inguinal hernias will usually present as a mess in the groin and are not associated with knee pain.

D. Spigelian hernias are palpable behind the rectus abdominus muscle. They are not associated with knee pain.

E. Umbilical hernias are palpable in the umbilicus upon exertion. They are not associated with knee pain.

447. **B.** Intrathecally administered baclofen can be used to treat spasticity in patients with multiple sclerosis.

A. Azathioprine is thought to reduce relapse rates in relapsing and unremitting multiple sclerosis.

C. Methotrexate is used to slow the progression of multiple sclerosis.

D. Immunoglobulin is used to reduce the overall level of disability but does not specifically target spasticity.

E. Interferon B is thought to reduce relapse rates in relapsing and unremitting multiple sclerosis.

448. **B.** This infant has bronchiolitis. This condition results from inflammatory obstruction of the small airways. It is common in the first 2 years of life. The treatment of choice is cold, humidified oxygen. Patients must remain well hydrated to prevent tachypnea.

A and **C.** Antibiotics have no therapeutic value unless there is a secondary bacterial pneumonia.

D. Bronchodilators may show the presence of hyperactive airway conditions.

E. Inhaled corticosteroids are unlikely to be of benefit in the patient with bronchiolitis.

449. **B.** The proper treatment for cholera is vigorous rehydration with oral and/or intravenous fluids along with tetracycline. *Vibrio cholerae* produces a heat-labile exotoxin that stimulates Gs protein, causing adenylate cyclase to be activated, which increases cyclic adenosine monophosphate causing a secretory diarrhea. Due to the patient's dehydration noted by laboratory studies and physical examination findings, hydration is of great importance in this patient. The rice-water appearance of the stool is characteristic of cholera. Gram-negative rods with motility may also be seen on stool examination.

A, C, D, and **E.** Metronidazole, trimethoprim, amphotericin B, and penicillin G are not appropriate treatments for *Vibrio cholerae* infection.

450. **B.** Nausea and vomiting are common complaints in pregnancy. The etiology is not well understood but appears to be related to increased levels of human chorionic gonadotropin levels. Nausea should be treated conservatively if possible. If persistent vomiting leads to weight loss, ketonuria, or electrolyte imbalance, hospitalization may be required.

A. Nausea and vomiting are unrelated to estrogen levels.

C. Nausea and vomiting are unlikely to be related to elevated progesterone levels.

D. Testosterone level elevation is unlikely to be associated with the symptoms of nausea and vomiting.

E. Thyroxine level changes are unlikely to be associated with nausea and vomiting.

451. **A.** This individual has brief reactive psychosis. This condition is defined by a symptom constellation of less that 1 month's duration and follows an obvious stress on the patient's life. Patients exhibit an increase in volatility and lability, confusion, disorientation, and affective symptoms. This condition is highly associated with individuals who have a preexisting personality disorder and those who have experienced a major life stressor such as a natural disaster.

B. Posttraumatic stress disorder occurs following a severe loss or stress such as rape, car accident, or natural disaster and is notable for marked anxiety, personality change, insomnia, and nightmares.

C. This patient has symptoms that are clearly identifiable with a psychiatric disorder.

D. Schizoaffective disorder is a vague and poorly defined disorder meant for people with evidence of both schizophrenia and major depression.

E. Schizophrenia is the most common psychotic disorder with varying degrees of severity. Affected individuals have an impaired sense of reality and may be confused and disoriented.

452. **A.** The film demonstrates a narrowed loop of ileum with a "cobblestone" appearance of the mucosa and deep "rose thorn" ulcers. These findings along with the history and physical examination point to Crohn disease as the correct answer. This type of inflammatory bowel disease involves transmural inflammation occurring anywhere in the gastrointestinal tract. The lesions are disseminated, giving rise to the term "skip lesions." The peak age of onset is between 15 and 30 years, with a second peak occurring between 50 and 80 years of age. It occurs equally in men and women. A typical history for Crohn disease is one of diarrhea with or without gross blood, abdominal pain, and weight loss. An associated fever is also a hallmark symptom, but is not present in this patient. The suggestion of a family history of inflammatory bowel disease further supports the diagnosis.

Figure 452

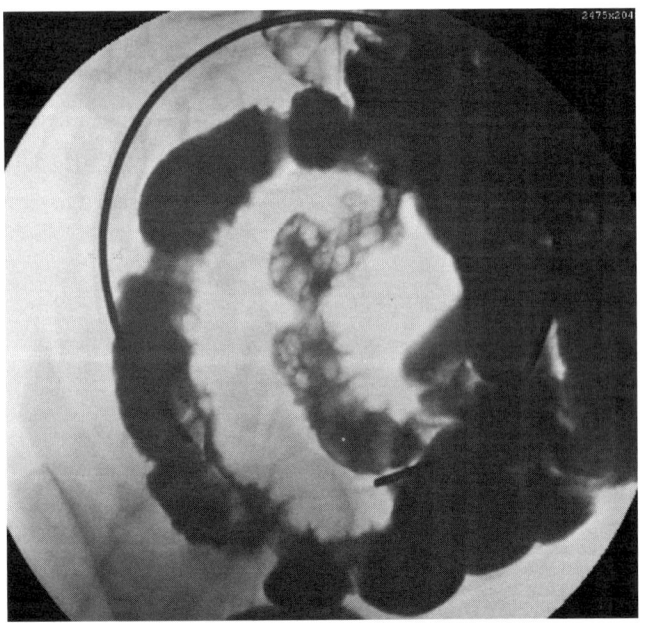

B. Although a patient with crampy abdominal pain may be considered to have irritable bowel syndrome (IBS) the additional symptoms of weight loss and anorexia are uncommonly associated with this syndrome. A patient with IBS will have no organic cause. The film of our patient clearly demonstrates a physical reason for her abdominal pain.

C. The typical history of appendicitis includes the acute onset of periumbilical pain that gradually shifts to right lower quadrant pain. The crampy nature of this patient's abdominal pain as well as the film and other signs and symptoms does not suggest appendicitis as the diagnosis.

D. Basic radiographs are usually used to make the diagnosis of small bowel obstruction. Upright films will show air-fluid levels perpendicular to the horizontal. CT scan with diluted barium or contrast will show discrepancy in the size of proximal and distal small bowel. Also, dilated loops of small bowel may be seen.

E. Although Crohn disease can affect any part of the gastrointestinal tract, ulcerative colitis is isolated to the colon. The involvement of the ileum makes Crohn disease a better diagnosis.

453. **A.** This patient likely has bladder cancer. This can frequently be associated with painless, gross, or microscopic hematuria in 85% of patients. The fact that this patient has a long history of cigarette smoking increases her risk for bladder cancer.

B. Bladder stone with obstruction is unlikely given the absence of voiding symptoms.

C. Chronic urinary retention is unlikely given the lack of irritative and obstructive voiding symptoms.

D. Interstitial cystitis is rarely associated with gross hematuria. Patients often complain of urinary urgency, frequency and chronic pelvic pain.

E. The absence of flank pain and colic make ureteral calculus disease less likely.

454. **E.** This patient has central sleep apnea. A permanent tracheostomy may dramatically improve patient symptoms in this condition. This is an effective long-term treatment for these patients.

A. Exercise is important for these patients but will require diet and dedicated efforts to be successful.

B. Hypnosis is unlikely to be of benefit in this patient.

C. Continuous positive airway pressure has a role in the management of obstructive sleep apnea.

D. Tonsilectomy is unlikely to benefit this patient with obstructive sleep apnea and normal throat examination findings.

455. **D.** Always initiate the advanced cardiac life support protocol in the proper order: ABCD—airway, breathing, circulation, deficits.

A. The airway must be managed first.

B and **C.** The airway must be managed first, then fluids can be administered.

E. The airway, breathing, and circulation must be managed before any attempt at surgical repair.

456. **E.** Patients with diabetic ketoacidosis (DKA) need rapid volume expansion and hyperglycemia correction by insulin replacement. Rapid decrease of serum glucose may lead to acute cerebral edema and should be avoided. Sodium chloride 0.9% should be rapidly infused with 1 L given in the first 30 minutes; 5% glucose should be added to the intravenous fluids once glucose levels decline to 250 to 300 mg/dL to prevent hypoglycemia.

A. Bicarbonate is not required to correct the pH unless it is below 7. Bicarbonate treatment presents the risk for alkalosis and hypokalemia.

B. Glucose should be added to the intravenous fluids once the serum glucose level decreases to 250 to 300 to prevent hypoglycemia.

C. Oral hypoglycemics are slow acting and have no role in the presence of DKA.

D. Potassium (K) should not be given until blood pressure is shown to be stable and urine output is adequate. A K level of 4.7 mEq/L is within the normal range.

457. **B.** The history of oral contraceptive use brings about the suspicion of a hepatic adenoma. In this case, the adenoma has ruptured. CT scan will confirm the diagnosis, and surgery will follow after stabilizing the patient.

A. This patient could be suffering from acute appendicitis, but her presentation of generalized abdominal pain and unstable vital signs are not classic for that diagnosis. Appendicitis can begin as generalized pain that later localizes to the right lower abdominal quadrant. Most often it presents with nausea and a persistent low-grade fever.

C. There is no evidence to suggest a ruptured spleen in this patient. There was no history of trauma, which is the most common cause.

D. Due to the absence of fever, a tuboovarian abscess is unlikely in this patient.

E. There is no evidence to suggest uremia in this patient.

458. **C.** Papules and pustules in the beard area typify pseudofolliculitis barbae, an inflammatory disorder of the hair follicles. Regular application of benzoyl peroxide, retinoic acid, or both may be helpful along with oral antibiotic therapy.

A. Amphotericin B is unlikely to be of value in the treatment of this condition.

B. Laser ablation is not a first-line treatment for this condition.

D. Surgical ablation is not an appropriate treatment for this condition.

E. Watchful waiting only if it involves growing a full beard might be of value if the offending hairs lift out of the dermis.

459. **E.** This patient has hand-foot-mouth disease. This condition is a viral exanthem that produces a vesicular rash on the hands, foot, and mouth. The condition is common in the summer months. Some lesions can be painful. The course of the illness is usually benign, and treatment is for symptoms only.

A. There is no indication to begin antibiotic therapy for hand-foot-mouth disease.

B. Corticosteroids are not indicated in the treatment of this viral condition.

C. Surgical excision has no role in the treatment of hand-foot-mouth disease.

D. Topical mupirocin is used to treat impetigo, a bacterial infection of the skin associated with crusted vesicopustular lesions.

460. **A.** This patient has primary dysmenorrhea. It is the most common gynecologic disorder among young women and occurs in approximately 50% of menstruating women. It can be severe in approximately 10% of patients. Treatment with nonsteroidal antiinflammatory agents can be helpful.

B. Secondary dysmenorrhea can be due to endometriosis or pelvic inflammatory disease.

C. Endometriosis is a cause of secondary dysmenorrhea.

D. Pelvic inflammatory disease is a cause of secondary dysmenorrhea.

E. Psychogenic factors can coexist with dysmenorrhea but are not thought to be related issues.

461. **B.** This patient exhibits signs and symptoms of Tourette disorder. Multiple motor and vocal tics occur several times daily. Simple motor tics can include eye blinking and facial grimacing. Simple vocal tics include coughing and grunting. Complex motor tics include hitting oneself and jumping, whereas complex vocal tics include repeating one's own words and repeating the words of others. Excessive swearing can also be noted. Eighty-five percent of patients improve with haloperidol and its associated sedative properties.

A. Clonidine is not as effective as haloperidol in the treatment of Tourette syndrome.

C. Pimozide is an antidopaminergic medication that is a second-line agent in the treatment of Tourette syndrome.

D. Propranolol is not recommended in the treatment of Tourette syndrome.

E. Thorazine is not recommended in the treatment of Tourette syndrome.

462. **D.** This patient has an abnormal Pap smear and should be referred for colposcopy. When the Pap smear suggests neoplasia, this is usually correct and intervention is required. Thus, follow-up Pap smears are not recommended until colposcopy has been performed.

A, B, C, and **E.** This patient needs colposcopy to evaluate the abnormal Pap smear results.

463. **C.** This is the presentation of acute pancreatitis. In this case, the pancreatitis is due to hypertriglyceridemia. These patients frequently present with the chief complaints of nausea, vomiting, and abdominal pain that is out of proportion to that found on physical examination. CT scan is not only helpful in confirming the diagnosis but also in establishing the severity of the attack. The CT Severity Index defines five grades of pancreatic inflammation based on CT findings. Grade A is a normal pancreas. Grade B shows focal or diffuse enlargement of the pancreas but no peripancreatic inflammation. Grade C shows peripancreatic inflammation and is associated with an increased risk for complication. Grade D shows intra- or extrapancreatic fluid collections, and grade E shows two or more large collections of gas or fluid in the pancreas or retroperitoneum. Our patient shows Grade C with an edematous pancreas and stranding (inflammatory changes) of the peripancreatic fat. When presented with a case of acute pancreatitis there are three basic levels of treatment. The first and foremost is intravenous hydration. Patient's with acute pancreatitis are usually dehydrated because of vomiting and anorexia. Intravenous hydration is essential because giving liquids by mouth would stimulate pancreatic secretions and thereby worsen the pain and inflammation. The next step would be to control the pain. Narcotic analgesics are indicated for this. Finally, the patient should not be allowed anything by mouth (NPO). This will prevent stimulation of the pancreas to secrete enzymes when food enters the small intestine.

Figure 463

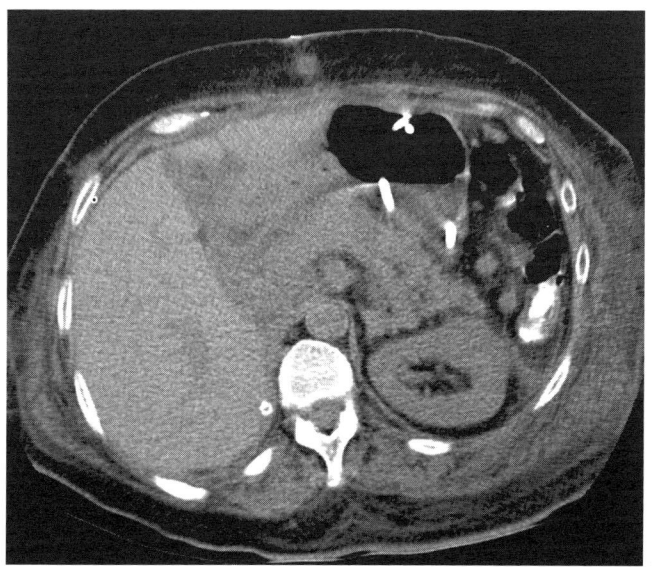

A. Although serum amylase is the most common laboratory test ordered to help make the diagnosis of acute pancreatitis, it is unnecessary in this patient. The history and physical are more than enough to suggest the diagnosis, which was confirmed by CT scan.

B. Although providing pain control and keeping a patient NPO is an extremely important step in the management of acute pancreatitis, the patient's fluid status should be tended to first.

D. Fluid restriction only is never indicated because all enteral feeds must be stopped to prevent pancreatic secretion and thereby further inflammation and pain.

E. Although providing pain control and keeping a patient NPO is an extremely important step in the management of acute pancreatitis, the patient's fluid status should be tended to first.

464. **E.** Osteomyelitis is normally caused by *Staphylococcus aureus* and involves the femur and tibia in over two thirds of cases. Physical examination may reveal soft tissue swelling, limited range of motion, and erythema. A history of fever is often noted. Initial radiographs may be normal, and definitive diagnosis is made by aspiration. Treatment consists of intravenous or high-dose oral antibiotics for 4 to 6 weeks.

A. *Escherichia coli* is an important cause of osteomyelitis in neonates.

B. Group A streptococcal osteomyelitis may also occur in children, but is less frequent than *Staphylococcus aureus*.

C. Group B streptococcal osteomyelitis is a less important cause in neonates.

D. Patients with sickle cell disease are particularly susceptible to *Salmonella* osteomyelitis.

465. **B.** Fibrocystic change is associated with breast tenderness and swelling premenstrually. Fluctuation in mass size and discomfort is related to the menstrual cycle. Patients with severe atypia or hyperplasia on biopsy are at risk for breast carcinoma. Treatment is largely symptomatic. Patients should be advised to perform monthly breast self-examination.

A. Fat necrosis is associated with ecchymosis, skin retraction, and local tenderness and may be related to breast trauma.

C. Galactocele is a cystic dilatation of a duct with a thick, inspissated milky fluid that occurs near the time of lactation.

D. Typically, scirrhous adenocarcinoma of the breast begins in the upper outer quadrant of the breast. It takes approximately 5 to 8 years for the typical breast cancer to become palpable (>1 cm in size).

E. Macromastia, usually unilateral, is an unknown disorder that may develop after pregnancy and often regresses with antiestrogen therapy.

466. **A.** The first step in sexual maturation in females begins between ages 10 and 11 in most girls. However, some girls will develop breast buds at age 8. There is a considerable range in the developmental cycle of young females, and this patient and her mother should be reassured accordingly.

B. Adult axillary hair growth typically occurs between the ages of 13 and 16.

C. Breast buds develop under the influence of estradiol and this typically occurs between the ages of 10 and 11.

D. Pubic hair development occurs under the influence of androgens and typically occurs between the ages of 10.5 and 11.5.

E. The growth spurt occurs under the influence of growth hormone and typically occurs between the ages of 11 and 12.

467. **B.** The classic findings for basilar skull fractures include raccoon eyes, Battle sign (postauricular ecchymosis that occurs as a result of basilar fractures), otorrhea, and rhinorrhea. Perhaps the most important consideration in a patient with a basilar skull fracture is to evaluate for cervical spine injury.

A. If the patient was unconscious, a CT scan would be in order.

C. There is no indication to intubate this patient.

D. Prophylactic antibiotics have not been shown to decrease the incidence of meningitis in patients with basal skull fractures.

E. This patient needs to be evaluated for a cervical spine injury. Waiting can make things worse.

468. **D.** Axis IV involves psychosocial and environmental problems.

A. Axis I includes clinical disorders such as schizophrenia.

B. Axis II includes personality disorders and mental retardation.

C. Axis III includes other medical conditions.

E. Axis V is the global assessment of functioning scale.

469. **A.** This patient has a gross abnormality of the placenta known as placentomegaly. In this condition, the placenta weighs at least 600 g. Possible causes of this condition include diabetes, anemia, and chronic infections. Blood group abnormalities and twin-twin transfusions can also contribute to the etiology of this condition.

B. Hyperglycemia, as seen with diabetes mellitus, is a likely cause of placentomegaly.

C. Chronic infection is a possible cause of this condition.

D. Blood group abnormality, not an increase in WBC count, can result in placentomegaly.

E. Percocet abuse can result in a newborn that is small for gestational age.

470. **D.** The most likely cause of these symptoms is polymyalgia rheumatica, which is characterized by pain and stiffness of the shoulder and pelvic girdles without objective findings of weakness or decreased range of motion. Patients classically present with difficulty arising from a seated position and lifting arms above their heads as well as systemic complaints of fever, malaise, and weight loss. This condition is typically seen in elderly women and is associated with anemia and an elevated erythrocyte sedimentation rate. Low-dose prednisone (5–20 mg daily) improves symptoms in most patients.

A. Patients with fibromyalgia have diffuse myalgias and weakness. They must have at least 11 of 18 "trigger points" that have reproducible pain with palpation. These patients do not respond to steroid therapy.

B. Osteoarthritis is a chronic, noninflammatory arthrosis of movable joints and display irregular joint space narrowing on x-ray. There are no systemic symptoms associated with osteoarthritis.

C. Osteosarcoma is the most common primary malignant tumor of the bone. It typically occurs in the distal femur, proximal tibia, and proximal humerus with metastasis to the lungs. It generally occurs in adolescent boys, and masses are typically seen on radiographs.

E. Rheumatoid arthritis is a chronic, destructive, systemic inflammatory arthritis characterized by involvement of both large and small joints. It most commonly involves joints of the wrists, metacarpophalangeal and proximal interphalangeal joints, but may also involve the ankles, knees, shoulders, hips, elbows, and cervical spine. Radiographs show soft tissue swelling, joint space narrowing, and erosions.

471. **E.** Because the patient has a right of privacy to his health, the physician should ask the family to leave in as humble and neutral a manner as possible so as not to give them a hint to what the test results may yield. Once the family has left the physician should ask the patient if it is ok if the family knows what the tests have shown, without telling the patient what the results are yet.

A. The physician should not give the family any clue as to what the tests have shown before the patient has said that it is ok if they are told.

B. Although this is not a horrible thing to say, it is not the most polite way of approaching such a delicate topic, and it hints to the family that the results are serious.

C and **D.** The physician has not yet asked the patient if the family can know the test results.

472. **E.** This patient is hemodynamically unstable. Severe head injury may have occurred. However, this does not explain the hypotension and tachycardia. Hemorrhage may be occurring from another site, such as a fracture of the lower extremity. This is a likely source for massive blood loss in this patient since the thigh has a lot of room to hold an expanding hematoma.

A. The lower extremity injury is the cause of hemorrhagic shock in this patient. Diffuse axonal injury would cause multiple neurologic (sensory and motor) deficits. Nothing in the presentation leads one to believe diffuse axonal injury has occurred.

B. The lower extremity injury is the cause of hemorrhagic shock in this patient. Epidural hematomas result most often from trauma. Patients present with the "lucid interval." That is, the patient is knocked unconscious immediately after the trauma, then quickly regains consciousness with the only symptom being a headache, but then slowly loses consciousness again within minutes to hours as the hematoma expands and increases intracranial pressure.

C. The lower extremity injury is the cause of hemorrhagic shock in this patient. Subdural hematoma is caused by the disruption of bridging veins between the dura and the cortical surface. Often, the bleeding is slow, so it may take weeks to months to show signs such as dementia.

D. The lower extremity injury is the cause of hemorrhagic shock in this patient. Subarachnoid hemorrhage is due most often to rupture of a Berry aneurysm in the circle of Willis. It is associated with sudden onset of "the worse headache of your life," nausea, vomiting, stiff neck, photophobia, and/or decreased mentation. CT scan can pick up about 90% of all spontaneous subarachnoid hemorrhages.

473. **C.** The patient described above is diagnosed with cluster headaches. This type of headache is most common in men in their twenties. The clinical picture is composed of periorbital headache of brief duration, ipsilateral Horner syndrome, conjunctival injection, ipsilateral tearing, and nasal congestion. Both abortive and prophylactic therapy are indicated.

A and **B.** Both abortive and prophylactic therapy is indicated.

D. There is no diagnostic test for cluster headaches, and therefore no further testing is needed.

E. Patients can be treated with both abortive and prophylactic therapy, and thus, the patient should be treated in this manner.

474. **A.** This patient has chronic myelogenous leukemia (CML). This condition is notable for clonal expansion of all hematopoietic cell types. Many clonal cells have the Philadelphia chromosome translocation (t9:22). Initial treatment consists of lowering the WBC count to less than 100,000 cells/mm^3 to decrease blood viscosity. Hydroxyurea and busulfan are the agents of choice for this condition.

B. Doxorubicin is a chemotherapeutic agent used in the treatment of acute lymphocytic leukemia.

C. Interferon is a less promising treatment option in the management of CML. It is also used in the treatment of metastatic renal cell carcinoma.

D. Methotrexate is used to treat non-Hodgkin lymphoma.

E. Radiation therapy to the lumbar spine is unlikely to be of benefit in the treatment of this patient.

475. **B.** This patient presents with a classic triad of syncope, angina, and dyspnea on exertion, which may be caused by hypertrophic obstructive cardiomyopathy, also known as obstructive hypertrophic subaortic stenosis. Aortic stenosis that is a normal part of aging is frequently termed aortic sclerosis. The diagnosis is clinical and confirmed by echocardiography.

A. Aortic regurgitation is seen with endocarditis, trauma, rheumatic fever, ventricular septal defect in children, tertiary syphilis, aortic dissection, Marfan syndrome, and congenital bicuspid aorta.

C. Patients with mitral stenosis usually have a prior history of rheumatic fever. Echocardiography findings include left atrial enlargement and subsequent right heart failure.

D. Mitral valve prolapse is a benign finding in young people.

E. Mitral regurgitation results in dilatation of the left atrium and may cause pulmonary edema.

476. **A.** It has been found that sexually active adolescent girls are approximately 10 times more likely to suffer PID than older women. Yearly risks of acquiring PID have been calculated at 12.5% for 15-year-old girls, 10% for 16-year-old girls, and 1.25% for 24-year-old women.

B and **C.** Adolescent girls who are sexually active have decreased economic resources and a decreased tendency to seek out early diagnostic screening and treatment services for sexually transmitted infections.

D. Adolescent girls who are sexually active have been shown to have little mucosal immunity to sexually transmitted infections. As a female ages, her mucosa obtains a greater inherent acquired immunity against contracting a sexually transmitted infection.

E. Adolescent girls who are sexually active tend to have sexual relationships with adolescent boys. Adolescent boys who are sexually active have been shown to have a high prevalence of gonococcal and chlamydial infections, those two organisms being the primary culprits in PID.

477. **E.** This patient has cystic fibrosis (CF) by evidence of failure to thrive, multiple respiratory tract infections, and a positive sweat Cl test result. These patients are particularly susceptible to *Pseudomonas aeruginosa* pneumonia. *Pseudomonas* is a gram-negative aerobic bacillus. This organism is common in CF patients. It is thought that the frequent colonization and persistent infection with *Pseudomonas* in CF patients may be related to the defective CFTR protein.

A. *Mycobacterium avium-intracellulare* is more common in more severely immunocompromised patients such as those with HIV.

B. Tuberculosis is unlikely in this patient because there is no history of exposure, and chest x-ray findings are not consistent.

C. *Mycoplasma pneumoniae* is unlikely in this patient. It is responsible for atypical community-acquired pneumonia common in older children and young adults.

D. *Pneumocystis carinii* is more common in more severely immunocompromised patients such as those with HIV.

478. **B.** Epidural hematoma has occurred in this patient. This injury occurs when a patient suffers an acute blow to the head that causes rupture or tearing of an artery, most commonly the middle meningeal. The artery is under pressure and bleeds quickly into the epidural space, a confined area due to the limited area of the cranium. Once enough blood accumulates, the pressure will cause brain matter to shift with concomitant uncal herniation and the resulting blown pupil (loss of the parasympathetic effects on cranial nerve III). These patients often present with a history of unconsciousness or drowsiness immediately after the trauma, which is followed by a brief period of lucidity in which the patient appears healthy. This lucid interval is unfortunately interrupted by sudden collapse or loss of consciousness.

A. This patient has evidence of an epidural hematoma. The neurologic symptoms show that a certain portion of the brain is compromised. No evidence of diffuse axonal injury, causing diffuse neuropathy, is suggested.

C. No information is given to suggest that a rupture of an arteriovenous malformation has occurred.

D. This patient has evidence of an epidural hematoma. Subarachnoid hemorrhages are most commonly caused by rupture of a Berry aneurysm in the circle of Willis. These are often described by the patient as "the worse headache of my life."

E. Subdural hematoma is a slower process and would not cause such an acute change in mental status. These hematomas are caused by rupture of bridging veins.

479. **E.** Thrombotic thrombocytopenic purpura (TTP) is due to a deficiency in von Willebrand factor–cleaving protease, in some cases due to an antibody directed against the protease. It is seen primarily in young adults between the ages of 20 and 50, and has a slight female predominance. Patients present with anemia, bleeding, or neurologic abnormalities. Neurologic symptoms often wax and wane over minutes and include headache, confusion, aphasia, and altered consciousness. Laboratory findings show anemia with hemolysis features, including fragmented RBCs on smear, elevated indirect bilirubin, elevated lactate dehydrogenase, and occasional hemoglobinemia/uria. Coagulation tests are normal. Renal function is usually preserved. Treatment is with plasmapheresis.

A. Evan syndrome is a combination of autoimmune thrombocytopenia and autoimmune hemolytic anemia. However, it differs from TTP in that peripheral smear will show spherocytes rather than fragmented RBCs.

B. Disseminated intravascular coagulopathy differs from TTP by the coagulation studies. They will show elevated prothrombin time, low fibrin, and high fibrin degradation products such as the D-dimer.

C. Hemolytic uremic syndrome (HUS) is distinct from TTP in that HUS usually has more renal failure and TTP has more neurologic findings.

D. Idiopathic thrombocytopenia purpura (ITP) usually occurs in childhood following an illness. It is an autoimmune disorder in which IgG autoantibody binds to platelets where they are then destroyed by the spleen. ITP can be easily differentiated from TTP by the absence of systemic illness in ITP.

480. **A.** Circumstantial speech has small tangents, but the speaker eventually gets to the point.

B. Echolalia is copying what someone else is saying; it can be mild, which leads to only repeating a few words.

C. Echopraxia is copying the movements and expressions of someone else.

D. Tangential speech leads from one tangent to another; the person never gets to the point.

E. Thought insertion is when a person is talking and an unrelated thought pops into the story. There is usually a pause and the person is usually unaware that there was an unrelated thought included.

481. **B.** This patient is suffering from postpartum psychosis. This syndrome occurs after childbirth and is characterized by severe depression and delusions. Most cases occur in the first week post partum. The etiology is secondary to underlying mental illness. In some cases, sudden change in hormone levels after parturition may contribute.

A. Treatment involves antidepressants and antianxiety agents. Psychotherapy also plays an important role in treatment.

C. This patient should be treated as an outpatient. There is no evidence to suggest instability or suicidal ideation.

D. Psychodynamic conflicts regarding motherhood, unwanted pregnancy and fears of motherhood are possible.

E. This condition is unrelated to an underlying systemic infection.

482. **C.** Inflammatory carcinoma in situ is an uncommon form of breast cancer occurring in only 3% of cases. It presents with a rapidly growing, sometimes painful mass that enlarges the breast. The overlying skin becomes erythematous, edematous, and warm. Often there is no distinct mass because the tumor infiltrates the involved breast diffusely. The diagnosis should be made when the redness involves more than one third of the skin over the breast and biopsy shows infiltrating carcinoma with invasion of the subdermal lymphatics. The inflammatory changes, often mistaken for an infection, are caused by invasion of the lymphatics, with resulting edema and hyperemia. Suspicion should be high when the lesion does not respond to antibiotics.

A. Cystosarcoma phyllodes arises from intralobular stroma. It usually must be differentiated histologically, but in larger tumors there can be leaflike bulbous protrusions.

B. Ductal carcinoma in situ (DCIS) involves malignant cells that lack the capacity to invade through the basement membrane but can spread throughout a ductal system to involve an entire sector of a breast. Erythema, edema, and breast enlargement are not usually symptoms of the disease.

D. Lobular carcinoma in situ (LCIS) almost never forms a mass and is usually detected incidentally on biopsies performed for other reasons. LCIS is unique in its ability to occur bilaterally in the other half of cases.

E. Paget disease/carcinoma of the breast is a type of infiltrating ductal carcinoma (DCIS). The ducts of the nipple epithelium are infiltrated, but often no gross nipple changes are present, and a palpable mass is often not present. There is usually itching or burning of the nipple, with superficial erosion or ulceration of the skin.

483. **C.** This patient likely has a follicular cyst. The most appropriate next step in the management of this patient is a pelvic ultrasound study to determine if the structure is more cystic or solid and to ascertain whether it is unilocular. A unilocular, cystic adnexal mass of 6 to 8 cm warrants close observation in a woman of reproductive age.

A. Oral contraceptives in this patient are not appropriate as the next step in management. A trial of oral contraceptives during a 60-day period of observation is appropriate in patients of reproductive age with cysts less than 6 cm in size. However, cysts of this size that do not resolve within 60 days despite close observation and gonadotropin suppression require a pelvic ultrasound study for further evaluation.

B. Obtaining a CA-125 level is not appropriate as the next step in management for this patient. A CA-125 level should be obtained for those patients who are at high risk for ovarian cancer. Ovarian tumors are malignant 15% of the time in menstruating women versus 50% of the time in postmenopausal women.

D. Surgical exploration is not appropriate as the next step in management of this patient. Laparoscopy is indicated for cystic adnexal masses of greater than 8 cm in women of reproductive age and for masses of greater than 4 cm in postmenopausal women.

E. It is not appropriate to wait and examine this patient after her next menses secondary to the size of the cystic mass. It is appropriate to wait and examine a patient after her next menses for a cystic mass that is less than 6 cm in diameter.

484. **D.** This patient has amnesic syndrome. The condition is associated with impaired short- and long-term memory with normal cognition. The most common form of amnesic syndrome is associated with thiamine deficiency associated with alcohol dependence. Treatment involves thiamine supplementation.

A. Amoxicillin would unlikely be of benefit in the management of amnesic syndrome.

B. Electroconvulsive therapy is not indicated in the management of this condition.

C. Labetalol is an antihypertensive agent. This patient has no evidence of hypertension.

E. This patient likely has thiamine deficiency and should be treated accordingly.

485. **A.** Using the Framingham criteria, this patient has congestive heart failure (CHF). To be diagnosed by this method you must have two major criteria or one major and two minor criteria. Our patient actually has three major criteria. She has paroxysmal nocturnal dyspnea (PND) as she describes waking up at nights gasping for air. Her second major criteria is the third heart sound. Lastly, her chest x-ray shows cardiomegaly. This is defined as a heart border that is greater than half the width of the mediastinum. Because she has given us a 5-year history of her PND, we predict that this is a chronic disease state. With chronic CHF, ventricular myocytes secrete brain natriuretic peptide in response to the high atrial and ventricular filling pressures; therefore, we would suspect this laboratory value to be elevated among all of the others.

Figure 485

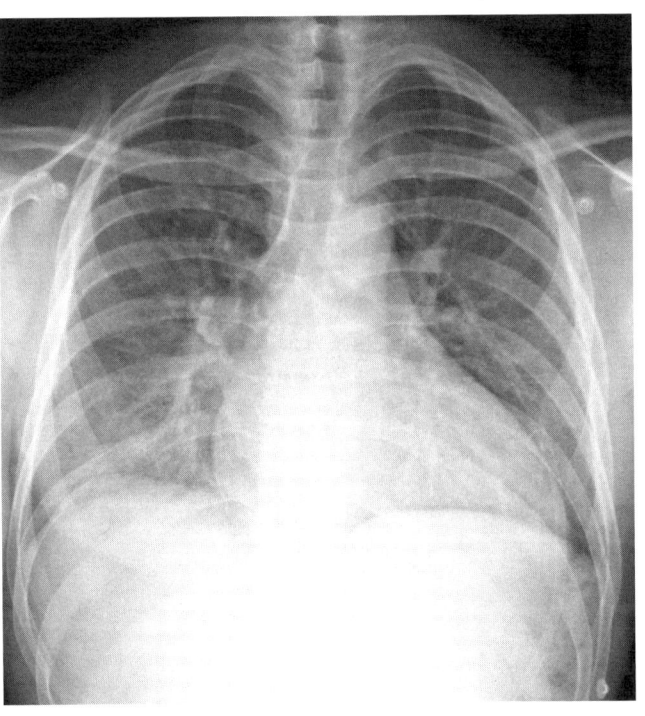

B–E. All of these enzymes are elevated in the case of acute myocardial infarction, which would most likely present with chest pain, dyspnea, and specific ECG changes such as ST segment elevation.

486. **B.** Suicide rates are highest in females, Native Americans, and the chronically ill patient. This patient has three risk factors: sex, race, and medical problems. Ingestion is the most common method of adolescent suicide.

A. This patient has a female risk factor.

C–E. This patient has a medical problem as a risk factor.

487. **B.** Fibroadenoma is the most common breast tumor in women, especially in the early twenties. It changes with the menstrual cycle and pregnancy, and disappears after menopause. Average size is 2 to 4 cm.

A. Cystosarcoma phyllodes is a rare, mostly benign, nonepithelial neoplasm of the breast that is sharply demarcated, has a smooth texture, is freely movable, and has an average size of 5 cm but can be as large as 30 cm. Median age of onset is in the fifth decade of life with more rapid growth. There is no cure if it is metastasized. Thirty percent of patients with metastasis die.

C. This is very unlikely in this age group and is less common than the fibroadenoma.

D. An intraductal papilloma usually presents as a bloody nipple discharge and appears as a small wart that projects into the ducts of the breast near the nipple. It usually occurs in women nearing menopause.

E. Simple cysts usually occur in women between the ages of 35 and 50 and appear as a fluid-filled sac on ultrasonography.

488. **D.** Tachycardia is the first sign of dehydration and can occur at less than 5% dehydration. This would be apparent on evaluation of vital signs, which should be performed in every patient. This may be unassociated with hypotension, which is a late finding in volume depletion states.

A. Dry mucous membranes are not found until the child is moderately dehydrated (5%–10%).

B. The respiratory rate is retained within the normal range early on in dehydration and does not increase until metabolic acidosis sets in.

C. Hypotension is a late finding that is indicative of a poor prognosis.

E. Urine output cessation (anuria) is a late finding and portends a poor prognosis.

489. **D.** This pair of people demonstrates signs of shared psychotic disorder, with the mother imposing her delusions on the daughter. In this situation, separation of the pair is critical and psychiatric evaluation is necessary.

A. This choice is not appropriate because it fails to address the daughter's delusions.

B. It is not appropriate to deny the girl birth control.

C. There is no evidence to suggest rape at this time.

E. This choice is not appropriate because it fails to address the daughter's delusions.

490. **E.** The response of the patient's fever and symptoms to heparin and the failed response to the antibiotics strongly suggests septic pelvic thrombophlebitis. The condition can be due to the Virchow triad (venous stasis, endothelial injury, and hypercoagulability). Venous thrombi usually develop in relatively small veins and then extend centrally as far as the inferior vena cava.

A. Antibiotics would most likely alleviate symptoms of acute endometritis.

B. Antibiotics would most likely alleviate symptoms of chorioamnionitis.

C. Antibiotics would most likely alleviate symptoms of pelvic abscess.

D. Antibiotics, analgesics, and hormonal agents would be of benefit in patients with pelvic inflammatory disease.

491. **E.** Yellow fever is caused by togavirus and is transmitted by *Aedes* mosquitoes. There is a vaccine available. It is endemic to Africa and South America. Symptoms include malaise, headache, retroorbital pain, fever, nausea, and photophobia. After a brief remission, patients may acquire symptoms again plus bradycardia, hypotension, jaundice, hemorrhage, and delirium. Laboratory values often include leukopenia, albuminuria, and hematuria. Eosinophilic intracytoplasmic councilman bodies are characteristic on liver biopsy.

A. Chagas disease is caused by *Trypanosoma cruzi*, which is a flagellated protozoan. The reduviid bug transmits it by injection of its feces.

B. Cryptosporidiosis is caused by *Cryptosporidium parvum* and presents as acute diarrhea. In immunocompetent patients, the disease is self-limiting. In malnourished children or immunocompromised patients, it presents as severe diarrhea. Supportive management is the only treatment.

C. Echinococcosis is caused by *Echinococcus granulosus*. It is acquired from ingesting material contaminated by feces of a carnivore that has eaten contaminated meat. The liver is the most common site of invasion.

D. Lymphatic filariasis is a chronic disease caused by filarial roundworms, which cause lymphatic obstruction.

492. **B.** The appropriate follow-up for someone who has had endometrial cancer is evaluation every 3 months for 2 years, then every 6 months for 3 years, then every year. Seventy-five percent of recurrences occur in the first 2 years after treatment, and 85% occur by the end of the third year. High-dose progestins are first-line treatment for recurrent and advanced disease, but the appropriate follow-up regimen should still be observed.

A. Estrogen replacement therapy is controversial in patients who have had endometrial cancer. It is only used in those patients who had minimally invasive and well-differentiated disease and only after they have been cancer free for 5 years.

C. Ninety percent of patients with endometrial cancer have irregular bleeding. On physical examination you should look for signs of metastases, which include lymphadenopathy, abdominal masses, hepatosplenomegaly, ascites, and pleural effusion.

D. Pelvic examinations are usually normal, but the cervical os may be patulous and the cervix may be firm and expanded in advanced disease. The uterus may be normal or enlarged. Postmenopausal bleeding may be caused by many things including endometrial atrophy (60% to 80%), exogenous estrogen use (15%–25%), endometrial cancer (10%), cervical or uterine polyps/fibroids (2%–12%), or endometrial hyperplasia (5%–10%).

E. Follow-up for endometrial cancer is required at the intervals mentioned above.

493. **C.** This child has evidence of a dog bite. The likely organism is *Pasteurella multocida*. This organism infects humans through direct inoculation by animal bites. Treatment of uncomplicated wounds is on an outpatient basis with penicillin V. More severe wounds may require intravenous antibiotics and débridement as necessary.

A. This patient has an uncomplicated dog bite and should do well on oral outpatient therapy.

B. This wound is uncomplicated. Intravenous therapy would be warranted for wounds with systemic toxicity and tendon/joint/bone involvement.

D. This therapy would be appropriate in patients who are allergic to penicillin.

E. Watchful waiting will be associated with a worsening of infection and may result in systemic complications such as meningitis.

494. **D.** In normal bereavement it is common for people to experience depressive symptoms after the loss of a loved one. If these symptoms persist for longer than 2 months, the diagnosis of major depressive disorder is usually given.

A. Bipolar disorder must include manic as well as depressive symptoms.

B. In dysthymic disorder, the depressive symptoms must last at least 2 years.

C. The presence of certain symptoms that are not characteristics of "normal" grief may also warrant a diagnosis of major depression. These include guilt, overwhelming thoughts of death, preoccupations of worthlessness, marked psychomotor impairment, marked functional impairment, or hallucinations.

E. In schizoaffective disorder, there must be delusions or hallucinations.

495. **A.** This patient has a *Trichomonas vaginalis* infection. These infections can induce cell changes in the Pap smear. Thus, this infection should be treated with metronidazole and the Pap smear repeated in 2 weeks. If the results are normal, usual follow-up is appropriate. If the results are abnormal, referral for colposcopy is appropriate.

B and **C.** This patient should be treated appropriately and have a repeat Pap smear in a timely fashion.

D. Colposcopy would be appropriate if the repeat Pap smear was abnormal after treatment with metronidazole.

E. This patient needs to be evaluated with colposcopy initially, assuming an abnormal repeat Pap smear.

496. **E.** Tricuspid regurgitation occurs due to incompetence of the tricuspid valve, resulting in back flow of blood into the right atrium. This is most commonly due to right ventricular dilatation secondary to left-sided heart conditions. Increased intensity of the pansystolic murmur may be heard on inspiration and is termed the Carvallo sign.

497. **D.** Mitral stenosis is an obstruction causing increasing left atrial pressures, resulting in increased pulmonary venous pressure. The final result is pulmonary edema, pulmonary hypertension, and right-sided heart failure. The enlarged left atrium can predispose patients to atrial fibrillation, which predisposes them to emboli. This condition occurs 15 to 40 years after rheumatic heart disease. The classic triad on physical examination is a diastolic rumble, opening snap, and loud S_1. Surgery is indicated for patients with moderate to severe stenosis. Balloon valvoplasty is the treatment of choice.

498. **B.** Aortic stenosis (AS) may be congenital in persons under age 30. Other causes include bicuspid valve, rheumatic heart disease, senile degeneration, peripheral pulmonary stenosis, or hypercalcemia. AS is almost always also associated with mitral valve pathology. Most cases are asymptomatic and are found incidentally. Exercise-related syncope may be present in as many as 25%. Pulsus tardus et parvus is a slow late carotid upstroke that is found in AS. A systolic ejection click may be present. The less audible the S_2, the more severe the stenosis. Surgical valve replacement is curative. Balloon valvoplasty may be used for those who cannot tolerate surgery.

499. **A.** Aortic regurgitation is diastolic backflow of blood into the left ventricle. Causes include rheumatic fever, congenital defects, trauma, endocarditis, degeneration, connective tissue diseases, or collagen vascular diseases. The classic murmur is a high-pitched, diastolic, decrescendo murmur. Patients may exhibit a de Musset sign, which is a nodding of the head. Overactivity of the neck vessels may be visualized. The Austin Flint murmur is the apical diastolic rumble. A Corrigan pulse is the sharp, rapid carotid upstroke followed by collapse. A pistol shot at the femoral artery is termed Duroziez murmur. Nailbed capillary pulsation with gentle nail pressure may be seen (Quincke pulse).

500. **C.** This patient has lower gastrointestinal bleeding. The differential diagnosis of this condition includes colorectal carcinoma. This must be carefully evaluated with endoscopy. With flexible sigmoidoscopy one can evaluate the sigmoid colon, where many carcinomas arise.

A. CT scan would not help with diagnosis of colon cancer.

B. If sigmoidoscopy is normal, then a colonoscopy would be indicated.

D. A barium enema may miss small colorectal carcinomas.

E. The patient is currently having bleeding, so repeating the test in a week will not be advisable. He needs to be further evaluated.

501. **D.** The etiology of constipation in pregnancy is multifactorial. Factors include reduced gut motility, mechanical obstruction by the uterus, and increased water resorption. Treatment includes limitation of iron therapy and psyllium supplementation.

A and **B.** Iron therapy is constipating and should be avoided in this patient.

C. Increasing fluid intake may serve to increase stool water, which may ease constipation.

E. Constipation in pregnancy can be debilitating and should be managed with increasing fluids and fiber in the diet as well as increasing physical activity.

502. **C.** This individual exhibits signs of functional encopresis. This condition is associated with at least 6 months of passage of feces in inappropriate places such as on the floor or into clothing. Fecal passage is involuntary or unintentional. This condition is associated with social embarrassment. Approximately 25% also have functional enuresis.

A. Anal fissures can occur with functional encopresis secondary to retention of feces and constipation. However, the incidence of this finding is less than 10%.

B. Anal fistulas are rarely seen in association with functional encopresis.

D. Hemorrhoids are uncommon findings in patients with functional encopresis.

E. It is important to rule out physical disorders such as aganglionic megacolon in patients with primary encopresis.

503. **A.** This patient has an adjustment disorder. This is a reaction to an identifiable psychosocial stressor that occurs within 3 months of the onset of the stress. In this patient, the stressor is the new job and the situations that evolve around the job. He has subsequently developed an impairment in social and occupational functioning.

B. Depression requires symptoms present for at least 2 weeks in the areas of mood, interest, loss of pleasure in daily activities, sleep disturbance, weight change, fatigue, concentrating ability, and feelings of worthlessness.

C. Dysthymia is a depressive syndrome where the patient is depressed most of the time but lacks symptoms to warrant a diagnosis of major depression.

D. Organic affective disorder includes endocrine and pharmacologic causes, which are not demonstrated by this patient.

E. This patient has no evidence of thyroid disease by history and examination.

504. **C.** Acute mesenteric adenitis occurs most often in childhood, especially in those patients with a recent upper respiratory tract infection. Generalized lymphadenopathy is noted in this condition. Thus, because this patient is 21 years of age, this particular entity is much less likely to occur than the other choices.

A. Acute appendicitis should be one of the most likely causes of this patient's symptoms. He has classical findings on physical examination, including an elevated WBC count, signifying infection.

B. Acute gastroenteritis can be associated with abdominal cramping and diarrhea, with relief of symptoms between the hyperperistaltic bowel waves.

D. Regional enteritis is associated with chronic abdominal pain but also anorexia, nausea, and emesis.

E. Testicular torsion can mimic the symptoms of acute appendicitis. Thus, it is important to perform a testicular examination on all patients with abdominal pain.

505. **E.** The functional outcome for a patient with a C1–C3 neurologic injury requires a great deal of dependence on others for care. Respiratory function at best will require mechanical ventilation with assisted cough.

A. Patients are dependent for bladder function.

B. Patients are dependent for bowel function.

C. Patients are dependent for dressing.

D. Patients are dependent for feeding.

506. **C.** This patient has an increased chance of recurrence and progression of superficial bladder cancer. Mitomycin should be administered intravesically to this patient. Although less effective than BCG, this therapy is associated with fewer major side effects. This would be important if this patient would like to continue working during therapy.

A. Full-dose BCG is associated with greater toxicities than mitomycin C.

B. Reduced-dose BCG is associated with greater toxicities than mitomycin C.

D. Radical cystectomy would require a 5- to 7-day hospital stay and is not indicated at this point because the patient only has superficial disease.

E. Watchful waiting is associated with a 50% to 70% chance of recurrence. Thus, intravesical treatment is appropriate for this patient.

507. **A.** Vitamin A is the most likely cause of toxicity in this man, especially due to his symptoms. Vitamin A toxicity is associated with hepatomegaly, hepatotoxicity, headache, vomiting, dry oral mucosa, papilledema, and joint pain. X-rays of joints will show hyperostosis in bones. Vitamin A toxicity is unlikely from eating normal foods alone. Taking either large amounts of multivitamins or eating polar bear liver (they concentrate the vitamin A in their livers in preparation for the decrease in food supply during winter). In fact, most older formulations of multivitamins have too much vitamin A because there is a thought that they increase men's risk for hip fractures if they take more than 5000 IU a day.

B. It would be hard to imagine ingesting more B vitamins or vitamin C that would cause such symptoms.

C. The B vitamins and vitamin C are renally excreted, so if too much is taken in, the excess is voided.

D. Megadoses of vitamin B_3 (niacin) are prescribed to lower cholesterol levels, which give side effects of flushing and pruritis, which may respond to treatment with ibuprofen.

E. Vitamin C toxicity can result in renal stones.

F. Vitamin K is not found in most multivitamins because the gastrointestinal flora synthesizes it naturally. Vitamin K is predominantly ingested through eating green leafy vegetables (spinach has the most).

508. **C.** This patient presents with the classic signs of a femoral hernia that has been strangulated. This type of hernia is more common in women than in men. The history of lifting heavy objects can tune the physician into thinking of a hernia of some sort. Femoral hernias occur in the femoral canal and the contents protrude posterior to the inguinal ligament, anterior to the Cooper ligament and medial to the femoral vein. Pain and a mass seen and felt in the groin strengthens the diagnosis. The distended abdomen suggests that the hernia may be strangulated, whereas the diffuse tenderness and skin color change support an ischemic necrosis picture caused by the strangulation. In cases such as these, emergent surgery is required to correct the hernia or resect any section of necrotic bowel (which has the risk for perforation).

A and **B.** Antibiotics are usually also given, but they are secondary to emergent surgery. Intravenous antibiotics are preferred over oral antibiotics.

D. Fine-needle aspiration could be considered in this case because of the finding of a mass. However, given the other symptoms, it would not be an appropriate first course of action.

E. Inguinal lymph node biopsy would be performed if a cancer were suspected. Without any complete blood count information or symptoms of weight loss or nausea, and with the symptoms strongly suggesting a hernia, one would not move to sample the lymph node first.

509. **C.** This diabetic patient who is otherwise in good health awakens to find that only one eye can perceive light. Such sudden and dramatic loss of vision usually reflects dense intraocular hemorrhage from previously unrecognized neovascularization.

A. This condition will present with slow loss of vision.

B. The funduscopic examination in this patient does not suggest retinal detachment.

D. There is no evidence to suggest infarction of the optic nerve.

E. This condition will present with slow loss of vision.

510. **D.** This patient has evidence of osteogenic sarcoma. He has the classic physical examination complaints of knee pain with some limited motion that is refractory to oral analgesic therapy. The film shows the characteristic periosteal lifting that occurs as the tumor invades the covering of the bone. Osteosarcoma is the most common malignant bone tumor and commonly involves the metaphysis of the long bones. Treatment involves limb amputation and/or radical dissection with or without adjuvant chemotherapy. Pulmonary metastasis is common, and the diagnosis carries a grave prognosis. Paget disease increases the likelihood of developing osteosarcoma in the future.

A. There is no evidence to suggest an arthritic component in this patient.

B. There is no evidence to suggest a meniscal tear.

C. This patient does not display features of Osgood-Schlatter disease, a common knee disorder that results from chronic avulsion and aseptic necrosis (due to infarction caused by interruption of arterial blood supply) of the tibial tubercle.

E. X-ray findings in this case do not reveal evidence of a stress fracture. These are fractures that result from abnormal stress on normal bone or normal stress on abnormal bone. Common sites for patients with normal bone (younger people) include the tarsal bones, metatarsals, and tibial shaft.

511. **C.** Lead time bias is when a time differential exists between diagnosis and treatment, which may result in higher survival rates being attributed to treatment instead of early detection.

A. A confounding variable affects both dependent and independent variables. It is related to both the disease in question and the risk factors leading to that disease.

B. Interviewer bias is when a subject may be swayed by an interviewer due to their tone of voice or attitude. Blinding or double blinding the study helps prevent this by keeping knowledge about subjects and their treatments unknown to the interviewer.

D. Recall bias deals with different abilities to remember details due to certain associations with those details. For instance, a mother may remember being exposed to a toxin after having a miscarriage, even though there was never an exposure. This may lead to certain risk factors being over- or underreported.

E. This is an example of lead time bias.

512. **E.** This patient has fibromyalgia, a common connective tissue disease seen almost exclusively in women 20 to 50 years of age and characterized by diffuse myalgias and weakness in the absence of signs of inflammation or objective weakness. Patients generally have complaints of depression, anxiety, and/or irritable bowel syndrome. Diagnosis is one of exclusion and is based on a minimum of 11 of 18 standard trigger areas with reproducible pain on palpation. Results of laboratory studies, physical examination, and radiographic examination are usually normal. There is no specific treatment for this disorder, and treatment is supportive with exercise, psychotherapy, and low-dose antidepressants.

A. Acetaminophen is unlikely to be of benefit in this case.

B. The symptoms would not be expected to respond to a change in antidepressant therapy.

C. Prednisone is unlikely to be of benefit in this case.

D. Nonsteroidal antiinflammatory medications would not be expected to significantly improve symptoms.

513. **A.** Of the substances listed, only alcohol has been consistently associated with a "syndrome" involving intrauterine growth retardation, abnormal facies, and cardiac abnormalities, most commonly atrial septal defects.

B. Cocaine has been associated with growth restriction, placental abruption, and central nervous system effects.

C. Marijuana has not been proven to be teratogenic.

D. Opioids are not proven to be teratogenic.

E. Although associated with intrauterine growth retardation and other problems of pregnancy, it does not fit with the presented case.

514. **C.** Necrotizing fasciitis can mimic cellulitis, but the area of erythema can be numb due to nerve destruction. This infection has an associated mortality rate of 30% and requires immediate surgical débridement and broad-spectrum antibiotics. It is usually caused by group A beta-hemolytic *Streptococcus*. In addition to the crepitus noted on physical examination, blisters can also be present.

A. Cellulitis would not present with numbness or crepitus.

B. Factitious disorder would not be likely in a febrile individual with an obvious pathology of the skin. In order to fake a fever, the patient would have been sweating profusely in order to increase her core temperature so much, and a woman with such a body habitus would be very winded after exercising so vigorously.

D. Shingles would present as exquisitely painful or itchy vesicular lesions localized to a single dermatome on half of the body. It can be found on more than one dermatome in the presence of an immunodeficiency.

E. Although a fungal infection would likely be found in this morbidly obese woman's skin folds, such an infection probably would not cause a fever, increased temperature to the touch, crepitus, or numbness. The lesion would more likely have a border of increased erythema.

515. **C.** This child has meconium ileus. The most appropriate treatment is nasogastric tube placement with fluids followed by Gastrograffin enema. With any evidence of bilious vomiting one must suspect bowel obstruction. In this case it may be from impacted stool due to another disease state such as cystic fibrosis. The appropriate treatment at this time is to decompress the gastrointestinal system and to try to hydrate the child in an attempt to correct any electrolyte deficits. The enema will be both therapeutic and diagnostic. Children with meconium ileus should always be worked up for cystic fibrosis. Consider ordering a sweat test if no bowel pathology is found.

A. There is no indication to administer oral hypertonic oral solutions.

B. Simethicone is not indicated in this patient. Simethicone is commonly used as an antiflatulent. Simethicone without the silica gel (Dimethicone) is commonly used as an ointment and skin protectant.

D. This patient also needs intravenous fluids in addition to nothing by mouth status.

E. This patient needs to be decompressed with a nasogastric tube.

516. **B.** Hodgkin lymphoma has a bimodal distribution, occurring at 15 to 30 years of age and after the age of 50. The most common presentation is painless, firm lymphadenopathy of, most commonly, the supraclavicular and cervical nodes. Approximately 30% of patients have systemic symptoms such as fever, night sweats, and weight loss. Diagnosis is confirmed by identification of Reed-Sternberg cells. Treatment depends on tumor staging, and an initial chest radiograph evaluates any possible mediastinal or hilar involvement, whereas a CT scan evaluates any retroperitoneal involvement.

A. Bone marrow biopsy is indicated if disseminated disease is suspected.

C. Multiagent chemotherapy is indicated in patients with stage 3 and stage 4 disease, and for patients with bulky disease.

D. Radiation of the involved lymph nodes is often used for local disease.

E. Radiation and chemotherapy are indicated for any secondary malignancy (acute myelogenous leukemia and/or non-Hodgkin lymphoma) that may occur.

517. **D.** Candidiasis is associated with variable amounts of white discharge, a vaginal pH of 4 to 5, and the presence of mycelia on potassium hydroxide microscopic preparations. Treatment is topical 2% miconazole nitrate suppositories for 3 to 7 days.

A. Acyclovir is the treatment for viral infections.

B. Erythromycin is ineffective in the treatment of candidiasis.

C. Metronidazole is the treatment of choice for bacterial vaginosis.

E. Tetracycline is the treatment of choice for *Chlamydia* infections of the vagina.

518. **D.** Intravenous TPA can be administered within 3 hours of the onset of symptoms resulting from an ischemic stroke. There are many exclusionary criteria that must be considered prior to administration of TPA. It is of primary importance to rule out hemorrhagic stroke. Intraarterial TPA can be administered within 6 hours, but intravenous TPA has a 3-hour time limit.

A, **B**, **C**, and **E**. This medication must be administered within 3 hours of the onset of symptoms.

519. **C.** The recurrent laryngeal nerve has been injured. Thyroidectomy is the treatment of choice for patients diagnosed with thyroid cancer. Although this is a rare complication (occurring in only 1% of patients) of the surgery, the recurrent laryngeal nerve injury soon becomes apparent when the patient assumes a husky and hoarse voice. This injury may cause temporary voice pathology lasting 6 to 12 months or it may be a permanent issue. This type of injury is more common when surgeons are dealing with large invasive or recurrent tumors.

A, **D**, and **E**. The recurrent laryngeal nerve has been injured in this patient.

B. The recurrent laryngeal nerve has been injured in this patient. The internal laryngeal nerve innervates the mucous membrane above the vocal cord and taste buds on the epiglottis.

520. **D.** This patient has evidence of hypertrophic obstructive cardiomyopathy (HOCM). Patients should avoid strenuous exercise. Beta blockers, verapamil, or diisopyramide can be used to reduce symptoms. Endocarditis prophylaxis is necessary in patients with outflow obstruction or mitral regurgitation.

A. Digitalis is a cardiac glycoside that increases contractility of the heart muscle. Digitalis is contraindicated in the management of HOCM.

B. Diuretics are absolutely contraindicated in patients with aortic stenosis. The patient's vasculature is maximally constricted in order to maintain an appropriate blood pressure. This patient is already experiencing syncopal episodes, and adding these drugs could easily precipitate shock.

C. Although this is an effective treatment, it is usually reserved for patients with severe cases who are poor surgical candidates and cannot tolerate the procedure for a mechanical or bioprosthetic valve.

E. This patient is symptomatic, and a form of treatment is available to help her.

521. **D.** This newborn has idiopathic infantile hypercalcemia (William syndrome). Patients can present with a history of poor feeding or constipation in the neonatal period. Mental retardation and congenital facial and cardiovascular abnormalities can result. Hypercalcemia is treated with a low-calcium diet (<100 mg/day) and, if necessary, hydrocortisone.

A. Calcitonin may be given subcutaneously for patients with primary hyperparathyroidism and hypercalcemia.

B. Furosemide is a treatment for hypercalcemia.

C. Hydrocortisone is a second-line treatment for infants with idiopathic infantile hypercalcemia.

E. Rehydration with 0.9% saline corrects the dehydration associated with hypercalcemia. This is usually given as an inpatient therapy.

522. **A.** This is the presentation and CT scan typical for acute appendicitis. The CT scan is diagnostic of this patient along with the positive rebound tenderness and the history of abdominal pain that starts in the periumbilical area and later moves to the right lower quadrant. The CT scan shows a thick-walled appendix in cross-section along with fat stranding (inflammation of the periappendiceal fat) both above and below. Other findings that suggest acute appendicitis are a target structure (concentric thickening of the inflamed appendiceal wall), appendicolith, abscess, and free fluid.

Figure 522

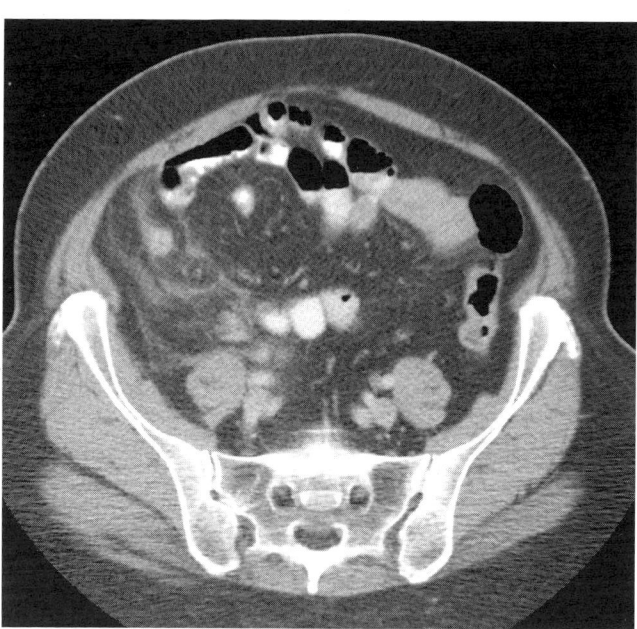

B. Because this patient presented within 24 to 72 hours of the start of symptoms, immediate appendectomy is indicated; however, in patients outside of this window, medical management may be considered. This is because immediate operation on these patients results in an increase in morbidity, including injury of adjacent structures in surgery. For this reason the initial management of these patients involves antibiotics, intravenous fluids, and bowel rest. The appendectomy can then be performed at a later time.

C. The control of pain is an important issue in a patient with acute appendicitis; however, immediate appendectomy is the treatment of choice in our patient.

D and **E.** Appendectomy is indicated in this patient.

523. **E.** Trigeminal neuralgia is characterized by stabbing pain that lasts approximately 30 seconds and is located along the distribution of the maxillary and/or mandibular division of the trigeminal nerve. Neurologic examination findings are usually normal. Treatment involves carbamazepine and is effective in 66% of patients.

A. Classic migraine begins early in life and is more common in women, especially those with a positive family history for migraine headaches.

B. Common migraine is also more common in women, with a more gradual onset of pain than in those patients with classic migraine.

C. Cluster migraine often occurs at night in young men and typically awakens the patient 2 to 4 hours after sleep onset.

D. Intracranial hypertension occurs in obese women under the age of 40. Typical patients have normal CT or MRI findings but have elevated cerebrospinal fluid pressure.

524. **B.** This newborn was connected to a single umbilical artery. The incidence of this condition is approximately 1% of newborns and is more common in infants of diabetic mothers and twins. The perinatal outcome is associated with problems of the newborn in 25% and can include central nervous system abnormalities and tracheo-esophageal fistula.

A. This condition is not associated with rectal fistula.

C. Ureteral fistulas occur in the setting of trauma or obstetric injury.

D. Urethral fistulas occur in the setting of trauma or surgical complications.

E. Vaginal fistulas can occur after childbirth in underdeveloped nations or surgical procedures in this country.

525. **E.** Ventricular septal defect is the most common congenital heart disease and accounts for 25% of all congenital heart disease. Clinical symptoms depend on the degree of shunting. Symptoms include dyspnea, tachypnea, poor feeding and growth, and diaphoresis. Cardiac examination reveals a pansystolic murmur that may have an associated thrill. ECG may reveal left atrial enlargement and left ventricular hypertrophy.

A. Dextrocardia is caused by formation of the cardiac loop to the left instead of to the right. This condition may be associated with situs inversus.

B. Ectopia cordis is a rare anomaly where the heart is located on the surface of the chest. The etiology of this defect is failure of the embryo to close in the midline.

C. Situs inversus results when the heart is located in the right side of the thorax. This condition is also known as transposition of the viscera.

D. Transposition of the great vessels occurs when the aorta arises from the right ventricle and the pulmonary arteries arise from the left ventricle. Oxygenation of the systemic blood occurs by a patent foramen ovale, ventricular septal defect, or a patent ductus arteriosus.

526. **D.** The pelvic inlet, determined by the distance between the sacral promontory and the inferior surface of the pubis, is the critical diameter necessary for passage of the fetal head.

A, **B**, **C**, and **E.** These are not the landmarks of the pelvic inlet.

527. **A.** With a low thyroid-stimulating hormone value, one must consider a benign adenoma, and a thyroid scan would tell if it was a hot nodule or not and rule out carcinoma. This would be an important step in the management of this patient.

B. Ultrasonography is mainly used for staging cancer spread.

C. Any nodule found on examination of the thyroid needs to be worked up now to rule out carcinoma.

D. A repeat fine-needle aspiration was just done and would not be helpful to repeat.

E. It would be important to determine the type of nodule before surgical resection is attempted.

528. **C.** Testing someone's judgment helps the physician understand the patient's ability to understand the outcome of a behavior.

A. This question does not test accuracy.

B. Insight is tested by asking the patient his three wishes, or why he is seeing the doctor. It helps the physician understand the patient's degree of awareness about being ill.

D. Reliability is also assessed throughout the interview and involves the capacity of the patient to report the situation accurately.

E. Thought process is not assessed with specific questions. It is assessed throughout the interview. It involves an inventory of the quantity of ideas, the speed that they arrive, their associations, and their relevance.

529. **B.** The patient is exhibiting hypocalcemia due to iatrogenic causes. There was likely accidental removal of the parathyroid glands during the thyroidectomy. The patient is not producing parathyroid hormone, which leads to hypocalcemia and hyperphosphatemia. She should be given calcium gluconate via intravenous, oral calcium supplements, and vitamin D preparations to help increase calcium levels of the blood. Hydrochlorothiazide, a calcium-sparing diuretic, can help the kidneys from excreting much needed calcium.

A. Furosemide is noted to cause hypocalcemia.

C. Phenytoin has been noted to cause hypocalcemia.

D. Phosphate supplementation would only further exacerbate hyperphosphatemia.

E. Rapid intravascular expansion has been noted to cause hypocalcemia.

530. **C.** Pseudogout is an acute to subacute episodic inflammation of a joint. A low-grade fever and polymorphonuclear leukocytosis are common. Large joints are usually involved, most commonly the knee. Pseudogout is often less intense than gout but may be similar in duration and joint involvement. Surgery, trauma, and stress may precipitate pseudogout as well as gout. Calcium pyrophosphate dihydrate crystals found in synovial fluid is diagnostic for pseudogout.

A. Gout is characterized by needle-shaped urate crystals free in synovial fluid or engulfed by phagocytes. Serum urate is elevated in 70% of patients. It may be precipitated by surgery, trauma, or stress.

B. Osteoarthritis has a more gradual onset and would not be associated with the laboratory values presented, especially the synovial fluid aspirate.

D. Rheumatoid arthritis usually has an insidious onset with inflammation in multiple joints. Four of the following criteria must be present to diagnosis rheumatoid arthritis: morning stiffness, arthritis of three or more joints, arthritis of hand joints, symmetric arthritis, rheumatoid nodules, positive rheumatoid factor, or radiographic changes.

E. There is no mention of trauma in the history and would not explain the laboratory values presented in the question.

531. **E.** Although it may be easier to accommodate the patient's family request and begin tube feedings or parenteral nutrition, it is more effective to educate the family about anorexia at the end of life. Simple compassionate acknowledgment of the family's fear and frustration can help resolve the conflict and better prepare for the inevitable death.

A–D. Education and discussion with the family will likely resolve this conflict as well as the associated fear and frustration.

532. **C.** This child has symptoms of genital pemphigoid. This condition can occur in early childhood and present with edema, erythema, erosion, and genital pain. Classic skin lesions are vesicular with blistering. Confirmation requires skin biopsy. The diagnosis requires a high index of suspicion.

533. **E.** Crohn disease is an inflammatory disorder of the gastrointestinal tract and can affect any site from the mouth to the anus. Perirectal involvement is common with this disease and can take many forms. Typical lesions include skin tags, fissures, fistulas, ulcerations, and abscess. Anal dilatation is also a common feature of this condition.

534. **A.** This patient has evidence of Behçet syndrome. This condition is characterized by recurrent oral and genital ulcers and relapsing uveitis. Most patients have oral ulcers. Genital ulcers may be deep and heal with scarring but are relatively painless. The diagnosis is made clinically.

535. **B.** This patient likely has peptic ulcer disease. This should be further evaluated with upper gastrointestinal endoscopy. The patient can then be treated with H2 blockers such as cimetadine.

A. This patient has guaiac-positive stools, and the cause of the bleeding must be determined.

C. Symptoms indicate an upper gastrointestinal bleed; thus, an upper gastrointestinal study should be performed.

D. There is no indication for surgical exploration at this time.

E. Testing for *Helicobacter pylori* is not indicated at this time, since his primary problem is gastrointestinal bleeding.

536. **E.** The most common cause of management failure in the use of medications such as miconazole in the treatment of candidiasis vaginitis is noncompliance. When a vaginal or vulvar medication is prescribed, noncompliance has been found to occur in 50% of patients. Higher compliance rates have been found to occur with use of oral preparations such as ketoconazole and fluconazole, which avoid the potentially messy creams and suppositories.

A. Resistance to azoles has been found within *Candida* strains. However, taking into account this patient's history of poor glucose regulation, it is more likely that this patient was noncompliant with her use of the previously prescribed miconazole.

B. Although underlying risk factors in the development of candidiasis vaginitis include diabetes mellitus and this may be a contributing factor to acquiring this pathology, the most likely cause of treatment failure is noncompliance.

C. Diagnosis of candidiasis is made by microscopically identifying the spores and pseudohyphae of *Candida albicans* in a KOH wet-mount preparation. This is currently the standard of care in diagnosing this pathology.

D. The imidazole creams, including miconazole, have been shown to be very effective in the treatment of candidiasis vaginitis and was an appropriate choice of treatment for this patient.

537.   **A.** This little girl is mimicking her dog's injury because she was stressed about his injury. Conversion disorder is a disturbance of bodily functioning that does not conform to current concepts of the anatomy and physiology of the central or peripheral nervous system. Paresthesias and anesthesia are common symptoms.

B. Factitious disorder implies that the patient is purposefully assuming the sick role. There is usually no precipitating event to explain this reaction. In this case, there is a precipitating event (dog accident).

C. Hypochondriasis requires that the patient be preoccupied with a fear of contracting an illness.

D. This is not a normal grief reaction.

E. Somatization disorders usually encompass multisystem complaints.

538.   **A.** *Trichomonas vaginalis* is a unicellular anaerobic protozoan with three to five flagella and is about the size of a WBC. Signs and symptoms usually include an unpleasant odor accompanied by a yellow or gray, frothy, profuse discharge. Vaginal pH is usually elevated to 6 or 7. The characteristic strawberry cervix, which is actually punctate hemorrhages, is only seen in about 10% of cases. Treatment is metronidazole.

B. Gonorrhea is a gram-negative diplococcus and is treated with ceftriaxone. It often presents with a purulent, diffuse urethral discharge along with burning on urination.

C. *Chlamydia* is an obligate intracellular bacteria. Presentation is similar to that of gonorrhea.

D. Syphilis is caused by *Treponema pallidum*. The primary stage is characterized by a painless ulcer or chancre. Inguinal adenopathy is often present.

E. Human papilloma virus causes genital warts. It is also associated with cervical cancer.

F. Herpes simplex virus causes herpes. The infection begins initially with fever, malaise, vomiting, and diarrhea. Within a few days, painful genital ulcers appear.

G. Bacterial vaginosis presents with a foul odor and vaginal irritation. The vaginal pH is usually 5 to 6. Clue cells and the whiff test are pathognomonic for bacterial vaginosis.

H. Although the patient should be tested for HIV due to the presence of another sexually transmitted disease, the presenting symptoms are not diagnostic of an immunodeficiency state.

I. Common symptoms of candidiasis include dysuria, vaginal and vulvar itching, and a cottage cheese–like discharge.

539.   **A.** With normal physical examination findings and lack of occult blood 1 month prior, the index of suspicion in a patient with an aortic graft must be heightened to include aortoenteric fistula. In this case, because the patient is "stable," an emergent aortogram may be obtained. A vascular surgeon should also be immediately contacted in case the patient has an immediate decompensation. Any suspicion of a vascular leak is an emergency until proven otherwise.

B. The diagnosis of aortoenteric fistula is not made by barium enema. The investigation for neoplastic processes does not preclude the immediate search for an aortoenteric fistula.

C. Colonoscopy is not a diagnostic method for aortoenteric fistula. In this case, colonoscopy should be delayed until a fistula is ruled out.

D. A patient with an aortic graft should never be only observed because the risk for a vascular bleed is significant.

E. Oral medications to loosen the bowels to reduce or prevent hemorrhoids is a reasonable first-line treatment in patients without a history of aortic reconstruction. However, in this case, one must search for a fistula immediately.

540.   **D.** Cells damaged during storage can lyse when infused, causing release of their intracellular potassium. The excess potassium causes a hyperkalemia, which can lead to cardiac arrhythmias.

A. ABO mismatch causes agglutination and can cause pain and immediate hemolysis. Fever, chills, oliguria, hemoglobinuria, and jaundice are also commonly seen. Arrhythmias are not seen because of ABO blood type mismatching.

B. Excessive citrate in the blood binds calcium and removes it from circulation, causing a hypocalcemia. However, during small/slow infusions (such as this one), the citrate gets metabolized and thus the plasma calcium level does not change significantly.

C. There is no indication that this patient has any type of hypovolemia following the blood transfusion.

E. Rh antigen mismatch causes agglutination, but it is less potent than the agglutination of ABO mismatch. Hemolysis will also occur, but it will usually take several days.

541.   **D.** This patient has a midpelvic contraction because the anteroposterior diameter of the pelvis is short, the ischeal spines are prominent, and the baby is large (4000 g). The best treatment at this time is cesarean section.

A. Nothing is gained by waiting, cesarean section is the best treatment for this patient.

B. Epidural anesthesia may result in further arrest in labor.

C. Oxytocin infusion will increase fetal distress by increasing tetanic contractions of the uterus.

E. This patient needs a cesarean section for treatment of midpelvic contraction.

542. **B.** If a pleural effusion is found on chest x-ray, then a diagnostic thoracentesis is indicated. Our patient's radiograph shows two clear indications of a left pleural effusion. First, there is significant blunting of the left costophrenic angle. Secondly, the top of the fluid level can be seen as it crosses the left posterior seventh rib. Other radiographic findings in pleural effusion consist of thickened pleura and fluid in the horizontal or minor fissures.

Figure 542 ··

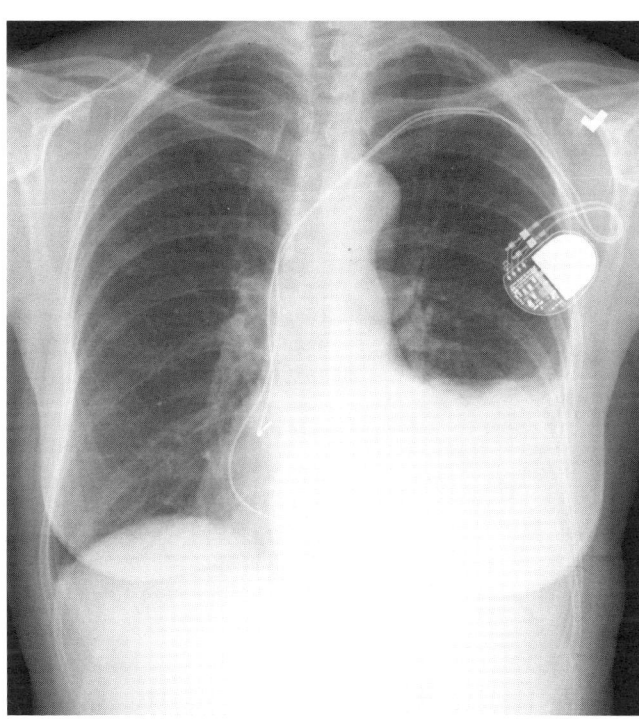

A. This scenario would increase the intravascular volume. Doing so would exacerbate any existing congestive heart failure, which would be quite harmful to this patient.

C. In general, bronchoscopy is not indicated for pleural effusion.

D. This scenario would increase the intravascular volume. Doing so would exacerbate any existing heart failure, which would be quite harmful to this patient.

E. An aggressive workup should be completed on a patient with chronic heart disease who has recently undergone a cardiac procedure. Observation is not the best course of action to take, especially because a complete and thorough history cannot be taken.

543. **D.** Nongestational choriocarcinoma is a germ cell tumor. Germ cell tumors are believed to come from totipotential germ cells that can differentiate into the yolk sac, placenta, and fetus (the three germ cell layers). Germ cell tumors are rapidly growing and usually occur in patients in their teens and twenties. Only 5% of germ cell tumors are malignant, and these are found most often in children and young women.

A. Epithelial tumors are slow growing and are usually found in women in their fifties. They are usually large and advanced at the time of diagnosis, with 75% of them spreading beyond the ovary at diagnosis. They have a poor prognosis. Eighty percent of patients with these tumors have an elevated CA-125 level. The CA-125 level is useful for monitoring treatment effectiveness, but it is not useful as a screening tool, partly due to the many other conditions that may cause it to increase. These tumors arise from the ovary surface mesothelial cells. There are six primary types: serous (40% malignant), mucinous (10% malignant), endometroid (20% malignant), clear cell (6% malignant), Brenner, and undifferentiated (10% malignant).

B. Granulosa-theca cell tumors and Sertoli-Leydig cell are both sex cord–stromal tumors. They are rare, usually bilateral, and typically affect women in their fifth to eighth decades of life. They arise from the sex cords of the embryonic gonad, before differentiation to female or male, or from the ovarian stroma (which may become an ovary or a testis). Both produce large amounts of hormone, with granulose-theca cell tumors producing estrogens and causing feminization, precocious puberty, and postmenopausal bleeding, and Sertoli-Leydig tumors producing testosterone and other androgens and causing virilization, including acne, deepened voice, hirsutism, and clitoromegaly. Ovarian fibroma is a stromal cell neoplasm, but it originates from mature fibroblasts and is not a functioning tumor. Meig syndrome is the combination of an ovarian tumor, ascites, and right hydrothorax.

C. Immature teratoma and dysgerminoma are the most common germ cell tumors. Less common ones include choriocarcinoma, embryonal cell carcinoma, endodermal sinus (yolk sac) tumors, and mixed germ cell tumors. Immature teratoma would be part of the differential diagnosis for this patient, but the tumor marker levels rule it out. Serum tumor markers for the different germ cell tumors are human chorionic gonadotropin (hCG), alpha-fetoprotein (AFP), lactate dehydrogenase (LDH), and CA-125. The different tumors have different positive serum tumor markers. Mixed germ-cell: hCG, AFP, LDH, and CA-125 positive. Embryonal carcinoma: hCG, AFP, and CA-125 positive. Endodermal sinus tumor: AFP positive. Dysgerminoma: LDH and CA-125 positive. Immature teratoma: CA-125 positive. Nongestational choriocarcinoma: hCG positive.

E. Squamous cell carcinoma can occur in the cervix and urinary bladder.

544. **D.** This patient is suffering from an acute dystonic reaction, a known side effect of antipsychotic medications, particularly haloperidol. The time course can be anywhere from 4 hours to 4 days after exposure to the antipsychotic. Muscle spasm may occur anywhere in the body, but is classically in the neck (torticollis). Intravenous diphenhydramine should be given immediately, because of its faster absorption than oral administration.

A. Benztropine is an anticholinergic used for parkinsonism-like symptoms.

B. Benztropine is an anticholinergic used for parkinsonism-like symptoms.

C. Dantrolene is a calcium channel blocker used for neuroleptic malignant syndrome.

E. Oral diphenhydramine will take a long time to be absorbed and improve symptoms of dystonia. Therefore, it should be administered in its intravenous form.

545. **C.** In the evaluation of the suicidal patient it is important to perform a careful medical history with some emphasis on the psychiatric history. Several psychiatric conditions are associated with an increased risk for suicide and an increased risk for successful suicide completion. Of the conditions listed in this question, patients with major depression have an increased risk for suicide, and nearly 20% of those patients will successfully commit suicide.

A and **B.** Patients with concurrent psychosis and personality disorders also have an increased risk for suicide, and nearly 10% of those patients will also successfully commit suicide.

D. Patients with panic disorder may also have an increased risk for suicide.

E. Patients with schizophrenia have a 10% increased risk for suicide.

546. **C.** 1600 mL. Maintenance fluid can be calculated by the patient's weight using the Holliday-Seger method. A child should receive 100 mL/kg for the first 10 kg of body weight. They should then receive 50 mL/kg for the next 10 kg of body weight and 20 mL/kg for every kilogram thereafter. In our example it would be (100 mL/kg × 10 kg) + (50 mL/kg × 10 kg) + (20 mL/kg × 5 kg) = 1600 mL.

547. **E.** This woman likely has interstitial cystitis. A disorder characterized by chronic pelvic pain and urinary symptoms such as urgency, frequency, and decrease in the force of stream. Nearly 75% of women complain of anterior vaginal wall tenderness, both on physical examination and during sexual intercourse. Pain is the most common sexual complaint in women with interstitial cystitis.

A. Women with interstitial cystitis complain of decreased sexual arousal when compared with age-matched controls.

B. Women with interstitial cystitis complain of slightly decreased sexual desire.

C. Young women with interstitial cystitis report no difficulties with lubrication. However, women over the age of 50 with interstitial cystitis do have decreased lubrication.

D. Women with interstitial cystitis have decreased ability to achieve orgasm when compared with age-matched controls.

548. **D.** This patient has evidence of ulcerative pyoderma gangrenosum. This condition is associated with systemic diseases such as ulcerative colitis. The lesions start as tender erythematous papules that become necrotic and tender.

A. Erythema is caused by bacterial organisms.

B. Erythema nodosum is associated with tender erythematous nodules over the shins and extensor surfaces.

C. Herpetiform dermatitis is associated with gluten-sensitive enteropathy.

E. This lesion is not characteristic of steroid-induced dermatitis.

549. **B.** This patient's presentation suggests the diagnosis of measles. The rash associated with measles is a confluent maculopapular erythematous rash that starts on the head and progresses caudally. Small red spots with blue centers on the buccal mucosa are known as Koplik spots and are seen early in the disease. Coryza, cough, and conjunctivitis are also common in measles.

A. Fifth disease, also known as erythema infectiosum or "slapped cheek" disease, is characterized by a reticular ("sandpaper") erythematous maculopapular rash that begins on the arms and spreads to the trunk and legs.

C. Roseola rash is also similar to measles, but the rash starts after an acute onset of high fever. This rash starts on the trunk and spreads peripherally.

D. Rubella's rash is similar to that of measles, but the rash does not coalesce and lasts approximately 3 days.

E. Varicella's rash is a pruritic teardrop-shaped vesicular rash that will break and crust. Lesions are typically is several stages of development, and the rash begins on the face and trunk and then spreads to the extremities.

550. **C.** Urine metanephrines/normetanephrines and vanilmandelic acid are sensitive for the detection of pheochromocytomas. Pheochromocytomas are usually unilateral, benign, and found in the adrenal gland. Symptoms include flushing, sweating, and hypertension.

A. MRI will not be as sensitive in detecting an adrenal pheochromocytoma because the adrenal gland may not be enlarged or abnormal in contour.

B. MIBG scan is only helpful in locating extraadrenal pheochromocytomas after the diagnosis has been made.

D. Sestamibi scan is used to detect an overactive parathyroid gland.

E. MRI of the head will be very low yield in this scenario.

551. **B.** One of the most frequent complaints of hospitalized patients and their families is the poor manner in which their prognosis was conveyed. Suggestions in giving bad news to patients includes the use of a quiet, safe room, sitting down close to the patient, being an attentive listener, and acknowledging the patient's fears and concerns. The physician should also answer questions concisely, honestly, and compassionately.

A. A complete discussion should be undertaken over multiple interviews.

C. The physician is responsible for delivering the bad news personally.

D. Technical jargon should be avoided.

E. Use of euphemism portrays false hope.

552. **E.** This patient presents with typical signs of cholelithiasis with secondary cholecystitis. Ultrasonography is the diagnostic imaging method of choice for detecting gallstones. This evaluation should reveal gallstones, thickening of the gallbladder wall, and the presence of pericholecystic fluid.

A. Administering antibiotics is not helpful in treating either cholelithiasis or cholecystitis. Ultrasonography is an appropriate imaging modality.

B. Angiography cannot demonstrate gallstones or inflammation of the gallbladder. There is no indication here for angiography based on the presentation.

C. CT of the abdomen is not optimal because gallstones cannot be visualized well. Also, with contrast the bile in the gallbladder shows up the same as gallstones; thus, the two cannot be differentiated.

D. MRI of the abdomen will not demonstrate gallstones.

553. **C.** This patient has dysfunctional uterine bleeding. This is defined as bleeding for which no specific cause has been defined. This is the case with this patient, who has already had a negative diagnostic laparoscopy, hysteroscopy, and biopsy.

A. Adenomatous hyperplasia is part of the differential diagnosis of dysfunctional uterine bleeding, but this patient has a negative endometrial biopsy.

B. Adenomyosis would be present on endometrial biopsy (which was negative in this patient).

D. Submucosal fibroma would be present on diagnostic laparoscopy.

E. Uterine polyps would be present on diagnostic hysteroscopy.

554. **B.** Arthritis of distal extremities, clubbing of digits, and periosteal bone formation are characteristic of hypertrophic osteoarthropathy. This disease process is related to intrathoracic malignancy. X-rays of distal extremities may suggest osteomyelitis but is bilateral. Management consists of treating the underlying disease.

A. Behçet syndrome is a chronic disorder that affects multiple systems. It is inflammatory, relapsing, and may involve skin, eyes, genitals, joints, central nervous system, and gastrointestinal tract. Painful oral ulcers are seen in almost all patients.

C. Osteomyelitis is an infection of bone and may be caused by aerobic bacteria, anaerobic bacteria, mycobacteria, and fungi. It affects the vertebrae and feet of diabetics. The metaphysis of the tibia and femur are most commonly affected in children.

D. Reiter syndrome is characterized by a urologic or gastrointestinal infection followed by arthritis. Urethritis, conjunctivitis, and skin lesions are associated with this disorder. Reiter syndrome can be sexually transmitted, usually after infection with *Chlamydia trachomatis*. It may also be contracted after infection with *Shigella*, *Salmonella*, *Yersinia*, or *Campylobacter*.

E. Four of the following criteria must be present to diagnose rheumatoid arthritis: morning stiffness, arthritis of three or more joints, arthritis of hand joints, symmetric arthritis, rheumatoid nodules, positive rheumatoid factor, or radiographic changes.

555. **E.** This patient has radiation proctitis. This condition is associated with diarrhea, rectal bleeding, tenesmus, rectal pain, and incontinence. Further complications of this condition include bleeding, stricture, and fistulas. Treatment involves bulking agents, antidiarrheals, and steroid enemas.

A. External hemorrhoids are abnormally dilated anal veins below the dentate line. They may show a skin tag and occasionally erode through the skin.

B. Acute onset of perirectal pain associated with straining and blood on the toilet tissue suggests the diagnosis of fissure-in-ano. Risk factors for the development of this condition include straining during bowel movements, constipation, and anal intercourse.

C. Fistula-in-ano describes perianal pain and a mass in the perianal skin associated with discharge of liquid from the perianal area.

D. Internal hemorrhoids are veins with mucosa above the dentate line. They are prone to prolapse and bleeding.

556. **E.** von Hippel-Lindau disease is an autosomal-dominant condition characterized by hemangioblastomas of the retina and central nervous system. Renal cell carcinoma can be found in 25% of cases. CT scans have been recommended to identify these tumors at a young age. Pheochromocytomas and pancreatic islet cell neoplasms are also common. Disease pathogenesis involves a defect in a tumor suppressor gene.

A. Autosomal-dominant polycystic kidney disease is a condition characterized by grossly enlarged cysts on the surface of the kidneys. Progressive renal decline often results in end-stage renal disease by 60 years of age.

B. Bartter syndrome is an autosomal-recessive disorder consisting of hypokalemia secondary to renal potassium wasting, metabolic alkalosis, and normal to low blood pressure. Diagnosis is made in childhood.

C. Neurofibromatosis 1 is characterized by multiple benign tumors called neurofibromas that occur on peripheral nerve sheaths. Pigmented lesions on the skin called café au lait spots also occur. This condition is caused from a mutation of a gene on chromosome 17 that encodes a tumor suppressor protein called neurofibromin.

D. Tuberous sclerosis is a multisystem disease commonly presenting with skin lesions, seizures, and mental retardation. Benign tumors of the central nervous system may also occur. Renal involvement is common, but benign angiomyolipomas rather than renal cell carcinoma are the characteristic tumors. Bilateral renal cysts are also common.

557. **B.** Maternal systemic lupus erythematosus increases the rate of abortion and may result in a perinate with cardiac arrhythmia, most notably complete heart block.

A. Coarctation of the aorta can result from embryonic exposure to hyperglycemia, as seen in maternal diabetes mellitus.

C. Transposition of the great vessels can result from embryonic exposure to hyperglycemia as seen in maternal diabetes mellitus.

D. Tricuspid atresia can result from embryonic exposure to teratogens.

E. Ventricular septal defect can result from embryonic exposure to hyperglycemia as seen in maternal diabetes mellitus.

558. **D.** Tuberous sclerosis is a progressive autosomal-dominant neurocutaneous disorder. Neuroimaging reveals distinctive periventricular knoblike areas of localized swelling (tubers). Mental retardation, seizures, and skin lesions are common findings. Skin lesions include ash leaf spots (flat, hypopigmented areas) and shagreen patches (areas of thickened skin).

A. Down syndrome is not associated with tuber formation or skin lesions.

B. Neurofibromatosis is characterized by Lisch nodules, neurofibromas, and café au lait spots.

C. Sturge-Weber disease is associated with a port-wine stain over the area innervated by the first division of the trigeminal nerve.

E. von Hippel-Lindau disease is characterized by retinal and central nervous system vascular hamartomas and renal cell carcinoma.

559. **B.** This patient's history should arouse suspicion of mental retardation. The DSM-IV criteria are (1) IQ of 70 or below, (2) deficits or impairment in adaptive functioning, and (3) onset before 18 years of age. Since he has exhibited deficits in adaptive function, an IQ test would likely confirm or exclude the diagnosis.

A. Admitting this patient is not warranted.

C. Reassurance may be inappropriate at this time, because an etiology has not been identified.

D. Behavior monitoring may be useful, but an IQ test should be done first.

E. This patient needs to be treated and evaluated.

560. **B.** Appendicitis is more common in the younger age group. It often starts as a vague epigastric pain that is followed by symptoms of nausea and vomiting. The pain then becomes sharp and migrates to the McBurney point in the right lower quadrant. Patients usually have an ongoing low-grade fever that does not go away. Rebound tenderness is seen in cases of peritonitis that can occur if the appendix ruptures (common with appendicitis). Pain on passive extension of the hip while lying on the left with the knee extended (positive Psoas sign) without pain during passive internal rotation of the hip (negative Obturator sign) suggests a retrocecally located appendix.

A. An infected appendix located in the anterior pelvis would be suggested by pain on passive internal rotation of the hip (positive obturator sign) and no pain on passive extension of the hip while lying on the left with the knee extended (negative psoas sign).

C. Cecal diverticula can cause right-sided lower quadrant abdominal pain; however, rebound tenderness, signs of peritonitis, and a low-grade fever are not likely symptoms.

D. Pancreatitis presents as a midepigastric pain that often radiates to the back. The patient can seem to have signs of a generalized peritonitis, but the patient with pancreatitis often is constantly moving.

E. Testicular torsion can produce a right lower quadrant pain. However, it is not likely to cause fever and an increased neutrophilia, making the diagnosis less likely.

561. **C.** Ethylene glycol is the major constituent of most antifreeze compounds and in the body is broken down to the highly toxic organic acids of glycolic and oxalic acids. The patient has likely ingested ethylene glycol as either an attempt to become intoxicated related to his history of alcoholism, to commit suicide related to his history of depression, or by accident working on farm machinery. Toxicity is characterized by increased serum osmolality or osmolar gap of greater than 50 mOsm/L, severe anion gap metabolic acidosis, and low calcium serum levels due to the formation of calcium oxalate crystals in plasma. The crystals are then found in the urine and cause acute renal failure as they exit the kidneys. Patients exhibit altered mental status, convulsions, tachypnea, and coma. The patient will need emergent dialysis to remove the parent compound and either ethanol or fomepizole to help reverse the effects of the substance.

A. Chlorinated insecticide poisoning is a logical consideration considering this patient works on a farm. These compounds are central nervous system stimulators that cause nervous irritability, muscle twitching, seizures, and coma. Arrhythmias and hepatic and renal damage may occur. Patients are usually given activated charcoal and diazepam or other anticonvulsants for seizures.

B. Ethanol intoxication would be a logical consideration considering the history of alcoholism. However, ethanol toxicity would show stupor, respiratory arrest, bradycardia, hypotension, and hypothermia. Patients may be areflexic or show no electroencephalographic activity. Calcium crystals and renal failure would not likely occur. Patients are usually given activated charcoal.

D. Methanol is commonly found in a variety of products, including solvents, cleaning solutions, and paint removers. It is sometimes ingested intentionally by alcoholic patients in an attempt to become intoxicated. Methanol is converted to the toxic organic acid called formic acid. Methanol resembles ethylene glycol in terms of its symptoms and laboratory data; however, it does not cause calcium crystal formation or renal failure and notoriously causes visual disturbances. The treatment strategy is also the same as for ethylene glycol.

E. Mushroom ingestion could include various species that all contain a potent cytotoxin called amatoxin. Abdominal pains, vomiting, and diarrhea are common symptoms. Massive liver necrosis is responsible for most mushroom-related fatalities.

562. **D.** Scaphoid fracture is usually seen in young adults who fall on an outstretched hand. Physical examination may reveal tenderness in the anatomic snuffbox. Radiographs may not reveal evidence of fracture. However, if fracture is suspected, plaster casting and repeat x-ray studies should be undertaken.

A. Endochondroma is a benign bone tumor that appears as a radiolucent metaphyseal lesion associated with a good prognosis.

B. Nonossifying fibroma is a benign bone tumor associated with late pathologic fractures.

C. Perilunate dislocations occur with wrist hyperextension. Radiographs may show disruption of the axial alignment of the lunate, radius, and capitate bones.

E. Smith fracture occurs with a fall on the dorsum of the wrist. This type of injury results from a radius fracture with volar angulation. Treatment strategies include closed reduction.

563. **C.** By keeping a pneumoperitoneum of lower than the approximate vena cava pressure, one decreases the chance for deep vein thrombosis. The use of elevated pneumoperitoneum causes pooling of blood in the lower extremities and deep vein thrombosis.

A. A dose of 50,000 to 70,000 units of heparin can be toxic, causing immediate hemorrhage. Some studies have advocated the use of low-dose subcutaneous heparin prior to surgery, but doses in this region are dangerous.

B. Warfarin has a paradoxic effect in the short term of creating a hypercoagulable state. In very rare cases this has caused skin sloughing.

D. The use of pneumatic compression devices has been shown to reduce the incidence of deep vein thrombosis. However, in this situation, maintaining a lower vena cava pressure is most important to prevent deep vein thrombosis.

E. The use of spinal anesthesia for an intraperitoneal operation is generally ill advised due to poor airway control. In this special case, the use of medication to cause an increased peripheral vasodilation will cause increased pooling of blood and possibly increase the risk for deep vein thrombosis.

564. **D.** 295 mL/h is the correct answer. In this question, you must first determine the maintenance fluid requirements. This would be 1000 mL for the first 10 kg (100 mL/kg × 10 kg), 500 mL for the second 10 kg (50 mL/kg × 10 kg), and 300 mL for the remaining 15 kg (20 mL/kg × 15 kg). 1000 + 500 + 300 = 1800 mL maintenance or 1800 mL/24 h = 75 mL/h. Next you must calculate the fluid deficit, which is 35 kg × 10% = 3.5 L or 3500 mL. Half of the deficit should be replaced over the first 8 hours and the remaining half over the next 16 hours. So, 3500 mL/2 = 1750 mL over the first 8 hours or 1750 mL/8 h = ~220 mL/h for the deficit. When we add maintenance to deficit we get 220 mL/h + 75 mL/h = 295 mL/h.

565. **E.** This patient needs surgical repair of the patent ductus arteriosus. Infants are unable to communicate pain or discomfort, and one of the most important things to remember about pediatric cardiovascular issues is to observe feeding activities. Feeding is the equivalent stress test and will key an astute physician to search for problems. Look for signs of distress during feeding.

A. This patient needs surgical repair of the patent ductus arteriosus.

B. A patent ductus arteriosus that has been watched and then treated medically needs to be closed surgically.

C. This patient needs surgical repair of the patent ductus arteriosus.

D. Treatment of choice for patent ductus arteriosus is surgical repair.

566. **C.** Peripheral vascular disease is an atherosclerotic disease of the arteries of the lower extremities affecting nearly 10 million people in the United States. Risk factors include hyperlipidemia, hypertension, smoking, and diabetes. The diagnosis is made clinically, and can be determined by calculating the ankle:brachial index (<1 with disease). Ultrasonography or MRI can aid in diagnosis. Presurgical visualization is best achieved with peripheral angiography. Treatment begins with the correction of all risk factors, including an exercise regimen, as well as antiplatelet therapy.

A. Thromboangiitis obliterans, also called Buerger disease, is described as intimal proliferation and thrombi in small to medium-sized vessels with inflammatory infiltrates that may involve upper or lower extremities. Findings include cool extremities and ulcerations. It is common in male smokers.

B. Lumbar spinal stenosis is known as pseudoclaudication, which is usually bilateral and also occurs with standing. Sitting or bending forward relieves symptoms.

D. This patient has risk factors for peripheral vascular disease, which may be unilateral or bilateral. In this case, findings are bilateral. There is no evidence to suggest popliteal arterial entrapment, which tends to be a unilateral process.

E. Thromboangiitis obliterans is also known as Buerger disease, a proliferative disease of the small vessels.

567. **C.** Cyclothymia has depressive and manic features either separately or intermingled. This disorder is more common in women and begins at about the age of 20. Affected individuals demonstrate job instability, occasional suicide attempts, and an increased risk for substance abuse.

568. **H.** Uncomplicated bereavement usually follows severe loss or trauma and may produce symptoms of a full depressive syndrome. Affected individuals are able to work through their problems and see them to resolution through the process of grieving.

569. **A.** This individual experiences features of the adjustment disorder with depressed mood. This condition often occurs after a readily identifiable stress (death of a loved one) and results in impaired functioning and improves as the stress disappears. These patients are somewhere in between sadness and major depression.

570. **D.** Dysthymia is a chronic disorder (>2 years) that commonly affects women in their late twenties. These individuals have depressive features that are worse as the day progresses. These individuals feel well in the morning, and symptoms appear as the day progresses. Sleep disorders are common. Predisposing factors to this condition include major loss in childhood such as death of a parent.

571. **B.** This patient has giardiasis, which is the most common parasitic disease in the United States. This disease is commonly associated with contaminated water. It is typical after a scenario such as return from camping with symptoms of watery diarrhea, foul smelling stools, abdominal pain, nausea, vomiting, and flatulence. Symptoms usually resolve in a week, but stool may be infected for additional time.

A. *Clostridium difficile* is associated with prolonged antibiotic use.

C. *Salmonella* is associated with eating undercooked meats.

D. *Shigella* is associated with eating undercooked meats.

E. *Vibrio cholerae* may result from travel to the Middle East, India, or Africa. It is also associated with eating undercooked shellfish.

572. **D.** Positive evidence of pregnancy includes detection of fetal heart rate. This can be detected by transvaginal ultrasonography after 4 weeks from the date of conception. After 6 weeks, transabdominal sonography can detect fetal heart tones.

A. Blue violet hue to the cervix (Chadwick sign) is probable evidence of pregnancy.

B. Cervical softening (Goodall sign) is probable evidence of pregnancy.

C. Cessation of menses is presumptive evidence of pregnancy.

E. Nausea is present in only 50% of pregnancies and is considered presumptive evidence of the pregnant state.

573. **E.** This patient has evidence of a Salter-Harris type V fracture. The Salter-Harris classification system serves to categorize fractures that involve the growth plate. The system is composed of five types of growth plate injuries labeled I through V. A Salter V injury carries the worst prognosis and results from a crush injury, which compresses the growth plate and can cause aberrant growth. The prognosis is good for types I through III, with IV and V having a much worse outcome.

A. A Salter-Harris I injury is a transverse fracture through the metaphyseal side of the growth plate.

B. A Salter II injury is a fracture that is partially through the growth plate but exits out the metaphysis.

C. A Salter III injury is partially through the growth plate but exits out the epiphysis.

D. A Salter IV injury is a fracture that passes through the metaphysis, the growth plate, and the epiphysis.

574. **B.** Aspergillosis usually affects patients who are profoundly immunodeficient. Patients with HIV infection are therefore at higher risk. Pulmonary aspergillosis is the most common site of infection and can lead to necrotic pneumonia. Pleuritic chest pain and an elevated lactate dehydrogenase usually accompany the disease, as does severe neutropenia. Cultures are usually not helpful. Amphotericin B should be started as soon as aspergillosis is suspected.

A. Anthrax is a gram-positive, spore-producing, aerobic rod. Signs and symptoms often include dyspnea, hemoptysis, chest pain, fever, nonproductive cough, and possibly black necrotic skin lesions.

C. Coccidioidomycosis occurs as a result of inhalation of *Coccidioides immitis*, which is a mold that grows in Central and South America. This is a common infection among HIV patients in endemic areas. Symptoms usually include respiratory illness and chills. Arthralgias and knee swelling are also common.

D. Cytomegalovirus is common in AIDS patients. Symptoms include fever, dyspnea, and dry cough. Chest x-ray may show interstitial infiltrates.

E. *Pneumocystis carinii* pneumonia is also common in AIDS patients with CD4 counts below 200 and is usually treated prophylactically with trimethoprim-sulfamethoxazole.

575. **C.** The surgery can go on as scheduled. The patient has a platelet count above 50,000/mm³, which is considered stable in terms of being a bleeding risk. The patient should have his surgery, but fresh frozen plasma should be ready on call. Patients will not bleed spontaneously until they reach a platelet count of 20,000/mm³ or below. At that point it would be absolutely contraindicated to have an operation.

A, B, D, and **E.** This patient can have surgery as scheduled. The platelet count is stable in terms of surgical risk.

576. **A.** From birth to approximately 1 week after birth, infants should receive between 6 and 10 feedings per day. The appropriate volume of fluid is 30 to 90 mL. The infant should be held during feedings and the bottle handled so that the formula fills the nipple.

B. This regimen is appropriate for a newborn who is 1 week to 1 month of age.

C. This regimen is appropriate for a newborn who is 1 to 3 months of age.

D. This regimen is appropriate for a newborn who is 3 to 6 months of age.

E. This regimen is appropriate for a newborn who is 6 to 9 months of age.

577. **A.** The diagnosis of syphilis is made by microscopically identifying the characteristic mobile spirochete on dark-field microscopy from material scraped or expressed from the base of the chancre.

B. The incubation period for this organism is 7 to 14 days, with a chancre appearing about 10 to 60 days after inoculation. This patient has likely become infected with syphilis within the past 4 weeks. Although the RPR and VDRL tests are good screening tests for syphilis, a serological test will likely be negative at this time.

C. Again, although the RPR and VDRL tests are good for screening, due to the fact that the patient has been inoculated with the organism within the past 4 weeks, the results of these serologic tests are likely to be negative.

D. A syphilitic chancre appears on the vulva about 10 to 60 days after inoculation. If untreated, the lesion will spontaneously heal in 3 to 9 weeks. If this patient were instructed to return only if the lesion did not resolve, the diagnosis and subsequent treatment of her syphilis would be missed and her disease would progress.

E. The next appropriate step in managing this patient would be to establish the diagnosis. Although tetracycline can be given to treat syphilis, the treatment of choice in an adult patient without a penicillin allergy remains penicillin G.

578. **C.** This patient has acute pancreatitis, which is best managed conservatively. The patient should not be allowed anything by mouth (NPO), and the pancreas should be given time to rest. Patients that are going to be made NPO for over 5 days can be fed via total parenteral nutrition.

A. The majority of pancreatitis cases can be managed conservatively. Thus, exploratory laparotomy is not necessary.

B. This patient should be managed conservatively with admission, NPO, and observation.

D. A low-fat diet is inappropriate because the pancreas will continue to secrete digestive enzymes if the patient in being fed.

E. Although an abdominal aortic aneurysm may cause epigastric tenderness, amylase and lipase should not be elevated.

579. **C.** This is a first-degree atrioventricular (AV) block, which is defined as a PR interval of greater than 0.2 seconds. This can be measured easily on ECG paper by a PR interval that is greater than one large block (note: one large block is made up of five smaller blocks). Interestingly, this type of AV block is present in 1.6% of the healthy adult population. The patient's history as presented shows her to be in excellent medical condition for a 90-year-old woman. Without symptoms, this finding is considered a normal variant.

A. Cardioversion with electronic defibrillators plays no role in the treatment of AV block, including first-degree AV block.

B. Atropine is not an approved therapy for AV block but can be used as a noninvasive intervention to help locate the site of the conduction delay. Atropine has a vagolytic effect that will improve the PR interval in most patients with first-degree AV block. This is because the conduction delay in most of these patients lies in the AV node.

D. Permanent pacing does not usually play a role in the treatment of first-degree AV block. Situations in which it should be considered in first-degree AV block are as follows: (1) if the block is located in the Infra-Hisian specialized conduction system, (2) patients with pacemaker syndrome, and (3) and patients with neuromuscular disease. The Infra-Hisian system is made up of the bundle branches, fascicles, and the terminal Purkinje network. Pacemaker syndrome is the constellation of symptoms that come from the lack of synchrony between the atria and ventricles. As one would expect, the symptoms are those of decreased cardiac output such as presyncope, syncope, and fatigue. Other symptoms include paranocturnal dyspnea and orthopnea. The decreased cardiac output comes from a decrease in stroke volume and from atrial contraction against closed AV valves.

E. Electrophysiologic studies are not indicated for first-degree AV block.

580. **E.** CT scan of the abdomen and pelvis is the test of choice in diagnosing renal calculi. No contrast is used because contrast can obscure the presence of stones. In addition, pelvic vein stones (phleboliths) can be confused with urinary tract calculi.

A. Uric acid stones are radiolucent and would not be visible on abdominal x-ray studies.

Figure 579

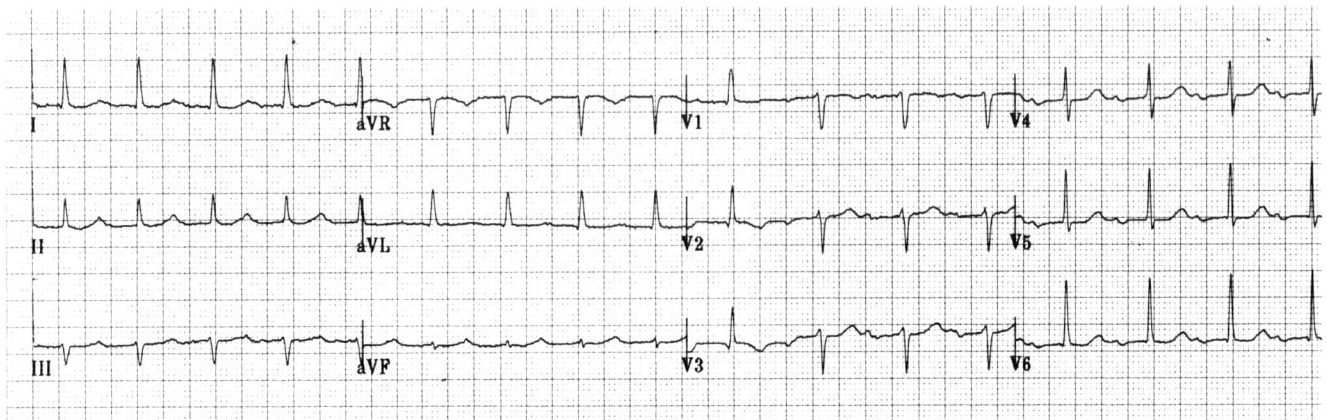

B. Renal ultrasonography may show the stone, but it is not as sensitive as a CT scan without contrast.

C. Intravenous pyelography is helpful but is not the test of choice because the patient is unnecessarily exposed to contrast.

D. CT scan with intravenous contrast is incorrect because the contrast will obscure the stone.

581. **C.** The clinical picture is consistent with a diagnosis of Ménière disease. The classic triad associated with Ménière disease is vertigo, tinnitus, and hearing loss. After several years, Ménière disease can result in permanent hearing loss. Several differentials must be considered with the above scenario. Cerebellar stroke is a possibility, albeit unlikely given the multiple recurrences of symptoms. Benign paroxysmal positional vertigo is also a possibility. Tumor and trauma must also be considered. In addition, loop diuretics, particularly furosemide, and aminoglycosides can lead to a similar clinical scenario.

A. Carbonic anhydrase inhibitors are used to treat Ménière disease. Acetazolamide is commonly used.

B and D. Beta blockers are not known to cause this clinical picture.

E. Carbonic anhydrase inhibitors are used to treat Ménière disease. Acetazolamide is commonly used.

582. **D.** Based on her symptoms and relief with calcium carbonate, the possibility of peptic ulcer disease is more possible than gallbladder disease. H2 blockers are a reasonable choice in a short course (4 weeks) for this patient. They may ultimately require an upper gastrointestinal endoscopy for confirmation of the diagnosis.

A. There is no reason for laparoscopic cholecystectomy at this time. There is no radiographic evidence of gallstone disease.

B. Diagnostic laparoscopy is not indicated unless the patient shows signs of an acute abdomen.

C. ERCP is indicated as a diagnostic and therapeutic tool for gallbladder disease, but not for ulcer disease.

E. Upper gastrointestinal endoscopy would be considered if the patient presented with bleeding or would be performed sometime later if the symptoms were to persist.

583. **E.** A special intraosseous catheter inserted into the anterior tibia will give prompt and reliable intravenous access in children. Little expertise is required to insert this catheter.

A. In situations where venous collapse may have occurred, finding a peripheral vein is often difficult.

B. In young children, the discovery of a vein on the back of the hand may take significant time and require some expertise due to the small caliber of these veins.

C. The femoral vein is close to the femoral artery in children, and percutaneous placement of an intravenous catheter is difficult.

D. While performing cardiopulmonary resuscitation in children, one should not stop to attempt to insert an internal jugular catheter. Children often have very large necks, making discovery of the vein difficult.

584. **D.** Lactate dehydrogenase levels are unchanged in the pregnant and nonpregnant states.

A. Alkaline phosphatase increases secondary to placental contribution.

B. Creatinine and blood urea nitrogen decrease in pregnancy.

C. Hemoglobin decreases, but this is due to an increase in plasma volume.

E. Blood lipids increase in pregnancy.

585. **B.** This patient has panic disorder with agoraphobia. These attacks tend to occur several times per week. This condition is chronic, with exacerbations and remissions, and has an excellent prognosis with therapy. Biologic theories for the cause of panic disorder include a hyperactive center in the temporal cerebral cortex.

A. Patients with panic disorder have increased norepinephrine metabolites. Experimental lactate infusion increases norepinephrine, which produces anxiety.

C. Gamma-aminobutyric acid inhibits central nervous system activity.

D. Patients with panic disorder have increased REM latency.

E. Urinary flow rate should be the same as patients without panic disorder.

586. **A.** This patient has postpartum mastitis. Breast-feeding is not contraindicated in mastitis without discharge; only if she had discharge should she stop breast-feeding. Antibiotics will be needed for the infection.

B. Breast biopsy is not indicated unless one suspects malignancy. Her signs support mastitis.

C. Fine-needle aspiration is not indicated in mastitis.

D and E. There is no discharge, so breast-feeding may continue.

587. **B.** Hydatidiform moles are characterized by proliferation of the trophoblast. They are most commonly recognized by the enlarged-for-dates uterus and continuous or intermittent bleeding in the first two trimesters. Clinical hyperthyroidism also can occur due to the binding of the human chorionic gonadotropin (hCG) molecule (with elevated levels of hCG) to the thyroid-stimulating hormone receptor site and by hyperfunction of the thyroid gland. An increase in blood pressure is also common. Ultrasonography will typically show a "snowstorm" pattern.

A. Adenocarcinoma of the endometrium is a common gynecologic malignancy. The most common presenting symptom is postmenopausal bleeding. The risk factors include unopposed estrogen exposure, nulliparity, chronic anovulation, and menopause after age 50. Other risk factors include diabetes mellitus, hypertension, cancer of the breast or ovary, and a family history of endometrial cancer.

C. This choice is unlikely because of the larger than expected uterus and bleeding. Although it is possible that her date was miscalculated, the clinical picture is more likely to be due to a molar pregnancy.

D. Placental abruption is associated with maternal cocaine abuse, but it would be unlikely to present this early in pregnancy. Half of all abruptions occur after the 30th week and are associated with severe abdominal pain and a firm, tender uterus.

E. Botryoid sarcoma is a soft tissue tumor found in children, classically described as grapelike clusters protruding from the vaginal orifice.

588. **B.** Germ cell tumor treatment involves complete surgical staging of the tumor, but because the tumor usually only involves one ovary at the time of diagnosis, only the involved ovary needs to be removed. Multidrug chemotherapy is effective against germ cell tumors. Radiation is not part of the treatment of germ cell tumors except in the case of dysgerminomas. They are extremely sensitive to radiation of the entire abdomen. These tumors are usually found in early stages and have a good prognosis. Five-year survival rates are as follows: dysgerminomas, 85%; immature teratomas, 70% to 80%; and endodermal sinus tumors 60% to 70%.

A. Chemotherapy is effective against germ cell tumors, and radiation is effective against dysgerminomas, but the involved ovary should still be removed.

C. Radiation therapy is not very effective. These tumors often recur. Overall, the 5-year survival rate is less than 20%.

D. Total abdominal hysterectomy and removal of the uterine tubes (TAHBSO) is the treatment for epithelial ovarian tumors and sex cord–stromal tumors. Epithelial

tumor treatment may also include omentectomy and cytoreductive surgery. Epithelial tumors are sensitive to cisplatin-based combination chemotherapy. Sex cord–stromal tumors are treated with TAHBSO. Postoperative pelvic radiation is used in early stages. Chemotherapy is not effective. Tumors usually recur, and recurrences may be found as long as 15 to 20 years after removal of the original tumor. The 5-year survival rate for stage I disease is 90%.

E. Watchful waiting is inappropriate for this patient.

589. **A.** de Quervain thyroiditis, also known as subacute thyroiditis, is precipitated by a viral upper respiratory infection. Histologically, it is defined by giant cell infiltration, polymorphonuclear leukocytes, and follicular disruption. Patients often complain of a sore throat, which is actually neck pain. The neck pain may shift from side to side before settling on one side. A low-grade fever is often seen. The disrupted follicles release thyroid hormone, causing hyperthyroidism. An asymmetric, firm, tender thyroid is characteristic. This disease is self-limiting. Treatment is usually high-dose aspirin or nonsteroidal antiinflammatory agents. Corticosteroids may be necessary in refractory cases.

B. Graves disease is characterized by hyperthyroidism plus goiter, exophthalmos, or pretibial myxedema. It is the most common cause of hyperthyroidism and is caused by an antibody against the thyroid-stimulating hormone receptor. Iodine, propylthiouracil, and methimazole are medical treatments. Surgery may be indicated after response failure to antithyroid drugs.

C. Hashimoto thyroiditis is chronic thyroiditis. It is characterized by lymphocytic infiltration of the gland due to autoimmune factors. A painless enlargement of the thyroid is often the presenting complaint. The goiter is usually nontender, firm, and rubbery. Other autoimmune diseases may be concurrent. Later in the disease the patient becomes hypothyroid.

D. Lymphocytic thyroiditis occurs mainly in women, especially 4 to 24 weeks postpartum. The thyroid is nontender. The patient experiences self-limited hyperthyroidism followed by hypothyroidism after depletion of thyroid hormone stores. Lymphocytic infiltration is seen on biopsy.

E. Medullary carcinoma usually presents as an asymptomatic thyroid nodule. It is found in patients with multiple endocrine neoplasia type IIA and IIB.

590. **B.** The infant mortality rate is obtained by dividing the total number of deaths within the first year of life by the number of live births. There were 13 deaths in the first year of life, and 1000 live births.

591. **E.** Whipple disease is a rare disease caused by *Tropheryma whippelii* and usually affects middle-aged men. Symptoms include abdominal pain, weight loss, diarrhea, malabsorption, and arthritis. The small intestine mucosa is always severely affected. Many antibiotics can be used to cure the condition, including tetracycline, chloramphenicol, ampicillin, penicillin, and trimethoprim-sulfamethoxazole.

A. Celiac disease is caused by gluten intolerance leading to chronic intestinal malabsorption. Symptoms are often secondary to deficiencies. Children fail to thrive and begin to pass pale, malodorous stools once they begin to consume foods containing gluten.

B. Crohn disease consists of transmural inflammation of the distal ileum and colon. This disease would not fit the clinical picture in the question.

C. Intestinal lymphangiectasia is a disorder that affects children and young adults. It is characterized by telangiectasia of the intramucosal lymphatics of the small intestine. Edema, diarrhea, vomiting, and abdominal pain are the usual presenting symptoms.

D. Tropical sprue is a malabsorptive disorder of unknown etiology. Presentation is usually the triad of sore tongue, diarrhea, and weight loss. Steatorrhea is often present along with abnormal D-xylose absorption.

592. **A.** This patient has evidence of chronic hypertension. Chronic hypertension in pregnancy is defined as a blood pressure of greater than 140/90 mm Hg either predating pregnancy or occurring before the 20 weeks' gestation.

B. Chronic hypertension with preeclampsia is defined as preexisting hypertension and a worsening of blood pressure after 20 weeks' gestation.

C. This patient has evidence of chronic hypertension.

D. Preeclampsia (pregnancy-induced hypertension) is a sustained increase in blood pressure after 20 weeks of pregnancy.

E. Transient hypertension (blood pressure >140/90 mm Hg) occurs in the immediate puerperium.

593. **C.** In an elderly patient with left lower quadrant pain one must consider the diagnosis of diverticulitis. In our case, we have a CT scan showing just that. It shows a thick-walled sigmoid colon with pericolic fat inflammation. Although a thickened bowel wall is found in 70% of patients with diverticulitis, 98% of patients will have pericolic fat inflammation. Our CT scan also shows colonic diverticula, which are present in 84% of patients with diverticulitis. This diagnosis is further supported by clinically correlating the CT scan with the history of painless rectal bleeding and abdominal pain out of proportion to physical examination findings.

Figure 593

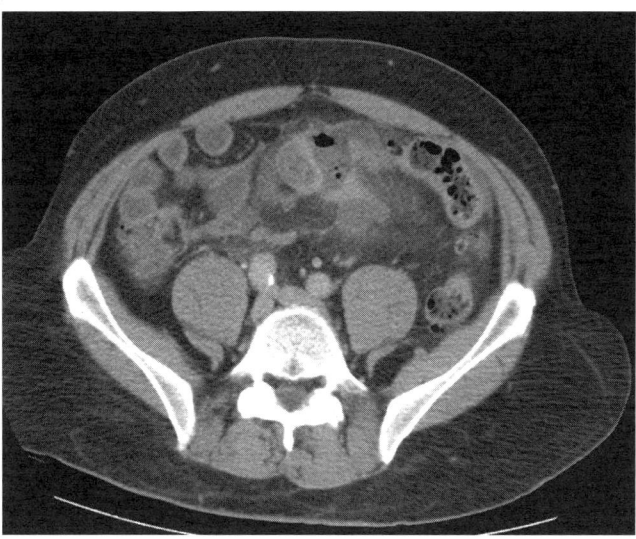

A. Bowel wall thickening on CT scan is present in 70% of patients with diverticulitis.

B. Colonic diverticula on CT scan are present in 84% of patients with diverticulitis.

D. Pericolic fluid collections on CT scan representing abscesses are present in 35% of patients with diverticulitis.

E. Soft tissue masses representing phlegmon (an acute, diffuse, and suppurative inflammation of loose connective tissue) are present on CT scan in 35% of patients.

594. **E.** This patient likely has a simple coryza caused by *Rhinovirus*. The virus can be isolated from nasal and respiratory specimens. Treatment is supportive. Interferon nasal spray, vitamin C, and zinc have been proposed as treatments but have received widespread acceptance among practitioners.

A. Amoxicillin is an antibiotic and unlikely to be of benefit in the treatment of a viral condition.

B. Doxycycline is unlikely to be of benefit in the treatment of simple coryza.

C. Erythromycin will neither treat nor prevent simple coryza.

D. Interferon-alpha nasal spray is a potential treatment of the common cold but is expensive and not widely available.

595. **D.** In a patient taking a neuroleptic antipsychotic, one must be wary about tardive dyskinesia. In this case, giving prochlorperazine, a second neuroleptic, may increase the risk for this serious side effect. Before prescribing any antiemetic, it is important to exclude emergent causes of nausea, such as appendicitis.

A. Cimetidine (Tagamet) is a blocker of stomach acid secretion. There is little or no antiemetic effect.

B. Metoclopramide (Reglan) is a good medication for the treatment of emesis. Few side effects are noted with the use of metoclopramide.

C. Ondansetron (Zofran) is a good antiemetic. However, it is cost prohibitive to use on a routine basis.

E. Trimethobenzamide (Tigan) works well to control nausea. Except for warnings about usage in children, there are few untoward side effects.

596. **E.** Pulmonary function tests (PFTs) would be valuable in this scenario to assess the patient's status for surgery. A patient with poor PFT values may not be able to have surgery because resection of lung tissue may exacerbate his already poor lung function to a level that requires a ventilator.

A. Bone scan would be appropriate for patients who report bony pain, have elevated alkaline phosphatase or calcium, or have abnormal physical examination findings.

B. Chest x-ray is not a suitable imaging test for lung cancer and would offer no benefit to this patient, who has likely already had a CT scan of the chest. Chest x-ray may be performed to evaluate for pleural effusion should there be evidence for that finding.

C. Liver ultrasonography may be appropriate with elevated liver function tests, abnormal findings on CT, asthenia, weight loss, or abnormal physical examination findings.

D. MRI or CT of the brain would be useful if the patient were describing central nervous system symptoms such as nausea, vomiting, headaches, seizures, altered mental status, or abnormal physical examination findings.

597. **C.** This patient has left ventricular heart failure. Dyspnea is a common symptom of congestive heart failure. Dyspnea initially is associated with exertion and then becomes present at rest later in the disease. Fatigue and lethargy are also common symptoms.

A. Asthma is not associated with nocturnal dyspnea, which is exhibited by this patient.

B. Cor pulmonale is associated with right-sided heart failure.

D. Right ventricular failure is associated with hepatic congestion and jugular venous distention, which are not present in this patient.

E. This patient has left ventricular heart failure.

598. **A.** It has been found that 20% to 30% of women develop uterine leiomyomas by 40 years of age. After cesarean section, they account for the most common indication for major surgery in women. However, if asymptomatic, the recommended management for uterine leiomyomas is careful observation of symptoms as well as size and growth of lesion.

B. Patients should not be placed on exogenous estrogen. Although the cause of uterine leiomyomas remains unclear, they are distinctly estrogen dependent. Exogenous estrogen could cause an enlargement of the lesion.

C. GnRH agonists are used in the management of uterine leiomyomas as an adjunct to surgery. Their effects are temporary and they are not appropriate as long-term management of asymptomatic individuals.

D. Because this patient is asymptomatic, hysterectomy is not indicated. Hysterectomy is the appropriate management of uterine leiomyomas when they cause such things as abnormal uterine bleeding resulting in anemia, severe pelvic pain, urinary frequency or retention, or rapid increase in size.

E. Because this patient is asymptomatic, surgical intervention is not indicated. Myomectomy is indicated if surgical intervention is appropriate and if future reproductive capability is desired.

599. **D.** This patient has evidence of subacute sclerosing panencephalitis. It is a slowly evolving inflammatory disease in adolescents appearing after an attack of measles. The electroencephalographic pattern is typical: periodic bursts of high-voltage slow waves followed by a flat pattern.

A. Diffuse flat waves are not characteristic of this condition.

B. High-voltage sharp waves are typical of subacute spongiform encephalopathy.

C. High-voltage slow waves are typical of subacute spongiform encephalopathy.

E. Transient low-voltage sharp waves are not characteristic of this condition.

600. **A.** This patient has folic acid deficiency. Megaloblastic anemia is associated with poor nutrition. Examination of the peripheral smear reveals macrocytic red blood cells. Treatment involves increased intake of fruits and vegetables.

B. Erythropoietin may be useful in the treatment of anemia states.

C. Plasmapheresis is not an appropriate treatment for folate deficiency.

D. Platelet transfusion will not benefit the patient with folate deficiency.

E. This patient has no evidence of deficiency of vitamin D.

601. **D.** This patient has major depression. He has had symptoms for at least 2 weeks and has deficits in the following areas: depressed mood, lack of interest or pleasure in the activities of daily living, weight change, and insomnia. Patients can also have feelings of worthlessness, decreased ability to concentrate, and suicidal ideation.

A. Adjustment disorder is associated with a recent onset and also tends to resolve quickly.

B. Dysthymia is a depressive syndrome where the patient has symptoms all the time but does not meet criteria for major depression.

C. Generalized anxiety disorder is associated with symptoms of anxiety. This patient does not exhibit signs of anxiety.

E. Organic affective disorders are associated with medications and conditions such as thyroid dysfunction. This diagnosis is unlikely because the patient is neither on medications nor has thyroid problems.

602. **D.** The patient presents with recurrence of a Bartholin duct cyst that may have progressed to an abscess given its size, persistence, and her low-grade fever. Incision and drainage is indicated for those cysts that are larger than 2 cm and those that are symptomatic. Antibiotic therapy is only recommended if culture grows *Neisseria gonorrhoeae*.

A. Antibiotic therapy as mentioned above would be recommended before incision and drainage.

B. The patient's history and previous occurrence that resolved makes neoplasm unlikely.

C. Neoplasia not likely given the patient's history; excision would be too aggressive at this time.

E. Warm compresses and sitz baths are not appropriate for larger and recurrent cysts or abscesses.

603. **C.** Before the implementation of antibiotic therapy for endometritis, cultures must be obtained from the likely sources of infection, including the blood, endocervix, uterine cavity, and urine. This allows antibiotic sensitivities to be established for second-line therapy in the event that first-line therapy of ampicillin, gentamicin, and clindamycin is not effective.

A. This patient is suffering from endometritis, a puerperal infection. Although broad-spectrum antibiotics, including ampicillin and gentamicin are effective first-line drugs for mild and moderate cases of endometritis, the most appropriate first step in this patient's treatment is to obtain cultures from possible sources of infection to determine appropriate second-line drugs in the event of failure of first-line drugs.

B. The addition of clindamycin to ampicillin and gentamicin is appropriate to target *Bacteroides fragilis*, a common pelvic pathogen that is resistant to ampicillin and gentamicin. However, this triple therapy is not the appropriate first step, for reasons mentioned above.

D. Helical CT of the chest is useful to establish or rule out the diagnosis of pulmonary emboli. Pulmonary embolism is an unlikely diagnosis with this clinical setting, including a blood oxygen saturation of 97% and respiration rate of 14 breaths/min.

E. Surgical exploration is not indicated in the setting of endometritis.

604. **D.** Tuberous sclerosis is characterized by cutaneous lesions, seizures, and mental retardation. The cutaneous lesions include facial angiofibromas, ash-leaf-shaped hypopigmented macules, shagreen patches (yellowish thickenings over the lumbosacral region), and depigmented nevi. Ninety percent of patients have benign tumors of the brain that can obstruct the foramen and produce hydrocephalus. Treatment is symptomatic, with anticonvulsants for seizures and shunting for hydrocephalus.

A. Central nervous system lymphoma usually occurs in immunocompromised patients, especially AIDS patients. It reveals a ring-shaped mass on MRI and often must be differentiated from toxoplasmosis, which occurs in this population as well.

B. A craniopharyngioma is a tumor that arises from remnants of the Rathke pouch, the mesodermal structure from which the anterior pituitary gland is derived. Such tumors can produce growth failure in children, endocrine abnormalities in adults, or visual loss in either age group. They are usually removed surgically.

C. Neurofibromatosis type 2 is a disease characterized by bilateral acoustic neuromas. Deafness usually begins in the third decade of life. Café au lait spots and peripheral neurofibromas occur more rarely than in neurofibromatosus type 1 (von Recklinghausen disease).

E. von Hippel-Lindau syndrome is characterized by retinal and central nervous system hemangioblastomas, which are slow-growing cystic tumors that may present at any age. Renal cell carcinoma, pheochromocytomas, and pancreatic islet cell neoplasms can also occur.

605. **E.** Patients with Rett disorder have a normal prenatal and perinatal development and normal head circumference at birth. Between the ages of 5 and 48 months, head growth decelerates; between 5 and 30 months, they experience a loss of previously acquired purposeful hand skills and develop stereotyped hand movements such as hand wringing or washing. They also have poorly coordinated gait or trunk movements, loss of social engagement, and severely impaired expressive and receptive language development. This disorder has only been reported in females. The characteristic head growth deceleration is unique to Rett disorder and distinguishes it from the other choices.

A. In contrast to Asperger disorder, Rett disorder is characterized by severe impairment in expressive and receptive language development.

B. Children with autistic disorder do not exhibit loss of hand skills or uncoordinated gait, and the social impairment is much more severe.

C. Although the symptoms of childhood disintegrative disorder are similar to those seen in Rett disorder, the onset is usually after at least 2 years of normal development.

D. There is no evidence to suggest that this patient has mental retardation.

606. **B.** Gross motor skills of the 2-year-old child include the ability to walk up and down stairs without help. Children are able to run well, open and close doors, and climb on furniture. The child is also able to turn pages one at a time, as well as remove his or her shoes and socks. Behavior patterns at this age also include the ability to stack a tower of cubes (up to seven cubes tall) and fold paper into a variety of shapes.

A, C, D, and **E.** This child has the gross motor skills of a 2-year-old.

607. **A.** Bacteremia implies the presence of viable organisms in a blood culture. In this case, gram-negative organisms have been cultured from both the aerobic and anaerobic bottles. The patient is not septic because vital signs are stable. There is no evidence of tachypnea, tachycardia, or hypotension. In this patient, the only clinical evidence of infection is the fever to 102.1°F and the positive blood culture.

608. **D.** This patient has a clinical picture compatible with sepsis syndrome. He has clinical evidence of infection such as tachypnea, tachycardia, and hyperthermia as well as decreased renal function, as evidenced by decreased urine output. This patient has decreased tissue perfusion, as evidenced by an elevated serum lactate level.

609. **A.** AFP is a useful tumor marker to monitor in hepatocellular carcinoma, testicular cancer, teratoembryonal carcinoma, and occasionally in gastric carcinoma. Up to 70% of patients with hepatocellular carcinoma will show elevated AFP levels, but it can also be elevated in chronic hepatitis.

B. hCG is useful in choriocarcinoma and testicular cancer.

C. 5-HIAA is useful in carcinoid syndrome.

D. CA-125 is useful in ovarian cancer.

E. CEA is useful in colon, lung, breast, and pancreatic cancer.

610. **C.** This patient has likely suffered an injury to the obturator nerve. This nerve originates from L2 to L4 and passes posterior to the iliac vessels and lateral to the hypogastric vessels. It can be injured during pelvic surgical procedures such as radical hysterectomy. Resultant injury leads to deficits in adduction of the leg, hip, and medial thigh; loss of power in external and internal rotation; and sensory losses.

A. Injury to this nerve results in sensory deficits in the labia majora.

B. Injury to this plexus would lead to profound deficits in the rectum, vagina, bladder, and uterus.

D. Injury to the sacral plexus would result in profound deficits in perineal sensation.

E. Injury to this nerve results in lower extremity weakness.

611. **B.** The diagnosis of acute closed angle glaucoma is suspected. With this condition, the pupils must not be dilated. The first step involves lowering intraocular pressure with a carbonic anhydrase inhibitor. All of the other parts of the physical examination listed above can be performed.

A, C, D, and **E.** This portion of the physical examination can be performed.

612. **E.** Mitral valve prolapse is commonly idiopathic. Pathophysiology relates to redundant mitral valve tissue with myxedematous degeneration and elongated chordae tendoneae. Asymptomatic patients without regurgitation do not require prophylactic treatment with antibiotics.

A. Amoxicillin is an appropriate prophylactic treatment for dental, respiratory, or esophageal procedures.

B. Clindamycin is an appropriate prophylactic treatment for patients undergoing dental, respiratory, or esophageal procedures who are allergic to penicillin.

C. Cefazolin is an appropriate prophylactic treatment for patients undergoing dental, respiratory, or esophageal procedures who are allergic to penicillin.

D. Vancomycin is an appropriate prophylactic treatment for gastrointestinal or urologic procedures in patients who are penicillin allergic. Amoxicillin and ampicillin are preferred agents.

613. **A.** This patient has evidence of idiopathic pulmonary fibrosis and restrictive lung disease. In restrictive lung disease, pulmonary function testing will indicate alteration in pulmonary functioning. Total lung capacity will decrease, as will residual volume and vital capacity. Detailed work history is important in these patients, who often have occupational exposures to substances such as asbestos, fumes, drugs, or radiation.

B. Forced expiratory volume will decrease in restrictive lung disease.

C. Residual volume will decrease in restrictive lung disease.

D and **E.** Vital capacity will decrease in restrictive lung disease.

614. **C.** The cross-match test is the last major test to be performed before surgery. A positive result is an absolute contraindication to transplantation. This test is performed by mixing recipient serum with donor cells. This test has helped to reduce the incidence of hyperacute rejection in the operating room.

A. ABO group matching is another essential element to finding an appropriate recipient for a donor organ.

B. In cadaveric transplantation, HLA typing is used more for allocation purposes and is not a contraindication to surgery.

D. Studies indicate that graft survival is highly correlated with HLA matching, but it is not a contraindication for surgery.

E. HLA typing is not a contraindication for surgery.

615. **E.** The height of the fundus can be used to estimate gestational age. When the fundus is palpable at the ensiform cartilage, the gestational age approximates term (36 weeks). There can be deviations from the expected growth rate and, thus, fundal height can be used along with traditional methods to determine the estimated date of confinement.

A. The fundus is still in the pelvis at 8 weeks' gestation.

B. The fundal height at 12 weeks is just above the pubic symphysis.

C. The fundal height at 16 weeks is about half the abdomen.

D. The fundal height at 20 weeks is at the level of the umbilicus.

616. **A.** Before deciding whether to correct Na balance, one must determine the corrected Na. To calculate the corrected Na, you add 1.6 mEq for each 100 mg/dL increase in glucose. This comes to $(4 \times 1.6 = 6.4)$ $6.4 + 132 =$ a corrected Na of 138.4. This value is normal and requires only observation.

B. Salt administration would alter the child's Na balance and may make him hypernatremic.

C. Salt restriction would alter the child's Na balance and make him hyponatremic.

D. Water administration would alter the child's Na balance and make him hyponatremic.

E. Water restriction would alter the child's Na balance and make him hypernatremic.

617. **D.** This patient may have malaria. Giemsa-stained thick and thin peripheral blood smears are the standard diagnostic tool for malaria and should be done quickly due to the life-threatening potential of the disease. Plasmodia in erythrocytes will be seen on the smear. Several smears should be performed over the first 36 hours after presentation if the initial smear is negative. The disease is acquired by being bit by *Anopheles* mosquitoes infected with one of several species of *Plasmodium*.

A. A chest x-ray would be appropriate if respiratory symptoms persist.

B. A CT may be helpful if central nervous system symptoms persist after the patient is stabilized but is not the first test to be ordered.

C. ELISA is not appropriate in the diagnosis of malaria.

E. Chloroquine is the proper treatment as long as the patient was not in an area where chloroquine resistance is common. In that case, mefloquine would be the treatment of choice.

618. **E.** This patient takes multiple medications that can be causing hallucinations. The most common cause of hallucinations in elderly patients is propranolol. Visual or auditory hallucinations are possible with this medication. Hallucinations may respond to antipsychotic medications.

A–D. Cimetidine, digoxin, hydrochlorothiazide, and ibuprofen are not associated with visual or auditory hallucinations.

619. **D.** All of the diagnoses listed are part of the differential for an ovarian mass; however, in a postmenopausal woman, the presence of an abdominal mass should be considered malignant until proven otherwise. Many features of this patient led to the diagnosis of malignancy. First, she is in the age group where the highest incidence of malignancy is found. Thirty percent to 60% of ovarian masses in this age group are malignant. Second, the presented history of weight loss, physical examination findings of cachexia and muscle wasting, and subsequent ultrasound findings are highly suggestive of malignancy. Also, the low prealbumin level, which is an indicator of malnutrition, lends to the diagnosis of malignancy. Third, the presence of a right-sided adnexal mass and an elevated CA-125 level suggests ovarian carcinoma as the etiology of the mass. CA-125 levels, while not specific for ovarian tumors, are often elevated in patients with this disease. Typically, the CA-125 level is measured to follow the course of the disease and response to treatments, much like prostate-specific antigen is followed in prostate cancer. Lastly, the pelvic ultrasound shows the most common findings with ovarian carcinoma, including a unilateral, complex (meaning both cystic and solid components) adnexal mass. To confirm the diagnosis, an exploratory laparotomy should be performed first. Upon confirmation, the patient should subsequently undergo tumor debulking, including a total abdominal hysterectomy and bilateral salpingo-oophorectomy.

Figure 619

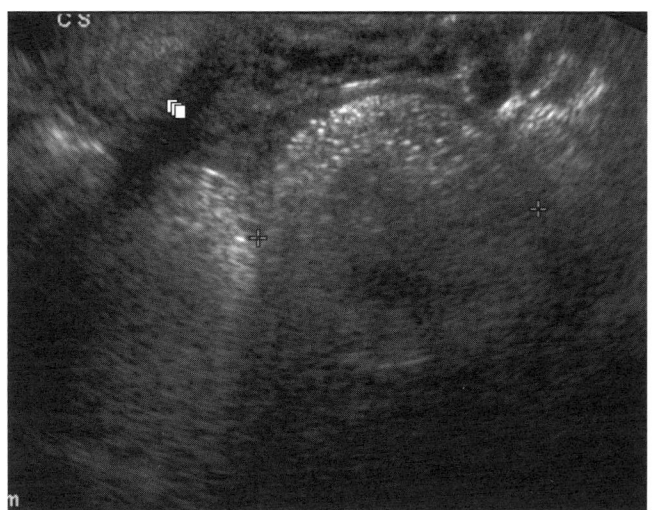

A. Although a hysterectomy and oophorectomy is the definitive treatment of a malignancy, confirmation of the diagnosis via an exploratory laparotomy should be performed first.

B and **E.** Serial ultrasonography and determination of CA-125 levels are the mainstay for postmenopausal women that have a simple unilateral cyst on ultrasonography that is less than 3 cm in diameter. The ultrasonographic appearance of a simple cyst is an anechoic fluid-filled cyst cavity and thin walls.

C. The ill nature of this patient demands for immediate action. A confirmatory diagnosis must be made, and serial pelvic examinations do not play a role in this process.

620. **C.** This patient likely has sarcoidosis. The combination of hilar and paratracheal adenopathy as well as parenchymal lung disease further suggest sarcoidosis. Other associations may include weight loss, fatigue, polyarthritis, uveitis, bony cysts, arrhythmias, erythema nodosum, splenomegaly, cholestasis, and hypercalcemia. The etiology is unknown. Noncaseating epithelioid granulomas are pathognomonic for the disease. Half of all cases are found incidentally on chest x-ray. The disease is most common in African Americans, Puerto Ricans, and West Indians. Women are more commonly affected than men.

A. Asbestosis is an interstitial lung disease for which this patient does not have a history of any exposure. In addition, it is usually discovered in a patient's lower lung lobes.

B. Blastomycosis is a fungal infection acquired by inhalation of spores from the soils of the Mississippi river and its tributaries. Patients show a mild symptomatic respiratory illness, a pneumonia with infiltrates on x-ray and possibly granulomas with calcifications, or a systemic infection in immunocompromised hosts. Diagnosis is made by placing intradermal antigenic preparations (similar to PPD) and noting a delayed type hypersensitivity reaction. Treatment is performed aggressively with itraconazole or amphotericin B.

D. This patient lacks a history of exposure that would make silicosis probable. However, silicosis does commonly involve the upper lung zones.

E. Tuberculosis is unlikely. The patient's history states that she has had a recent negative PPD test result.

621. **C.** This patient has a retropharyngeal abscess (RPA). An emergent otolaryngology consult is necessary for the abscess to be drained. This is considered to be a surgical emergency. Airway compromise is possible.

A. A cricothyrotomy is only performed in patients with signs of upper airway obstruction who cannot be intubated.

B. It is difficult to intubate when the upper airway is distorted. Prophylactic intubation is not required unless an interhospital transfer is planned.

D. The safety of the procedure is unclear, and this procedure does not have a role in the diagnosis or treatment of an RPA.

E. Tracheostomy is a last resort in definitive airway management in patients with RPA and respiratory distress.

622. **A.** This patient has evidence of basilar artery syndrome. This is a combination of brainstem syndromes characterized by paralysis or weakness of all extremities, diplopia, paralysis of conjugate and lateral gaze, blindness, coma, and sensory loss.

B. Unilateral medullary syndrome typically does not produce bilateral deficits.

C. Infarction of the cerebellar peduncle will result in cerebellar ataxia, which has not been demonstrated in this patient.

D. Infarction of the medial lemniscus is characterized by syringomyelic sensory loss.

E. Unilateral pontine syndrome does not explain the bilateral deficits seen in this patient.

623. **C.** Treatment of ALL consists of induction chemotherapy, consolidation, and maintenance chemotherapy. Induction typically lasts 4 weeks, during which time maximum log kill is achieved. Consolidation involves a one-time dose of intrathecal methotrexate, which prevents leukemic relapse within the central nervous system. Maintenance therapy follows and normally lasts 2 years.

A. Bone marrow transplantation is considered if chemotherapy fails to produce remission, or if the patient relapses.

B. The consolidation phase is performed prior to the maintenance phase.

D. Intravenous antibiotics are given if the patient becomes febrile or has other signs of infection.

E. ALL must be treated with antileukemic therapy for the patient to be cured.

624. **D.** Minute ventilation increases because of increased tidal volume with the same or slightly increased respiratory rate.

A. Blood pressure decreases, especially in the second trimester.

B. Creatinine decreases as glomerular filtration rate increases.

C. Free thyroxine remains normal.

E. There is actually a respiratory alkalosis secondary to hyperventilation in pregnancy.

625. **C.** This patient has Ewing sarcoma. This condition most commonly affects the femur and is associated with pain, fever, and tenderness with a massive soft tissue component. The treatment of choice is chemotherapy and radiation. Radiation therapy is high dose and may have side effects of poor bone growth, fibrosis, or secondary osteosarcoma.

A. Intravenous antibiotics are useful in the treatment of osteomyelitis, which is part of the differential diagnosis of this condition.

B. Oral antibiotics may actually improve symptoms associated with Ewing sarcoma, but only transiently.

D. Surgical excision is not an appropriate treatment for Ewing sarcoma.

E. Surgical resection and pelvic reconstruction is not appropriate for these patients, especially due to the high rate of relapse and metastasis.

626. **D.** This patient has had the hepatitis B vaccination in the past. This is recognized by the presence of HBsAb in the absence of other markers. The hepatitis B vaccine is made of surface antigen particles so patients produce antibodies toward the surface antigen but are seronegative for surface antigen.

A. In acute hepatitis B infection, HBsAg is detectable. In 90% of patients this antigen will be cleared by the production of HBsAb. The following 10% are chronic carriers and are at risk for developing chronic active hepatitis. HBcAb becomes positive later in the acute phase. HBcAb does not mean recovery from hepatitis B infection.

B. In chronic hepatitis B, patients fail to clear HBsAg after production of HBsAb. This occurs in about 10% of patients.

C. HDAg is negative. Patients should be tested for hepatitis D in the presence of hepatitis B.

E. If the patient had hepatitis B but is now recovered, he would be positive for HBsAb and HBcAb.

627. **A.** Patients with Asperger disorder show sustained impairment in social interactions, and repetitive patterns of behavior and activities. There is no delay in language development.

B. There is delay in language development with autistic disorder.

C. Pervasive developmental disorder requires a profound delay in communication skills.

D. There is no delay in communication skills as would be seen with schizoid personality disorder.

E. Tourette disorder is characterized by outbursts of language.

628. **C.** This patient has an auricular hematoma. These injuries are common in high school and college wrestlers or football players. The injury occurs when an opponent's forearm rakes the patient's ear and disrupts the perichondrium. Hematoma forms between the perichondrium and the cartilage. Needle aspiration and application of a pressure dressing is the initial treatment to maintain blood supply to the perichondrium and prevent cartilage necrosis.

A. Intravenous antibiotics are not the treatment of choice for auricular hematoma because there is no indication for underlying infection.

B. Intravenous corticosteroids are not the treatment of choice for auricular hematoma.

D. Although pressure dressing is important in the treatment of auricular hematoma, this should be performed following needle aspiration of the hematoma.

E. Suturing a red Robinson catheter to the helix of the affected ear may promote drainage, but there may be an increased risk for subsequent infection.

629. **D.** This patient has pyloric stenosis, and ultrasonography of the pylorus will confirm your diagnosis. Another good diagnostic tool is an upper gastrointestinal series.

A. Plain films will not show the pylorus.

B. Colonoscopy is incorrect because it will not give any information on the upper digestive tract.

C. CT scan is not as sensitive for measuring the diameter of the pylorus as ultrasonography is.

E. Upper gastrointestinal endoscopy is an unnecessary invasive test.

630. **A.** Atrial septal defect is a high-flow, low-pressure, left-to-right shunt. There is intraatrial communication through which blood flows down the path of least resistance. Physical examination may reveal a pulmonic ejection murmur at the left sternal border with fixed, wide splitting of the second heart sound. A soft midsystolic rumble over the tricuspid valve may also be noted. Older children may present with ostium segundum defects and are often asymptomatic with mild exercise tolerance.

631. **B.** This individual has symptoms of coarctation of the aorta. Congestive heart failure, cyanosis, poor feeding, and failure to thrive are common presentations. Examination of blood pressure in all four extremities will reveal decreased blood pressure distal to the coarctation. Associated findings may include a systolic ejection murmur that radiates to the back and faint femoral pulses.

632. **A.** The axillary nodes drain 97% of the breast on the ipsilateral side. They also drain the ipsilateral supraclavicular and jugular nodes. The axillary nodes are classified into three levels. Level I nodes are lateral to the pectoralis minor muscle, level II nodes are deep to the pectoralis minor, and level III nodes are medial to the pectoralis minor.

B. The interpectoral nodes (Rotter nodes) are between the pectoralis major and pectoralis minor. They provide lymphatic drainage for the ipsilateral breast.

C. The internal mammary glands drain 3% of the ipsilateral breast. They mainly drain the upper and lower inner quadrants.

D. The axillary nodes drain the supraclavicular nodes.

E. The thoracic nodes drain the internal chest wall.

633. **C.** The patient is showing characteristic symptoms of schizophrenia: auditory hallucinations, delusions, poor school performance and emotional expression, disorganized speech, and symptoms lasting greater than 6 months. The most appropriate treatment is the antipsychotic haloperidol.

A. Clozapine could be used, but should generally be reserved as a second-line treatment because of the accompanying risk for agranulocytosis.

B. Diazepam would merely sedate the patient without treating his symptoms.

D. Psychotherapy is not generally as effective as pharmacotherapy in schizophrenia.

E. Reassurance is not appropriate for schizophrenia; more acute treatment is recommended.

634. **B.** This patient presents with noncardiac chest pain. The most common cause is gastroesophageal reflux, but it has been ruled out with normal endoscopy and biopsy. The second most common cause is esophageal spasm; thus, a motility test is indicated.

A. CT would not help to show esophageal spasm.

C. MRI would not help to show esophageal spasm.

D. pH probe is not indicated because reflux has been ruled out with normal endoscopy.

E. Upper gastrointestinal series will not add any more useful information that would be different from the endoscopy that was already performed.

635. **D.** This patient has an irreducible inguinal hernia. You can try to reduce the hernia in the office and schedule a hernia repair electively. If the hernia cannot be reduced in the office, surgery will need to be scheduled as soon as possible.

A. One should attempt to reduce the hernia first and save the patient from an emergent surgery.

B, C, and **E.** This is an emergency and the herniated intestine can strangulate if the hernia is not reduced in a timely fashion.

636. **A.** This patient had clubfoot. This is a disorder of the foot characterized by metatarsal adduction, malrotation of the calcaneus under the talus, and plantar flexion of the ankle. Cast correction is effective in approximately 33% and is a reasonable first-line approach. However, this patient may require surgical release of all bony alignments and tendon contractures.

B. Exercises to improve foot flexion may be appropriate in the treatment of flatfoot.

C. Orthotic shoes may help in the management of flatfoot.

D. Complete release of all bony attachments and tendon contractures may be required in the management of clubfoot. However, amputation is rarely required.

E. Watchful waiting would be associated with a progression of symptoms and is not an appropriate option for this patient.

637. **D.** This patient has hypertension and is pregnant. Her hypertension is stable; therefore, her antihypertensive medication should be discontinued. She should be followed at regular intervals for blood pressure checks. Therapy should be reinstituted if the diastolic pressure is greater than 100 mm Hg in the second trimester.

A. It is appropriate to stop antihypertensive therapy at this time.

B. Methyldopa should not be instituted in this patient at this time.

C. This patient is normotensive and can have the antihypertensive medication stopped at this time.

E. This patient is normotensive, and it is appropriate to stop amiloramide.

638. **B.** Biopsy is mandatory in this situation and will most likely show distinctive pagetoid cells. This description is classic for Paget disease of the breast (unrelated to Paget disease of the bone). It is a primary ductal carcinoma that secondarily invades the epithelium of the nipple and areola, although it has also been associated with lobular carcinomas. Treatment is dependent on the extent of the underlying tumor. Mastectomy is usually indicated because of the rich network of lymphatics underneath the nipple-areola area.

A. This reaction is unlikely to be caused by an allergy because it appears to be localized to just one part of the body.

C. This lesion may represent carcinoma and should be promptly evaluated and undergo biopsy.

D. This lesion should be examined via biopsy.

E. Local treatment is not very helpful and only delays definitive treatment.

639. **E.** The concentration of glycosylated hemoglobin reflects glucose concentration during the half-life of the RBC. The average life span of an RBC is 120 days. Thus, the half-life is 60 days and reflects the hemoglobin A1C level.

640. **C.** In assessing the patient's risk for violence, several factors should be ascertained. Demographic information is important. For example, male patients, those between age 15 and 25, lower socioeconomic status, and limited social supports place patients at risk for violent behavior. Past history is important, and the physician should determine some of the following information: past history of violence, impulse discontrol, gambling, substance abuse, and prior suicide attempts.

A. Typical age of the suicide victim is age 15 to 25.

B. Suicide victims often have poor impulse control.

D. There is no specific correlation between anorexia nervosa and increased suicide risk.

E. Lower socioeconomic status may correlate with suicide risk.

641. **C.** Pulmonary embolism (PE) is an acute, life-threatening event that demands immediate treatment. This is especially true in our patient, who survived the first PE because most of these patients will die during the treatment period from a second PE. We see the classic ECG changes associated with PE in our patient's reading. There is a large S wave in I, ST depression in II, and large Q waves in III. Some ECGs, including this one, will also show T wave inversion in V_1–V_4. The treatment of PE starts with anticoagulation with intravenous heparin.

Figure 641

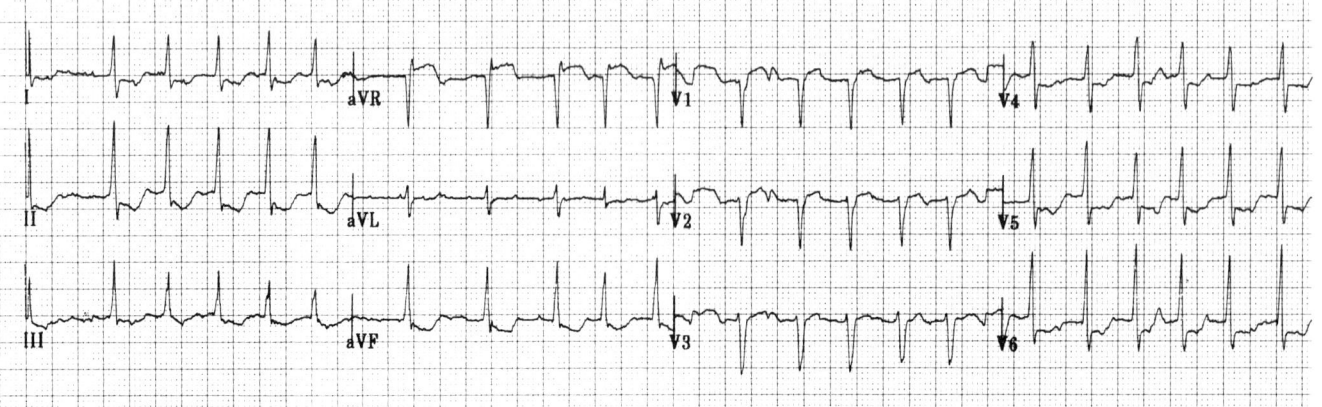

A. Aspirin is not indicated for anticoagulation in cases of acute pulmonary embolism.

B. Celecoxib is not indicated for anticoagulation in cases of acute pulmonary embolism.

D. If the patient has some contraindication to anticoagulation, then an inferior vena caval filter should be inserted.

E. Intravenous heparin must be started first because of its immediate anticoagulation effect. This anticoagulant state will be maintained with oral warfarin. Warfarin should be overlapped with heparin for 4 to 5 days or the amount of time it takes to maintain an international normalization rate (INR) of 2.0 to 3.0 (therapeutic INR). It is possible to start the two drugs together, but some clinicians prolong the initial heparin-only phase in cases of massive PE.

642. **D.** A post-term pregnancy is one that persists beyond 42 weeks (294 days) from the onset of a menstrual period. The incidence of postterm pregnancy is approximately 5% to 10%. If this woman would have had prenatal care, a more accurate determination of her due date could have been made.

643. **C.** This patient is in unstable condition with hypotension probably secondary to hemorrhagic shock. Fluid resuscitation with intravenous fluids is necessary. Two large-bore intravenous lines should be started as soon as possible.

A, B, D, and **E.** First the patient needs to be stabilized before diagnostic examinations are ordered to find the cause of hypotension.

644. **A.** This patient likely has multiinfarct dementia. Neurologic signs are usually present. Treatment is to identify and reverse the cause of the strokes. Hypertension, diabetes, and cardiac disease must be treated.

B. Antidepressants can be used in these patients, but some can develop side effects from the medication.

C. Prednisone has no role in the treatment of multiinfarct dementia.

D. Thiamine has no role in the treatment of multiinfarct dementia.

E. Tolterodine is an anticholinergic agent used in the management of urge urinary incontinence.

645. **C.** This patient has evidence of infection by *Enterobius vermicularis* (pinworm). The diagnosis is made by identifying eggs on microscopic examination of adhesive tape applied to the perineal skin. Treatment is with mebendazole. All members of the household should be treated. Repeat treatment in 2 to 3 weeks may be necessary to prevent recurrence.

A. Amoxicillin will not treat pinworm infections.

B. Erythromycin will not effectively treat nematode infections.

D. Mebendazole, not metronidazole, is the most appropriate treatment for pinworm infections.

E. Trimethoprim is an inappropriate choice for nematode infections.

646. **D.** Although the patient has multiple risk factors for a physiologic cause for his impotence, the laboratory values are all within normal limits and the NPT test showed that he is able to obtain an erection. So since his NPT result was normal, this indicates a high likelihood of emotional and psychological causes for the impotence.

A, B, C, and **E.** These are used in those patients with true erectile dysfunction as a result of a physiologic abnormality.

647. **A.** This woman has clinical features of interstitial cystitis and has microhematuria. The microhematuria needs to be further evaluated with studies of the upper and lower urinary tract. The upper tract can be evaluated with ultrasonography, CT scan, or intravenous pyelography. The lower tract can best be evaluated with diagnostic cystoscopy.

B. There is no indication to perform diagnostic laparoscopy in this patient.

C. Hysteroscopy is not indicated in this patient. She has no history of vaginal bleeding.

D. MRI is not indicated in this patient. A better study would be ultrasonography or CT scan.

E. Transvaginal ultrasonography is unlikely to add any additional information useful for the management of this patient.

648. **C.** This patient has hypertension. The goal of antihypertensive treatment is to reduce blood pressure to below 140/90 mm Hg in patients under the age of 60 years. This patient will need pharmacologic and nonpharmacologic therapies, including weight reduction, reduction of smoking and alcohol use, and exercise.

A, B, D, and **E.** The goal of blood pressure reduction in this patient should be below 140/90 mm Hg.

649. **D.** This patient needs to undergo surgical placement of an external fixator. When any patient presents in a trauma situation, the airway, breathing, and circulation (ABC's) must always take priority. Chest, spine, and pelvic films will help establish further points of treatment. This patient is unstable and displaying signs of shock, and operative stabilization is the treatment of choice for pelvic hematoma. As a general rule the patient must always be stabilized with fluids and, if necessary, blood, before any surgical procedure.

A. This patient has an unstable pelvic hematoma and is hemodynamically unstable. Waiting is not an option.

B. This patient is unstable and requires immediate surgical intervention.

C. When a pelvic hematoma is found and the patient is stable, drainage is not recommended due to the complexity of the pelvic anatomy. It is thought only more harm is done.

E. The bleeding source is not in the gastrointestinal tract. Endoscopy is not necessary in this patient.

650. **D.** The criteria for pica include: persistent eating of non-nutritive substances for at least 1 month, the eating is inappropriate to developmental level, the behavior is not part of a culturally sanctioned practice, and if the eating behavior occurs during the course of another mental disorder (e.g., mental retardation), it is sufficiently severe to warrant independent clinical attention.

A. There is no evidence of binge eating or methods to control weight gain that would characterize bulimia.

B. There is no evidence to suggest enuresis.

C. There is no evidence to suggest a feeding disorder of childhood.

E. Rumination disorder is the repeated regurgitation and rechewing of food after eating.

651. **D.** Even with appropriate antibiotic therapy, the mortality rate for bacterial meningitis approaches 10% for *Haemophilus influenzae*. Poor prognosis is associated with several factors, including young age and long duration of illness prior to effective antibiotic therapy. Thus, good prognostic indicators include a child of older age and one who is placed on appropriate antibiotics early in the course of disease. Relapse may occur 3 to 14 days after treatment and is usually due to the same pathogen.

A. A high number of organisms and quality of antigen in the cerebrospinal fluid (CSF) implies a poor prognosis for this condition.

B. Patients with AIDS have a poor prognosis when afflicted with bacterial meningitis.

C. Late-onset seizures imply neurologic compromise and is a poor prognostic indicator.

E. The presence of gram-negative enteric bacteria or the presence of pneumococci in the CSF implies a poor prognosis in this condition.

652. **E.** This patient has physiologic discharge. If the patient is asymptomatic, only microscopy should be performed. Vaginal cultures are not recommended in this patient. Treatment should be supportive and requires observation.

A. This patient has no evidence of a bacterial vaginosis.

B and **C.** This patient has no evidence of a vaginal fungal infection.

D. This patient has no evidence of a bacterial infection or a sexually transmitted disease by either history or physical examination.

653. **C.** This patient has reported a case of colorectal cancer in an immediate family member. Therefore, cancer screening of the colon should begin before the typical age of 50. Generally it is recommended for patients to be screened 10 years prior to the age of onset of the family member's cancer. In this case it would be age 45.

654. **D.** The patient is experiencing carcinoid syndrome, which is the result of a carcinoid tumor secreting excess serotonin into the blood stream. Serotonin is then metabolized to 5-HIAA, creating elevated plasma and urinary levels of the compound. Midgut carcinoid tumors are more prone to produce carcinoid syndrome than other areas of the gastrointestinal tract. Diagnosis can be made by showing elevated 5-HIAA in the urine.

A. The erythrocyte sedimentation rate is a nonspecific test the results of which are commonly elevated in anemia or inflammatory states.

B. HLA-B27 testing is a genetic test that is positive in many patients with various diseases including Reiter syndrome and ankylosing spondylitis.

C. SPEP/UPEP are assays commonly used in multiple myeloma to assess for monoclonal gammopathy and Bence Jones proteinuria. Patients with this disease have back pain, bone fractures, hypercalcemia, and frequent infections due to a plasmacytosis of the bone marrow. Bone marrow biopsy confirms the diagnosis.

E. Pheochromocytomas are tumors of chromaffin cells and are involved in the excess production of catecholamines. These commonly take place in but are not confined to the adrenal medulla. Most patients experience hypertension with episodes of headache, profuse sweating, palpitations, apprehension, and feelings of impending doom. Diagnosis revolves around obtaining 24-hour values for urine VMA, metanephrines, or catecholamines.

655. **B.** A more accurate history may be obtained with the parents not present. Thus, asking her about drug use without first asking the parents to leave the room would not be appropriate.

A. The patient should not be admitted to the psychiatric ward unless it is established that she has a substance abuse disorder for which she requires medical attention.

C. This question is not appropriate at this time.

D. Mentioning the results of the urine test in front of her parents would violate the patient's confidentiality.

E. A physical examination would not be warranted at this time.

656. **C.** Coumadin is a medication used as an anticoagulant for patients with deep venous thrombosis. This agent is a potential teratogen and is associated with nasal hypoplasia, stippled epiphyses, growth retardation, and mental retardation. Fetal bleeding is also possible.

A. Clear cell carcinoma of the vagina is associated with maternal use of diethylstilbestrol.

B. Congenital heart disease can be associated with maternal use of anticonvulsants during pregnancy.

D. Neonatal jaundice is associated with maternal use of sulfonamides during pregnancy.

E. Staining of the newborn's teeth is associated with maternal use of tetracycline during pregnancy.

657. **A.** The goal of treatment is to restore a connection between the femoral head and the acetabulum. Treatment varies with the patient's age and degree of instability. The brace is worn until the clinical and radiologic examination findings are normal. Children over 6 months of age are too old to wear a brace.

B. Closed reduction should be attempted only in children over 6 months of age, for whom the brace is too big.

C. Most unstable hips in neonates spontaneously resolve in the first 2 to 4 weeks after birth. Observation and reexamination is recommended in neonates 3 to 4 weeks of age.

D. Closed reduction should be attempted first; open reduction should be attempted only when closed reduction is unsuccessful.

E. Open reduction with pelvic osteotomy should only be undertaken if the diagnosis is made after the deformity has occurred, which is usually in children over 2 years of age.

658. **D.** Pancreatic cancer has been associated with depression, impaired glucose tolerance, and migratory thrombophlebitis, which is the probable cause of the leg pain described by the patient. Diarrhea is also common due to maldigestion. Cancer of the head of the pancreas can cause jaundice from biliary obstruction. The Courvoisier law suggests that a palpable gallbladder signifies obstruction by a neoplasm. Weight loss is a late finding, which is suggested by the patient's lack of appetite.

A. Acute cholecystitis usually occurs following a fatty meal and produces right upper quadrant pain, nausea/vomiting, and fever. A palpable gallbladder and jaundice may be present.

B. Choledocholithiasis is the most common cause of obstructive jaundice and should be considered in this patient. Right upper quadrant pain is more suggestive of this disorder, but epigastric pain may occur as well. Migratory thrombophlebitis, glucose intolerance, palpable gallbladder, and diarrhea point more toward pancreatic cancer.

C. Hepatocellular carcinoma would more likely show hepatomegaly, ascites, cachexia, and weakness.

E. A peptic ulcer may create epigastric pain after eating but would not create the other symptoms mentioned above.

659. **E.** Pyloric stenosis is the most common congenital obstruction of the stomach and intestines. The clinical symptom of projectile vomiting in the second week of life is caused by hyperplasia of the gastric antrum. The midgastric "olive" may be palpable on physical examination. Diagnosis is confirmed via ultrasonography, which reveals a dilated gastric bulb and hypertrophy of the antrum.

A. The physical examination findings do not suggest abscess formation. There is no evidence of peritoneal signs on physical examination. The infant is afebrile.

B. Chalasia describes gastroesophageal reflux across a dilated lower esophageal sphincter, made worse with Valsalva maneuvers.

C. Esophagitis may result from gastroesophageal reflux, as a result of infection or extension of a retropharyngeal abscess.

D. Children may swallow a number of small objects that become lodged in the esophagus. Symptoms include dyspnea, drooling, dysphagia, and coughing.

660. **B.** This patient has evidence of dysfunctional uterine bleeding by history. Physical examination findings are unremarkable. Endometrial biopsy reveals glandular hypertrophy and an increase in stromal ground substance. This is a typical finding in the late proliferative phase of the menstrual cycle.

A. This phase is noted for tubular glands that are straight and narrow.

C. The biopsy provides no evidence of neoplastic gland formation.

D. There is no sonographic evidence of a pelvic mass with clusters of cysts other than the small ovarian cyst.

E. The biopsy provides no evidence of neoplastic gland formation.

661. **B.** Increasing age increases the risk for suicide. Religion also can affect the risk for committing suicide. More strict feelings against suicide, as in Catholicism, can decrease a person's risk. The more education a person receives, the higher their risk for committing suicide. The majority of people who have committed suicide have a mental illness, mainly mood disorders and alcoholism. Having a terminal disease increases the risk for committing suicide.

662. **B.** In this patient, a constellation of typical symptoms involving sore throat, fatigue, lymphadenopathy, and fever in a college-age student provide the clinician with a rather interesting differential diagnosis: reactive lymphadenopathy, leukemia, lymphoma, infectious mononucleosis (Epstein-Barr virus), and thyroid disorders can all present with these symptoms. A CBC with a differential count in this case will lead the clinician to suspect bacterial causes if leukocytes predominate or viral causes if lymphocytes predominate.

A. Abdominal CT is not likely to add any useful information to the differential diagnosis of this patient.

C. Lymph node biopsy will help the clinician to ascertain the possibility of leukemia versus lymphoma versus reactive lymphadenopathy. However, this should be done following a complete laboratory analysis and possibly a course of antibiotics.

D. MRI of the abdomen is not likely to reveal any useful information to assist with the diagnosis of this patient.

E. Abdominal ultrasonography is not likely to add any further useful information to the differential diagnosis of this patient.

663. **B.** This patient should have a fine-needle aspiration biopsy. This is warranted even though mammography did not visualize the 2-cm mass. It is important to understand that mammography misses 10% of masses that are noticed on physical examination.

A. CA-125 is not used to screen for breast cancer.

C. One must rule out carcinoma and should not wait for the mass to change size.

D. Repeating mammography in 6 months is not of value because any mass found during examination needs to be worked up now to rule out carcinoma.

E. Tamoxifen is indicated for treatment of patients with breast cancer. At this point, no diagnosis of cancer has yet been made.

664. **C.** Chronic lymphocytic leukemia (CLL) is most common in men over the age of 60 years. It is often diagnosed with incidental blood tests or assessment of generalized lymphadenopathy. Symptomatic patients complain of fatigue, weight loss, loss of appetite, and abdominal fullness due to hepatosplenomegaly. Sustained lymphocytosis and greater than 30% lymphocytes in the bone marrow are characteristic of CLL. Anemia is common due to abnormal hematopoiesis. Median survival length is about 10 years. Chemotherapy, corticosteroids, and radiotherapy are all used in the treatment of CLL.

A. Acute lymphoblastic leukemia (ALL) is the most common malignancy in children. It has a smaller second peak in adulthood. Remission occurs in greater than 95% of children and greater than 70% of adults. Treatment involves vincristine, etoposide, cyclophosphamide, and/or methotrexate. Radiotherapy may be used in patients at high risk for central nervous system involvement.

Table 661					
	INCREASING AGE	BEING CATHOLIC	HIGHER EDUCATION	HAVING A MENTAL ILLNESS	HAVING A TERMINAL ILLNESS
A.	Increased risk	Increased risk	Increased risk	Increased risk	Increased risk
B.	Increased risk	Decreased risk	Increased risk	Increased risk	Increased risk
C.	Increased risk	Decreased risk	Decreased risk	Increased risk	Increased risk
D.	Decreased risk	Decreased risk	Increased risk	Increased risk	Increased risk
E.	Increased risk	Decreased risk	Increased risk	Increased risk	Decreased risk

B. Acute myelogenous leukemia (AML) incidence increases with age. AML responds to fewer drugs than ALL, and the goal of initial treatment is to induce remission. Remission rates are 50% to 85%, with a lower chance of remission in patients over 50 years of age.

D. Malignant transformation of pluripotent stem cells leads to chronic myelogenous leukemia (CML). It is characterized by increased production of granulocytes, especially in the bone marrow. The diagnosis of CML is similar to that of CLL and is often found during an incidental CBC. The Philadelphia chromosome is present in nearly all patients which a reciprocal translocation between chromosomes 9 and 22. Treatment usually consists of palliation and not cure.

E. Myelodysplastic syndrome is usually seen in patients over 50 years of age. Ineffective myelopoiesis occurs due to hypercellular bone marrow. Clonal proliferation of hematopoietic cells is characteristic of this disease. The patient often presents with nonspecific symptoms.

665. **B.** Odds ratio is determined by the ratio of people who are smokers with lung cancer multiplied by the number of people without lung cancer who are nonsmokers. This number is divided by the number of people who are nonsmokers with lung cancer multiplied by the number of smokers without lung cancer. Thus, (45)(90)/(5)(60) = 13.5. The risk for lung cancer is 13.5 times higher in people who smoke that in those who do not smoke.

666. **A.** Although angiotensin-converting enzyme (ACE) inhibitors are contraindicated in bilateral renal artery stenosis, this patient presents with unilateral renal artery stenosis resulting from fibromuscular dysplasia. This condition causes secondary systemic hypertension. The affected kidney becomes ischemic due to the hyperplasia and fibrotic thickening in the renal artery. Renin is secreted from the ischemic kidney, causing elevated plasma renin. Surgically correcting the condition is possible with stenting and balloon angioplasty.

B. ACE inhibitors are the preferred treatment for this patient.

C. Simvastatin is not appropriate treatment for this patient.

D. Diet and exercise will not improve the pathophysiology in fibromuscular dysplasia.

E. This patient should be treated to decrease her blood pressure to appropriate levels.

667. **E.** Spironolactone, a potassium-sparing diuretic, inhibits the aldosterone receptor in the collecting tubule cells of the nephron. This reduces the expression of Na^+/K^+ ATPase in these cells. As a result, K is not moved into the cells where it subsequently would move down its concentration gradient flowing into the urine. Instead, this ion remains in the interstitium/blood, and at toxic levels, hyperkalemia results. The ECG reflects this electrolyte imbalance with peaked T waves in the majority of leads.

Figure 667

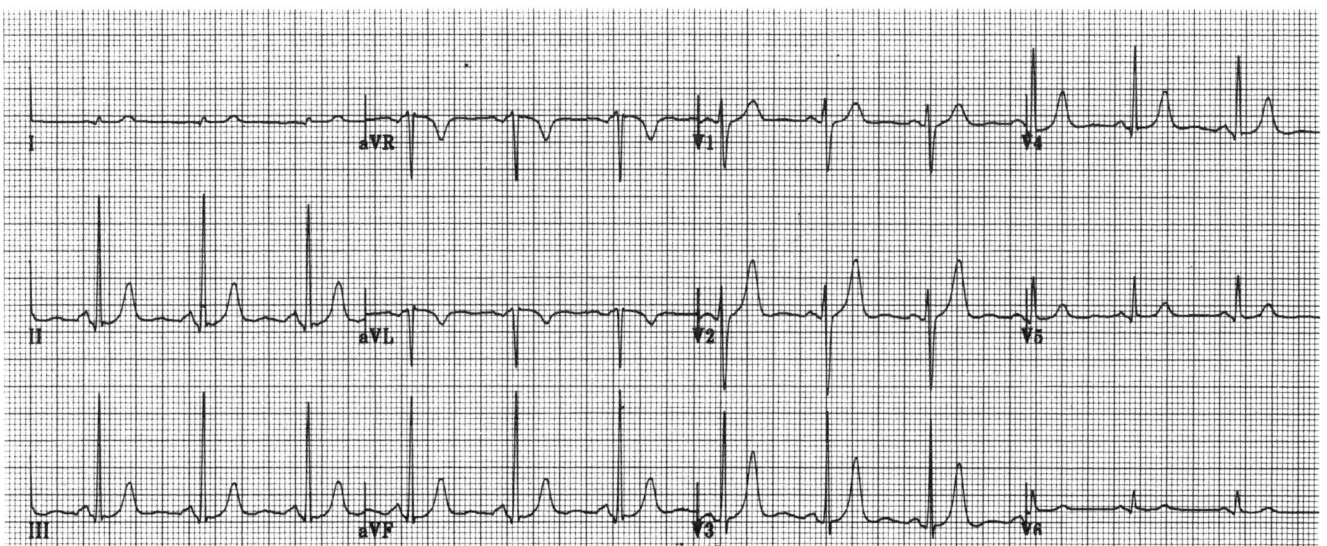

A. Acetazolamide belongs to the carbonic anhydrase inhibitor class of diuretics. By inhibiting this enzyme it prevents resorption of CO_2 in the proximal tubule cell. Without CO_2 to combine with H_2O and form H_2CO_3, no H^+ will be formed from the dissociation of this week acid. Consequently, Na^+ will not be resorbed via the cotransport of protons into the urine. The excess Na is reabsorbed in the collecting tubule in exchange for K, thereby facilitating a significant wasting of K. At toxic levels, hypokalemia will result.

B. Furosemide and ethacrynic acid, both loop diuretics, inhibit the $Na^+/K^+/2Cl^-$ transporter in the thick ascending limb of the loop of Henle. This prevents the resorption of these three ions. Hence, K remains in the urine and is excreted. Loop diuretic toxicity manifests as hypokalemia.

C. Furosemide and ethacrynic acid, both loop diuretics, inhibit the $Na^+/K^+/2Cl^-$ transporter in the thick ascending limb of the loop of Henle. This prevents the resorption of these three ions. Hence, potassium remains in the urine and is excreted. Loop diuretic toxicity manifests as hypokalemia.

D. By inhibiting the NaCl transporter in the distal convoluted tubule, Na is not resorbed. The mechanism for hypokalemia is then the same as for the loop diuretics.

668. **D.** This patient has had an incomplete abortion. This is evident because of the physical examination findings of incomplete removal of the placental tissue. Dilation and curettage is indicated to remove all placental tissues.

A. Antibiotic therapy is indicated after the retained products of conception have been removed.

B. Corticosteroid therapy is unlikely to be of benefit in the patient with an incomplete abortion.

C. Ergonovine infusion can be used if all of the products of conception have been removed.

E. This patient needs surgical intervention to remove the retained products of conception. Failure to do so can result in infectious complications.

669. **C.** In this trauma setting, one must rule out intraabdominal hemorrhage as the cause of hypotension with diagnostic peritoneal lavage (DPL). Patients with abdominal trauma can have no physical findings during abdominal examination, and his altered level of consciousness with alcohol intoxication could mask the abdominal signs.

A. This procedure would be too invasive and would be indicated if DPL were positive.

B. Arteriogram of the aorta is not indicated unless aortic rupture is suspected.

D. CT scan of the chest would not be indicated with a normal chest x-ray.

E. The patient is still volume depleted, and one would want to maintain the intravenous fluids.

670. **D.** This child may have Meckel diverticulitis. A technetium 99 pertechnetate scan can identify ectopic acid–secreting cells found in the vestigial remnant of the omphalomesenteric duct or Meckel diverticulum. This condition is described as a 5-cm anomalous pouch that projects from the antimesenteric border of the ileum and is located approximately 100 cm from the iliocecal valve. The pouch may be lined by ileal or ectopic (gastric or colonic) mucosa.

A. Abdominal ultrasonography is used to identify an inflamed appendix. Technetium 99 pertechnetate scans are unlikely to assist with the diagnosis of appendicitis.

B. Hirschsprung disease can be identified either by anal manometry (showing failure of the internal sphincter to relax upon balloon distention) or by a rectal biopsy (showing aganglionic segments).

C. Malrotation may be visualized by an upper gastrointestinal series with small bowel follow through showing abnormal position of the ligament of Treitz and cecum.

E. Pyloric stenosis is diagnosed by ultrasonography demonstrating the hypertrophic pylorus. A palpable olive-sized motile mass may also be palpated.

671. **A.** This patient has evidence of lead intoxication. This condition is more common in children than adults. Neuropathic syndromes such as radial palsy can occur. Treatment of lead poisoning involves chelation therapy.

B. Mercury intoxication presents with symptoms of tremor, ataxia, and confusion.

C. Methotrexate toxicity includes focal necrotic lesions of the brain and spinal cord.

D. Thallium toxicity includes an acute sensory polyneuropathy.

E. Vincristine toxicity includes paresthesias in the feet, legs, and hands.

672. **D.** Mesenteric angiography will help you diagnose mesenteric ischemia in this patient. Mesenteric ischemia is classically associated with periumbilical pain out of proportion to tenderness. Nausea, vomiting, GI bleeding and altered bowel habits can be identified. Thumbprinting is a classical finding on imaging studies and is due to submucosal edema.

A. Barium swallow will not show decreased blood flow through the ischemic segment of intestine.

B. CT scan will not demonstrate mesenteric ischemic changes.

C. Flat and upright x-ray will not demonstrate bowel ischemia.

E. Upper endoscopy will not show the ischemic intestinal segment.

673. **B.** This patient's examination findings and positive hepatitis C status increase his risk for cancer. For this reason, screening should be undertaken. This disease is common in intravenous drug users. Hepatitis C is caused by a flavivirus. The incubation period is approximately 8 weeks. The clinical course is usually mild and marked by fluctuating elevations of serum aminotransferase levels. Approximately 20% of cases lead to cirrhosis.

A. Bone marrow is not necessary because the thrombocytopenia is not secondary to bone marrow failure.

C. Hepatitis B, not hepatitis C, is usually associated with hepatitis D.

D. Liver biopsy is not indicated at this time.

E. Splenectomy should be avoided in patients with portal hypertension.

674. **A.** The patient has demonstrated the criteria for diagnosis of pelvic inflammatory disease (PID), including abdominal tenderness, cervical motion tenderness, adnexal tenderness, and purulent cervical discharge. Because she is an adolescent and compliance with treatment and follow-up are an issue, she should be admitted to the hospital for observed treatment. In-hospital treatment for PID in a person without a penicillin allergy consists of cefoxitin for 48 hours with a concomitant course of doxycycline for a 14-day course.

B. Although the definitive diagnosis of PID is made via laparoscopy, this procedure is no longer the standard of care secondary to invasiveness and cost. Laparoscopy is typically used in practice when appendicitis cannot be ruled out by clinical examination.

C. Although it is true that women with PID should be tested for chlamydial and gonococcal infections prior to starting antibiotic treatment, empiric antibiotic regimens should be started prior to obtaining the results. Although adjunctive antiinflammatory treatments to reduce fibroblast proliferation and scarring of the fallopian tube have been proposed, none have proved to be consistently beneficial in human studies.

D. For nonhospitalized patients, the recommended treatment of PID is ceftriaxone and probenecid followed by doxycycline for 14 days. However, in the case of patients with whom compliancy is an issue, such as adolescents, nonhospitalized treatment is not appropriate.

E. This patient has met the criteria for diagnosis of PID and should be treated. Although a temperature of or greater than 38.0℃ is a confirmatory finding of PID, it is not necessary for the diagnosis. In fact, fever is seen in only 20% of women with PID.

675. **E.** Wegener granulomatosis is a vasculitis that is found in middle-aged adults. A triad of necrotizing granulomatous vasculitis involving the upper respiratory tract, lower respiratory tract, and focal segmental glomerulonephritis characterizes it. Its onset may be insidious or abrupt. Presenting symptoms are usually nonspecific complaints with a history of recurrent sinusitis. Bloody nasal discharge is common. Pulmonary complaints may range from asymptomatic to chest pain, dyspnea, or hemorrhage. Renal involvement is usually seen with hematuria, proteinuria, and RBC casts. Cutaneous findings are also common. C-ANCA is positive in 80% of patients, and p-ANCA is positive in a minority.

A. Churg-Strauss syndrome involves the lungs, which helps differentiate it from polyarteritis nodosa. Patients often have a history of asthma or allergies. It develops in middle age and affects men more than women. Constitutional symptoms occur first, followed by cutaneous, pulmonary, neurologic, abdominal, and renal complaints.

B. Giant cell arteritis is also known as temporal arteritis. It usually begins gradually but may have an abrupt onset. Headaches, scalp tenderness, jaw claudication, vision loss, and sore throat are common complaints. Diagnosis is made by temporal artery biopsy.

C. Polyarteritis nodosa usually affects the skin, nerves, gastrointestinal tract, and kidneys, but may affect any organ of the body. Skin manifestations include palpable purpura, ulcers, and livedo reticularis. Joint pain is also common. Multiple mononeuropathies are common, as are sharp pain or paresthesias in peripheral nerve distributions.

D. Takayasu arteritis is a chronic vasculitis that affects the aorta and its branches. It is usually seen in Asian women. Asymmetrically reduced or absent pulses are seen in almost all patients. Hypertension is common due to renal artery stenosis. Bruits may be heard over the carotid and subclavian vessels.

676. **D.** Laparoscopic cholecystectomy is a clear alternative in the management of uncomplicated biliary lithiasis. The most common postoperative complication in this series was phlebitis, which occurred in approximately 4% of patients. Overall, complications occurred in 14% of patients in the laparoscopic group as compared with 23% of patients in the open cholecystectomy group.

A. Adynamic ileus is more commonly seen in patients who undergo open cholecystectomy.

B. Diarrhea is a rare side effect of both laparoscopic and open cholecystectomy.

C. Foreign body is essentially a complication of open cholecystectomy.

E. Residual lithiasis is a rare complication of both open and laparoscopic cholecystectomy.

677. **E.** This patient likely has an inferior wall myocardial infarction and has presented to the emergency department promptly. He should receive immediate thrombolytic therapy with streptokinase. This therapy may reduce infarct size and mortality rate, especially when administered within the first 6 hours after symptoms begin.

A. This patient has a myocardial infarction and needs immediate therapy.

B. Heparin infusion is useful in patients with acute myocardial infarction and left ventricular thrombi, deep venous thrombosis, or anterior wall myocardial infarction.

C. Lidocaine is an antiarrhythmic. This patient needs immediate thrombolytic therapy.

D. Morphine is important to reduce pain associated with acute myocardial infarction. However, this patient needs immediate thrombolytic therapy.

678. **B.** Duct ectasia is associated with multicolored, sticky discharge. The incidence is approximately 1% and typically occurs in women over the age of 40. Symptoms include tender breast masses, nipple retraction, and enlarged axillary lymph nodes.

A. A breast abscess is associated with purulent discharge.

C. Intraductal papilloma and invasive papillary cancer are associated with bloody discharge.

D. Pituitary adenoma as well as pregnancy, hypothyroidism, acromegaly, stress, and medications such as antihypertensives, oral birth control pills, and psychotropic drugs are associated with galactorrhea.

E. Tuberculosis is not typically associated with tender breast masses and nipple retraction.

679. **A.** Countertransference is defined as the reaction the psychiatrist has to the client, which can be influenced by other relationships and experiences in the therapist's life.

B. Projection is perceiving and reacting to unacceptable inner impulses and their derivatives as though they were outside the self.

C. Reaction formation is the transformation of an unacceptable impulse into the opposite.

D. Transference is the experience of the patient and how that influences his or her attitudes toward the therapist.

E. Triangulation is the aligning of two people in a conflict against a third.

680. **F.** *Rotavirus* is the most important cause of severe diarrhea in children under 3 years of age worldwide. Typical symptoms include persistent diarrhea, vomiting, and low-grade fever. This condition is more common in colder months. Treatment involves fluid replacement.

681. **E.** Norwalk-like viruses are food- and waterborne agents that cause 33% of epidemics of nonbacterial diarrhea in developed countries. Disease occurs in older children and can even affect adults. Disease distribution is year-round. Treatment is supportive since this disease is mild.

682. **G.** Shigellosis is the cause of diarrhea in this individual. This diarrhea is transmitted by person-to-person mechanisms. Clinical manifestations range from mild watery diarrhea to severe dysentery accompanied by fever and diarrhea. Diagnosis of shigellosis is based on the finding of fecal leukocytes and culture of the organism in the stool. Treatment includes intravenous fluid replacement and antibiotics such as trimethoprim-sulfamethoxazole.

683. **I.** *Vibrio parahemolyticus* causes disease in association with consumption of raw or undercooked seafood. Clinical presentation can include acute watery diarrhea, abdominal cramps, nausea, and vomiting after an incubation of 4 hours to 4 days. Diagnosis is made by culture of the organism on special media and must be suspected on the basis of exposure to seafood. Treatment involves fluid repletion and antibiotics (tetracycline).

684. **D.** Paget disease of the nipple involves eczematous changes in the skin of the nipple. These changes include scaling, crusting, erosion, ulceration, and discharge. A breast mass may be present. Paget disease is often present in conjunction with ductal carcinoma in situ (DCIS) or invasive carcinoma of the subareolar region.

A. DCIS, or intraductal carcinoma, is a premalignant lesion. The malignant epithelial cells proliferate in the mammary ducts. It is usually found in women in there fifties. These lesions may sometimes be palpated, but DCIS is usually (80%) found by mammography. The mammogram findings show clustered microcalcifications. It is diagnosed by needle or excisional biopsy. The lesions are usually unilateral. DCIS is more common than lobular carcinoma in situ. Treatment is wide-margin excision of the microcalcifications or simple mastectomy, depending on the extent of the disease. The yearly recurrence rate is 5%, with half of the recurrent disease being DCIS and half being invasive carcinoma.

B. Inflammatory breast carcinoma is responsible for 1% to 4% of breast cancer and is extremely aggressive. Skin changes associated with it are warmth, erythema, edema, and induration called peau d'orange. It is also associated with dermal lymphatic invasion and axillary lymphadenopathy. Distant metastasis is present in 17% to 36% of cases.

C. Infiltrating ductal carcinoma accounts for 80% of breast cancer. Its subtypes are less common, but more favorable, and they include medullary, colloidal, tubular, and papillary carcinoma. None of them are associated with the skin changes described in the question.

E. Tuberculosis is unlikely to occur in this presentation.

685. **D.** Pneumopericardium, air within the pericardial sac, is suggested by the radiographic findings of an air-tissue interface along the left cardiac border. In addition, an enlarged cardiac silhouette with normal pulmonary vasculature indicates pericardial disease. This may be caused by gas-producing organisms in an infection, or from air entering from around the pulmonary veins.

A. Although anxiety can cause shortness of breath, the culmination of findings is significant enough to allow for the diagnosis of pneumopericardium.

B. Pneumothorax is air in the pleural space causing a subsequent collapse of the lung. Typical presentation is pain and shortness of breath, with dyspnea, tachypnea, and/or tachycardia. A thin, radiolucent pleural line is seen on chest x-ray.

C. A continuous diaphragm sign (right and left hemidiaphragms look continuous) is seen with pneumomediastinum. There is mediastinal air below the heart and along the edge of the diaphragm.

E. Tension pneumothorax would occur after trauma. This patient has no history of trauma.

686. **A.** Patients with anorexia nervosa must have a body weight that is less than 85% of what is expected, display an intense fear of gaining weight, and show a disturbance in body image, and in postmenarchal females, there must be amenorrhea (i.e., the absence of at least three consecutive menstrual cycles). The disease may be further characterized by the presence or absence of binge eating or purging behavior (binge eating/purging type or restricting type, respectively).

B. Body dysmorphic disorder should only be considered as an additional diagnosis in anorexia patients if the distortion is unrelated to body shape and size.

C. Bulimia is similar to anorexia, but the distinction is that patients with bulimia nervosa are able to maintain body weight at or above a normal level.

D. Superior mesenteric artery syndrome is a medical condition characterized by postprandial vomiting secondary to intermittent gastric outlet obstruction, and should be distinguished from anorexia nervosa, although it may develop in anorexia patients because of their emaciation.

E. This patient meets the criteria for anorexia nervosa.

687. **B.** The treatment of choice for hypercholesterolemia is dietary modification. Patients should reduce fat calories. Exercise, reduction of smoking, and alcohol intake are also important measures. Drug therapy is a second-line consideration.

A, C, D, and **E.** These options are all second-line agents in the management of hypercholesterolemia.

688. **A.** A child who is less than 4 weeks of age who has otitis media may not have a fully developed immune system to combat the infection. Therefore, hospitalization and observation for sepsis is recommended. Broad-spectrum intravenous antibiotics are instituted upon admission.

B. Outpatient therapy is appropriate for older children with uncomplicated infections.

C. Outpatient observation until positive cultures return is not prudent in a neonate who is acutely ill.

D. Percutaneous antibiotic therapy is costly and requires the presence of nursing personnel to administer the medications.

E. Watchful waiting is not appropriate for a neonate who is acutely ill.

689. **B.** This patient has a small-for-gestational-age baby who has not been moving well for the past several hours. Results of the contraction stress test are positive, and the biophysical profile is poor. The best treatment for this patient is immediate cesarean section.

A. Antihypertensive agents will lower blood pressure and can compromise blood flow through the placenta.

C. Furosemide will compromise uteroplacental blood flow and is not indicated in this patient.

D. Oxytocin gel will delay delivery in a baby who already has a poor biophysical profile and a positive contraction stress test result.

E. Prostaglandin gel will delay delivery. This baby needs to be delivered as soon as possible.

690. **B.** This patient has acute mania. He has an abnormally elevated irritative mood. He has feelings of inflated self-esteem and grandiosity. He has decreased need for sleep, flight of ideas, distractibility, and sexual indiscretion. These symptoms cause impairment in occupational and social functioning.

A. Attention deficit disorder occurs in younger patients.

C. This patient has no evidence of an organic brain deficit. He has no history of drug dependency.

D. Schizoaffective disorder is unlikely because the patient's delusions are associated in time with affective symptoms.

E. Schizophrenia is less likely because of the good premorbid functioning.

691. **C.** This patient has radiographic evidence of a dermoid cyst. This is a common adnexal mass. In preadolescent females, ovarian cysts are the most common cause of an abdominal mass. With the ultrasonographic appearance of a simple, uniloculated, low echogenic (low brightness) mass, an ovarian cyst becomes the most likely diagnosis. Almost all cysts found in this age group will resolve spontaneously; therefore, follow-up ultrasonography in 4 to 8 weeks is usually sufficient to monitor the cyst's reduction. It is also standard in case any complication may arise, with ovarian torsion being the most likely complication.

Figure 691

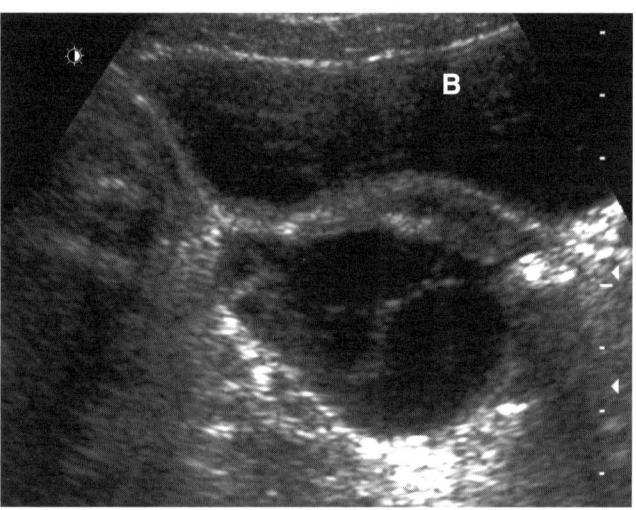

A. Although ovarian cysts may be detected on physical examination, ultrasonographic documentation of its reduction and absence of complications is essential.

B. Oophoropexy is the surgical procedure that is performed for ovarian torsion. After the ovary is untwisted, the surgeon uses this technique to fix the ovary in the desired position so that torsion does not recur.

D. When there is ovarian torsion, some surgeons are proponents to not only performing oophoropexy to the involved ovary but also to the contralateral, uninvolved ovary. This is considered acceptable by some because of the theoretic propensity to torsion on the contralateral side; however, there is no agreed-upon standard for this treatment for ovarian torsion at this time.

E. Even though most ovarian cysts in this age group spontaneously regress, the chance that the patient may develop complications warrants further follow-up.

692. **D.** This patient has evidence of herpes zoster. This condition is characterized by intense ear pain and the appearance of grouped vesicles. Treatment involves systemic corticosteroids such as methylprednisolone and oral acyclovir. Pain control is important because these lesions are typically quite painful.

A. Acyclovir should be given with a corticosteroid for maximal benefit in this condition.

B. Metronidazole has no role in the treatment of this condition.

C. Methylprednisolone should be given with acyclovir for maximal benefit in this condition.

E. Tetracycline has no role in the treatment of this condition.

693. **E.** This woman has classic symptoms of a urethral diverticulum. These include dysuria, urinary dribbling, and dyspareunia. Physical examination reveals a bulge in the anterior vaginal wall along the course of the urethra. Treatment involves surgical excision.

A. There is no evidence to suggest a Bartholin cyst in this patient.

B. This mass is in the anterior vaginal wall. There is no evidence of bladder prolapse.

C. This mass is in the anterior vaginal wall. Rectoceles produce a posterior vaginal wall defect.

D. Spasm of the levator muscles produces pain with palpation in the lateral vaginal walls. There are no associated cystic lesions.

694. **D.** This woman has a threatened abortion. The cervix is not dilated and there has been no passage of tissues. This condition occurs during the first 20 weeks of pregnancy. Mild abdominal cramping accompanies the bleeding.

A. Incomplete abortion is when there has been partial but incomplete expulsion of the products of conception from the uterine cavity.

B. Inevitable abortion occurs when bleeding or rupture of the membranes is associated with cramping and dilatation of the cervix.

C. Missed abortion is death of the fetus or embryo without the onset of labor or the passage of tissue for a prolonged period of time.

E. Spontaneous abortion is the broad term used to describe all the above entities. The more descriptive term should be used when clinically known.

695. **B.** A null hypothesis usually says that the results of a test are by chance. If you want to show that a screening test works, then the null hypothesis says it does not work. We do not accept the null hypothesis. We either reject it or we fail to reject it.

A. Null hypothesis is usually rejected when the p value is less than or equal to 0.05, meaning the test is statistically significant because the likelihood that the results occurred by chance is less than or equal to a 1 in 20 occurrence. A type I error is rejecting the null hypothesis when it is really true, or assuming a drug works when it does not. The probability of a type I error is given by the p value.

C. A type II error occurs when you fail to reject the null hypothesis when it is really false. Increasing the power of the test decreases the chance of a type II error.

D. There is risk for both type I and type II errors.

E. There is no such error as a type III error.

696. **E.** This patient's symptoms and laboratory results are the classic appearance of a "VIPoma," which include watery diarrhea, hypokalemia, and achlorhydria. Laparotomy is indicated because laboratory values of vasoactive intestinal peptide (VIP) levels are not reliable, so even if they are in the normal range, one cannot rule out a VIPoma, and laparotomy would still need to be performed to search for the tumor. Laparotomy would also be therapeutic in this case if the tumor is located.

A. Checking gastrin/VIP levels is not reliable, so a negative result, even if repeated, will not rule out a VIPoma. A gastrinoma is not likely since he would have had symptoms of excess gastric acid production and the presence of peptic ulcers that tend to perforate.

B. He has no symptoms associated with either an insulinoma (hypoglycemia) or a glucagonoma (hyperglycemia/diabetes).

C. Colonoscopy would not be of use yet because his symptoms are not only diarrhea, he has no abdominal pain, and there is no blood in his stool.

D. Esophagogastroduodenoscopy would not be of much help because he has no complaints of pain, dysphagia, or heartburnlike symptoms.

697. **C.** The primary treatment for vaginal carcinoma is by radiotherapy which will shrink large tumors rather well. Following radiotherapy, it is possible that chemotherapy or surgical excision will be viable options. This cancer typically occurs in women over the age of 40 with classical symptoms of vaginal bleeding and urinary symptoms from compression on the bladder.

A. Intravenous chemotherapy provides poor results for patients with vaginal carcinoma.

B. Intravesical chemotherapy is appropriate for carcinoma in situ of the bladder.

D. Surgical excision, although an appropriate additional therapy for this condition, should be attempted after radiotherapy.

E. Watchful waiting is an inappropriate strategy for the management of vaginal carcinoma.

698. **A.** The first steps in the evaluation of the patient with decreased responsiveness is assessment. Always assess airway, breathing, and circulation first. All other answers are actions that should be taken as well, but not as the first option.

B–E. This is secondary to the primary patient survey.

699. **E.** Gross motor skills of the 5-year-old child include the ability to skip with alternation of feet and jumping over low obstacles. This age also marks the time that children can spread butter or jelly with a knife and tie their own shoes. The 5-year-old child is able to draw a triangle from copy and can dress and undress. Domestic role playing is also evident at this age.

A. A child of this age may be able to walk with assistance.

B. A child of this age can walk alone.

C. A child of this age can pedal a tricycle.

D. A child of this age can walk and run well.

700. **A.** The patient has hypertension that is refractory to most medical treatments, a history of vascular disease, and a chronically elevated creatinine level. This most likely reflects renal artery stenosis caused from atherosclerotic renal disease. Renal artery stenosis causes refractory hypertension that over time can lead to diastolic heart failure. The elevated creatinine level likely signifies reduced flow to the kidneys. Angiotensin-converting enzyme inhibitors are useful in the treatment of systolic heart failure but have been proven to decrease renal perfusion in the case of renal artery stenosis.

B. Aspirin is an important medicine for this patient to help prevent myocardial infarct. Aspirin is less likely than other nonsteroidal antiinflammatory agents to cause renal damage.

C. A beta blocker is a good antihypertensive agent that is also useful for this patient's diastolic heart failure to help slow heart rate and increase filling time.

D. A calcium channel blocker is good for hypertension as well as diastolic heart failure to slow heart rate and increase filling time.

E. A thiazide diuretic is a good treatment for hypertension. However, thiazide diuretics can become ineffective if the glomerular filtration rate falls below 30 mL/min. This could potentially occur in this patient, but stopping the drug is not an immediate concern.

701. **E.** The patient is suffering from neuroleptic malignant syndrome, which is most often precipitated by neuroleptic phenothiazines. Some more commonly prescribed medications of this class include thioridazine, haloperidol, chlorpromazine, and fluphenazine.

A. This clinical picture is not typical for alcohol ingestion.

B. This clinical picture is not typical for benzodiazapine ingestion.

C. Cocaine ingestion may result in a similar consternation of symptoms, but the fact that he has a history of schizophrenia raises the suspicion that a phenothiazine is the precipitating factor.

D. This clinical picture is not typical for ethylene glycol ingestion.

702. **B.** Dextrose is available as a 5% solution in saline or water. This intravenous fluid provides 170 kcal/L and contributes approximately 280 mOsm to a solution. Infusion of dextrose can fuel the production of lactic acid in ischemic organs such as this individual who has renal insufficiency and stroke. Thus, serum lactate levels will increase. Serum osmolarity also will increase because this fluid is hyperosmolar.

703. **A.** Ringer lactate is a balanced electrolyte solution that substitutes K and calcium for some of the Na in isotonic saline. Lactate is added as a buffer. The added K can be detrimental to patients with renal insufficiency. Serum calcium levels may also increase due to the added calcium.

704. **D.** Hetastarch is a synthetic starch that was introduced as an inexpensive alternative to albumin. This solution is cleared by the kidneys, and the largest particles can take several weeks to clear. Thus, elevations in serum creatinine are possible. Serum amylase levels can increase to three times normal and is a normal response to degradation of Hetastarch and does not indicate pancreatitis. Serum lipase must be used to diagnose and follow pancreatitis when Hetastarch is used.

705. **E.** Drug interactions are important to consider in patients who are taking antiretroviral agents. Patients who are taking zidovudine and trimethoprim-sulfamethoxazole are at increased risk for developing neutropenia. It is important to be aware of this interaction when treating such patients.

A–D. Anemia, headache, malaise, and nausea are typical side effects of zidovudine.

706. **A.** Calcium must be supplemented during pregnancy to meet fetal needs and preserve maternal calcium stores. Milk is the recommended substance to promote calcium stores because it is inexpensive and provides 1 g of calcium and 33 g of protein per quart. The pregnant patient requires an additional 400 mg of calcium above the 800 mg required by nonpregnant individuals.

B. Fourteen milligrams of niacin is required daily by the nonpregnant patient, whereas 16 mg is required in the pregnant state.

C. Eight hundred milligrams of vitamin A is required daily in the nonpregnant state, whereas 1 g is required in the pregnant state.

D. Two hundred milligrams of vitamin D is required daily in the nonpregnant state, whereas 400 mg is required in the pregnant state.

E. Eight milligrams of vitamin E is required daily in the nonpregnant state, whereas 10 mg is required in the pregnant state.

707. **D.** Wilms tumor is the most common kidney tumor in children and can be associated with genitourinary anomalies, hemihypertrophy, and sporadic aniridia. Patients are approximately 3 years of age at diagnosis and present with an abdominal mass that does not cross the midline. Associated symptoms can include nausea and vomiting. Ultrasonography can show an intrarenal mass, whereas CT scan may reveal a heterogeneous mass arising from the kidney.

A. The differential diagnosis of this condition does not include gastrointestinal causes. Therefore, barium enema is not a useful study.

B. Bladder tumors or lesions are not likely in this age group. Therefore, cystoscopy is not indicated.

C. Retrograde urethrography is indicated in patients with significant voiding symptoms to evaluate the contour of the urethra.

E. Ureteral pathology is rare in children. Thus, retrograde ureteroscopy is not indicated in this patient.

708. **E.** Sodium bicarbonate is the best choice because alkalinization of the urine is the best method to expel salicylates from the body. Intravenous fluids with sodium bicarbonate (three ampules 50 mEq in 1 L of D5W, or two ampules in 1 L D5¼NS) are administered at 100 to 250 mL/h. Urine pH should be maintained at or above 7.5 to 8.0. The fluid infusion also helps increase diuresis. Hemodialysis may be required if severe alkalemia develops (pH > 7.55).

A. Dialysis is useful in all-out renal failure. However, dialysis should not be performed in this case until other options were first explored or if the pH alteration was quick and severe.

B. Ethanol infusion is the treatment for overdose on ethylene glycol or methanol. It helps decrease the accumulation of toxic metabolites. Fomepizole has been shown to be a safe alternative to ethanol infusion.

C. Insulin is an appropriate treatment for diabetic ketoacidosis. A continuous infusion is performed until the metabolic acidosis is resolved. Intravenous fluids, bicarbonate, and K would also be useful in this setting.

D. N-acetylcysteine is the antidote for acetaminophen toxicity, not salicylates.

709. **B.** The systolic blood pressure of 140 mm Hg in this community is 2 standard deviations above the mean of 120 mm Hg. The area under the curve between 2 and 3 standard deviations is about 2.35% plus about 0.15% (everything above 3 standard deviations). Thus, a total of 2.50% of the people will have blood pressures at or above 140 mm Hg.

710. **E.** Viral gastroenteritis can cause more than a week of diarrheal symptoms, which are worsened by lactose ingestion. Viruses such as Norwalk and *Rotavirus* will cause the initial bouts of diarrhea, which also causes atrophy of the jejunal brush border, resulting in decreased ability to digest the lactose, causing increased pulling of water into the gastrointestinal lumen. It should be recommended to this patient that he avoid lactose-containing products for a week or two after his diarrheal symptoms have resolved, thus giving his brush border the chance to replenish.

A. *Bacillus cereus* infection consists of copious diarrhea within hours of eating rice that has been left at room temperature.

B. This patient has neither been drinking from possible contaminated sources of water with *Giardia*, nor has he experienced the symptoms of greasy, bulky, and malodorous stools.

C. Irritable bowel syndrome usually consists of diarrhea or constipation associated with abdominal pain that is immediately resolved with defecation. The individual will report no weight loss and a considerable amount of stress/anxiety in his or her life. If not resolved with anticholinergics or antidiarrheals such as loperamide, it is recommended to switch to an anticholinergic agent such as amitriptyline.

D. While his symptoms of cramping, gas, and diarrhea exacerbated with milk ingestion mimic those of a lactose deficiency, they will only be transient while his cold persists and a week or two afterward.

711. **B.** This child has gastroesophageal reflux. Eighty-five percent of infants with chalasia present during the first week of life, and symptoms may improve as the child becomes more upright by age 2. Diagnosis is made by barium swallow and pH probe tests. Medical management includes metoclopramide to increase the tone of the lower esophageal sphincter.

A. Cimetidine may be used when gastroesophageal reflux is complicated by esophagitis.

C. Postprandial placement in the prone position with the head at a 30-degree angle may improve reflux.

D. In cases refractory to medical management, a surgical fundoplication may control reflux in 90% of cases.

E. Thickening of feeds may reduce reflux in children with chalasia.

712. **C.** Hepatocellular adenoma is a rare benign tumor that is associated with both oral contraceptive and anabolic steroid use. Presenting symptoms include abdominal pain and/or a palpable abdominal mass. Thirty percent of patients can present with an intraperitoneal hemorrhage (seen as free fluid in the abdomen on CT scan).

A. Hemangiomas are benign lesions that require no treatment. These tumors are not known to bleed spontaneously.

B. Hepatic abscess is most often the result of a previous peritonitis. They do not usually bleed.

D. Metastatic adenocarcinoma is usually seen as multiple lesions on the liver. They are painless and do not bleed.

E. Hepatic cysts mostly do not rupture and would not cause an intraperitoneal hemorrhage.

713. **D.** This patient has aortitis that is a late consequence of infection, which may occur many years after the primary stage of syphilis infection. In this condition, the aortic root becomes weakened and dilated. Degeneration and fibrosis of the outer two thirds of the vessel media can be found. The intima becomes fibrosed, resulting in ostial stenosis and causing myocardial ischemia, and may affect the femoral arteries, causing claudication symptoms.

A. This patient's condition is the result of syphilic exposure.

B. Myocardial infarction is most commonly caused by atherosclerosis. ECG would most likely show ST segment elevation, peaking of T waves, or Q waves.

C. Rheumatic heart disease involves the aortic valve in 20%. This patient does not meet the Duckett-Jones criteria requiring two major or one major and two minor conditions.

E. This patient presents with more physical findings than would be expected with unstable angina.

714. **E.** The patient is suffering from high anion gap acidosis. Ethylene glycol ingestion causes an alcohol-intoxicated state as well as calcium oxalate crystals in the urine due to its conversion to calcium oxalate formic acid.

A. Acetaminophen overdose usually does not show a high anion gap acidosis, and signs and symptoms, when they occur after 24 hours, are more consistent with liver failure.

B. Cocaine overdose would reveal pinpoint pupils with jugular venous distention.

C. Diabetic ketoacidosis is a cause of high anion gap acidosis. However, the patient would not generally have a normal serum glucose level.

D. Ethanol ingestion, similar to ethylene glycol ingestion, would cause a high anion gap acidosis, but calcium oxalate crystals are more commonly seen with antifreeze ingestion.

715. **E.** This patient has evidence of a post–subarachnoid block headache (spinal headache). The incidence approaches 50% with large-gauge epidural needles. Treatment includes bed rest, liberal use of intravenous fluids, and epidural blood patch.

A. Liberal use of pain medications is encouraged. Acetaminophen is unlikely to relieve this type of pain.

B. Amoxicillin is not indicated in the management of postsubarachnoid headache.

C. Bed rest would be encouraged in this patient.

D. Liberal use of IV fluids (100 mL/h) would be recommended in this patient.

716. **B.** The macroscopic finding indicates creeping fat, and microscopic findings indicate noncaseating granulomas, which are pathognomonic for Crohn disease. This disease can manifest anywhere from the mouth to the anus, although most patients will have ileal or ileal and cecal disease.

A. Crohn disease increases the risk for colon cancer slightly, but biopsy did not reveal cancer.

C. Ischemic bowel would show necrotic tissue rather than the findings of inflammation.

D. Tuberculosis is unlikely to affect the colon, and the patient has no other findings of infection.

E. Ulcerative colitis would have mucosal bleeding without significant bowel wall thickening.

717. **B.** This is a classic case of appendicitis. This patient should be taken to the operating room for exploratory laparotomy and possible appendectomy by either the laparoscopic or traditional open approach.

A. Appendicitis is a clinical diagnosis. A negative CT scan should not deter you from surgically exploring this patient.

C. This patient should not be observed. The story is classic for appendicitis.

D. Hospital discharge may result in a patient with a perforated appendix.

E. Barium enema has no role in the patient with appendicitis. However, this test may be useful in a child with intussusception.

718. **B.** This is a controversial issue. Some physicians will do a needle biopsy during the initial office visit. However, the board answer is to perform mammography first so that you have a baseline mammogram to compare all subsequent mammograms with. A biopsy will need to be performed after mammography is completed.

A. This patient should have a mammogram before any intervention (biopsy or aspiration).

C. This patient should have an imaging study and possibly a biopsy to further evaluate this mass.

D and **E.** This is an appropriate step after mammography.

719. **C.** Senekot works by inducing peristalsis. This agent may increase gastrointestinal transit time and improve constipation in this patient.

A. Docusate sodium is a stool softener and will not increase gastrointestinal transit time.

B. Mineral oil is an osmotic agent.

D. Increased amounts of simple carbohydrates can lead to constipation, and it is recommended that children with constipation limit simple carbohydrates while increasing fiber intake.

E. Vincristine is an anticancer drug that causes constipation.

720. **D.** The patient described above is manifesting signs and symptoms of urinary stress incontinence. Sudden increases in intraabdominal pressure resulting from coughing and straining are resulting in involuntary loss of urine. The most accepted theory for this pathology is that the proximal urethra drops below the pelvic floor secondary to pelvic relaxation defects. Risk factors for urinary stress incontinence include vaginal childbirth, aging, chronic cough, heavy lifting, and estrogen deficiency.

A. Although polyuria does occur with the use of hydrochlorothiazide secondary to its diuretic properties, the history described by the patient above is one of stress incontinence with involuntary urine loss secondary to a sudden increase in intraabdominal pressure.

B. Urinary tract infections (UTIs) can manifest themselves as cystitis or inflammation of the urinary bladder. And although urinary incontinence can, at times, result from cystitis, without symptoms of dysuria, urgency, or nocturia her symptoms are less likely to be a result of a UTI.

C. Detrusor insufficiency or detrusor areflexia can be caused by autonomic neuropathy. However, these two entities result in overflow incontinence that manifests as frequent or constant urinary dribbling. Autonomic neuropathy in this patient is unlikely secondary to her history and the fact that her diabetes is of relatively new onset and is controlled by diet and exercise, which remarks on its low severity stage.

E. Urinary fistulas will cause total urinary incontinence, which manifests as painless and continuous vaginal leakage of urine. Within the United States, 95% of vesicovaginal fistulas result from pelvic surgery and/or pelvic irradiation. Fistulas resulting from obstetric trauma rarely occur in this country as opposed to developing countries, where obstetric trauma is the most common cause of urinary fistulas.

721. **D.** Fractures of the hip are described in reference to the major structure the fracture line passes next to or between. Because this fracture occurs between the greater and lesser trochanters of the femur it is called an intertrochanteric fracture. The radiograph shows a fracture line running from the greater to the lesser trochanter. In an elderly patient with a fall and hip pain, a radiograph of the hip is essential because of the high incidence of fracture in this population.

Figure 721

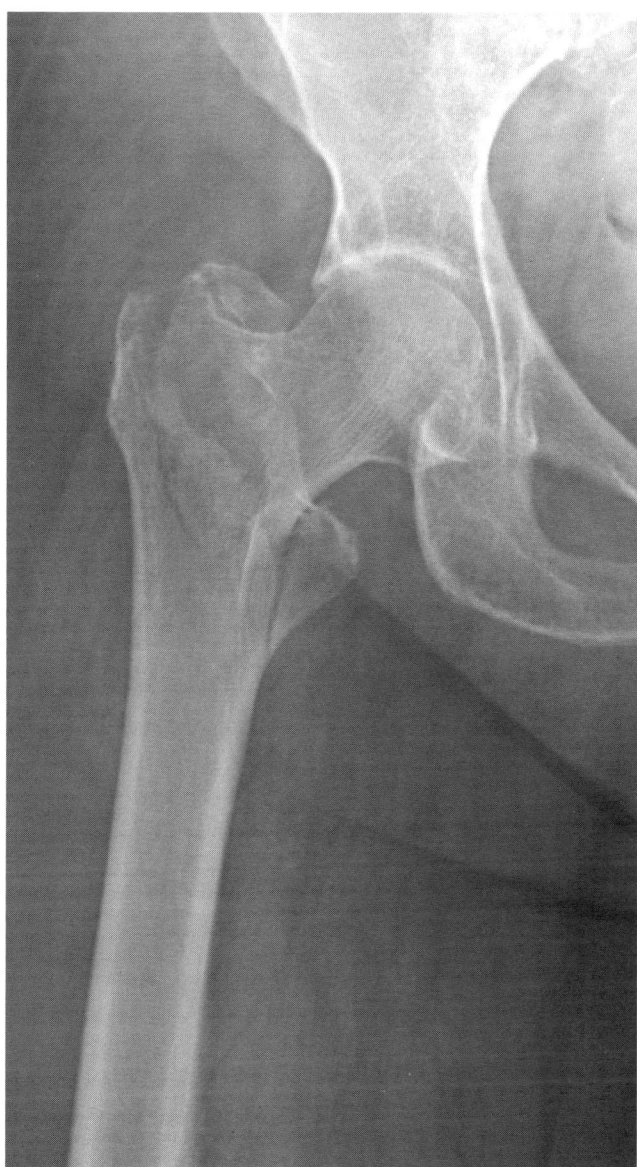

A. There is no fracture of the femur diaphysis (shaft of a long bone).

B. There is no fracture of the femoral neck (the stretch of bone that connects the femoral head to the intertrochanteric segment of the femur).

C. There is no fracture line in the femoral head, which rules out a femoral head fracture.

E. Subtrochanteric fractures are located at the superior portion of the femur diaphysis but below the lesser trochanter.

722. **B.** Erythromycin is the correct treatment of choice for atypical pneumonia. Atypical community-acquired pneumonia is most often caused by *Mycoplasma pneumoniae* followed by respiratory syncytial virus. Erythromycin is effective against *Mycoplasma* and should be used when it is suspected as the causative agent. Alternative therapies include tetracycline and erythromycin.

A. Acyclovir is indicated in cases of viral pneumonia. It can also be used in lung infections caused by herpes simplex, herpes zoster, or varicella. Cytomegalovirus pneumonia is treated with ganciclovir.

C. Penicillin is the drug of choice for patients with aspiration pneumonia.

D. Although nearly all patients with atypical pneumonia will recover without antibiotic treatment, antibiotics decrease the length of fever and pulmonary infiltrates, accelerating symptomatic recovery.

E. Trimethoprim is the drug of choice against *Pneumocystis carinii* pneumonia.

723. **C.** You calculate the perinatal mortality rate by adding the number of stillbirths and the number of neonatal deaths (deaths within the first 28 days of life), and dividing this by the total number of births, including the stillbirths: (45 stillbirths + 6 neonatal deaths) / (45 stillbirths + 1000 live births) = 51/1045.

724. **C.** An excisional biopsy is the necessary treatment in a number of cases. These include failure of needle aspiration to obtain fluid, the discovery that the mass is solid, the fluid obtained is bloody, the mass does not go away after it is aspirated, the mass remains after two aspirations, or the fluid reaccumulates within 2 weeks of aspiration. The mass should be excised with a 1-cm margin to decrease the risk for recurrence.

A. This procedure would not provide any new information about the lesion, and waiting could put the patient at risk if the lesion were malignant.

B. The mass should be removed with a 1-cm edge of normal tissue. By doing this, further surgery can be avoided if the mass is found to be malignant.

D. This lesion requires that an excisional biopsy be performed. Mammography is a screening tool. The American Cancer Society dictates that every woman should have a baseline mammogram at ages 35 to 39, a mammogram every 2 years at ages 40 to 50, and annually after 50 years of age. Architectural distortion, linear-branched patterns of microcalcifications, a spiculated mass, asymmetric fibrosis, increased vascularity, and distorted subareolar duct patterns are mammography findings that suggest malignancy.

E. This lesion requires excisional biopsy to rule out malignancy.

725. **E.** Ophthalmia neonatorum refers to a red eye that occurs within the first 21 days of life. Eighty percent of neonatal red eyes are from chemical irritation after silver nitrate prophylaxis. *Chlamydia trachomatis* is the most common infectious agent, but *Neisseria gonorrhoeae* is the most damaging agent. It normally occurs 2 to 5 days after delivery, and must be treated with emergency topical and intravenous penicillin to prevent blindness.

A. Observation would be appropriate if red eyes occurred within the first 24 hours and subsequently resolved (due to silver nitrate).

B. Oral erythromycin alone is not sufficient for treatment.

C. Saline eye drops would not treat the infection.

D. Topical tetracycline and oral erythromycin is the treatment of choice for *Chlamydia trachomatis* infection.

726. **E.** Physical examination findings suggest Cushing syndrome, and testing for urinary cortisol is used to screen for the presence of a cortisol-producing adrenal tumor.

A. A normal glucose level makes this test unuseful.

B. MRI will not help with the diagnosis of the mass.

C. Biopsy would be used if cancer is suspected with metastasis and used for staging.

D. An aldosterone-secreting mass is unlikely in this patient.

727. **C.** The patient is diagnosed with Bell palsy, which is unilateral paresis in the distribution of the facial nerve from an undetermined cause. Leading theories pin herpes simplex virus type 1 as the underlying cause. For this reason, antiviral agents such as acyclovir can be used in treatment. Other theories of etiology encompass autoimmune inflammation and vascular ischemia. Because of this, steroids have also been used in treatment. Greater than two thirds of patients diagnosed with Bell palsy will recover completely regardless of the treatment regimen used. Some patients have autonomic dysfunction, motor spasms, or paresis as sequelae.

A, B, D, and **E.** Nearly 66% of patients with Bell palsy will recover completely.

728. **A.** This patient appears to be suffering from an anterior wall myocardial infarction. The presence of Q waves and ST elevation in leads V_1 through V_4 confirm the diagnosis. This patient should have immediate administration of streptokinase, since his symptoms have lasted less than 6 hours.

B. Chest wall pain should not produce ECG abnormalities.

C. Inferior wall myocardial infarction would produce ST elevation and Q waves in leads II, III, and AVF.

D. This patient does not have myocardial ischemia.

E. Pericarditis presents with ST elevation in all leads of the ECG.

729. **C.** This individual likely has a femoral stress fracture. This condition is usually seen in high-mileage long-distance runners and is characterized by a persistent, vague thigh pain. Treatment involves walking with crutches and avoidance of weight bearing.

A. Arthroscopy is not indicated in the treatment of a femoral stress fracture.

B. Corticosteroids are not indicated in the initial treatment of a femoral stress fracture.

D. Dimethylsulfoxide is not indicated in the treatment of a femoral stress fracture.

E. Although watchful waiting is an appropriate selection, this patient should not continue with his running regimen.

730. **A.** This patient has hypotonic labor. Performing an amnionotomy may assist with progression of labor. This will cause rupture of the membranes that were intact. The patient should be placed in a lateral position to allow the amnionic fluid to drain.

B. Oxytocin should be administered after the amnionic membranes are ruptured.

C. There is no indication for an epidural anesthetic at this time.

D. Jogging around the hospital may theoretically assist with rupture of membranes, but amniotomy is a more prudent selection.

E. This patient has already walked around the floor without a response (progression of labor).

731. **B.** This patient likely has a thrombosis of the middle cerebral artery. He should have a CT scan of the head to differentiate ischemic stroke from hemorrhagic stroke. This will provide information as to the further treatment of this patient and the possible role of thrombolytic therapy.

A. Angiography is contraindicated in the acute phase of stroke.

C. Digital subtraction angiography will not help with diagnosis of acute stroke.

D. Lumbar puncture will not help with the diagnosis of acute stroke.

E. MRI is not as good as CT scan in the differentiation between ischemic and hemorrhagic stroke.

732. **C.** This patient may have an uncomplicated skin infection. This patient is an outpatient and is well outside the window of serious complications from the surgery. This may be a superficial infection due to the common gram-positive skin organisms. Good oral gram-positive coverage can be attained by first using cephalexin.

A. Ampicillin is given intravenously only; therefore, it is less likely to be given on an outpatient basis.

B. Clindamycin is appropriate for anaerobic infections.

D. Ketoconazole is an antifungal agent.

E. Metronidazole is appropriate for anaerobic organisms.

733. **C.** This child has a foreign body lodged in his nose. Clinical history usually reveals a persistent purulent nasal discharge. The foreign body may be obscured by nasal secretions. Treatment involves removal with a grasping forceps.

A. Direct laryngoscopy would be important for a foreign body of the larynx or trachea.

B. Flexible laryngoscopy would be important for a foreign body of the larynx or trachea.

D. The foreign body needs to be removed. There is no indication for corticosteroid therapy.

E. Watchful waiting is inappropriate. The foreign body needs to be removed.

734. **B.** Cigarette smoking is a preventable cause of small-for-gestational-age babies. It is more common than alcohol or illicit drug use among women. Birth weight can be reduced by as much as 200 g in pregnant women who smoke.

A. Cigarette smoking among pregnant women is more common than alcohol abuse.

C. Hypertension can cause small-for-gestational-age babies, but this patient is not hypertensive.

D. Smoking is more common than illicit drug use among pregnant women.

E. Maternal malnutrition is an uncommon cause of small-for-gestational-age babies.

735. **C.** This ECG demonstrates the digitalis effect. This is seen with both therapeutic and toxic levels of the cardiac glycosides. It shows up on ECGs as a gradual downward curve of the ST segment. The lowest part of this segment will be curved below the baseline. In this case, we can assume it is not toxic because the patient is asymptomatic and there are no other signs of toxicity on ECG.

A. Digoxin does not typically cause atrial fibrillation, even at toxic levels; however, it can cause many different arrhythmias, some being deadly. This list includes atrial and junctional tachyarrhythmias, ventricular bigeminy, ventricular trigeminy, and ventricular fibrillation. The latter is a common cause of mortality in toxic patients.

B. The digitalis effect is not present on ECG unless there is an adequate or toxic dose.

D. Any patient taking digoxin should be evaluated for digoxin-related toxicity. Digoxin and the cardiac glycosides have many effects at toxic levels. These include abdominal and neurologic symptoms such as nausea, vomiting, abdominal pain, headache, weakness, drowsiness, confusion, and visual disturbances. Significant cardiac effects include a host of arrhythmias (see explanation to choice A). None of these are shown in this ECG, however.

E. Hypokalemia, not hyperkalemia, sensitizes the myocardium to the effects of digoxin; therefore, serum electrolytes must be monitored in these patients.

736. **C.** This patient has panic disorder with agoraphobia. These attacks tend to occur several times per week. This condition is chronic with exacerbations and remissions and has an excellent prognosis with therapy. Medication is essential for panic disorder. Tricyclic antidepressants such as imipramine are good choices for these patients and often produce a response within 2 to 3 weeks.

A. Alprazolam is a medication used in the treatment of panic disorder but is associated with depression, addiction, and the need for frequent dosing.

B. Clonazepam, not clonidine, is useful in the management of panic disorder with agoraphobia.

D. Propranolol is also a possible treatment for panic disorder but is not as effective as imipramine.

E. Trazodone is a serotonin reuptake inhibitor that has unproven benefits in the management of panic disorder.

737. **E.** This patient has evidence of chylomicronemia syndrome. Clinical features include acute pancreatitis, xanthoma, lipidemia retinalis, dementia, and dyspnea. Treatment includes removal of medications that could raise triglyceride levels such as beta blockers and cimetidine.

A. Dietary fats should be restricted in this patient.

B. Heparin should be avoided in this patient because it may cause bleeding into the pancreatic bed.

C. Lipid emulsion should be avoided in this patient.

D. Plasmapheresis is unnecessary in this patient.

Figure 735

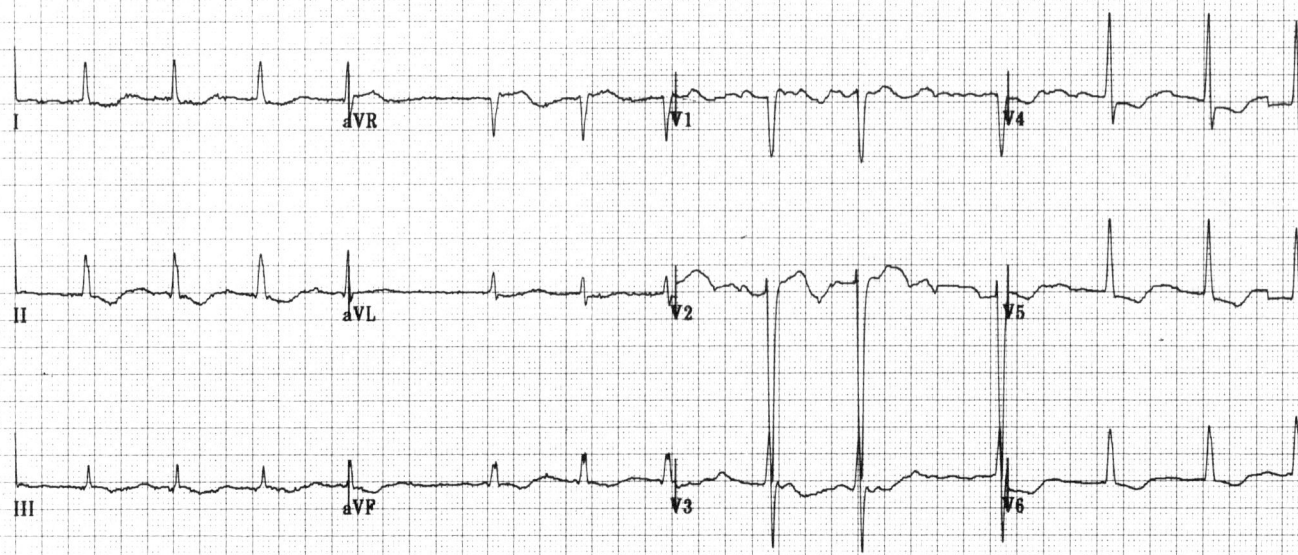

738. **E.** The location of the wound indicates a zone II injury, and no diagnostic evaluation is needed. Patients with these injuries need to be sent to the operating room for exploration with tests.

A–D. This selection would be indicated in zone I and III injuries.

739. **B.** This patient has narcolepsy with cataplexy. Patients should avoid precipitating stimuli. Narcolepsy with cataplexy is best treated with imipramine. Patients may also benefit from planned daytime naps.

A. Corticosteroids are of no benefit for the patient with narcolepsy with cataplexy.

C. Methylphenidate is an appropriate treatment for sleep attacks.

D. Tonsilectomy would be indicated for obstructive sleep apnea secondary to tonsilar hypertrophy.

E. This patient needs a comprehensive treatment plan, including daytime naps, avoidance of dangerous occupations, and imipramine.

740. **E.** This child likely has cataracts. This condition is due to an opacification of the crystalline lens of the eye. Visual acuity testing should be performed in this patient. The treatment of partial cataracts includes patching and mydriatics.

A. CT scan of the head is unlikely to provide additional useful information in the case of cataracts.

B. MRI of the head is unlikely to provide additional useful information in the case of cataracts.

C. Ocular ultrasonography should be performed in the case of total lens opacity.

D. Vertebral artery angiography is unlikely to provide any additional information in this case.

INDEX

✺ TEST 1   ANSWER SHEET

BLOCK 1

1. _____
2. _____
3. _____
4. _____
5. _____
6. _____
7. _____
8. _____
9. _____
10. _____
11. _____
12. _____
13. _____
14. _____
15. _____
16. _____
17. _____
18. _____
19. _____
20. _____
21. _____
22. _____
23. _____
24. _____
25. _____
26. _____
27. _____
28. _____
29. _____
30. _____
31. _____
32. _____
33. _____
34. _____
35. _____
36. _____
37. _____
38. _____
39. _____
40. _____
41. _____
42. _____
43. _____
44. _____
45. _____
46. _____

BLOCK 2

47. _____
48. _____
49. _____
50. _____
51. _____
52. _____
53. _____
54. _____
55. _____
56. _____
57. _____
58. _____
59. _____
60. _____
61. _____
62. _____
63. _____
64. _____
65. _____
66. _____
67. _____
68. _____
69. _____
70. _____
71. _____
72. _____
73. _____
74. _____
75. _____
76. _____
77. _____
78. _____
79. _____
80. _____
81. _____
82. _____
83. _____
84. _____
85. _____
86. _____
87. _____
88. _____
89. _____
90. _____
91. _____
92. _____

BLOCK 3

93. _____
94. _____
95. _____
96. _____
97. _____
98. _____
99. _____
100. _____
101. _____
102. _____
103. _____
104. _____
105. _____
106. _____
107. _____
108. _____
109. _____
110. _____
111. _____
112. _____
113. _____
114. _____
115. _____
116. _____
117. _____
118. _____
119. _____
120. _____
121. _____
122. _____
123. _____
124. _____
125. _____
126. _____
127. _____
128. _____
129. _____
130. _____
131. _____
132. _____
133. _____
134. _____
135. _____
136. _____
137. _____
138. _____
139. _____

BLOCK 4

140. _____
141. _____
142. _____
143. _____
144. _____
145. _____
146. _____
147. _____
148. _____
149. _____
150. _____
151. _____
152. _____
153. _____
154. _____
155. _____
156. _____
157. _____
158. _____
159. _____
160. _____
161. _____
162. _____
163. _____
164. _____
165. _____
166. _____
167. _____
168. _____
169. _____
170. _____
171. _____
172. _____
173. _____
174. _____
175. _____
176. _____
177. _____
178. _____
179. _____
180. _____
181. _____
182. _____
183. _____
184. _____
185. _____

✸ TEST 1   ANSWER SHEET

BLOCK 5	BLOCK 6	BLOCK 7	BLOCK 8
186. _____	233. _____	279. _____	325. _____
187. _____	234. _____	280. _____	326. _____
188. _____	235. _____	281. _____	327. _____
189. _____	236. _____	282. _____	328. _____
190. _____	237. _____	283. _____	329. _____
191. _____	238. _____	284. _____	330. _____
192. _____	239. _____	285. _____	331. _____
193. _____	240. _____	286. _____	332. _____
194. _____	241. _____	287. _____	333. _____
195. _____	242. _____	288. _____	334. _____
196. _____	243. _____	289. _____	335. _____
197. _____	244. _____	290. _____	336. _____
198. _____	245. _____	291. _____	337. _____
199. _____	246. _____	292. _____	338. _____
200. _____	247. _____	293. _____	339. _____
201. _____	248. _____	294. _____	340. _____
202. _____	249. _____	295. _____	341. _____
203. _____	250. _____	296. _____	342. _____
204. _____	251. _____	297. _____	343. _____
205. _____	252. _____	298. _____	344. _____
206. _____	253. _____	299. _____	345. _____
207. _____	254. _____	300. _____	346. _____
208. _____	255. _____	301. _____	347. _____
209. _____	256. _____	302. _____	348. _____
210. _____	257. _____	303. _____	349. _____
211. _____	258. _____	304. _____	350. _____
212. _____	259. _____	305. _____	351. _____
213. _____	260. _____	306. _____	352. _____
214. _____	261. _____	307. _____	353. _____
215. _____	262. _____	308. _____	354. _____
216. _____	263. _____	309. _____	355. _____
217. _____	264. _____	310. _____	356. _____
218. _____	265. _____	311. _____	357. _____
219. _____	266. _____	312. _____	358. _____
220. _____	267. _____	313. _____	359. _____
221. _____	268. _____	314. _____	360. _____
222. _____	269. _____	315. _____	361. _____
223. _____	270. _____	316. _____	362. _____
224. _____	271. _____	317. _____	363. _____
225. _____	272. _____	318. _____	364. _____
226. _____	273. _____	319. _____	365. _____
227. _____	274. _____	320. _____	366. _____
228. _____	275. _____	321. _____	367. _____
229. _____	276. _____	322. _____	368. _____
230. _____	277. _____	323. _____	369. _____
231. _____	278. _____	324. _____	370. _____
232. _____			

BLOCK 9	BLOCK 10	BLOCK 11	BLOCK 12
371. _____	417. _____	463. _____	510. _____
372. _____	418. _____	464. _____	511. _____
373. _____	419. _____	465. _____	512. _____
374. _____	420. _____	466. _____	513. _____
375. _____	421. _____	467. _____	514. _____
376. _____	422. _____	468. _____	515. _____
377. _____	423. _____	469. _____	516. _____
378. _____	424. _____	470. _____	517. _____
379. _____	425. _____	471. _____	518. _____
380. _____	426. _____	472. _____	519. _____
381. _____	427. _____	473. _____	520. _____
382. _____	428. _____	474. _____	521. _____
383. _____	429. _____	475. _____	522. _____
384. _____	430. _____	476. _____	523. _____
385. _____	431. _____	477. _____	524. _____
386. _____	432. _____	478. _____	525. _____
387. _____	433. _____	479. _____	526. _____
388. _____	434. _____	480. _____	527. _____
389. _____	435. _____	481. _____	528. _____
390. _____	436. _____	482. _____	529. _____
391. _____	437. _____	483. _____	530. _____
392. _____	438. _____	484. _____	531. _____
393. _____	439. _____	485. _____	532. _____
394. _____	440. _____	486. _____	533. _____
395. _____	441. _____	487. _____	534. _____
396. _____	442. _____	488. _____	535. _____
397. _____	443. _____	489. _____	536. _____
398. _____	444. _____	490. _____	537. _____
399. _____	445. _____	491. _____	538. _____
400. _____	446. _____	492. _____	539. _____
401. _____	447. _____	493. _____	540. _____
402. _____	448. _____	494. _____	541. _____
403. _____	449. _____	495. _____	542. _____
404. _____	450. _____	496. _____	543. _____
405. _____	451. _____	497. _____	544. _____
406. _____	452. _____	498. _____	545. _____
407. _____	453. _____	499. _____	546. _____
408. _____	454. _____	500. _____	547. _____
409. _____	455. _____	501. _____	548. _____
410. _____	456. _____	502. _____	549. _____
411. _____	457. _____	503. _____	550. _____
412. _____	458. _____	504. _____	551. _____
413. _____	459. _____	505. _____	552. _____
414. _____	460. _____	506. _____	553. _____
415. _____	461. _____	507. _____	554. _____
416. _____	462. _____	508. _____	555. _____
		509. _____	

BLOCK 13	BLOCK 14	BLOCK 15	BLOCK 16
556. _____	602. _____	649. _____	695. _____
557. _____	603. _____	650. _____	696. _____
558. _____	604. _____	651. _____	697. _____
559. _____	605. _____	652. _____	698. _____
560. _____	606. _____	653. _____	699. _____
561. _____	607. _____	654. _____	700. _____
562. _____	608. _____	655. _____	701. _____
563. _____	609. _____	656. _____	702. _____
564. _____	610. _____	657. _____	703. _____
565. _____	611. _____	658. _____	704. _____
566. _____	612. _____	659. _____	705. _____
567. _____	613. _____	660. _____	706. _____
568. _____	614. _____	661. _____	707. _____
569. _____	615. _____	662. _____	708. _____
570. _____	616. _____	663. _____	709. _____
571. _____	617. _____	664. _____	710. _____
572. _____	618. _____	665. _____	711. _____
573. _____	619. _____	666. _____	712. _____
574. _____	620. _____	667. _____	713. _____
575. _____	621. _____	668. _____	714. _____
576. _____	622. _____	669. _____	715. _____
577. _____	623. _____	670. _____	716. _____
578. _____	624. _____	671. _____	717. _____
579. _____	625. _____	672. _____	718. _____
580. _____	626. _____	673. _____	719. _____
581. _____	627. _____	674. _____	720. _____
582. _____	628. _____	675. _____	721. _____
583. _____	629. _____	676. _____	722. _____
584. _____	630. _____	677. _____	723. _____
585. _____	631. _____	678. _____	724. _____
586. _____	632. _____	679. _____	725. _____
587. _____	633. _____	680. _____	726. _____
588. _____	634. _____	681. _____	727. _____
589. _____	635. _____	682. _____	728. _____
590. _____	636. _____	683. _____	729. _____
591. _____	637. _____	684. _____	730. _____
592. _____	638. _____	685. _____	731. _____
593. _____	639. _____	686. _____	732. _____
594. _____	640. _____	687. _____	733. _____
595. _____	641. _____	688. _____	734. _____
596. _____	642. _____	689. _____	735. _____
597. _____	643. _____	690. _____	736. _____
598. _____	644. _____	691. _____	737. _____
599. _____	645. _____	692. _____	738. _____
600. _____	646. _____	693. _____	739. _____
601. _____	647. _____	694. _____	740. _____
	648. _____		